Spinal Cord Injury

Functional Rehabilitation

Second Edition

Spinal Cord Injury

Functional Rehabilitation

Second Edition

Martha Freeman Somers, MS, PT

Department of Physical Therapy
Duquesne University
Pittsburgh, PA

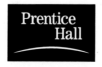

Prentice Hall, Upper Saddle River, New Jersey 07458

Library of Congress Cataloging-in-Publication Data:

Somers, Martha Freeman.
    Spinal cord injury : functional rehabilitation / Martha Freeman Somers.—2nd ed.
      p. cm.
    Includes bibliographical references and index.
    ISBN 0-8385-8616-3 (hard cover)
     1. Spinal cord—Wounds and injuries—Patients—Rehabilitation.   2. Spinal cords—Wounds
and injuries—Physical therapy. I. Title.

    RD594.3 .S63 2001
    617.4'82044—dc21

                                           00-057434

Publisher: Julie Alexander
Executive Editor: Greg Vis
Acquisitions Editor: Mark Cohen
Production Editor: Andover Publishing Services
Production Liaison: Janet Bolton
Director of Manufacturing and Production: Bruce Johnson
Managing Editor: Patrick Walsh
Manufacturing Buyer: Ilene Sanford
Art Director: Marianne Frasco
Marketing Manager: Kristin Walton
Editorial Assistant: Melissa Kerian
Interior Design: Eve Siegel
Cover Art: Martha and Dave Somers
Illustrations: Susan Gilbert
Composition: North Market Street Graphics
Printing and Binding: Courier Westford

Notice: The author and the publisher of this volume have taken care that the information and recommendations contained herein are accurate and compatible with the standards generally accepted at the time of publication. Nevertheless, it is difficult to ensure that all the information given is entirely accurate for all circumstances. The publisher disclaims any liability, loss, or damage incurred as a consequence, directly or indirectly, of the use and application of any of the contents of this volume.

Prentice-Hall International (UK) Limited, *London*
Prentice-Hall of Australia Pty. Limited, *Sydney*
Prentice-Hall Canada Inc., *Toronto*
Prentice-Hall Hispanoamericana, S.A., *Mexico*
Prentice-Hall of India Private Limited, *New Delhi*
Prentice-Hall of Japan, Inc., *Tokyo*
Prentice-Hall Singapore Pte. Ltd.
Editora Prentice-Hall do Brasil, Ltda., *Rio de Janeiro*

10

ISBN 0-8385-8616-3

To Dave and Jess, my two greatest blessings.

Contents

CHAPTER 12
WHEELCHAIRS AND WHEELCHAIR SKILLS

CHAPTER 13
AMBULATION

The following additional material is available on the publisher's web site,
www.prenhall.com/somers.

CHAPTER 14
BOWEL AND BLADDER MANAGEMENT

CHAPTER 15
ARCHITECTURAL ADAPTATIONS

APPENDIX A
SOLUTIONS TO PROBLEM-SOLVING EXERCISES

APPENDIX B
SPINAL SEGMENT INNERVATION OF THE EXTREMITIES

Preface

Spinal cord injury causes a host of physical and psychosocial problems that can interfere with an individual's health, feelings of well-being, and participation in activities and relationships within the family and community. The goal of rehabilitation after spinal cord injury is to enable the person to resume and then continue a lifestyle that is healthy, fulfilling, and integrated with his or her family and community. Physical therapists play a central role in this process, working with recently injured people and their families to maximize physical capabilities and mobility, and to develop the knowledge and skills needed to remain healthy. Three major elements are required for a therapist to fulfill this role most effectively.

The first requirement is a basic understanding of spinal cord injuries and issues relevant to disability. Pertinent areas of knowledge include the disablement process, pathology, mechanisms of injury, physical sequelae, medical and surgical management, the prevention and management of complications, psychosocial impact, disability-related civil rights, functional potentials, equipment options, and wheelchair-accessible architectural design. This knowledge base is needed for optimal program planning and implementation.

The second requirement is a knowledge of the physical skills involved in functional activities and the process involved in acquiring these skills. It is not enough merely to know the eventual outcome, which may take months to accomplish. The therapist must know how to design and implement therapeutic programs to develop the needed strength, flexibility, and motor skills involved in functional activities. Many a therapist has been baffled when faced, on the one hand, with a text that explains the maneuvers that a person with a spinal cord injury performs during functional tasks and, on the other hand, with a newly injured person who can barely

remain conscious while sitting upright, much less even begin to perform the skills shown in the book.

The third major element required for effective participation in rehabilitation is an approach to the individual that promotes self-respect and encourages autonomy. Unfortunately, this element is often overlooked. Although we health professionals have as our stated goals the independent functioning of our patients, we often unwittingly encourage dependence. Many practices in health care serve to encourage "compliance" and to discourage autonomous behavior. If the rehabilitation effort is to be successful, the social environment of the rehabilitation unit must be structured in a way that fosters the development of self-reliant attitudes and behaviors.

In order to prepare readers to work effectively with people who have had spinal cord injuries, a text must encompass all of the elements described above. *Spinal Cord Injury: Functional Rehabilitation* was written to provide such a comprehensive treatment of the subject. The reader will gain a broad knowledge base relevant to spinal cord injuries and will develop an understanding of both the physical skills required for functional activities and the therapeutic strategies for achieving these skills. As importantly, the reader will gain an appreciation for the importance of psychosocial adaptation after spinal cord injury and will develop some insight into the impact that rehabilitation professionals can have in this area.

CHANGES IN THE SECOND EDITION

In the years since the publication of the first edition, a number of developments have occurred in the area of rehabilitation after spinal cord injury. Clinical and basic science research has deepened our understanding of the neuropathological changes associated with spinal cord injury, factors associated with neurological return, and appropriate interventions for spinal cord injury and its sequelae. Several new clinical practice guidelines now exist describing optimal care in a variety of areas relevant to spinal cord injury. Finally, health care delivery has changed dramatically in recent years as funding sources have shortened the time allotted to acute care and inpatient rehabilitation.

This edition was written to reflect all of these changes. It provides updated information from clinical and basic science research, uses terminology and presents interventions that are consistent with published clinical practice guidelines, and includes strategies for delivering quality rehabilitative services in today's health care environment.

This edition also reflects feedback from a variety of clinicians, academic faculty, and students. Thanks to suggestions from these sources, the book now contains chapters on skin care and respiratory management. Additional content areas that have been added or expanded in the text include the Nagi Model of Disablement, complications and their prevention and management, interventions appropriate for individuals with incomplete spinal cord injuries, post-discharge follow-up, community reintegration, erectile dysfunction, infertility, functional potentials, precautions, strategies for enhancing motor learning, and detailed information on muscle innervation.

In addition to providing content that was not presented in the first edition, the second edition has several features that are designed to enhance learning and the development of clinical problem-solving skills. These new features include chapter openers presenting schematic representations of each chapter's content and its relevance to the disablement process, problem-solving exercises presented as boxed materials in each chapter, and bulleted summaries that highlight major points in each chapter.

Portions of this edition are included on the web site for this book (www.prenhall.com/somers) instead of in the text itself. This arrangement made it possible to provide readers with important additional content without increasing the length (and therefore cost) of the book. The web site includes two full chapters (Chapter 14, Bowel and Bladder Management, and Chapter 15, Architectural Adaptations) and two appendixes (A, Solutions to Problem-Solving Exercises, and B, Spinal Segment Innervation of the Extremities).

Martha Somers

A Few Words about Words

"What's in a name? A rose by any other name would smell as sweet."
William Shakespeare

Maybe so, Bill, but I bet if you labeled that rose "radioactive," not too many people would get close enough to take a whiff.

Language has a profound impact on attitudes and values. Our perceptions of and judgments about others are both expressed and perpetuated by the words that we use. The health care system in the United States is replete with the use of dehumanizing language. Health professionals label people by their diagnoses, calling people "paras," "quads," "cords," and so on. When we do this, we define people by their disabling conditions, reducing them to one-dimensional shadows of people. (How can a *person* be a *spinal cord*?)

Another common practice among health professionals involves referring to people as "patients" when this term no longer applies. Most of us think of ourselves as *patients* only while we are utilizing the services of another clinician. As soon as we walk out of the health professional's office, we cease being *patients* and revert to our accustomed roles. When thinking/writing/speaking about people with disabling conditions, however, we often refer to them as *patients* whether or not they are utilizing the services of health professionals. The implication is that they remain *dependent* on health professionals indefinitely. Once a patient, always a patient.

In writing this text I have attempted to avoid language that dehumanizes people who have spinal cord injuries. Instead of labeling people by their diagnoses, I have chosen language that affirms their personhood. Thus rather than referring to "a C6 tetraplegic," for example, I have referred to "a person (or individual) with C6 tetraplegia."

In like manner, I gave much thought to eliminating the word "patient" from the text. "Patient" has implications of dependency and powerlessness. Another word may more appropriately convey the role of the person undergoing rehabilitation. But what word to use? "Client" evokes images of business suits and impersonal, formal interactions. I personally like "student," but I didn't think it would fly. Readers, especially health professional students, may find the term confusing. For lack of a better term, I have retained the word "patient" but have attempted to avoid its overuse.

And then there's gender. The world is inhabited by both males and females. Both genders sustain spinal cord injuries, and both genders are involved in their rehabilitation. But hundreds of pages of "he or she," "himself or herself," and "his or her" would have been confusing in places and tiresome throughout. I know, because I tried it. I also tried achieving gender-neutrality by using plural pronouns, but that approach yielded equally unacceptable results. In the interest of retaining clarity and readability, I settled on the following solution: Each chapter contains either male or female pronouns, and the chapters alternate between the two. The one exception is Chapter 5, which addresses sexuality and sexual functioning. I chose to refer to both genders throughout this chapter in an attempt to counteract the tendency of some rehabilitation professionals to ignore or to minimize the impact of spinal cord injury on the sexual functioning of women.

As a result of my attempts to minimize the use of "patient," achieve gender neutrality, and affirm the sexuality of women with spinal cord injuries, I may at times have resorted to some verbal gymnastics. I beg the reader's indulgence if I did so.

Martha Somers

Acknowledgments

I am deeply grateful to the following people for their assistance and support:

- Andrea Behrman, James Tomlinson, and Anne Thompson, who reviewed large portions of the manuscript and provided extremely useful suggestions.
- Terri Wubben and Marion Johnson, who were instrumental in providing me with opportunities to expand my clinical experience.
- Kathy Brown, who generously gave me full access to her library.
- Mary Hudak and Mary Massery, who taught me much of what I know about the respiratory component of rehabilitation.
- Andrea Behrman, who introduced me to body-weight-supported treadmill training.
- Pat Crist and Jane Wetzel, who reviewed parts of the manuscript and made a number of helpful suggestions.
- Carol Probst and Mary Hudak, who always found just the right word or phrase when I asked for help with wording.
- Jen Tanzilli and Dale Kreller, who helped me with some of the new illustrations for this edition.
- Mary Schmidt Read, who suggested that I ask for feedback from therapists at Model Spinal Cord Injury Centers. Thanks also to Sherri Barash, Claire Beekman, Amy Hammond, and Sarah Morrison, who provided that feedback.
- The numerous family, friends, and colleagues who provided suggestions, information, reference material, technical assistance, and encouragement in the writing of this edition. In this group are included Dave Somers, Carol Probst, Sue Perry, Bob Morgan, Rege Tourocy, Rick Clemente, Tammy McClafferty, Lisa Saladin, Nigel Shapcott, Cliff Pohl, Fran Huber, Sue Polich, Bonnie Dowdell, Gayle Sligar, Carol Rigg, Julia Freeman-Woolpert, Robert Somers, Dave and Connie Freeman, and the "gourmet ladies."
- Former students who provided feedback on the first edition. These include Beth Attenberger, Jeannine Moyer, and Elizabeth Anderson. Many more students provided helpful suggestions, but I have managed to lose my list. I could try to blame it on Y2K, but the truth is that I simply lost track of the various scraps of paper on which I had written the names.
- Mark Cohen of Prentice Hall and Susan Hunter and Niels Buessem of Andover Publishing Services, who used just the right combination of patience and prodding during the writing and production of this edition.
- Susan Gilbert, whose illustrations are still one of the best features of the book.
- Most of all, thanks to Dave and Jess Somers for making it possible for me to write this edition. I could not have done it without their understanding and support.

Reviewers

Anne W. Thompson, PT, EdD
Assistant Professor
Department of Physical Therapy
Armstrong Atlantic State University
Savannah, Georgia

Wen Ling, PhD, PT
Associate Professor and Chair
New York University
Department of Physical Therapy
New York, New York

Jennifer S. Stith, PhD, PT
Associate Director for Professional Education
Program in Physical Therapy
Washington University
Saint Louis, Missouri

Andrea L. Behrman, PhD, PT
Department of Physical Therapy
University of Florida
Gainesville, Florida

James D. Tomlinson, MS, PT
Department of Physical Therapy
Beaver College
Glenside, Pennsylvania

Nancy Fell, PT, MHS, NCS
Assistant Professor
Department of Physical Therapy
University of Tennessee at Chattanooga
Chattanooga, Tennessee

1

Introduction

Pathology ◄─► Impairment ◄─► Functional Limitation ◄─► Disability

Damage to the spinal cord has profound and global effects. Paralysis of voluntary musculature can lead to reduced mobility as well as impairment of vocational, avocational, and self-care abilities. Spinal cord injury can also affect the functioning of the sensory, respiratory, cardiovascular, gastrointestinal, genitourinary, and integumentary systems. A host of debilitating and potentially life-threatening physical complications can result.

The psychosocial sequelae of spinal cord injury are equally important. Bodily changes, altered sexual functioning, impaired mobility, incontinence, and functional dependence all constitute seemingly overwhelming losses with which people with spinal cord injuries must come to terms. Moreover, spinal cord injuries cause previously "normal" people to become "handicapped" and thus to become subject to society's prejudices regarding people with disabilities.

Although spinal cord injury is one of the most serious injuries that a person can survive, it is possible to return to a healthy, fulfilling, and productive life after even the most severe of cord injuries. Achieving this outcome, however, is a monumental task. To the health professional unfamiliar with spinal cord injuries, it may seem daunting. With such a broad array of physical and psychosocial problems that can result from spinal cord injury, where should the health care team focus its attention? Perhaps the process of rehabilitation following spinal cord injury can be better understood using the Nagi model of disablement.

NAGI MODEL OF DISABLEMENT

Over the past several decades, the Nagi model of disablement[8, 9] has gained wide acceptance as a useful tool for conceptualizing disability and the process of disablement.[3, 4, 5, 7, 12, 13] This model is summarized in Figure 1–1. Simply stated, a pathological process at the cellular level ("pathology") can cause abnormalities or losses in the body's gross structure or function at the tissue, organ, or body system level ("impairments"). These impairments can lead to a reduced ability to perform functional tasks ("functional limitations"), which in turn can result in limitations in the individual's ability to participate in social roles ("disability"). Pathology, impairment, and functional limitations are attributes of the individual; one can determine their extent by examining the person with the disabling condition. In contrast, disability results from the interplay between the individual and his environment. A reflection of the person's ability to function in the context of his social and physical environment, disability results from "the gap between a person's capabilities and the demands of the environment."[12]

The process of disablement is more complex than the schematic representation of Nagi's model may imply. Instead of a unidirectional progression from pathology to disability, disablement can include a cycle of increasing pathology, impairment, functional limitation, and disability

1

	Definition	Examples
Pathology	Interruption or interference with normal cellular processes, and efforts of the organism to regain normal state.	Spinal cord damage and secondary neural tissue destruction. Vertebral injury.
Impairment	Anatomical, physiological, mental, or emotional abnormalities or loss. (Loss at the tissue, organ, or body system level.)	Paralysis, sensory impairment, abnormal muscle tone, joint contractures, pain, cardiopulmonary deconditioning due to inactivity.
Functional Limitation	Limitations in performance at the level of the whole organism or person.	Limitations in performance of tasks such as walking, climbing, reaching, transfers, and other physical tasks such as driving a car.
Disability	Limitations in performance of socially defined roles and tasks expected of an individual within a sociocultural and physical environment (work, home, school, recreation.) Roles include those within the family, peer group, community, work, and other settings. Influenced by the characteristics of both the individual and the social and physical environment.	Limitations in ability to return to work, participate in social activities, function as a parent or spouse, participate in sports. Example: unable to return to work or recreational activities due to environmental barriers or social stigma.

Pathology ⟶ Impairment ⟶ Functional Limitation ⟶ Disability

Figure 1–1.   Nagi's Model of Disablement. (*Sources:* references 4, 5, 7–9, 12.)

due to the development of secondary conditions such as pressure ulcers or joint contractures. Moreover, a person's perceptions of and responses to his condition impact on the process of disablement. For example, emotional responses to spinal cord injury can influence motivation, which in turn can affect performance in functional tasks and socially defined roles. Additional factors that can influence the course of disablement include the availability of quality medical and rehabilitative services, access to equipment, the responses of significant others (family, friends, coworkers, employers) to the disabling condition, and the prevalence of architectural or social barriers in the individual's environment.[4–8, 10, 12] Because of the many factors that modify the course of disablement, identical pathologies in different people can result in widely divergent levels of disability. For example, one individual with a spinal cord injury could eventually return to live at home and resume the roles of spouse, parent, and breadwinner. Another person with identical damage to his spinal cord could wind up living in a skilled nursing facility, divorced from his wife, estranged from his children, and unable to return to work.

Health professionals have a powerful influence on the degree to which pathology leads to disability. Medical and rehabilitative interventions can be provided at any point in the disablement process (Figure 1–2). Applying Nagi's model to program planning, health professionals identify which impairments lead to functional limitations, and which functional limitations lead to increased disability. They then work with patients and their families to minimize impairments and maximize functional capacity. Health professionals can also enhance their patients' ability to function in their home and work environments by providing appropriate equipment and guidance regarding architectural adaptations. They can also reduce disability by preventing secondary conditions through proper medical care, education and training of the patient and family, and provision of appropriate equipment. Finally, rehabilitation professionals can reduce disability by working with patients, significant others, and the community at large to promote healthy responses to the disabling conditions.

REHABILITATION FOLLOWING SPINAL CORD INJURY

Goals of Rehabilitation

The ultimate goal of rehabilitation after spinal cord injury is to minimize disability. This involves enabling the person with a spinal cord injury to return to as healthy, fulfilling, and independent a lifestyle as possible. It also involves facilitating his return to performance of accustomed tasks and roles in his family and in society. Accomplishing these outcomes requires psychosocial, sexual, vocational, and avocational adjustment; the acquisition of functional skills, appropriate

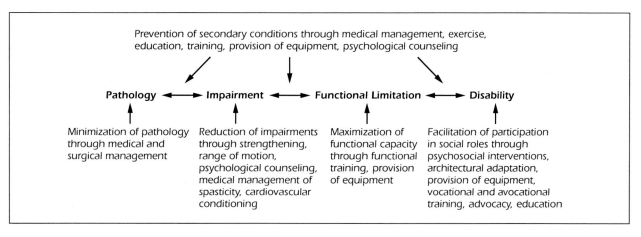

Figure 1–2. Medical and rehabilitative services for minimization of disability following spinal cord injury. Bidirectional arrows between the stages of disablement reflect the potential cycle of increasing pathology, impairment, functional limitation and disability due to the development of secondary conditions such as pressure ulcers or joint contractures.

PROBLEM-SOLVING EXERCISE 1–1

Your patient has been admitted to your facility for outpatient rehabilitation. During your initial examination, you find that she has the following problems:

- She has no voluntary motor function in her lower extremities.
- She is unable to walk.
- She has not been able to return to her job.
- She has tight hamstrings.
- She requires assistance to transfer in and out of bed, is unable to perform uneven transfers, and cannot negotiate uneven terrain, ramps, or curbs in her wheelchair.
- She cannot take care of her infant son.
- Her diagnosis is transverse myelitis.
- She is currently living with her parents. She cannot stay in her own home with her husband and son because there are steps at the home's entrance and the bathroom door is too narrow for a wheelchair.

Classify each of the problems listed above as pathology, impairment, functional limitation, or disability.

equipment, and the knowledge and behaviors required for health maintenance; and the appropriate adaptation of the person's physical environment.

Psychosocial adjustment. To return to a happy and fulfilling life following spinal cord injury, an individual must come to terms with his losses and formulate a new identity. He must also learn how to cope in a society in which he is now a member of a devalued minority. In terms of disability and quality of life, this psychological and social adjustment may be the most crucial area of growth after spinal cord injury.

Sexual adjustment. Many of the social roles that are typically performed in the family and in society include an element of sexuality. To return to full participation in social and sexual relationships, a person with a spinal cord injury needs to adjust to the changes in sexuality and sexual functioning that the cord injury brings.

Vocational and avocational adjustment. In many instances, paralysis makes it impossible or impractical to return to a job held prior to the spinal cord injury. Recreational activities enjoyed prior to the injury may also be impossible or impractical. Return to an independent and fulfilling lifestyle with full participation in socially defined roles requires adaptation in both of these areas.

Functional skills. During rehabilitation, a person with a spinal cord injury learns how to perform a variety of physical activities. Through functional training, he gains skills required for self-care and mobility in the home and community. By maximizing his functional skills, he can enhance his capacity to perform socially defined roles and tasks.

Equipment. Following spinal cord injury, equipment can have a significant impact on function and health. Thus, equipment procurement is an important aspect of disability prevention. Following spinal cord injury, the rehabilitation team and the patient work together to identify and obtain the equipment needed to maintain health, maximize functional independence, and enhance the performance of socially defined roles.

Health maintenance. Health maintenance is an active process after spinal cord injury. Virtually constant vigilance is required to avoid complications such as pressure sores and urinary tract infections. If an individual is to stay healthy after spinal cord injury, he must learn how his body works, how to prevent and detect complications, and what to do when complications occur.

Architectural adaptation. The presence of architectural barriers in the physical environment increases disability by limiting mobility and function. By providing guidance and advocacy regarding architectural adaptations, the rehabilitation team can enhance a person's ability to perform socially defined roles in his home and the community.

Services Required

Spinal cord injury necessitates specialized and comprehensive rehabilitation services; a multidisciplinary team is required to enable people to achieve their optimal levels of health and functioning. Rehabilitation involves the coordinated efforts of counselors, nurses, occupational therapists, physical therapists, physicians, recreation therapists, rehabilitation engineers, respiratory therapists, speech therapists, and vocational counselors. To maximize outcomes, each of these professionals should have expertise in rehabilitation after spinal cord injury. Because of the specialized services required, general hospitals are not able to provide the comprehensive care needed for rehabilitation following spinal cord injury. For this reason, patients who receive care in specialized centers are likely to have better outcomes.[2, 11, 14]

Fostering Independence Following Spinal Cord Injury

One of the major ways in which a rehabilitation program reduces disability is by maximizing the individual's capacity to function independently. That involves developing independence from family members, independence from friends, and independence from the rehabilitation team.

Requirements for independent functioning. There are three basic requirements that must be met for a person to function independently: knowledge, ability, and attitude.

Knowledge is critical to self-direction. Knowledge in the following areas will promote independence after spinal cord injury: the body's functioning following spinal cord injury, prevention and management of complications, treatment alternatives, legal rights, equipment options, architectural accessibility, and the services and resources available in the community. Armed with this knowledge, a person with a spinal cord injury can be self-reliant.

A variety of abilities are required for independent functioning. Physical abilities enable people to perform functional tasks without assistance. If a person lacks the physical capacity to perform a given activity, autonomous functioning requires the ability to gain and direct assistance from another person. Other abilities involved in independent functioning include skills in problem solving, social interaction, and self-advocacy.

Finally, an independent attitude is essential for autonomy. A person with significant impairments and functional limitations will not function independently unless he is motivated to do so.

Fostering independence. A rehabilitation program must address each of these areas—knowledge, ability, and attitude—if the person with a spinal cord injury is to function as independently as possible. The first two requirements, knowledge and ability, may be most readily achieved. Educational and training programs can be implemented to provide information and develop skills.

The development of an independent outlook can be more problematic. It is an area more likely to be neglected and most easily undermined. By virtue of the types of people who enter health professions, and the training that we receive, health professionals tend to be good at taking care of people. Because of this, we can inadvertently develop a *dependent attitude* in our patients. This happens when we feed them, bathe them, dress them, and push their wheelchairs even when they are capable of doing these things for themselves. It happens when we make decisions for them or "protect" them from full knowledge of their physical conditions. When we do these things, we communicate to our patients that they are dependent and that they need our help.

To foster an independent attitude, the rehabilitation team must emphasize the patient's autonomy and personal responsibility. From the day of injury onward, the person with a spinal cord injury should be included in decision making and self-care as much as possible. He should be provided with all relevant information and work as a partner with clinicians to set goals, solve problems, and make decisions. To the extent possible, the patient should be responsible for the rehabilitation program—taking initiative, directing, and participating fully in it.

Autonomous behaviors do not always appear spontaneously when a patient is given the opportunity to direct his care. A variety of factors can cause initial reluctance or inability to participate actively in rehabilitation. Some people with spinal cord injuries learn dependence after their injuries when they are placed in the role of dependent and passive patient. Some feel incapable of self-direction because of their preexisting beliefs about people with disabling conditions. Others may simply feel overwhelmed. Finally, a certain number may have been passive and dependent prior to their injuries. Whatever the cause of a patient's reluctance or inability to participate actively in his program, the rehabilitation team must work with him to encourage and develop the capacity to take responsibility for himself.

ON YOUR MARK, GET SET, GO

One of the greatest challenges facing health professionals today is that of adapting to a rapidly changing health care environment. The reduction of time allotted to inpatient care is one of the more profound changes that have occurred in health care. In the not-too-distant past, a person who sustained a spinal cord injury could spend months in an acute care hospital, followed by months in an inpatient rehabilitation facility. The process of recovery and adaptation began in the acute hospital and continued in the rehabilitation setting when the patient was determined to be ready for the rigors of rehabilitation. Inpatient rehabilitation continued until the patient reached, or at least approached, his maximal functional potential. Prior to discharge, there was time for physical and psychological healing, comprehensive patient and family education, and extensive training in functional skills. Equipment procurement could be delayed until significant time had been spent in rehabilitation and the patient's definitive equipment requirements could be determined.

In today's health care environment, a person who becomes injured or ill moves as rapidly as possible through intensive care, floor-level care, and rehabilitation. People with spinal cord injuries now often arrive at rehabilitation facilities while they remain medically and orthopedically unstable, and have not had adequate time to begin the process of adapting psychologically to their losses. Although they may not be ready to participate fully in rigorous therapeutic programs when they arrive, patients are expected to complete their rehabilitation in as short a time as possible. As a result, people with spinal cord injuries may leave inpatient rehabilitation facilities without having reached their potentials.[1]

Health professionals must accommodate to the time constraints imposed by funding sources. With shortened time allotted to inpatient stays in hospitals, more emphasis must be placed on rehabilitation in outpatient clinics, extended care facilities, and in the home. The inpatient stay should be seen as the beginning phase of rehabilitation, with significant continued progress expected in appropriate alternative settings following discharge. Immediately after discharge from inpatient rehabilitation, therapy in the home will allow patients to continue to develop skills and utilize them in their home environments. Outpatient therapy makes it possible for patients to utilize their developing functional skills at home between therapy sessions. Their performance at home can provide information that is helpful in program planning.

Although therapy at home and in outpatient settings can be beneficial, the inpatient phase of rehabilitation remains critical. It is during inpatient rehabilitation that the foundation is laid for physical, functional, psychological, and social adaptation. Patients who have orthopedic or medical restrictions that temporarily prevent full participation in rehabilitation may benefit from discharge to other settings (home or extended care facility, as indicated) with readmission to rehabilitation facilities when they are ready to participate in their programs.

In the face of shrinking lengths of stay, goals must be prioritized carefully during each phase of rehabilitation, with greatest priority given to those goals that are critical to survival. When patients are discharged home prior to achieving independent functioning, it is imperative to provide them and their caregivers the education and training needed to enable them to remain healthy and continue to progress after discharge.

SUMMARY

• Spinal cord injury has a profound impact on a person's ability to care for himself, to move from place to place, and to participate in his accustomed social, vocational, and avocational activities. Injury to the spinal cord also makes a person vulnerable to social discrimination and a variety of physical complications.

• The Nagi model is a useful tool for conceptualizing disability and the process of disablement. In this model, a pathological process at the cellular level ("pathology") can cause abnormalities or losses in the body's gross structure or function at the tissue, organ, or body system level ("impairments"). These impairments can lead to a reduced ability to perform functional tasks ("functional limitations"), which in turn can result in limitations in the individual's ability to participate in social roles ("disability"). Using this model, health professionals can minimize disability through a variety of interventions at each of the stages in the disablement process.

• The ultimate goal of rehabilitation after spinal cord injury is the minimization of disability. Interventions are aimed at enhancing psychological, social, sexual, vocational, and avocational adjustment; maximizing functional independence; and developing the knowledge, skills, and behaviors that will be required to remain healthy in the years to come.

• During rehabilitation, *how* things are done can be as important as *what* is done. Services should be delivered in a manner that affirms and fosters autonomy of patients undergoing rehabilitation.

• Spinal cord injury necessitates specialized and comprehensive rehabilitation services. In the past, these services were delivered primarily in inpatient settings. In recent years, inpatient stays have been shortened dramatically. This change has necessitated a continuation of the rehabilitation process in outpatient clinics and in the home.

2

Spinal Cord Injuries

Pathology ◄─► Impairment

Every year an estimated 10,000 people[a] in the United States sustain spinal cord injuries.[125] Presently, there are approximately 183,000 to 230,000 people with spinal cord injuries alive in this country.[76]

In the United States, motor vehicle accidents are the most common cause (37.2 percent) of spinal cord injury. Motor vehicle accidents are followed by acts of violence (26.8 percent), falls (21.0 percent), and sports injuries (7.1 percent). The remaining 7.9 percent of spinal cord injuries result from a variety of other causes.[125] The incidence of the different causes of cord injury varies with gender, race, age, employment status, and marital status, being influenced by the activities and hazards prevalent in each population.[57, 76, 91, 147]

A large majority of spinal cord injuries (approximately 80 percent) are sustained by males. Most are between 16 and 30 years of age at the time of injury.[76, 125] Nineteen is the most common age of injury.[76] The prevalence of spinal cord injuries among young males is not the result of any anatomic or physiologic vulnerability peculiar to this population. It is simply due to the fact that these are the people who are most prone to participating in such high-risk activities as driving too fast (and too drunk), joining gangs, riding motorcycles, playing football, and diving into unfamiliar waters where stumps and boulders are hidden beneath the surface.

ANATOMY REVIEW

An understanding of spinal cord injuries and their management requires a basic knowledge of the anatomy of the vertebral column, spinal cord, the cord's vascular supply, and spinal nerves.

Vertebral Column

Most spinal cord injuries are the result of trauma to the vertebral column, which contains 7 cervical, 12 thoracic, 5 lumbar, 5 sacral, and 4 coccygeal vertebrae. The cervical, thoracic, and lumbar vertebrae are separated by intervertebral disks and are connected and stabilized by ligaments. The sacral and coccygeal vertebrae are fused.

A typical vertebra consists of a body, located anteriorly, and an arch. The spinal cord is encased within the vertebral foramen, formed by the vertebral bodies and arches. Figure 2–1 illustrates the components of a vertebra.

The vertebral column is stabilized by ligaments. The anterior longitudinal ligament is attached to the anterior aspect of the vertebral bodies and intervertebral disks, and limits extension. The posterior longitudinal ligament is attached to the posterior aspect of the vertebral bodies and intervertebral disks, and limits flexion.[143, 177] The ligamenta flava, supraspinous ligament (C7 and below), ligamentum nuchae (cervical region), interspinous ligaments, and articular capsules stabilize the posterior arch.[48, 52, 143]

The three-column model of the spine (Figure 2–2) helps to understand the degree of instability

---

[a] This number does not include people who die at the scene of the accident.

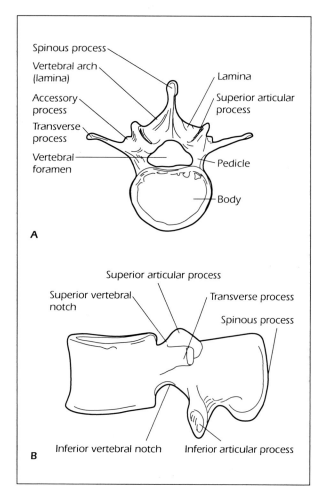

Figure 2–1. Components of a vertebra. **(A)** Superior view. **(B)** Lateral view.

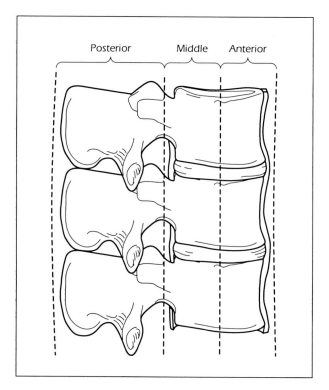

Figure 2–2. Three-column model of the spine.

that results from different ligamentous or boney injuries. This model was first proposed for the thoracolumbar spine[52] but is also applicable to the cervical region.[2, 80] In this model, the spine is conceptualized as consisting of three columns. At a given spinal segment, the anterior column consists of the anterior part of the vertebral body, the anterior longitudinal ligament, and the anterior anulus fibrosus.[b] The middle column includes the posterior wall of the vertebral body, the posterior longitudinal ligament, and the posterior anulus fibrosus. The posterior column consists of the vertebral arch and the supraspinous ligament, interspinous ligament, capsule, and ligamentum flavum. Each column contributes to the overall stability of the spinal column. Instability of the spine occurs only when two or more columns sustain damage.[52]

---

[b] The anulus fibrosus is the fibrous outer portion of the intervertebral disk.

Spinal Cord

The spinal cord extends from the medulla oblongata just above the foramen magnum to the level of the L1 or L2 vertebra.[27, 48, 160, 177] It is located within the vertebral foramen, also called the vertebral canal. The cord is protected by the vertebral bodies anteriorly, and by the vertebral arches laterally and posteriorly.

Seen in transverse section, the spinal cord has an H-shaped area of gray matter centrally (Fig-

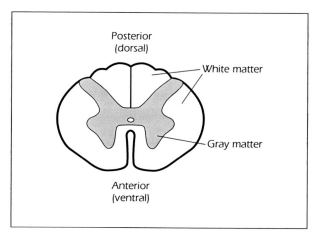

Figure 2–3. Schematic cross-section of the spinal cord.

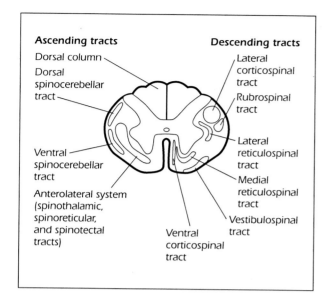

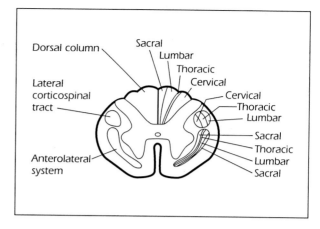

Figure 2–5. Somatotopic organization of the spinal cord (depicted on the right).

Figure 2–4. Major ascending and descending fiber tracts in the spinal cord. Ascending tracts are shown on the left; descending tracts are shown on the right.

ure 2–3). This gray matter is composed of cell bodies, small projection fibers, and glial[c] cells.[160] The dorsal (posterior) horn of the gray matter is predominately sensory. The ventral (anterior) horn contains the bodies of lower motor neurons innervating skeletal muscles.

The gray matter of the spinal cord is surrounded by white matter consisting of ascending and descending fibers, the axons of motor and sensory neurons. Fibers carrying similar sensory information or motor functions travel together in tracts (Figure 2–4 and Table 2–1). Additionally, the fibers within at least some tracts are organized somatotopically: fibers are grouped with others traveling to or from the same cord segment (Figure 2–5).[27, 48]

Vascular Supply

The spinal cord receives its blood supply from a single anterior spinal artery and from two posterior spinal arteries. The anterior and posterior spinal arteries travel the length of the cord.[27]

The anterior and posterior spinal arteries supply circulation to the cord through two arterial systems, the centrifugal and centripetal arterial systems. The centrifugal system arises from the anterior spinal artery and supplies the central region of the cord. The centripetal system arises from the anterior and posterior spinal arteries and supplies the peripheral region of the cord. The distribution of these two arterial systems overlaps.[159]

Centrifugal system. The anterior spinal artery gives rise to small branches that enter the anterior median fissure of the cord. These vessels, called sulcal arteries, supply the central portion of the spinal cord. This area includes most of the gray matter and approximately the inner half of the posterior, lateral, and anterior white matter.[159]

Centripetal system. The anterior spinal artery also gives rise to pial arteries. The pial arteries and branches of the posterior spinal arteries travel circumferentially around the outer surface of the cord and supply its peripheral regions. The area of the spinal cord supplied by the pial and posterior spinal arteries includes part of the dorsal horns, most of the posterior columns, and the outer portions of the lateral and anterior white matter.[159]

In the cervical region, the anterior spinal artery is supplied primarily by the vertebral arteries and the intracranial vessels from which they arise. The posterior spinal arteries in this region are supplied by the vertebral arteries or the posterior inferior cerebellar arteries. In the thoracic, lumbar, and sacral regions, the anterior and posterior spinal arteries are fed by segmental radicular arteries that arise from the aorta.[27] The largest of these arteries, the vessel of Adamkiewicz, supplies the anterior spinal artery at some point

---

[c] Glial cells are the non-neuronal supporting cells of the nervous system.

TABLE 2–1.   MAJOR SPINAL PATHWAYS

| | **Motor Tracts** | |
Name	Travels in Cord Ipsilateral or Contralateral to Muscles It Innervates	Type of Control
Lateral corticospinal	Ipsilateral	Voluntary motion, especially precisely controlled movements of the distal limbs
Ventral corticospinal	Contralateral	Voluntary motion of axial musculature; minimal clinical significance due to small size
Rubrospinal	Ipsilateral	Voluntary motion of the upper extremities, especially precisely controlled movements of the distal musculature
Vestibulospinal	Bilateral	Posture and balance
Lateral and medial reticulospinals	Ipsilateral	Posture, balance, modulation of spinal reflexes, axial and proximal limb motions; in performance of motor tasks, complements actions driven by corticospinals

| | **Sensory Tracts** | |
Name	Travels in Cord Ipsilateral or Contralateral to Areas It Innervates	Type of Control
Anterolateral system (spinothalamic, spinoreticular, and spinotectal tracts)	Contralateral	Pain, temperature, and crude touch
Dorsal column	Ipsilateral	Proprioception, vibratory sense, deep touch, and discriminative touch
Dorsal spinocerebellar	Ipsilateral	Unconscious proprioception from trunk and lower extremities
Ventral spinocerebellar	Bilateral	Unconscious proprioception from trunk and lower extremities

Sources: references 27, 108, 174.

between T8 and L4. It is an important contributor to spinal circulation.[48, 116, 118]

Spinal Nerves

There are 8 cervical, 12 thoracic, 5 lumbar, 5 sacral, and 1 coccygeal pairs of spinal nerves. Each spinal nerve has a dorsal (sensory) and a ventral (primarily motor) root that arise from a single cord segment. The C1 through C7 spinal nerves exit the vertebral foramen above the cor-respondingly numbered vertebrae. The C8 spinal nerve exists below the C7 vertebra. (There are 8 cervical nerves and only 7 cervical vertebrae.) The spinal nerves of T1 and below exit below the correspondingly numbered vertebrae (Figure 2–6).[27, 48]

Because the spinal cord is shorter than the vertebral column, the nerve roots must travel cau-dally before exiting the vertebral canal. Distal to the conus medullaris, the nerve roots form the cauda equina (Figure 2–6).

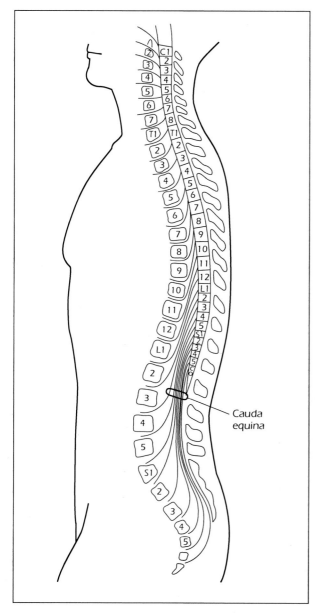

Cauda
equina

Figure 2–6. Schematic diagram of the spatial relationship of the vertebrae, spinal cord, nerve roots, and cauda equina.

MECHANISMS OF VERTEBRAL INJURIES

Most spinal cord injuries occur as the result of direct or indirect trauma to the vertebral column. Approximately 10 percent of these spinal cord injuries occur with no detectable vertebral injury. In adults, this is most likely to occur in individuals with preexisting narrow spinal canals or spondylosis.[39, 142] Children can sustain spinal cord injury without any detectable damage to the vertebral column because their spinal columns are more mobile than those of adults.[130]

Most injuries of the vertebral column involve either a single level or a limited number of contiguous vertebrae. In 3 percent to 5 percent of cases of vertebral injury, however, the spinal column sustains damage at two or more levels that are separated by undamaged vertebrae. The secondary level of injury is often located at the rostral or caudal extremes of the spine. Multiple noncontiguous vertebral injuries are associated with severe trauma. They occur most commonly in association with injuries of the upper and middle thoracic spine.[39, 142] Noncontiguous injuries rostral to a known injury are a matter of concern because if undetected and not treated properly, they may result in higher damage to the spinal cord with resulting paralysis and sensory loss at a higher level. Caudally located noncontiguous injuries can impact on muscle tone and bowel, bladder, and genital functioning.[18]

Spinal column injuries are rarely caused by direct trauma to the vertebrae; most result from forces that create violent motions of the head or trunk.[142] The magnitude and direction of the traumatic force determines the type and extent of boney and ligamentous damage. The degree to which the vertebrae, soft tissues, or both impinge upon the cord, the cord's vascular supply, or the spinal nerves determines the extent of neurological damage that results.

Laboratory studies have demonstrated that forces applied in different directions lead to distinct patterns of boney and ligamentous damage. Other factors that affect vertebral injury include the position of the person's head, neck, and trunk at the time of injury; the magnitude, rate of application, and duration of injuring force; and the point of application of the injuring force.[42, 114] Outside of the laboratory, most injuries probably result from a combination of forces. Moreover, the forces involved in a given person's injury are usually unknown; they can only be inferred from a history of the accident and the pattern of vertebral and ligamentous injury found. Despite these limitations, information gleaned from laboratory studies is useful for understanding the causative mechanisms of vertebral column injury.[80, 118, 142]

Cervical Injuries

Because of its relatively poor mechanical stability, the cervical spine is more vulnerable to trauma than other areas of the vertebral column.[118, 177] Moreover, injury to the spine in this region is likely to result (40 percent incidence) in damage to the cord.[39] As a result of these factors, a disproportionate number (approximately 52 percent) of spinal cord injuries occur in the cervical region.[125]

Most survivors of cervical spinal cord injuries have cord damage at the lower cervical levels; vertebral fractures at C1 and C2 are rarely associated with significant neurologic deficits.[39] This is largely due to a combination of two factors. The vertebral canal is large at the craniovertebral junction, with the spinal cord occupying only 50 percent of the available space. Thus, it is possible for 50 percent of the canal's area to be intruded upon by displaced boney elements without damage to the spinal cord. In addition, when the spinal cord *is* injured at this level, the injury is not likely to be survived. Complete cord injuries at C1 and C2 interrupt the diaphragm's innervation, making survival possible only if resuscitation is provided immediately.[67, 118, 142]

The forces most frequently causing vertebral injury in the cervical spine are flexion, vertical loading, and extension. These forces may be accompanied and modified by rotation, lateral flexion, or both.

Flexion.   Flexion injuries of the cervical spine have the highest incidence of neurological injury.[118] This type of injury is most commonly the result of rapid deceleration, as occurs in head-on collisions.[160]

When the neck is flexed violently, the vertebral column is subjected to compression force anteriorly and distraction force posteriorly.[39, 80] Hyperflexion can result in damage to soft tissue, vertebrae, or a combination of the two.[80] With the exception of clay-shoveler fractures,[d] the posterior ligamentous complex sustains damage in all flexion injuries.[39, 80]

Compression of the anterior aspect of the vertebral column can result in collapse of the anterior aspect of a vertebra, called a wedge fracture (Figure 2–7).[39, 42, 80] This type of fracture is usually stable[39] and typically does not result in neurological injury.[42]

A more serious injury that can result from compression of the anterior aspect of the vertebral column is a teardrop fracture. In this injury, a fragment is split from the vertebral body anteriorly. Flexion teardrop fractures are associated with severe ligamentous disruption[80] and are often accompanied by a sagitally oriented fracture of the vertebral body with posterior displacement of the boney fragments into the neural canal (Figure 2–8).[42] Severe damage to the cord typically results from flexion teardrop fractures.[42, 80, 142]

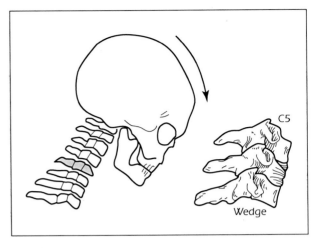

Figure 2–7.   *Wedge fracture resulting from flexion injury to the cervical spine.*

Damage to the ligaments stabilizing the cervical spine can also have grave results. When posterior distractive forces resulting from hyperflexion, possibly in combination with rotation,[5, 42] cause total disruption of the intervertebral ligaments and intervertebral disk, the vertebrae are free to dislocate. Typically, distraction and shearing forces drive the superior vertebra forward. The dislocated vertebra's inferior facets lodge in front of the superior facets of the subjacent vertebra, and the facets "lock" (Figure 2–9). A dislocation with bilateral locked facets is extremely unstable and usually results in severe neurological damage.[5, 39, 80, 142]

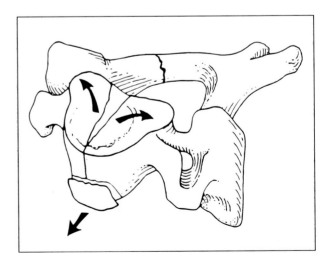

Figure 2–8.   *Flexion teardrop fracture accompanied by sagittally oriented fracture of the vertebral body with posterior displacement of the boney fragments into the neural canal. (From Crowell, R., Edwards, W., & White, A. [1989]. Mechanisms of injury in the cervical spine: Experimental evidence and biomechanical modeling. In H. Sherk, E. Dunn, & F. Eismont [Eds.], The Cervical Spine [2nd ed.] [p. 72]. Philadelphia: Lippincott. Reproduced with permission of Lippincott Williams & Wilkins.)*

---

[d] A clay-shoveler fracture is an avulsion fracture of the spinous process of C6, C7, or T1.[80]

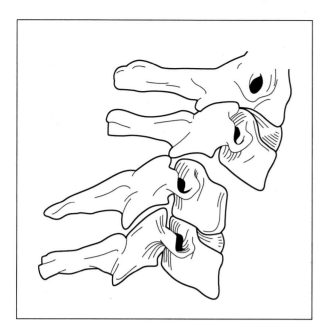

Figure 2–9. Bilateral facet dislocation.

Some patients with posterior ligamentous disruption present initially without neurologic deficits. If the injury is not recognized and stabilized, however, the vertebrae can subsequently sublux and cause spinal cord injury.[5]

Flexion with rotation. Flexion and rotation forces, possibly in combination with lateral flexion and shearing,[39] can result in the dislocation and locking of a single facet joint (Figure 2–10). This displacement is made possible by disruption of the facet joint capsule and posterior ligaments.[138] Unilateral facet dislocations can be associated with fractures of the pedicle or lamina.[5]

Unilateral facet dislocations are usually stable,[39, 80] but can be unstable due to significant ligamentous damage.[5] This type of injury is associated with neurological damage, usually Brown-Séquard syndrome or nerve root damage, approximately 30 percent of the time.[39, 80]

Vertical compression. Axial loading through the straightened (slightly flexed) cervical spine results in burst fractures.[42, 80] Burst fracture in the cervical spine is most often the result of striking the head while diving into shallow water (Figure 2–11). In this type of accident, a burst fracture occurs most frequently at C4 or C5, with complete tetraplegia resulting.[24]

A burst fracture is a comminuted fracture of the vertebral body; the vertebral body is crushed. Neurological damage occurs when boney fragments are driven posteriorly into the spinal canal (Figure 2–12). Burst fractures are accompanied by fractures of the vertebral arch.[80] The stability of a burst fracture in the cervical spine depends on the extent of injury to the posterior elements of the spine.[5]

Extension injuries. Extension injuries often occur when someone strikes his chin or forehead in a fall (Figure 2–13) or is struck from behind when riding in a vehicle. The most common location for an extension injury is C4-5.[24]

When the neck is extended violently, the cervical spine is subjected to distraction force anteriorly and compression force posteriorly.[39] These

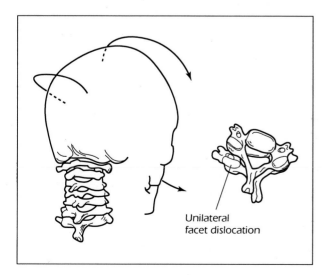

Figure 2–10. Unilateral facet dislocation resulting from combined flexion and rotation of the cervical spine.

Unilateral facet dislocation

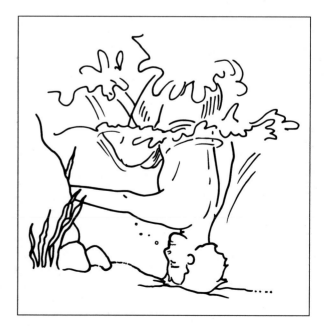

Figure 2–11. Common mechanism of injury of burst fracture in cervical spine: striking head while diving into shallow water.

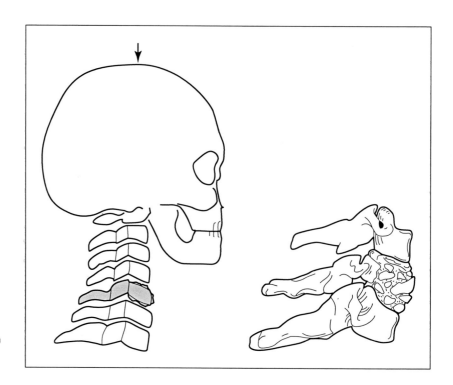

Figure 2–12. Burst fracture resulting from compression (axial loading) of the cervical spine.

forces can result in boney or ligamentous damage or both.

The posterior compressive forces involved in an extension injury can result in fractures on one (unilateral) or both (bilateral) sides of the vertebral arch, often in two adjacent vertebrae. A unilateral fracture is most common.[2, 39] When a bilateral fracture occurs, the vertebral body can dislocate.[80]

Severe anterior distractive forces can cause rupture of the anterior longitudinal ligament and discovertebral bond. A small fragment of the anterior vertebral body may be avulsed in the process (Figure 2–14). When hyperextension results in severe ligamentous disruption anteriorly, the superior vertebra dislocates posteriorly. This injury is called a hyperextension dislocation, sprain, or strain. The spinal cord is compressed by the vertebral body and disk fragments anteriorly and the ligamentum flava and laminae posteriorly (Figure 2–15).[39, 73, 80]

When the cervical spine is hyperextended, neurological damage can occur without any boney or ligamentous damage. This occurs most frequently in the presence of osteophytic changes or a congenitally small canal.[133] Spinal cord damage

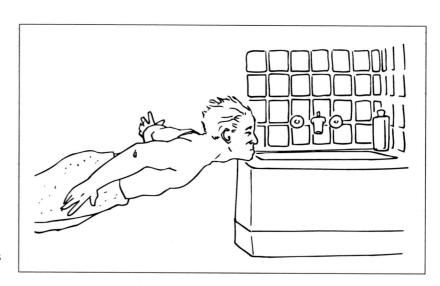

Figure 2–13. Common mechanism of extension injury in cervical spine: person falls and strikes chin or forehead.

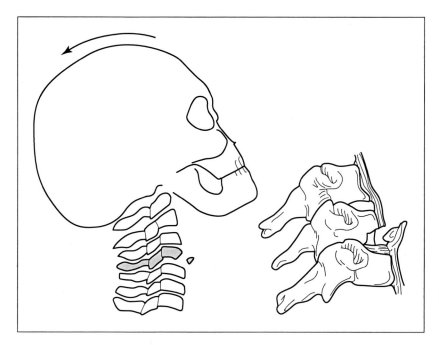

Figure 2–14. Hyperextension injury with severe anterior distractive forces causing rupture of anterior longitudinal ligament and avulsion of anterior fragment from vertebral body.

secondary to hyperextension injury is often confined to the central aspect of the cord.[5]

Hyperextension of the cervical spine is most likely to lead to cord damage if the person is elderly. Degenerative changes in the vertebrae of people in this age group make them more vulnerable to extension injuries. Osteophytes projecting posteriorly from the vertebral bodies can impinge upon the spinal cord when the neck is hyperextended by a relatively mild force. Because of the mild trauma involved, cervical cord injury can be overlooked by examining physicians. Symptoms

may be attributed to hysteria, malingering, cerebrovascular accident, or other neurological or cardiovascular disorder.[41, 133]

Lateral flexion.   Violent lateral flexion leads to compression on one side of the vertebral column and distraction on the other. The compressive forces, occurring on the side toward which the spine laterally flexes, can result in lateral wedging of the vertebral body and fracture of the vertebral arch. Distractive forces on the contralateral side can cause ligamentous disruption. Lateral flexion

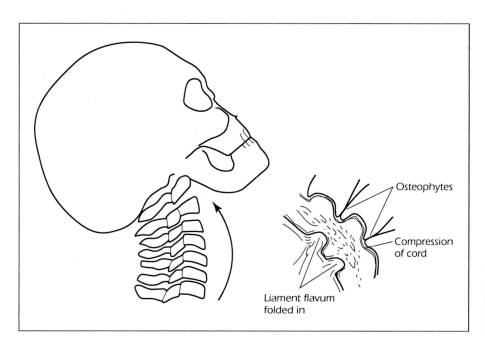

Osteophytes

Compression of cord

Liament flavum folded in

Figure 2–15. Hyperextension sprain. The spinal cord is compressed by the vertebral body, disk fragments, or osteophytes anteriorly and/or the ligamentum flavum and laminae posteriorly.

injuries can lead to severe spinal cord damage and are often associated with brachial plexus injuries.[2]

Pure lateral flexion injuries are rare.[2] More commonly, lateral flexion combines with and modifies the effects of other forces to produce spinal injury.[39, 80]

Thoracic Injuries

The rib cage provides the T1 through T10 spine with great stability. As a result, extreme violence is required to injure the spine in this region. Thoracic spinal cord injuries are less common than cervical injuries, but are more likely to be complete[67, 91, 168] and are less frequently associated with any subsequent return of motor or sensory function below the lesion.[58, 168] These findings are probably due to the magnitude of force required to injure the thoracic spine, the small size of the vertebral canal in this region, and the relatively poor vascular supply of the upper thoracic cord.[67, 118] Trauma to the lower thoracic spine can injure the vessel of Adamkiewicz, a major source of the thoracolumbar cord's vascular supply. The resulting neurological damage can ascend as high as T4.[118]

Thoracic injuries are often caused by gunshot wounds, vehicular accidents, and falls.[118] The most common site of injury to the thoracolumbar spine is the T12-L1 junction.[177] This is where the relatively rigid thoracic spine meets the relatively flexible lumbar spine.[39, 73]

The spatial arrangement of boney and neural tissue in the low thoracic and upper lumbar regions is such that vertebral injury can result in diverse patterns of neurological damage. All of the lumbar and sacral cord segments lie between the upper border of the T10 vertebral body and the level of L1 or L2. Additionally, spinal nerves from higher levels lie adjacent to the cord within the vertebral canal in this region as they travel caudally before exiting. As a result, the neural canal at a given vertebral level may enclose more than one cord level as well as spinal nerves from several higher levels (Figure 2–16). Vertebral damage can result in trauma to any or all of this neural tissue or in no neurological damage.

The basic mechanics of vertebral and ligamentous injury of the spine, described earlier in this chapter in reference to cervical injuries, are similar throughout the spinal column. For example, extreme motions in the sagittal or frontal planes cause compression of the vertebrae in the direction of the motion and distraction of the opposite boney and ligamentous elements. The patterns of injury typical of the thoracic spine are described below.

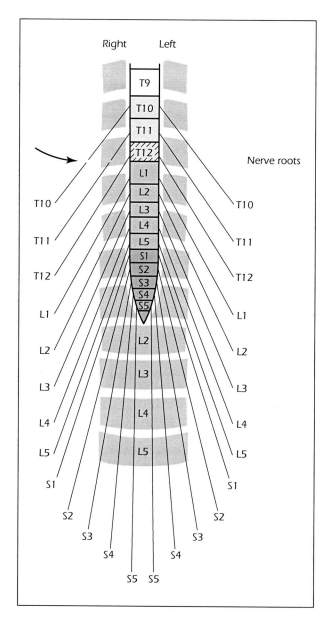

Figure 2–16. *Vertebral injury has resulted in damage to the T10 and T11 nerve roots on the right, plus the T12 level of the spinal cord.*

Flexion. Most fractures of the thoracic vertebrae are wedge compression fractures caused by compression of the anterior aspects of the vertebral bodies (Figure 2–17). The thoracic region may be prone to this type of fracture because the normal kyphotic curve converts vertical compression forces to flexion.[39] The incidence of neurological damage occurring with this type of injury varies with the severity of the fracture.[118]

In severe cases of flexion injury, a wedge compression fracture is combined with damage to the posterior ligamentous or boney elements or both.[52, 118] The posterior damage is caused by distraction forces created when the vertebra pivots on its intact middle column.[52]

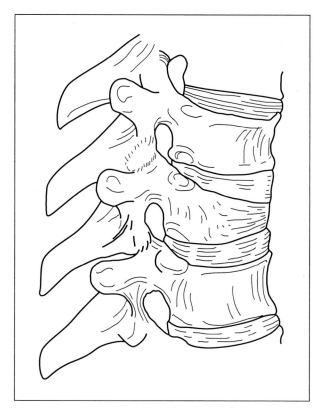

Figure 2–17. Wedge fracture resulting from flexion of the thoracic spine *(ribs not included in figure)*.

Flexion with rotation. When rotation is combined with flexion (Figure 2–18), rotational shearing is added to the anterior compressive and posterior distractive forces created by flexion. This combination of forces can disrupt all three columns of the spine. Flexion-rotation injuries can lead to fracture dislocations with anterior compression of the vertebral body, damage to the anterior longitudinal ligament, disruption of the disk, a horizontal fracture (slice fracture) through the vertebral body, and fractures of the posterior arch. Fractures of transverse processes and ribs are frequently associated with these injuries. Neurological damage is common following flexion-rotation injuries, resulting from dislocation of the vertebrae, entry of boney fragments into the spinal canal, or both.[39, 52, 118]

Vertical compression. The thoracic spine can be subjected to vertical compression when a person is struck by a falling object or falls and lands on his upper thoracic spine, buttocks, or feet. Falls most frequently result in burst fractures of T10, T11, or T12.[24, 118]

Burst fractures of thoracic vertebrae are similar to cervical burst fractures. The vertebral body is crushed, and the laminae fracture. Retropulsion

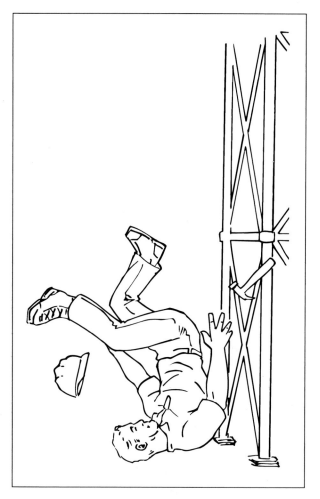

Figure 2–18. Flexion-rotation injury caused by fall onto upper back and one shoulder.

of boney fragments into the vertebral canal often leads to cord damage.[52, 93, 118]

Extension or lateral flexion. The thoracolumbar spine is rarely injured by isolated extension or lateral flexion forces.[39, 118, 177] When injuries occur from these forces, they involve disruption of the anterior ligaments and lateral wedging of the vertebral body, respectively.[52, 118]

Lumbar Injuries

The lumbar region of the spinal column is of intermediate stability: it is more flexible than the thoracic spine but less flexible than the cervical spine. Although it lacks the stability provided by the thoracic cage, the lumbar spine is supported by strong paraspinal and abdominal musculature.[39]

Common causes of injury to this region include falls, vehicular accidents, gunshot wounds, and direct impact from heavy objects.[118, 138] Injury occurs most frequently at the thoracolumbar junction.

Neurological damage resulting from trauma to the lumbar spine is usually incomplete.[67] This is due, in part, to the relatively good vascular supply and large vertebral canal in this region. In addition, caudal to L1 or L2, the cord is not present in the vertebral canal. The cauda equina, the sole neurological element within the neural canal in this region, is less sensitive than the spinal cord to trauma.[118, 177] Because nerve roots exit at each level, the vertebral canal of the more caudally located vertebrae contains less neurologic tissue. Thus in injuries at lower levels, a greater degree of encroachment into the spinal canal by boney elements is possible without neurological damage.[93, 137]

Flexion. The mechanism and patterns of injury from violent flexion of the lumbar spine are comparable to those of flexion injury in the thoracic spine. Wedge compression fractures due to flexion, often not associated with neurologic damage, are frequent at L1.[52]

Flexion with rotation. The orientation of the intervertebral facet joints in the lumbar spine (Figure 2–19) provides a good deal of anteroposterior stability. The limited mobility allowed by these joints, combined with strong joint capsules, makes pure dislocation rare in the lumbar region.[39, 177] Violent flexion-rotation is more likely to result in fracture dislocation, as occurs in the thoracic spine. These fracture dislocations usually result in neurological injury.[16, 39]

Flexion with distraction. Combined flexion and distraction forces are typical of, but not limited to, "seat-belt injuries" associated with lap belts that are worn without shoulder restraints. In this type of injury, the lumbar spine is flexed violently about a fulcrum located at the anterior abdominal wall. Flexion about this anteriorly located fulcrum results in extreme distractive forces on the middle and posterior columns of the spine.[39, 52, 114]

Spinal column damage in this type of injury can occur at one or two levels.[52] It can be limited to the ligaments and disks or include vertebral fractures.[39, 114] The boney fractures and ligamentous tears associated with flexion-distraction injuries are horizontally oriented (Figure 2–20). The posterior aspect of the vertebral body, annulus fibrosus, vertebral arch, and posterior longitudinal ligament can be torn by the distractive forces. In addition, the anterior aspect of the vertebral body can com-

press. Disruption of the middle and posterior columns allows dislocation or subluxation to occur.[52] From 15 percent[39] to 27 percent[114] of these injuries result in neurological damage. Associated abdominal injuries are common.[114, 138]

Shear. A horizontally-directed force, such as occurs when a person is struck from behind by a heavy object or falls onto an uneven surface, causes shearing of the spine (Figure 2–21). This force can cause total disruption of the ligaments, with resulting dislocation of the vertebrae and severe neurologic damage. Shear forces can also cause fractures of the vertebral body and the posterior arches.[39] Injuries caused by shear forces are the most unstable spinal injuries.[114]

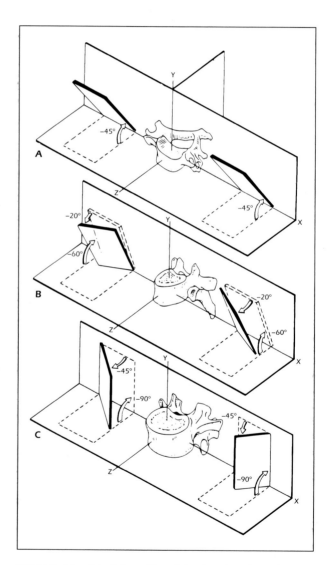

Figure 2–19. *Orientation of facet joints (rough estimates).* **(A)** Cervical. **(B)** Thoracic. **(C)** Lumbar: vertical orientation of facet joints makes pure dislocation in the lumbar region rare. *(From White, A. & Panjabi, M. [1978]. Clinical Biomechanics of the Spine [p. 30]. Philadelphia: Lippincott. Reproduced with permission of Lippincott Williams & Wilkins.)*

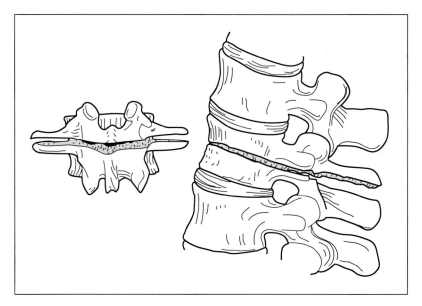

Figure 2–20. Flexion-distraction injury of the lumbar spine. Boney fractures and ligamentous tears associated with these injuries are horizontally oriented.

Vertical compression. As is true in more rostral regions of the vertebral column, violent force directed through the long axis of the lumbar spine can cause burst fractures. In this region, burst fractures are usually caused by falls.[118] About 50 percent of people sustaining burst fractures in the thoracic or lumbar spine sustain neurological damage, usually incomplete.[52]

Associated Injuries

Traumatic spinal cord injuries often occur with additional injuries sustained at the same time. Some of the more common associated injuries include fractures, pneumothorax, hemothorax, head injury, brachial plexus injury, and peripheral nerve injury.[76] These injuries can delay and pro-

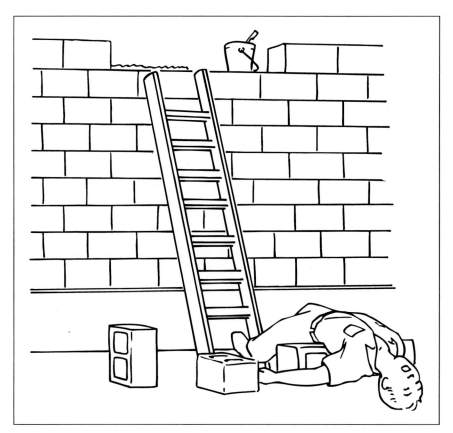

Figure 2–21. Fall onto uneven surface causes shearing of the spine.

long rehabilitation, and in some cases, limit patients' ultimate functional outcomes.

NEUROPATHOLOGY

When spinal cord injury occurs as a result of vertebral injury, the cord typically sustains damage as a result of impingement by boney or soft tissue structures. This occurs, for example, when vertebrae dislocate or a vertebral body bursts. The spinal cord can also be damaged by direct insult from a foreign body such as a bullet or knife. Gunshot wounds can damage the cord without the bullet entering the spinal canal; in these cases, a concussive shock wave damages the cord. In both penetrating and nonpenetrating injuries, more severe disruption of the spinal canal leads to more severe neurological damage.[169]

The spinal cord does not have to be severed for irreversible damage to occur. In fact, actual anatomic transection of the cord is rare.[118, 158] This is an important point to remember when educating people about their injuries. Often, patients are told that their spinal cords were "bruised" instead of severed, and they interpret this fact to mean that they will recover from their paralysis. Trauma that results in "bruising" or hemorrhaging in the spinal cord, however, can (and *often* does) cause neurological damage that is just as complete and just as permanent as when the cord is severed.

Not all spinal cord damage occurs as the result of physical trauma to the cord itself. The spinal cord can also be damaged by interruption of its vascular supply. The cord's vascular supply can be disrupted by vertebral trauma, surgery, gunshot or knife wounds, or various other causes.

Although most spinal cord injuries occur as a result of trauma, the cord can be damaged by a variety of nontraumatic causes. Examples include spinal hematoma, infection, arachnoiditis, radiation, spondylosis, rheumatoid arthritis, neoplasm, and interruption of the cord's vascular supply due to surgery, cardiac arrest, or aortic aneurysm.[177]

Pathological Changes

Blunt trauma to the spinal cord results in some primary destruction of neurons at the level of injury. This neuronal damage is most severe in the cell bodies but can also occur in the axons.[83] The neurologic damage that results from trauma to the spinal cord is due only in part to the initial trauma to the neurons themselves. Most of the damage to the cord is caused by secondary sequelae[e] of the initial trauma.[40, 84, 152, 182]

Typically, the spinal cord sustains a contusion as the result of impingement by displaced bone, soft tissues, or both. Within hours following the initial trauma, a process of progressive tissue destruction is initiated within the cord. These secondary reactions lead to ischemia, edema, demyelination of axons, and necrosis of the spinal cord.[22, 158, 170]

The injured spinal cord can look undamaged on visual examination soon after injury.[177] Microscopic examination within the first few hours following injury, however, reveals patchy hemorrhage, tissue laceration, edema, and necrosis, most prevalent in the central gray matter. Tissue destruction spreads outwardly into the white matter, as well as rostrally and caudally as time passes.[106, 129, 159, 177] Axons located peripherally in the cord are more likely to survive. Of those that survive, many remain nonfunctional as a result of demyelination.[181]

The process of secondary tissue destruction may last from several days[181] to 4 weeks[183] after the initial trauma. The extent of destruction that ultimately occurs is dependent on the severity of the initial trauma,[50] with some modification by the therapeutic interventions administered to limit the progression of the lesion.

The secondary tissue destruction initiated by trauma to the spinal cord can progress up and down the cord from the site of the initial trauma. The resulting area of cord necrosis is commonly spindle shaped, tapering in its rostral and caudal extensions.[83] The area of maximal cord damage usually spreads over one to three segments; however, the tissue destruction can spread over several segments, leading to the formation of cystic cavities.

Gross edema of the spinal cord can also occur following trauma. As the cord swells, it becomes compressed within the meninges, and further damage to the cord occurs.[83]

As the primary and secondary reactions to trauma subside, the necrotic region of the spinal cord is gradually resorbed and replaced by scar tissue, cysts, or cavities.[40, 69, 83]

---

[e] The following description of the pathological changes associated with spinal cord injury is based primarily on studies of blunt trauma to the cord as occurs when boney elements impinge on the cord as a result of vertebral injury. However, research indicates that the same process of secondary progressive tissue destruction occurs with any injury to the spinal cord, including cord damage from ischemia, slow compression,[182] contusion, or transection.[183]

Underlying Mechanisms of Secondary Tissue Destruction

Despite extensive research in recent years, the mechanisms underlying the secondary tissue destruction initiated by spinal cord injury remain only partially understood. Initial trauma to the cord appears to set off a multifactorial process that expands the area of cell death and damage. The mechanisms involved in this process include ischemia, inflammation, disruption of ion concentrations in the injured tissues, and apoptosis (Figure 2–22). Each of these pathologic processes and the cell damage and death that they cause leads to the release of substances that stimulate additional secondary tissue damage, creating an escalating cycle of tissue destruction.

Ischemia. Blood flow diminishes in the traumatized area of a spinal cord following injury. This reduction in circulation occurs rapidly in the gray matter. In severely traumatized cords, blood flow in the white matter falls after a 2- to 3-hour delay. It may not diminish at all in the white matter of less severely traumatized cords.[182]

One of the primary causes of interrupted blood supply to the damaged segment of the cord appears to be injury to the anterior sulcal arteries and arterioles, which provide circulation to the central part of the spinal cord.[159] In addition to disrupting circulation to the gray matter, damage of the arterioles within the gray matter disrupts circulation to the adjacent ascending and descending tracts. This happens because the sulcal arterioles pass through the gray matter on their way to the surrounding white matter.[159]

The blood supply to the spinal cord is disrupted both by mechanical trauma[f] to the vasculature[159,] and vasospasm. The arterioles arising from the anterior sulcal arteries constrict progressively during the first 24 hours after injury.[7] Vasoconstrictive substances such as norepinephrine, serotonin, histamine, and prostaglandins in the injured cord may contribute to this vasospasm and the resulting ischemia.[7,128] Additional possible causes of vasospasm include mechanical stimulation and the presence of vasoconstrictive substances formed during the breakdown of erythrocytes following hemorrhage.[7]

Disruption of the venous system in the damaged region of the cord may also contribute to

[f] This mechanical disruption includes rupture or compression of blood vessels, and intravascular thromboses.[7]

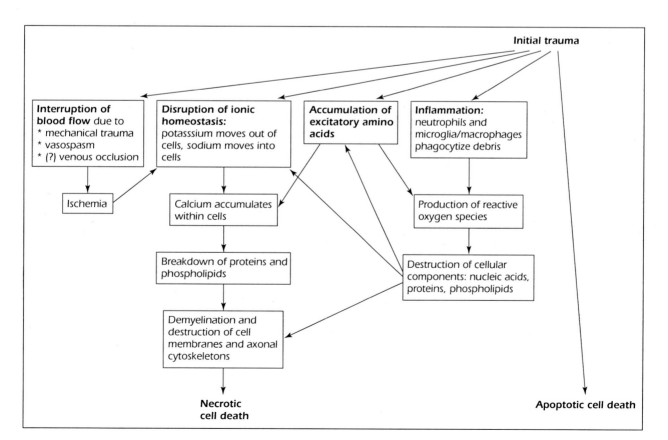

Figure 2–22. Secondary tissue destruction initiated by spinal cord injury.

ischemia.[7, 159] Other possible causes of ischemia in the injured spinal cord include thromboses, metabolic disturbances, and elevated pressure due to edema.[182]

The central nervous system is very intolerant to ischemia; as little as 15 to 30 seconds of anoxia can cause irreversible damage in the neurons.[184] When the blood supply to the injured portion of the spinal cord is interrupted, lack of oxygen and nutrients interferes with normal cellular functioning in this area. Ion derangement (described later in this chapter) quickly follows, initiating a cascade of metabolic events that lead to cell death.[155]

Inflammation. Inflammation plays a significant role in the secondary tissue destruction that occurs after spinal cord injury. Cells that are damaged in the initial trauma release proinflammatory substances that attract neutrophils to the injured area within a few hours of the injury. These inflammatory cells apparently contribute to the expansion of the area of tissue damage for 24 to 48 hours after the initial trauma. Microglia and macrophages arrive at the injury site slightly after neutrophils.[30, 184] These cells have been found at the level of the initial injury from 6 to 48 hours after the injury[30] and in areas containing degenerating fiber tracts rostral and caudal to the lesion for up to 8 weeks after the initial injury.[184]

Neutrophils, microglia, and macrophages phagocytose debris in the damaged area, releasing reactive oxygen species and a variety of other substances that damage surrounding healthy tissue, expanding the area of tissue necrosis.[20, 30, 152] Reactive oxygen metabolites damage cells by attacking cellular components such as nucleic acids, proteins, and phospholipids.[155] The breakdown products of these reactions can further disrupt cell functioning, contributing to the development of ion imbalance.[152]

Although inflammation contributes to the process of tissue destruction that follows spinal cord injury, it may also play a role in protecting some of the surviving neurons and promoting tissue repair.[30, 183, 184]

Ion derangement. Disruption of cell membranes in the injured area of the spinal cord results in abnormal concentrations of potassium and sodium: potassium moves out from the neurons into the extracellular space, and sodium accumulates within the cells. This derangement causes a loss of neuronal excitability because neurons require a normal ion balance to generate action potentials.[155] More importantly, a high concentration of sodium within the neurons results in

a shift in calcium, a key factor in secondary tissue destruction following spinal cord injury.[8]

Calcium ions accumulate in injured cells after a spinal cord is traumatized. The influx of calcium results from the abnormally high sodium concentration within the neurons and the collapse of the membrane potential.[155] Neurotoxic transmitters, particularly glutamate, contribute to this shift of calcium into the neurons.[31, 50, 64, 152, 157, 158, 175]

Concentration of calcium within neurons is one of the most important contributors to secondary tissue destruction following spinal cord injury.[87, 99, 155] The abnormal concentration of calcium within the damaged cells disrupts their functioning and causes breakdown of protein and phospholipids, with resulting demyelination, destruction of the cell membrane and axonal cytoskeleton, and cell death.[9–11, 84, 99, 155, 182] The metabolic by-products of this deranged cell functioning and membrane destruction may contribute to further membrane destruction and the development of ischemia and edema.[182]

Apoptosis. Apoptosis is a form of cell death (programmed cell death) that occurs normally during embryonic development and has recently been found to occur as a pathological process following central nervous system damage. It is an active process performed by individual cells, in contrast to the passive death of groups of cells as occurs in necrotic[h] cell death.[63, 104]

Both neurons and supporting cells within the spinal cord tissue undergo apoptotic cell death.[104] It is not yet known what initiates this "intrinsic suicide mechanism."[63] It begins at the level of the initial injury within 4 to 6 hours of the trauma, and runs its course at this level within 24 hours.[104]

Apoptosis occurs for a more prolonged period of time (up to 3 weeks) in areas of the spinal cord rostral and caudal to the site of the initial injury.[63, 148] It occurs in oligodendrocytes[i] associated with the myelin sheaths of degenerating ascending white matter tracts rostral to the site of the injury, and descending tracts caudal to the injury.[63, 148] Apoptotic oligodendrocyte cell death may cause demyelination of surviving axons, interfering with their subsequent functioning.[63, 148]

---

[g] Calcium overload is involved in cell death of both glial cells and neurons.[155]

[h] Mechanical disruption of injured cells and the secondary pathological processes described previously lead to necrosis.

[i] Oligodendrocytes are glial cells that form the myelin sheaths surrounding axons.

Effect of Compression on Recovery of Function

Spinal cord trauma does not always result in complete disruption of the cord at the level of lesion. Incomplete lesions are common, with surviving neurons passing through the damaged portion of the cord. If this undamaged neural tissue is subjected to chronic compression, however, it may survive but not resume functioning while subjected to the compression.[22]

Spinal Shock

Spinal shock is a transient phenomenon that occurs after trauma to the spinal cord. During spinal shock, the cord *temporarily* ceases to function below the lesion. Spinal reflexes, voluntary motor and sensory function, and autonomic control are absent[j] below the level of lesion.[48] The cause of spinal shock is unknown. Neurons below the lesion may become hyperpolarized, losing their excitability due to the absence of facilitation from descending tracts.[102]

Spinal shock usually resolves within a few weeks of injury,[48, 38, 177] but can take months to resolve completely.[102]

Spinal Cord Function below the Lesion

As spinal shock passes, the cord gradually resumes functioning below the lesion. This return of function is evidenced by resumption of spinal reflexes caudal to the lesion. Voluntary motor function, sensation, and supraspinal influences on the spinal autonomic centers may also resume as spinal shock resolves, if surviving descending or ascending fiber tracts traverse the level of the lesion. (Preservation of voluntary motor control, autonomic control, and perception of sensory stimuli can occur if the brain and the spinal cord caudal to the lesion remain "connected" by some surviving and functioning neurons that span the damaged segment of the cord. If this "connection" does not exist, the portion of the cord caudal to the lesion will function but will not communicate with the brain. In these cases, the individual will exhibit spinal reflexes below the lesion but will lack voluntary motor control, autonomic control, and sensation below the lesion.)

Neurological Return

Neurological return refers to a resumption of *voluntary motor function or sensation* that has been lost as the result of a spinal cord injury. For example, individuals may regain the ability to voluntarily contract one or more muscles that had been paralyzed, or regain the ability to feel a pin or cotton ball contacting their skin in one or more areas that had been anaesthetic. This resumption of motor or sensory function below the level of the lesion is evidence of at least some "connection" between the brain and the muscles or dermatomes that resume functioning. In contrast, the return of reflexive functioning below the lesion is *not* considered to be neurological return. For example, the onset of spasticity[k] below the lesion without any gains in sensory ability or *voluntary* motor function is not classified as neurological return. The presence of spasticity gives evidence of functioning of the spinal cord below the lesion, but it does not demonstrate a "connection" between the brain and the muscles.

Most neurological return following spinal cord injury occurs within the first postinjury year.[61, 166] It typically occurs most rapidly during the first 6 months after injury, then continues at a slower pace for up to 2 years.[61] In unusual cases, neurological return can occur for 5 or more years after injury.[135] People with incomplete injuries tend to exhibit motor return earlier than do people with complete injuries.[107]

Mechanisms of neurological return. Neurological return after spinal cord injury can occur as a result of resumed functioning within either the nerve roots or the spinal cord itself. The first of these is referred to as nerve root return or root recovery. It may be the most common source of neurological return, possibly occurring after all traumatic spinal cord injuries.[157] *Nerve root return* occurs as a result of resumed functioning or regeneration of nerve roots that were damaged during the initial trauma. (In traumatic spinal cord injuries, nerve roots are frequently damaged as they exit the spinal canal or as they travel caudally within the canal before exiting.) The reason that nerve root return occurs so frequently is that the nerve roots are more resistant to trauma and have a greater capacity for recovery and regeneration than do neurons within the spinal cord.[157]

The mechanisms of neurological return resulting from *improved functioning in the spinal cord* itself are not fully understood. Possible causes include resolution of the hemorrhaging, ischemia, edema, inflammation, and ion derangement associated with spinal cord trauma; relief of compression

---

[j] Sacral reflexes occasionally persist during spinal shock, particularly in people who have high cervical lesions.[8]

[k] Spasticity, an involuntary motor response, is discussed later in this chapter.

on the spinal cord; regeneration and regrowth of neurons and glial cells; remyelination of axons; and sprouting from intact axons.[102, 157, 185] Adaptive alteration in the functioning of surviving neurons may also play a role in neurological return following incomplete injuries. These changes in neural activity could include the activation of previously inactive neurons, increased sensitivity of receptors to neurotransmitters, increased density of receptors in postsynaptic neurons, and altered responsiveness of neurons below the lesion.[102, 185]

Predictors of return. Perhaps the most central question for patients, their families, and health professionals is how much recovery of motor function will occur after a spinal cord injury.[l]

Unfortunately, it is not possible to predict with certainty the neurological return that any individual will experience. The degree of completeness of the lesion may, however, provide some (albeit limited) prognostic information.[58, 77, 107, 166] The likelihood of experiencing significant return varies with the extent of neurological preservation evident below the lesion at the time of the initial admission.[58, 107] Examination at 72 hours[173] or 1 month postinjury may have better predictive value[169] due to the effects of spinal shock at the time of the initial evaluation.

Both spared motor function below the lesion and pin prick[m] in the sacral region[167] or the extremities[131] are indications of greater likelihood of experiencing significant motor return. Table 2–2 presents research findings on motor return after spinal cord injuries.

Neurological Deterioration

Deterioration of neurological function, evidenced by reduced sensation or muscle strength, can also occur soon after injury. This deterioration, which is exhibited by approximately 2 percent to 5 percent of people with spinal cord injuries, has been associated with sepsis, intubation, early surgical intervention, and ankylosing spondylitis.[65] Additional causes of neurological deterioration include vertebral instability and the development of a post-traumatic cyst.[59]

In many cases, the lost function is regained within a year. This is particularly true when the deterioration was relatively minor.[65]

CLASSIFICATION OF SPINAL CORD INJURIES

In the past, communication regarding spinal cord injuries was hampered by the lack of a universally accepted system of terminology.[32] In recent years, this problem has been reduced with the use of the classification system published by the American Spinal Injury Association (ASIA) and endorsed by the International Medical Society of Paraplegia.[n]

This book uses terminology that is consistent with this classification system.

Tetraplegia Versus Paraplegia

Damage to the nervous tissue contained within the cervical region of the spinal canal causes tetraplegia.[o]

"Tetraplegia" refers to impairment or loss[p] of motor and/or sensory function in the upper and lower extremities, trunk, and pelvic organs.[4]

Damage to the nervous tissue contained within the thoracic, lumbar, or sacral regions of the spinal canal causes paraplegia. Motor and sensory function is normal in the upper extremities. Depending on the level of lesion, paraplegia can involve impairment or loss of motor and/or sensory function in the trunk, lower extremities, and pelvic organs.[4]

Neurological Level of Injury

The neurological level of injury is defined as the most caudal level of the spinal cord that exhibits intact sensory and motor functioning bilaterally. To determine an individual's neurological level of injury, the clinician tests sensitivity to light touch and pin prick at key points in each dermatome

---

[l] A closely related question is the prognosis of regaining the capacity for functional ambulation. This issue is addressed in Chapter 13, Table 13–16.

[m] The association between spared pin prick and subsequent motor return may be due to the fact that the lateral spinothalamic tract (carrying pain information) and the corticospinal tract (carrying motor commands) lie relatively close to each other in the white matter of the spinal cord.[88]

[n] The International Standards for the Neurological and Functional Classification of Spinal Cord Injury[4] is revised periodically. Clinicians and researchers should use the most current version.

[o] "Quadriplegia" is synonymous with "tetraplegia." The latter word is recommended, however, because it is etymologically compatible with "paraplegia." ("Tetra" and "para" have Greek roots, whereas "quadri" has Latin roots.)

[p] In this context, "loss" refers to an *absence* of motor function (0/5 strength) or sensory function (anesthesia). "Impairment" refers to *a reduction* in motor or sensory function or altered sensory function, such as hyperesthesia. This is not to be confused with "impairment" as defined in the Nagi model of disablement, a broader definition that would include both of the above.

TABLE 2–2.   FACTORS ASSOCIATED WITH MOTOR RETURN

Factor	Subjects	Outcomes
Frankel Grade[a] at time of admission	5658 patients with spinal cord injury admitted to Regional Spinal Cord Injury Centers within 24 hours of injury[58]	Percent progressing to higher Frankel Grade[a] by discharge[b] <table><tr><th>Initial Grade</th><th>Percent progressing to Higher Grade</th><th>Percent progressing to Frankel D or E</th></tr><tr><td>A</td><td>10.7</td><td>2.8</td></tr><tr><td>B</td><td>43.9</td><td>28.3</td></tr><tr><td>C</td><td>54.6</td><td>54.6</td></tr><tr><td>D</td><td>6.5</td><td>6.5(E)</td></tr></table>
Presence or absence of early motor return in muscles initially testing 0/5	32 patients with tetraplegia, Frankel[a] A & B[173]	Motor return in zone of partial preservation[c] • ≥1/5 strength regained by 1 month postinjury: 86% regained ≥3/5 by 1 year • ≥2/5 strength regained by 3 months post injury: 100% regained ≥3/5 strength by 1 year
Motor function at 1 month postinjury	54 patients with traumatic incomplete paraplegia[166]	Strength in individual lower extremity muscles • 1/5 to 2/5 strength at 1 month postinjury: 85% recovered to ≥3/5 by 1 year • 0/5 strength at 1 month postinjury: 26% recovered to ≥3/5 by 1 year
Motor function at 1 month postinjury	50 patients with traumatic incomplete tetraplegia[167]	Strength in individual upper extremity muscles • 2/5 strength at 1 month postinjury: 100% recovered to ≥3/5 by 1 year • 1/5 strength at 1 month postinjury: 73% recovered to ≥3/5 by 1 year • 0/5 strength at 1 month postinjury: 20% recovered to ≥3/5 by 1 year Strength in individual lower extremity muscles • 2/5 strength at 1 month postinjury: 97% recovered to ≥3/5 by 1 year • 1/5 strength at 1 month postinjury: 77% recovered to ≥3/5 by 1 year • 0/5 strength at 1 month postinjury: 24% recovered to ≥3/5 by 1 year
Pin prick sensation at the time of initial examination	59 patients with complete and incomplete tetraplegia and paraplegia[131]	Return of functional strength in muscles initially testing 0/5 • Dermatomes with spared pin prick sensation: 85% of the corresponding myotomes regained ≥3/5 strength • Dermatomes without spared pin prick sensation: 1.3% of the corresponding myotomes regained ≥3/5 strength

[a] The Frankel Scale is presented in Table 2–4.

[b] Progress from A to B, C, or D; from B to C, D, or E; etc.

[c] *Note:* the definition of "Zone of Partial Preservation" was changed in the 1996 version of the International Standards for Neurological and Functional Classification of Spinal Cord Injury[4] to include sparing in complete injuries only. Previous definitions included motor and sensory sparing in both complete and incomplete injuries.

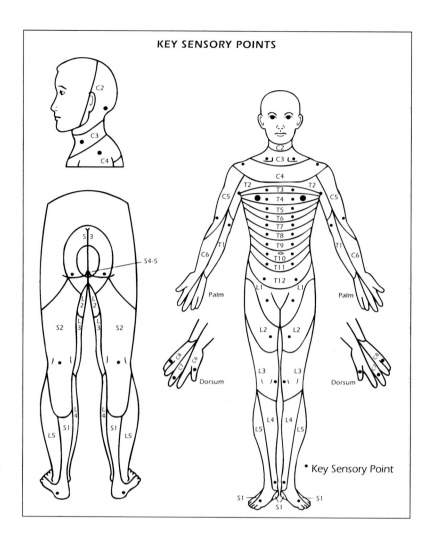

Figure 2–23. Key sensory points used to identify neurological level of injury. (Reproduced with permission from the American Spinal Injury Association [1996]. Standard Neurological Classification of Spinal Injury Patients.)

(Figure 2–23) and strength in key muscles (Table 2–3) that are representative of specific cord segments.

The key sensory points are well demarcated; each is innervated by a single spinal cord segment. As a result, the sensory ability at a key point provides a good representation of the functioning in the sensory portions of its corresponding cord segment. In contrast, muscles receive innervation from more than one spinal cord level. Thus, the strength of a given muscle is a reflection of the functioning of two or more cord segments. A lesion in the caudal segment innervating a muscle will cause reduced strength in that muscle.[q]

For the purposes of identifying the neurological level of injury, *a key muscle is defined as demonstrating intact innervation from the* *cord segment that it represents*[r] *if (1) it exhibits 3/5 or greater strength and (2) the next more rostral key muscle exhibits 5/5 strength.* If the next more rostral key muscle tests less than 5/5 but the examiner judges that its reduced performance in the manual muscle test is due to factors such as pain or disuse rather than spinal cord damage, this muscle can be assigned a grade of 5/5 for the purposes of determining neurological level.[4]

Certain spinal cord levels do not have myotomes that are readily testable using a manual muscle test. When classifying a spinal cord injury within these levels of the spinal cord (C1–C4, T2–L1, and S2–S5), the motor level is presumed to be the same as the sensory level.[4]

Sensory and motor examinations often reveal differences in the lowest level of intact cord

---

[q] For example, the biceps brachii receives C5 and C6 innervation, and normal functioning of this muscle involves intact innervation from both of these cord segments. A cord lesion that disrupts the functioning of the C6 level of the cord will result in a reduction of biceps strength.

[r] Key muscles are identified with the more rostral of the spinal cord segments from which they receive innervation. For example, the biceps brachii, which is the C5 key muscle, receives innervation from both C5 and C6.

TABLE 2-3.   KEY MUSCLES FOR IDENTIFICATION OF NEUROLOGICAL LEVEL OF INJURY

Motor Level	Key Muscles
C1–C4	Sensory level
C5	Biceps, brachialis
C6	Extensor carpi radialis longus and brevis
C7	Triceps
C8	Flexor digitorum profundus, middle finger
T1	Abductor digiti minimi
T2–L1	Sensory level
L2	Iliopsoas
L3	Quadriceps
L4	Tibialis anterior
L5	Extensor hallucis longus
S1	Gastrocnemius, soleus
S2–S5	Sensory level

Source: reference 4.

functioning. For example, an individual may exhibit intact motor function through the C5 myotome bilaterally but intact sensory function only through the C4 dermatomes. In cases such as this, it is more appropriate to report separate motor and sensory levels rather than a single neurological level of injury.[4] In this example, the patient exhibits a C5 motor level and a C4 sensory level.

Frequently, the motor function, sensory function, or both differ between the right and left sides of the body. When this is the case, it is best to report right and left motor and sensory levels[s] rather than a single neurological level.[4] This reporting gives a more complete picture of the patient's neurological functioning.[t]

Complete Versus Incomplete Lesion

A person is said to have a complete spinal cord injury if both sensory and motor function are

---

[s] This will involve reporting four levels: right sensory, left sensory, right motor, and left motor.
[t] Additional documentation involves generating motor and sensory scores. Motor and sensory scores, as well as additional components of an examination, are presented in Chapter 8.

absent in the lowest sacral segments of the spinal cord (S4 and S5). To test sensory and motor function in S4 and S5, the examiner inserts a finger into the patient's anus. Absent sensory function is evidenced by the patient's inability to feel the insertion of the examiner's finger into the anus. Absent motor function is evidenced by an inability to voluntarily contract the external anal sphincter around the examiner's finger.[4]

With an incomplete lesion, some sensory and/or motor function is preserved below the level of the lesion, *including sensory and/or motor function in the lowest sacral segments.*[4] (Function in the lowest sacral segments is defined as described above.)

Zone of Partial Preservation

The term zone of partial preservation is used only with complete injuries. It refers to partial preservation (sparing) of sensory and/or motor function in segments caudal to the neurological level.[4]

ASIA Impairment Scale

Varying degrees of sensory and voluntary motor function can be seen caudal to incomplete spinal cord lesions. At one end of the spectrum, an individual with an incomplete injury can have sparing of sensation or motor function in the lowest sacral segments with no other sensory or motor function below the lesion. At the other end of the spectrum, an individual can retain near-normal motor and sensory function caudal to the lesion. Thus two people with incomplete C6 tetraplegia, for example, could have markedly different motor and sensory function preserved below their lesions. The ASIA impairment scale, presented in Table 2–4, allows clinicians and researchers to communicate more effectively about the clinical presentations of people with spinal cord injuries.

CLINICAL SYNDROMES

Incomplete lesions of the spinal cord can result in a variety of patterns of motor and sensory loss. The clinical presentation is determined by the location and pattern of neurological damage. The three incomplete spinal cord injury syndromes are Brown-Séquard, anterior cord, and central cord. Two additional syndromes result from lesions of the conus medullaris and the cauda equina.

PROBLEM-SOLVING EXERCISE 2–1

Your patient sustained a T10 wedge compression fracture 2 weeks ago. His motor and sensory function have not changed since he was admitted to the hospital: his strength is normal (5/5) in both upper extremities and absent (0/5) in his lower extremities. On the right side of his body, his sensation (pin prick and light touch) is intact in the C1 through the T11 key sensory points, impaired in T12, and absent below. On the left, his sensation is intact in the C1 through the T12 key sensory points, impaired in L1 and L2, and absent below. He does not have any sensation around his anus, and cannot contract it voluntarily.

- Classify the injury: complete versus incomplete, ASIA Impairment Scale, neurological level of injury.
- This patient wants to know about his potential for regaining the use of his legs. What is the likelihood that he will experience motor return? Should you give him a definite answer about whether his legs will resume functioning?

Brown-Séquard Syndrome

When one side of the spinal cord is damaged, the resulting clinical picture is called Brown-Séquard syndrome (Figure 2–24). True hemisection of the spinal cord is rare, but it is common in incomplete lesions for one side of the cord to sustain more damage than the other.

People with Brown-Séquard syndrome exhibit more severe motor and proprioceptive deficits on the side of the lesion and more severe loss of sensitivity to pin prick and temperature on the contralateral side.[4] At the level of the lesion, the skin is anesthetic ipsilaterally. Spasticity is likely to be present below the lesion ipsilaterally.[48, 116, 177]

Brown-Séquard syndrome frequently occurs as a result of traffic accidents or penetrating (stab or gunshot) injuries.[145] When it is caused by vertebral injury, this syndrome is often associated with unilateral facet locks or burst fractures.[142]

People with Brown-Séquard syndrome are likely to experience neurological return and achieve functional independence during rehabilitation.[145]

Anterior Cord Syndrome

Anterior cord syndrome (Figure 2–25) includes preserved proprioception combined with variable loss of motor function and pain and temperature sensation.[4] It results from damage to the anterior and anterolateral areas of the cord, with preserva-

TABLE 2–4.   THE ASIA IMPAIRMENT SCALE AND FRANKEL GRADING SCALE[a]

ASIA Impairment Scale	Frankel Scale
A Complete: No sensory or motor function is preserved in S4–S5.	**A** Complete.
B Incomplete: Sensory function is preserved below the neurological level *and includes S4–S5.*	**B** Incomplete, preserved sensation only.
C Incomplete: Motor function is preserved below the neurological level. More than half of the key muscles below the neurological level are <3/5 strength.[b]	**C** Incomplete, preserved motor nonfunctional. Minimal voluntary motor function preserved.
D Incomplete: Motor function is preserved below the neurological level. At least half of the key muscles below the neurological level are ≥3/5 strength.[b]	**D** Incomplete, preserved motor functional. "Functionally useful" voluntary motor function preserved.
E Normal. Sensory and motor function is normal.	**E** Complete return.

[a] The ASIA Impairment Scale[4] is based on the Frankel Scale.[3]
[b] Voluntary motor function is present in the anus and/or more than three levels below the motor level.

tion of the posterior columns. This damage can occur due to trauma to the cord itself, damage of the anterior spinal artery, or both.[177] This syndrome results most often from flexion teardrop fractures and burst fractures.[80, 142]

Central Cord Syndrome

Central cord syndrome (Figure 2–26) results from damage to the central aspect of the spinal cord with sparing of the peripheral portions of the cord. This syndrome almost always occurs in the cervical region. People with central cord syndrome exhibit more pronounced weakness in their upper extremities than in their lower extremities, and sparing of sensation in the sacral region.[4] Many also have sparing of sacral motor function.[144]

Central cord syndrome may result when the process of central hemorrhage and necrosis (secondary tissue destruction) described earlier in the chapter does not progress peripherally to full destruction of the cord segment. An alternative explanation for the pattern of central damage with peripheral sparing is that it results from damage to the sulcal arteries, which supply the central portion of the spinal cord.[159]

This syndrome is most common in older people following extension injuries to the neck.[118, 142, 144] It can occur at any age, however, and can follow flexion injury. This syndrome often results from relatively minor trauma (especially in the elderly) with no evidence of vertebral trauma.[118]

People with central cord syndrome are likely to experience neurological return and achieve functional independence during rehabilitation.[144]

Conus Medullaris Syndrome

Conus medullaris syndrome results from damage to the sacral cord and lumbar nerve roots within

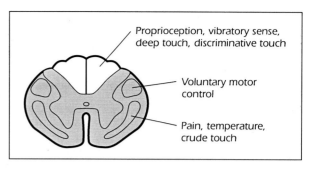

Figure 2–25. Area of spinal cord damage in anterior cord syndrome.

the spinal canal. Most people with conus medullaris syndrome exhibit flaccid paralysis of their lower extremities and have areflexic bowels and bladders. Some individuals retain sacral reflexes.[4]

Cauda Equina Syndrome

Cauda equina syndrome results from injury to the cauda equina, the lumbar and sacral nerve roots within the spinal canal caudal to the spinal cord. People with cauda equina injuries exhibit flaccid paralysis of their lower extremities and have areflexic bowels and bladders.[4]

PHYSICAL EFFECTS OF SPINAL CORD INJURIES

The location and extent of damage to neural tissue determines the motor, sensory, and autonomic effects produced by spinal cord injury. Complete spinal cord injury effectively disconnects the brain from the body below the lesion, disrupting supraspinal control of all of the various systems innervated below the lesion (Figure 2–27).

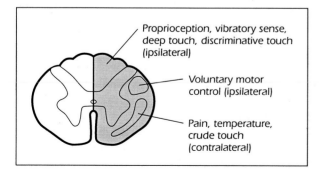

Figure 2–24. Area of spinal cord damage in Brown-Séquard syndrome. Proprioception, vibratory sense, deep touch, discriminative touch, and voluntary motor control are lost ipsilateral to the lesion. Pain, temperature and crude touch are lost contralateral to the lesion.

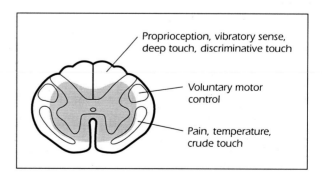

Figure 2–26. Area of spinal cord damage in central cord syndrome. The clinical picture resulting from central damage in the cord is due to the somatotopic organization of fibers within the tracts (see Figure 2–5).

PROBLEM-SOLVING EXERCISE 2–2

You have three patients who have spinal cord injuries with a C5 neurological level of injury. Their clinical presentations are as follows:

Patient #1 has (bilaterally) normal strength in her biceps, 2/5 strength in her radial wrist extensors, and 0/5 strength in all other key muscles. Pin prick is intact in the C1 through C5 key sensory points, impaired in C6 and C7, and absent below. Proprioception is normal in the upper and lower extremities.

Patient #2 has normal strength in her biceps bilaterally. Her radial wrist extensors test 2/5 on the right and 1/5 on the left. Her triceps test 1/5 on the right and 0/5 on the left. All other key muscles in the upper extremities test 0/5. The key muscles in both of her lower extremities test 4/5 to 5/5.

Patient #3 has 4/5 to 5/5 strength in the key muscles of his right upper and lower extremities. His left biceps exhibits normal strength. All other key muscles in the left extremities test 1/5 to 3/5. Below the lesion, pin prick is impaired or absent on the right side of his body and intact on the left. Proprioception is intact in the right extremities and impaired on the left.

- What are the names of the clinical syndromes exhibited by the three patients?
- Explain the neuroanatomical bases of each patient's clinical presentation.

Primary Effects

Voluntary motor function. Paralysis of the voluntary musculature is the most obvious effect of a spinal cord injury. Damage of descending motor tracts, anterior horn cells, or nerve roots leads to an impaired capacity to contract the skeletal muscles at or below the level of the lesion. This paralysis results in a loss of control over the trunk and extremities, affecting the ability to manipulate the environment and move in space.

Damage that occurs at or peripheral to the anterior horn cell is a lower motor neuron lesion and results in flaccid paralysis of muscles innervated by that cord segment. Damage to descending tracts is an upper motor neuron lesion and results in spastic paralysis of muscles innervated by cord segments caudal to the lesion.[48] Most spinal cord injuries are a combination of upper and lower motor neuron lesions, because both gray and white matter are disrupted at the level of the lesion.[116]

Fortunately, most people with spinal cord injuries experience some recovery of motor function in the months and years after injury. The majority exhibit significant recovery in musculature innervated by cord segments one or more levels caudal to their neurologic level of injury.[60, 61, 107, 135, 182]

Muscle tone. During the period of spinal shock immediately following cord injury, muscles inner-

vated below the lesion are areflexive. As time passes, spinal shock resolves and reflexes return. Reflexive functioning is weak at first but becomes stronger with time,[85] commonly progressing to spasticity. Spasticity is more prevalent in people with cervical and upper thoracic lesions and in those with incomplete lesions,[103, 112, 140] particularly ASIA B and C.[111, 112]

Spasticity is a velocity-dependent increase in muscle tone in response to passive movement.[68, 110] (Passive stretching of a spastic muscle elicits an involuntary contraction of that muscle, with higher velocity motion eliciting stronger contraction.) The elevated muscle tone that frequently occurs after spinal cord injury also includes clonus, increased deep tendon reflexes, and abnormal reflexive responses to cutaneous stimuli.[85, 110, 117, 120, 180] Reflexive responses to cutaneous stimulation may appear to be spontaneous "spasms" because the stimuli by which they are elicited can be so subtle as to go unnoticed by the clinician.[180]

Spasticity, clonus, increased deep tendon reflexes, and spasms result from upper motor neuron damage. The underlying neurological mechanism or mechanisms of these hyperreflexive responses are as yet unknown. Possible causes include a loss of inhibition from higher centers, loss of descending facilitation of afferents from Golgi tendon organs, sprouting of new synaptic terminals within the spinal cord caudal to the lesion, and hypersensitivity of neurons caudal to the lesion in response to their reduced input.[85, 102, 110, 120, 153, 177, 180]

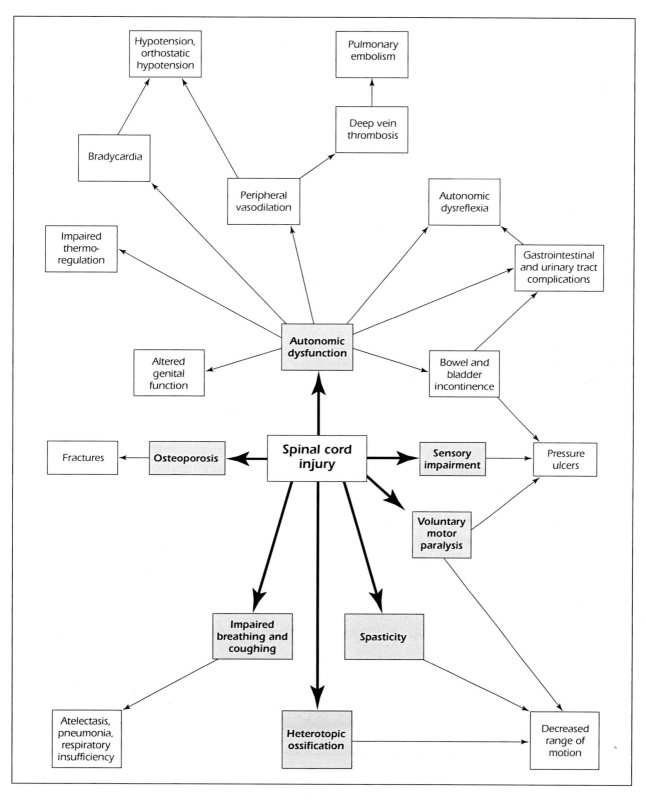

Figure 2–27.   Schematic representation of the physical effects of spinal cord injury.

Spinal cord injury can also result in flaccid paralysis with deep tendon reflexes and reflexive response to passive stretch diminished or absent. Flaccid paralysis frequently occurs with lower lesions, due to lower motor neuron damage of the conus medullaris or cauda equina.[112] Flaccid paralysis can also occur with higher lesions, in muscles innervated by anterior horn cells or nerve roots that are damaged.[19]

Sensation. Sensation is disrupted in most spinal cord injuries. A loss of sensation can lead to discoordination of body movements, vulnerability to trauma, and impaired body awareness. As is true with voluntary motor function, sensory ability usually improves as time passes after spinal cord injury.[182]

Breathing and coughing. Normal breathing and coughing involve coordinated action of the diaphragm, accessory muscles, intercostals, and abdominal musculature. Spinal cord injuries above T12 interrupt innervation to some or all of these muscles. Respiratory impairments can range in severity from difficulty in clearing secretions to the inability to breathe.[u]

Bowel and bladder function. Voluntary control of urination and defecation requires an intact sacral cord in communication with the brain. As a result, most spinal cord injuries lead to a loss of voluntary bowel and bladder control.[v]

Genital function. The genitals receive their innervation from the thoracolumbar and sacral regions of the spinal cord. Spinal cord injury alters the functioning of the genitals, disrupting sexual responses mediated by the brain and the spinal cord. Fertility is unchanged among women with cord injuries. Men are likely to be infertile.[w]

Cardiovascular function. Vasomotor centers in the medulla normally control the cardiovascular system. By reflexively adjusting the sympathetic and parasympathetic outflow to the heart and peripheral vasculature, the vasomotor centers control blood pressure, heart rate, and distribution of blood flow.[27, 75] Sympathetic outflow, arising from spinal segments T1 to L2 or L3, causes an increase in heart rate and increased contractility of the cardiac musculature. Parasympathetic outflow, transmitted through the vagus nerve from the brainstem, slows the heart rate and slightly reduces ventricular contractility.[27, 26, 109] The autonomic nervous system also controls vascular tone. Table 2–5 presents the effects of sympathetic and parasympathetic stimulation on the heart and peripheral vasculature.

When spinal cord injury blocks communication between the brainstem and the thoracic spinal cord, sympathetic input to the heart is lost and parasympathetic input remains. This disruption of the normal balance of sympathetic and parasympathetic control results in bradycardia and bradyarrhythmias. Loss of sympathetic outflow also causes dilation of the peripheral vasculature below the level of the lesion, resulting in hypotension.[34, 75, 100, 113, 118] The loss of sympathetic reflexes that normally modulate blood pressure during postural changes causes orthostatic hypotension: blood pressure drops when the individual moves from horizontal to an upright position. Symptoms of orthostatic hypotension include loss of vision, dizziness, ringing in the ears, nausea, and loss of consciousness.[34, 127, 177]

Bradycardia, bradyarrhythmias, hypotension, and orthostatic hypotension are usually significant only in people with lesions above T6.[25, 34, 100, 177] These cardiovascular effects are transient, resolving[x] within a few weeks of injury.[34, 100, 124, 134, 177] Both a compensatory reduction in parasympathetic outflow[78] and the return of sympathetic spinal reflexes[75] may contribute to the return of more normal cardiovascular function.

Although the parasympathetic/sympathetic imbalance that follows spinal cord injury resolves to some degree within a few weeks of the injury, cardiovascular control does not return to normal. Injuries that lie rostral to or within the region of thoracolumbar sympathetic outflow interfere with the brain's communication with sympathetic neurons caudal to the lesion, disrupting normal cardiovascular reflexes.[134] Cardiovascular responses to exercise are impaired, resulting in reduced exercise tolerance and, in some cases, exercise-induced hypotension.[46, 66, 75, 82, 94]

Another lasting effect of cervical and high thoracic spinal cord injury is reduced venous return to the heart. This probably results from a

---

[u] Chapter 7 addresses the respiratory sequelae of spinal cord injuries in depth.

[v] Complete descriptions of bowel and bladder function, complications, and care following spinal cord injury are presented in Chapter 14 (www.prenhall.com/somers).

[w] Sexuality, sexual functioning, and sexual rehabilitation strategies are addressed in Chapter 5.

---

[x] Hypotension frequently continues[126] but does not tend to be as severe as during the early phase after injury.[75]

TABLE 2–5.   CARDIOVASCULAR RESPONSES TO AUTONOMIC STIMULATION

	Response to Parasympathetic Stimulation	Response to Sympathetic Stimulation
Heart	Reduced heart rate Reduced contractility Reduced cardiac output	Increased heart rate Increased contractility Increased cardiac output

Peripheral vasculature supplying
  Skeletal muscles
  Skin
  Viscera
	——
	Face: vasodilation
	Vasodilation
		Vasodilation
		Vasoconstriction
		Vasoconstriction

Sources: references 26, 27, 109.

combination of reduced tone in the peripheral vasculature due to lower sympathetic input, loss of reflexive redistribution of blood flow during exercise, loss of the normal muscular pumping action in the lower extremities due to paralysis, and altered intrathoracic and intra-abdominal pressures due to impaired respiratory musculature.[75, 82, 123, 134] The reduction in venous return to the heart leads to reduced stroke volume and cardiac output in people with *tetraplegia*. Exercise capacity is reduced, and the left ventricle of the heart atrophies.[66, 75, 92, 123] People with *paraplegia* also exhibit a reduction in stroke volume. Their cardiac output tends to be lower than normal,[46] but it can be adequate during exercise due to a higher heart rate.[75, 82, 123]

Reduced cardiovascular fitness typically occurs following spinal cord injury. It results from impaired autonomic control (described in the preceding paragraphs), combined with limited skeletal musculature available for exercise.[46, 66, 81] A sedentary lifestyle also contributes to this deconditioning.[46, 66, 134, 165]

Thermoregulation.   Normally, when a person's core temperature falls, peripheral vasoconstriction and shivering serve to raise the temperature. When the core temperature rises above normal, peripheral vasodilation and sweating cause greater dissipation of heat with a fall in core temperature resulting.[21, 27]

Thermoregulation involves both the autonomic and somatic nervous systems. The sympathetic nervous system (T1–L2 or L3) is involved in the regulation of body temperature through its influence on peripheral vascular tone and perspiration.[26] The somatic system controls shivering.

Spinal cord injury that interrupts the cord's communication with the hypothalamus disrupts thermoregulation. Soon after injury, *hypo*thermia is likely to occur as a result of peripheral vasodilation, which allows loss of heat through the superficial vessels. When reflexive tone eventually returns in the peripheral vasculature, this problem resolves.[118] Although shivering remains absent below the level of lesion,[21] the tendency toward hypothermia is replaced by a tendency toward *hyper*thermia. This is because sympathetic control of the apocrine (sweat) glands is lost. Below the level of lesion, sweating does not occur in response to a rise in body temperature.[118]

Complications

A variety of complications can result from spinal cord injury. With proper management, the incidence and severity of most of these complications can be minimized.

Pressure ulcers.   Pressure ulcers are among the most common complications of spinal cord injury.[45, 96, 122, 176, 179] Pressure ulcers are localized areas of tissue necrosis that can occur when soft tissues are subjected to prolonged unrelieved pressure. People with spinal cord injuries are prone to developing this complication because of a combination of (1) motor and sensory impairments that cause the skin to be subjected to prolonged unrelieved pressure and other damaging forces, plus (2) skin and circulatory changes that make the skin more vulnerable to these damaging forces.

Vulnerability to the development of pressure ulcers begins at the time of injury and continues for the remainder of the individual's lifetime. A variety of serious medical, functional, and social problems can result from this complication. Chapter 6 addresses pressure ulcers in greater depth.

Respiratory complications. Respiratory complications are the most common cause of death following spinal cord injury.[54–56, 91, 95] These complications occur as a result of a reduction in both inspiratory and expiratory ability. Impaired functioning in the muscles of inspiration causes reduced ventilation of the lungs and atelectasis. Weakness in these muscles also makes them more likely to fatigue, which can lead to ventilatory failure.[53] Ineffective coughing allows secretions to build in the lungs, with atelectasis, pneumonia, and respiratory insufficiency resulting.[25, 113, 163, 177] Chapter 7 addresses the respiratory sequelae of spinal cord injuries in greater depth.

Decreased range of motion. Any condition that causes joint immobilization can result in reduced joint range of motion and muscle flexibility. People with motor paralysis are vulnerable to contractures due to the simple fact that their muscles do not actively move their joints. Range limitations are especially likely to develop when muscle strength imbalance, spasticity, gravity, or a habitual posture causes one or more joints to remain in a particular position for extended periods without intermittent motion out of the position. Contractures tend to develop more rapidly when edema is present.[44]

Reduced range of motion can seriously impair a person's functional capacity and can create cosmetic problems. Moreover, deformity can increase vulnerability to pressure ulcers by altering pressure distribution in sitting and by limiting the number of postures available for pressure relief when lying in bed.

Heterotopic ossification. Heterotopic ossification, also called ectopic bone formation, is the formation of new bone within muscles or other connective tissue. It occurs following 16 percent to 53 percent of all spinal cord injuries, most frequently in the hips, knees, and elbows. When heterotopic ossification develops, it usually first appears from 1 to 4 months after the injury and matures 12 to 18 months later. Heterotopic ossification can restrict joint motion and lead to

impaired functional status and pressure ulcers.[70, 71, 98, 111, 177] The cause of heterotopic ossification following spinal cord injury is unknown. Advanced age, complete lesions, male gender, and spasticity have been identified as risk factors.[98, 111]

Osteoporosis and fractures. Following spinal cord injury, osteoporosis develops below the lesion. It develops in the extremities innervated below the lesion but not in the spine.[90, 156] This reduction in bone mass is the result of loss of both calcium[34] and collagen[141] from the bones. Osteoporosis following spinal cord injury is likely the result of venous stasis and a loss of muscular action and weight bearing.[97]

Bone mass is lost most rapidly in the first few months after spinal cord injury.[51, 139] The rate of decline in bone mineral density slows after this point, but it can continue for many years.[13, 156] Osteoporosis tends to be more severe in the lower extremities and with complete injuries and flaccid paralysis.[51]

Osteoporosis is of concern because it increases the likelihood of fractures. Estimates of the incidence of pathologic fracture rates among people with spinal cord injuries range from 1.4 percent to 6 percent.[111] The following characteristics are associated with higher incidence of fractures due to osteoporosis after spinal cord injury: motor complete injuries (Frankel A or B), paraplegia, white race, greater time since injury,[111] and female gender.[101, 111]

Pain. Pain is a significant problem for many people with spinal cord injuries.[6, 89, 96, 172] It can occur during the acute phase after injury or as a chronic problem in the months and years that follow.

Shoulder pain occurs frequently during the acute postinjury phase, particularly in people with tetraplegia. This pain may be caused by impaired functioning in the upper extremity and shoulder girdle musculature that results in abnormal stresses being placed on the joints and soft tissues during activity.[111, 150] Additional possible sources of shoulder pain during the early postinjury period include nerve root impingement, referred pain from the cervical injury,[150] and abnormal stresses placed on the shoulders because of poor positioning in bed.

Chronic pain is often the result of overuse. When spinal cord injury results in significant loss of voluntary motor function, the upper extremities are used during transfers, ambulation, wheelchair propulsion, and activities such as rolling and assuming a sitting position. This heavy use of the upper extremities subjects the joints and soft tissues of the arms and shoulder girdles to higher than normal levels of stress. As a result, shoulder pain and carpal tunnel syndrome are common problems among people with long-standing injuries.[74, 149] The incidence of these problems increases with time after injury.[74, 132, 149] This increase may be due to a combination of chronic overuse and age-related degenerative changes.

Another type of pain, central neuropathic pain, results from damage to the spinal cord itself rather than the nerve roots or any musculoskeletal structures. Central neuropathic pain can be constant or intermittent, and can occur spontaneously or in response to sensory stimulation.[62] The cause of central neuropathic pain is not yet known.

Gastrointestinal complications. From 2.2 percent to 22 percent of people with spinal cord injuries develop stress ulcers in the stomach or duodenum during the acute phase following injury.[17, 146, 151] The cause of this complication is unknown. Possible contributing factors include shock, emotional stress, circulating catecholamines, steroid therapy, mechanical ventilation, and unopposed parasympathetic input to the stomach causing increased gastrin production.[17, 25, 34, 72, 146]

Gastrointestinal (GI) bleeds are most likely to occur during the first month after injury.[105, 177] Additional GI complications of spinal cord injury include paralytic ileus, gastric dilation, fecal impaction, bowel obstruction, superior mesenteric artery syndrome,[y] pancreatitis, esophagitis, gallstone disease, chronic constipation, and hemorrhoids.[28, 34, 36, 49, 72, 146, 177]

Urinary tract complications. Urinary tract complications were the leading cause of death after spinal cord injury until relatively recently. Advances in urologic management practices have significantly reduced the mortality rate in recent years.[54, 55, 91] Abnormal bladder function following spinal cord injury, combined with improper management, can lead to urinary retention, bladder infection, and reflux of urine into the ureters. Kidney and bladder stones, hydronephrosis, pyelonephritis, kidney failure, septicemia, and death can result.[1, 25, 28, 59, 79]

Deep vein thrombosis and pulmonary embolism. Deep vein thrombosis (DVT) is a common complication following spinal cord injury, particularly in the acute phase after injury. Various studies have reached conflicting conclusions about the frequency of this complication, with deep vein thrombosis found in 10 percent to 100 percent of subjects tested.[35, 113, 124, 136, 164]

Several factors combine to promote the development of blood clots in the deep veins after spinal cord injury. Peripheral vasodilation, absent or reduced lower extremity muscular function, and immobility lead to venous stasis. Hypercoagulability, trauma, and sepsis may also play a role.[25, 35, 113, 121, 161, 164, 177] Factors associated with higher risk for the development of deep vein thromboses include male gender, complete lesions, and paraplegia.[136, 164] The incidence of this complication is highest between 72 hours and 2 weeks after a spinal cord injury.[35] It is rare in chronic spinal cord injury.[136]

Thrombi in the deep veins are potentially life-threatening. An estimated 2 percent to 16 percent of people with spinal cord injuries die of pulmonary emboli within the first 3 months of injury.[161] After that point, pulmonary embolization rarely occurs.[177]

DVTs are also problematic because they can progress to post-thrombotic syndrome. This syndrome includes chronic edema, induration, pain, and skin ulceration.[35]

Autonomic dysreflexia. People with spinal cord lesions above the T6 level[z] can experience autonomic dysreflexia as a result of a "disconnection" between the brain and the sympathetic neurons in the thoracolumbar spine.[43, 126] This phenomenon, also called autonomic hyperreflexia, occurs in 10 percent to 85 percent of people with spinal cord injuries above T6.[33, 89, 162] It is characterized by a sudden increase in blood pressure, bradycardia, a pounding headache, and flushing and profuse sweating above the level of the lesion (Figure 2–28). It is often accompanied by anxiety. Additional signs and symptoms that can occur include flushing or sweating below the lesion, piloerection ("goose bumps") above or sometimes below the lesion, blurred vision, spots in the visual fields, nasal congestion, and cardiac arrhythmias. Occasionally, autonomic dysreflexia occurs without any symptoms.[37]

Autonomic dysreflexia occurs when a noxious stimulus below the lesion triggers an excessive sympathetic response. Possible causes of this exaggerated sympathetic response include loss of descending inhibition from the medulla, sprouting of new synaptic terminals within the spinal

---

[y] In this syndrome, the superior mesenteric artery compresses the duodenum.

[z] Autonomic dysreflexia has been reported in patients with lower lesions. However, it is more typically associated with lesions above T6.[21, 134]

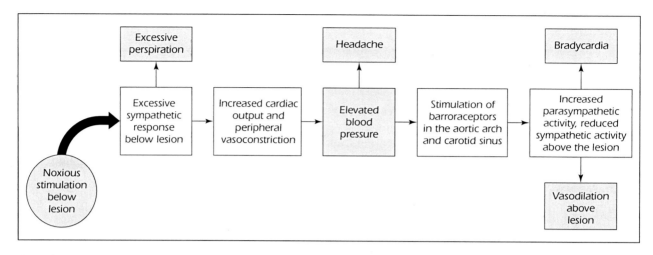

Figure 2–28.   *Schematic representation of autonomic dysreflexia. Clinical signs and symptoms are in darkened boxes.*

cord caudal to the lesion, and hypersensitivity of the sympathetic neurons.[21, 33, 171] Hypertension results when increased sympathetic outflow causes an increase in cardiac output and peripheral vasoconstriction. The hypertension stimulates baroreceptors in the aortic arch and carotid sinus, triggering increased parasympathetic activity that slows the heart.[aa]

Vasodilation above the lesion also occurs as a compensatory mechanism in response to the elevated blood pressure.[21, 23, 34, 37, 43, 134, 154, 162]

Autonomic dysreflexia occurs after spinal shock has resolved, usually first appearing about 6 or more months after the injury. This complication is more prevalent among people with tetraplegia than among those with paraplegia, and in people with complete lesions.[21, 34, 43, 113, 124, 136, 186]

Any noxious stimulus below the lesion can cause autonomic dysreflexia. Common origins of this noxious stimulus include bladder or rectal distension, urinary tract infection, and bowel impaction. A large variety of other stimuli have been reported to trigger autonomic dysreflexia, including *but not limited to* range of motion exercises, cutaneous stimulation, muscle spasm, pressure ulcers, fractures, ingrown toenails, functional electrical stimulation, electroejaculation, epididymitis or vaginitis, scrotal compression, sexual intercourse, labor, surgical and diagnostic procedures, and abdominal conditions such as appendicitis.[21, 33, 34, 37, 43, 113, 115, 124] The elevation in blood pressure that occurs with autonomic dysreflexia

can lead to renal failure, cardiopulmonary failure, loss of consciousness, seizures, hypertensive encephalopathy, retinal hemorrhage, apnea, aphasia, cerebrovascular accidents, coma, and death.[21, 33, 115, 162]

Cardiovascular disease. In recent decades, advances in medical management and rehabilitation have led to a reduction in deaths from complications of spinal cord injury. As people with spinal cord injuries are living longer, cardiovascular disease has become more prevalent in this population.[75, 134, 165] The risk of morbidity and mortality from ischemic heart disease is now comparable to[29, 56, 86] or higher than[14, 15, 54, 178] that of the general population.

Several factors may contribute to the development of cardiovascular disease following spinal cord injury. These include a sedentary lifestyle, higher proportion of body fat relative to lean body mass, lipid abnormalities, altered glucose metabolism, and the increased prevalence of diabetes.[12, 15, 47, 75, 97, 134, 165]

SUMMARY

- Most spinal cord injuries occur when direct or indirect forces applied to the vertebral column cause violent motion, resulting in failure of the ligamentous or boney elements or both. With disruption of the vertebral column, the spinal cord is traumatized.

- The neurological damage that results from spinal cord injury is due only in part to the initial trauma to the neurons themselves. Most of the damage to the cord is caused by secondary sequelae of the initial trauma, an escalating

---

[aa] In some cases, tachycardia (increased heart rate) occurs instead of bradycardia. The different clinical pictures occur because both parasympathetic and sympathetic stimulation to the heart are increased in autonomic dysreflexia.[21]

cycle of tissue destruction involving ischemia, inflammation, ion derangements, and apoptotic cell death.

- The motor, sensory, and autonomic effects of a spinal cord injury vary widely, depending on the level of the lesion and pattern of neurological damage. The American Spinal Injury Association and International Medical Society of Paraplegia have developed and adopted a classification system to facilitate communication about spinal cord injuries.

- Depending on the site and extent of a spinal cord lesion, it can result in paralysis, abnormal muscle tone, and sensory loss, as well as impaired control of the respiratory, gastrointestinal, genitourinary, cardiovascular, and thermoregulatory systems. A variety of debilitating and potentially fatal complications can result.

3

Medical and Surgical Management

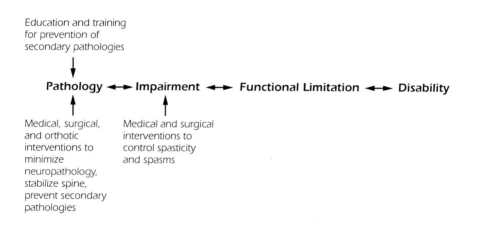

Education and training for prevention of secondary pathologies

Pathology ←→ Impairment ←→ Functional Limitation ←→ Disability

Medical, surgical, and orthotic interventions to minimize neuropathology, stabilize spine, prevent secondary pathologies

Medical and surgical interventions to control spasticity and spasms

Following injury to the vertebral column or spinal cord, specialized management is imperative. The effects of spinal trauma can be lessened or worsened by the first aid and subsequent medical and surgical interventions provided. At the accident site, care must be taken to avoid causing additional neurological damage. At the hospital, operative or nonoperative measures or both are taken to stabilize the spine to preserve neurological functioning. From the time of injury on, proper medical management is required to prevent a host of secondary complications. In the absence of appropriate fracture management and medical care, a cycle of worsening pathology is virtually inevitable, resulting in unnecessary disability or death.

EMERGENCY MANAGEMENT

Prehospital Care

The first aid treatment that people receive following spinal cord injury is crucial to their health and neurological integrity. Stabilization of the injured spine is of particular importance: if the vertebral column is allowed to move, the cord can sustain additional damage. Probably most rehabilitation personnel have had patients with spinal cord injuries tell them of being pulled out of cars or dragged up beaches by friends immediately after their accidents. Some neurological damage is even caused by emergency medical service personnel, but that problem has decreased as training and handling techniques have improved.[33, 155, 174]

Unless an individual has received specialized training in the emergency handling of people with spinal cord injuries, she should not attempt to move someone who might have sustained a cord injury.[a] The only exception to this rule is when trained personnel are not available and failure to move the injured person would lead to death, as when she is lying with her face under water.

In an emergency situation, a person should be treated as though she has a spinal cord injury if there is *any* reason to believe that there is a *possibility* of an injury of the spinal cord or spinal column. People who exhibit any of the following characteristics after a traumatic event (vehicular

---

[a] Health professionals are no exception.[155]

accident, fall, physical attack, diving accident, etc.) should be assumed to have a possible spinal injury: neck or back pain or tenderness; impairment due to drugs or alcohol;[b] motor or sensory deficits, however minor; paresthesias; head injury, unconsciousness, or decreased level of consciousness; and concomitant serious injury.[126, 177] Proper handling of people displaying any of these characteristics will prevent much unnecessary neurological damage.

Emergency management involves measures to enhance both survival and neurological integrity. Emergency medical personnel must first ensure that ventilation and circulation are adequate, avoiding unnecessary motion of the spine while doing so.[7, 8, 13, 37, 108, 109] Intubation or ventilation with an air-mask bag unit may be necessary if either associated injuries or cord damage above C5 significantly impair breathing.[33, 134]

The spine must be immobilized before the injured person is moved, and must remain immobilized during transport and emergency treatment until spinal column injury has been ruled out. Possible spinal injury necessitates stabilization from the head to below the buttocks.[110] A variety of techniques and devices are available for vertebral immobilization.[7, 13, 33, 79, 94, 96, 102, 134, 155]

Once the patient's spinal column has been stabilized and adequate ventilation and circulation have been assured, the injured person can be taken by ambulance or helicopter to a trauma center. Ideally, the patient is taken to a center that specializes in spinal cord injury care, as these centers have better outcomes.[3, 32, 45, 50, 174, 175]

Hospital Care

When someone with a known or suspected spinal injury arrives at the hospital, the trauma team works to discover and treat any life-threatening conditions and to preserve neurological function. All noncritical associated injuries are given lower priority.[155] During all procedures, care is taken to avoid motion in the spine.

The establishment of adequate ventilation, oxygenation, and circulation are of highest priority. Respiratory status is evaluated and arterial blood gasses are monitored. Intubation and ventilation are performed if indicated.[13, 37, 134, 155] The trauma team controls hemorrhaging from associated injuries and monitors for and treats cardiac

arrhythmias or hypotension.[37, 58, 146, 155, 181] In addition to enhancing the patient's survival, these measures may help prevent additional neurological damage that could result from inadequate perfusion of the spinal cord with oxygenated blood.[37, 114]

Once the priority survival needs have been addressed, a neurological examination can be performed. The neurological evaluation should include assessment of level of consciousness and cranial nerve function, because the patient may have sustained a head injury during the accident. Sensation, voluntary motor function, and reflexes[c] should also be evaluated thoroughly.[30, 37, 60, 109, 110, 155, 159] This baseline data will influence decisions regarding fracture management and will make it possible to detect any future improvement or deterioration in neurological status.[d]

Radiologic investigation is performed to detect spinal column damage, to determine whether these injuries are stable, and to determine the extent to which the spinal canal is compromised.[40] The radiologic examination should cover the entire spine, as this will make it possible to detect multiple spinal injuries.[31, 37, 120]

Standard x-rays are typically performed initially, while the spine is still immobilized.[33, 94, 102, 134] The cervical spine series should include a lateral view encompassing C1 through the C7-T1 junction, an anteroposterior view, and an open-mouthed odontoid view. Flexion–extension views may also be indicated[e] in some cases.[75, 109] Both anteroposterior and lateral views should be taken in the thoracic and lumbar regions of the spine.[109]

In addition to standard x-rays, computerized tomography (CT) scans and magnetic resonance imaging (MRI) may be performed. CT scans frequently reveal fractures that are not evident on radiographs. For this reason, they are indicated when there is continued suspicion of spinal column injury despite negative radiographs, when

---

[b] Although drug- or alcohol-induced impairment is not a sign of spinal injury, it can make these signs difficult or impossible to detect.

[c] The examination of sensation, voluntary motor function, and reflexes should include the anus, as it receives sacral innervation. Anal sensory and motor function provide information on the integrity of both the sacral cord and the ascending and descending tracts that link it with the brain. The International Standards for Neurological Classification of Spinal Injury Patients[1] should be used for the sensory and voluntary motor examinations. These standards are presented in chapters 2 and 8.

[d] During the acute period after a spinal cord injury, a person's neurological status may deteriorate due to progression of the lesion. For this reason, neurological status should be assessed frequently during this period.[110] Deterioration may indicate the need for a change in surgical or nonsurgical interventions.

[e] Radiographs taken with the spine flexed and extended are controversial, since these motions can cause additional neurologic damage.[131]

the x-rays reveal abnormal or ambiguous findings, or when they do not provide adequate visualization of the spine.[37, 75, 109, 118, 143] An MRI may also be performed, because it provides superior visualization of spinal cord compression, as well as morphologic changes in ligamentous, hematologic, intervertebral disk, and spinal cord tissue following trauma to the vertebral column.[35, 58, 59, 97, 124]

Additional emergency procedures include obtaining a complete medical history, evaluation and initial management of gastrointestinal and urinary systems,[f] and a complete evaluation for associated injuries.[30, 159] Finally, administration of methylprednisolone has become standard procedure in the emergency care of people with spinal cord injuries.[31, 58, 114, 132, 181] Treatment with high doses of this medication, *initiated within 8 hours of injury*, enhances recovery of both motor and sensory function whether the lesion is clinically complete or incomplete.[21–23] This beneficial effect occurs in people with blunt injuries, but not in people who sustain penetrating spinal cord injuries such as those caused by gunshot wounds.[86, 139] Although treatment with methylprednisolone leads to improved neurological outcomes in people with blunt spinal cord injuries, these beneficial effects are *statistically* significant but are fairly limited clinically.[58] In recent years, research has focused on finding additional interventions that will enhance neurological functioning after spinal cord injury. Blood volume augmentation and elevation of patients' mean arterial blood pressure may improve outcomes by enhancing blood flow to the spinal cord, reducing posttraumatic ischemia of the neural tissue.[169] A variety of pharmacological therapies aimed at reducing secondary tissue destruction and enhancing axonal regeneration within the spinal cord are also under investigation in both humans and animals.[20, 21, 56, 67, 68, 71, 81, 114, 138, 161]

Another area of research, performed to date on animals, is transplantation: tissues or cells are inserted into or near the damaged portion of the cord. Depending on the type of transplantation performed, this transplanted material can provide a bridge for axonal regeneration, create chemical and mechanical conditions conducive to this regeneration, create conditions beneficial to surviving neurons, and even provide new neurons to the damaged portion of the cord.[36, 71, 182] Additional lines of research include enhancing neuronal survival and regeneration using neurotrophic growth

factors, antibodies for growth-inhibiting factors, and electrical stimulation.[26, 106, 160]

FRACTURE MANAGEMENT

The primary goal of spinal fracture management is minimization of the neurological damage caused by vertebral injury. This process begins at the site of the accident, with careful handling and stabilization of the spine when injury is suspected. At the scene, during transport, and in the emergency room, extreme care is taken to avoid moving the spine while evaluations and treatments are being administered. The spine is evaluated (using x-ray, CT scan, and/or MRI, as indicated) as soon as is feasible in the hospital, and any vertebral column injuries found are reduced and stabilized. This early detection, reduction, and stabilization of vertebral injuries serves to optimize the ultimate neurological outcome of the injured person.

In addition to the initial preservation of neurological function, fracture management interventions are aimed at minimizing deformity and stabilizing the injured spine to prevent the late development of spinal deformity.[174] Fracture management regimens include the use of traction, positioning, surgery, orthoses, or any combination thereof for restoration of vertebral alignment, stabilization of the injured spine, and elimination of impingement upon neural tissue.

Nonsurgical Management

When radiologic examination reveals vertebral angulation or subluxation in the cervical region, the spine is usually realigned as soon as possible using skeletal traction.[142] Since this alignment decompresses the spinal cord, it may increase the patient's chances of neurological recovery.[28, 60, 120] In the cervical region, skeletal traction is achieved with a halo device or tongs that are affixed to the skull (Figure 3–1). The halo or tongs are attached through a pulley system to weights that apply traction to the cervical vertebrae. Reduction is confirmed by x-ray. Failure to achieve optimal alignment through traction may make surgery necessary.[28, 33, 82, 114, 120] In some instances, a cervical spine that will not reduce with traction can be realigned through nonsurgical manipulation.[37, 121]

In the treatment of thoracic and lumbar injuries, initial conservative (nonoperative) management generally involves careful positioning in a bed (either standard or rotating bed) or Stryker

---

[f] Gastrointestinal and urinary management are addressed below and in Chapter 14 (www.prenhall.com/somers).

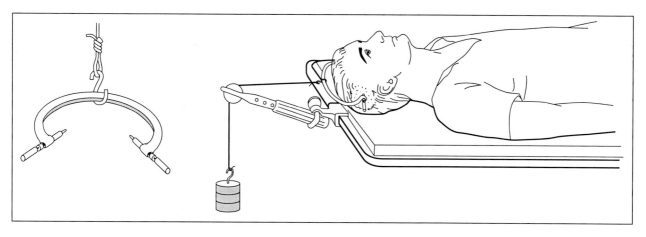

Figure 3–1. *Cervical skeletal traction using tongs.*

frame[g] (Figure 3–2). Pillows placed under the patient can position the spine in slight extension or flexion. The nature of the spinal column injury determines the optimal position. With some high thoracic injuries, reduction can be achieved using skeletal traction applied through the skull.[120]

In some cases, the injured spine is managed definitively through nonsurgical reduction and stabilization. Conservative management is particularly appropriate in instances of either stable or multiple-level vertebral injuries. Surgical stabilization of multiple-level injuries results in severe restriction of spinal motion, potentially interfering with functional status.[120]

When nonsurgical management techniques are used as the definitive treatment, the patient may be immobilized initially in traction or with bed positioning.[h] This treatment is followed by immobilization of the vertebral column in a spinal orthosis for a period of weeks or months. The length of time that a patient spends in traction, positioned in bed, or immobilized in an orthosis varies with the nature of the injury and the physician's philosophy.[54, 120, 172] At the end of the period of orthotic stabilization, the injured region of the patient's spine is evaluated radiologically. Persistent instability may make surgical stabilization necessary.[33, 52, 120]

Surgical Management

Indications for surgical intervention include an unstable fracture, a fracture that will not reduce without surgery, gross spinal malalignment, evidence of continued cord compression in the presence of an incomplete injury, deteriorating neurological status, and continued instability following conservative management (Figure 3–3). Open reduction and internal fixation may be done to restore optimal vertebral alignment and to stabilize the injured portion of the spine. Surgery may also be performed for decompression of neural tissue through removal of any boney fragments, soft-tissue structures, or foreign bodies impinging on the cord. Finally, surgery is often performed to enable the patient to get out of bed earlier, thus reducing hospitalization time and avoiding the physical and psychological deterioration that can come from prolonged bedrest.[25, 33, 35, 47, 102, 118, 120, 123, 149, 172]

Surgery may be performed within the first 24 hours after admission to the hospital or following a period of days or weeks of skeletal traction or positioning in bed. The optimal timing of surgery is a matter of debate. Early surgery makes it possible for patients to begin out-of-bed activities[i] and rehabilitation earlier[178] and may lead to superior neurological outcomes.[123, 149] On the other hand, early surgery may result in increased incidence of neurological deterioration.[57] Regardless of its timing, cervical spine surgery is often preceded by closed reduction (using skeletal traction, as described in the previous section) that is achieved as soon as possible after the injury.

---

[g] Use of a Stryker frame is controversial due to its ineffectiveness in stabilizing the spine and its potential for compromised respiratory function during prone positioning.[110, 116, 154] Positioning in a standard bed is also controversial, as significant vertebral motion can occur during log rolling.[117]

[h] Certain *stable* fractures without neurological deficit can be managed without these restrictions, with the patient allowed out of bed without an orthosis and participating in activities as tolerated.[150]

---

[i] This early mobilization may help prevent the numerous complications that can result from prolonged bed rest.[178]

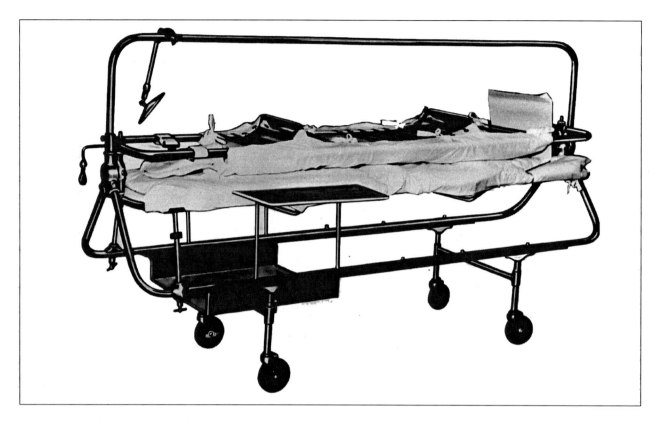

Figure 3–2.   Stryker Wedge Turning Frame (Photograph courtesy of Stryker Corporation, 2725 Fairfield Road, Kalamazoo, MI 49002.)

During surgery, bone fragments, soft-tissue structures, or foreign bodies that are impinging on the cord are removed, and the spinal column is aligned and stabilized. Depending on the type of surgery performed, various internal fixation devices may be used to enhance stability. The spine is often fused, using a bone graft with bone harvested from an iliac crest or fibula, or from vertebral spinous processes.[41, 93, 120, 121, 142, 168]

A variety of different surgical procedures can be used to achieve decompression, reduction, and stabilization. The surgical approach to the spine may be anterior, posterior, or combined anterior and posterior. The divers instruments used to stabilize the spine include devices that distract or compress the spine while immobilizing it. Other internal fixation devices immobilize the spine without distraction or compression. Factors influencing the surgical approach and internal stabilization device chosen include the level and type of spinal column injury, extent of spinal instability present, number of vertebral levels requiring stabilization, location of bone or soft tissue encroaching on the spinal canal, extent of neurological impairment, length of time that has passed since the injury, and preference of the surgeon.[17, 25, 33, 54, 84, 93, 118, 120, 121, 149, 168] Post-surgical

management depends on the nature of the injury and the surgery performed. In some instances, orthotic stabilization is not necessary.[27, 142] In other cases, an orthosis is required post-surgically to provide stability to the spine while it heals. When this is the case, the spine is typically immobilized with an orthosis for 6 weeks to 3 months postoperatively to allow boney fusion to occur.[27]

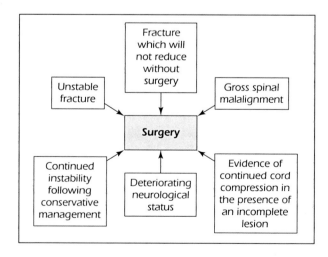

Figure 3–3.   Indications for surgical management of spinal injury.

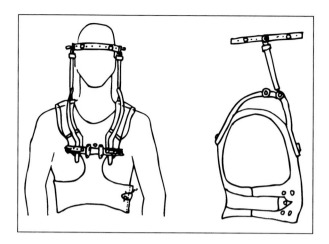

Figure 3–4. Halo orthosis. (Reproduced with permission from *Spinal Orthotics* [1983]. Sidney Fishman, Ph.D, & Norman Berger [Eds.]. New York: Prosthetic-Orthotic Publications.)

Spinal Orthoses

Spinal orthoses are often used to stabilize the spine for a variable period of time following spinal injury. This orthotic stabilization promotes fusion, prevents deformity, reduces pain, and protects neurologic tissue from further damage. Spinal orthoses may be used either after or in lieu of surgical stabilization.

The various designs of spinal orthoses differ in the degree to which they stabilize the vertebral column and the direction of motion that they can control. Orthotic selection is influenced largely by the motion restriction that the spine requires. This, in turn, will depend on the nature of the injury and surgery performed.[27, 131]

Cervical orthoses. An assortment of cervical orthoses are available. The halo, Minerva, poster-type, and a number of different hard collars are commonly used for stabilization of the cervical spine.

Halo. A halo orthosis consists of a metal ring that encircles the skull and is attached via metal bars[j] to a prefabricated adjustable plastic vest lined with sheepskin (Figure 3–4). The "halo" portion of the orthosis is attached to the skull with screws, which are called "pins."

With the *possible* exception of the Minerva, the halo is the orthotic device that is most effective in preventing cervical motion. It is particularly effective in limiting rotation and lateral

flexion of the entire cervical spine and flexion and extension in the higher cervical levels.[92, 167, 171] The halo provides maximal stabilization, but not complete immobilization, of the cervical spine. It allows some gross motion as well as "snaking," flexion or extension at one cervical level with compensatory opposite motion in adjacent segments.[14, 78, 167] Halo orthoses are appropriate for people who require maximal cervical stabilization to allow healing. The high degree of stabilization afforded by a halo apparatus makes it possible for the wearer to get out of bed and initiate functional training earlier than would otherwise be possible. This may result in earlier home visits and discharge.[66, 74, 135] Unfortunately, although halo orthoses make earlier mobilization possible, they make functional training more difficult because they limit shoulder motions and raise the wearer's center of gravity.[122, 129]

Complications experienced by people wearing halo devices include loss of reduction, pin loosening, infection at the pin sites (in turn occasionally resulting in septicemia, osteomyelitis, and subdural abscess), pressure ulcers in the skin underlying the vest, skin rash under the vest, injury of the supraorbital or supratrochlear nerve, dural penetration, dysphagia, disfiguring scars, pin discomfort, and temporomandibular joint dysfunction.[18, 29, 43, 65, 66, 74, 100, 176] Proper application, care, and monitoring can minimize the occurrence and severity of these complications.

The majority of complications associated with halo orthoses originate at the pins. Pin loosening is of concern for two reasons: it can result in loss of stability, and it often precedes infection at the pin site. Pins that loosen should be tightened or replaced with a pin in a different site. Proper hygiene at the pin sites will minimize the occurrence of infection. When an infection occurs, it should be treated early.[18, 19, 52, 65, 66]

Complications involving the skin underlying the vest can also be minimized with proper care and monitoring. The skin over the scapulae, ribs, acromion processes, and spinous processes are at greatest risk. These areas should be checked frequently when possible. The liner between the skin and vest should be kept dry and changed monthly.[129]

A halo should be comfortable. If pain occurs, the health care team should investigate the cause. Pain at the pin sites is likely to be caused by loosening or infection. Pain in the trunk is likely to be due to excessive pressure from the vest.

Despite the complications that halos can cause and the functional limitations that they impose, most people tolerate these orthoses well.

---

[j] Some orthoses include rings, pins, and bars that are made of carbon fiber or titanium. These materials allow magnetic resonance imaging.[27]

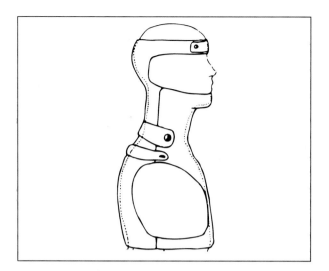

Figure 3–5. Minerva orthosis. (From Fishman, S., Berger, N., Edelstein, J., & Springer, W. [1985]. Spinal orthoses. In: American Academy of Orthopedic Surgeons: *Atlas of Orthotics: Biomechanical Principles and Application* [2nd ed.]. Princeton: C.V. Mosby Company. Reproduced with permission from C.V. Mosby Company.)

Halos remain a popular orthotic option for people who require maximal stability of their cervical spines.

Minerva.   The thermoplastic Minerva body jacket (TMBJ, or Minerva) is a custom-molded orthosis that encases the chin and the posterior aspect of the skull and extends caudally either to the inferior costal margin or to enclose the pelvis, depending on the stability required. A headband encircles the skull to hold the head in place (Figure 3–5).

Like the halo, the Minerva restricts cervical motion in all planes.[133, 167] Neither the halo nor the Minerva provides perfect immobilization of the cervical vertebrae; both allow some gross motion and "snaking." The Minerva orthosis has been reported[k] to provide better stabilization of the cervical spine than does the halo, except between C1 and C2.[14]

As is true with halo orthoses, the excellent stability afforded by Minerva orthoses allows early initiation of functional training. Because the Minerva allows good range of motion in the shoulders, it does not interfere as much with functional progress. Minervas are also reported to be more comfortable and cosmetically acceptable than halos.[14, 122]

Fewer complications are associated with Minerva orthoses than with halos. Since a Min-

erva is not screwed into the wearer's skull, it does not cause any pin-related problems. The Minerva's design may also reduce skin complications. Custom molding can result in better pressure distribution than is achieved with the prefabricated halo vest. Additionally, half of a Minerva can be removed at a time (with the wearer positioned in prone or supine) for skin inspection, bathing, and cleaning of the orthosis. If an area of excessive pressure is noted, the orthosis can be modified.[122]

Poster-type orthoses.   Several different designs of poster-type orthoses are used for restriction of cervical motion. These orthoses consist of pads at the chin and occiput, supported by two to four posts that are attached to anterior and posterior thoracic components.

The SOMI (sterno-occipital-mandibular-immobilizer) is an example of a poster-type orthosis. It is made of a padded metal sternal plate to which are attached three adjustable uprights that are connected to occipital and mandibular supports (Figure 3–6). It is most effective in restricting flexion between C1 and C5.[167] The motion restriction provided by the SOMI orthosis is less than that provided by halo and Minerva orthoses.[92, 142]

When someone wearing a SOMI moves between supine and upright postures, the position of the mandibular support should be adjusted. Proper adjustment is required for both comfort and optimal restriction of cervical motion.[129]

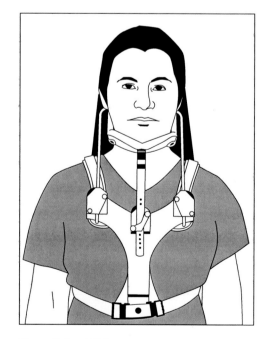

Figure 3–6. SOMI orthosis.

---

[k] In the study cited, the measurement of cervical motion allowed by the Minerva was done 3 weeks after measurement with the halo.[14]

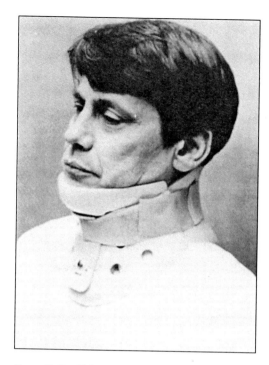

Figure 3–7. *Philadelphia collar. (From Fishman, S., Berger, N., Edelstein, J., & Springer, W. [1985]. Spinal orthoses. In: American Academy of Orthopedic Surgeons: Atlas of Orthotics: Biomechanical Principles and Application [2nd ed.]. Princeton: C.V. Mosby Company. Reproduced with permission from C.V. Mosby Company.)*

Cervical collars. There are a number of different cervical collars that can be used to stabilize the spine. Most are made of either rigid plastic or semirigid foam reinforced by rigid plastic struts. A typical cervical collar consists of two halves that encircle the neck and are joined by velcro straps. The anterior portion of the collar cups the mandible and extends to the upper chest. The posterior portion cups the occiput and extends to the upper back (Figure 3–7).

Cervical collars limit cervical spine motions to varying degrees, depending on their design. Soft collars, made of foam rubber, do not limit motion to any significant degree. Other collars, such as Philadelphia or Miami J collars, provide some motion restriction. This restriction is provided primarily in flexion and extension of the middle and lower cervical spine. No cervical collar can effectively immobilize the spine.[2, 27, 90, 148, 167] For this reason, they should not be used in the presence of significant vertebral instability.

Thoracolumbosacral Orthoses. There are several different types of thoracolumbosacral orthosis. Three designs are described in this section: molded plastic body jackets, Jewett orthoses, and Knight-Taylor orthoses.

Molded plastic body jacket. A molded plastic body jacket encases virtually the entire trunk (Figure 3–8). It is made of two pieces of rigid plastic that are molded to fit the individual[l] and attached to each other with velcro straps. The abdominal area may be covered or exposed. (A window in the abdominal region makes assisted coughing possible.)

Molded plastic body jackets provide maximal stability to the trunk, limiting motion in all planes.[61, 133, 144] A thigh extension (spica) may be included in the orthosis if immobilization is required at L5 or lower levels[27, 52, 167] although the effectiveness of this extension has been questioned.[4] Immobilization of vertebral levels higher than T7[27] or T8[167] requires the inclusion of anterior shoulder outriggers[27] or a cervical extension.[167]

The locations of the inferior and superior borders of the anterior portion of the jacket determine the degree to which the orthosis restricts hip and shoulder motion. If the jacket is shaped appropriately in these regions, hip flexion should be possible to at least 90 degrees,[m] and shoulder motions should be unrestricted. As rehabilitation progresses, hypertrophy of the shoulder musculature may necessitate trimming of the jacket's superior border.[129] A cotton T-shirt worn under the orthosis will absorb perspiration to increase comfort and prevent skin maceration. When the wearer is prone or supine, half of the orthosis can be removed to allow inspection and washing of the skin and cleaning of the orthosis.[129]

Jewett. A Jewett orthosis is a prefabricated orthosis made of a metal frame to which pads are attached (Figure 3–9). The suprapubic, sternal, and thoracolumbar pads exert forces on the trunk that restrict flexion and encourage hyperextension of the lower thoracic and upper lumbar spine.[61, 133, 167] Extension is free at all levels. Rotation and lateral flexion are controlled to an intermediate degree at best, depending on the amount of hyperextension[n] that the orthosis maintains.[61, 133] Improper adjustment of the orthosis can result in loss of vertebral stabilization and pressure on the throat or genitals when sitting.

---

[l] Prefabricated versions are also available. They are less expensive than custom-molded body jackets, but they are also less comfortable and less effective in immobilizing the spine.[27]

[m] In some instances, the inferior trim line needs to be lower in order to provide adequate immobilization of the spine. Hip flexion may then be limited to a greater degree. A thigh extension will also restrict hip motion.

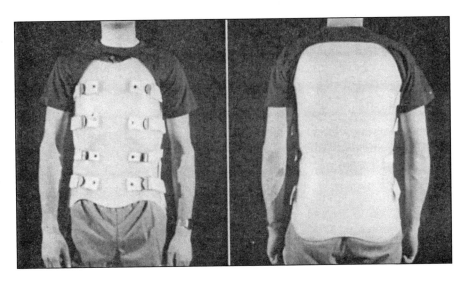

Figure 3–8.   Molded plastic body jacket. (From Fishman, S., Berger, N., Edelstein, J., & Springer, W. [1985]. Spinal orthoses. In: American Academy of Orthopedic Surgeons: *Atlas of Orthotics: Biomechanical Principles and Application* [2nd ed.]. Princeton: C.V. Mosby Company. Reproduced with permission from C.V. Mosby Company.)

Jewett braces are less effective than molded body jackets in preventing flexion, extension, rotation, and lateral flexion.[27] For this reason, they are not appropriate orthoses for unstable spines.[167]

Knight-Taylor.   The framework of a Knight-Taylor orthosis consists of pelvic and thoracic bands worn posteriorly, connected to two pairs of vertical uprights. Axillary straps encircle the shoulders from behind. An abdominal support is attached to the lateral uprights (Figure 3–10).

In the thoracic region, Knight-Taylor orthoses allow unrestricted rotation and provide an intermediate degree of restriction of flexion, extension, and lateral bending. A cervical extension should be added if motion restriction is required above T8.[167] Lumbar rotation is restricted to an intermediate extent. Motions in other planes are effectively restricted in the lumbar spine. In the lumbosacral region, flexion and extension are essentially unrestricted, rotation is limited to an intermediate degree, and lateral flexion is effectively restricted.[61, 133]

Management Differences

There is no generally agreed-upon protocol for the management of spinal column injuries. Decisions regarding surgical versus nonsurgical management, surgical procedure, timing of surgery, choice of orthoses, and duration of orthotic wear are influenced by the philosophy of the institution and the surgeon involved.[25, 54, 73, 83, 120, 149, 162]

---

n The hyperextension of the spine places the vertebrae in a close packed position. With the vertebrae "locked" in this manner, lateral flexion and rotation are restricted to some degree.[61, 133]

MEDICAL MANAGEMENT

Spinal cord injury can affect the functioning of virtually every system in the body. A variety of debilitating and potentially lethal complications can result. With proper medical management involving the coordinated efforts of a multidisciplinary team, many of these complications can be prevented. Without proper management, unnecessary morbidity and mortality are virtually inevitable. For this reason, specialized care is essential.

Bladder care

During the period of spinal shock, the bladder will not empty spontaneously. Bladder distention, urinary reflux, and kidney failure can result if the bladder is not drained by catheterization. An indwelling catheter is usually inserted upon admission to the hospital. In many centers, the indwelling catheter is removed within a few days, and the bladder is drained using intermittent catheterization. As the acute phase after injury passes, the patient and health care team work together to establish a permanent program for emptying the bladder at planned intervals and preventing incontinent episodes between times. For more information, see Chapter 14 (www.prenhall.com/somers).

Gastrointestinal care

During spinal shock, gastric dilation and paralytic ileus may develop. This is of particular concern because of the potential threat to the patient's already compromised respiratory system: diaphragmatic movements are inhibited by this distention, and vomiting and aspiration may occur.

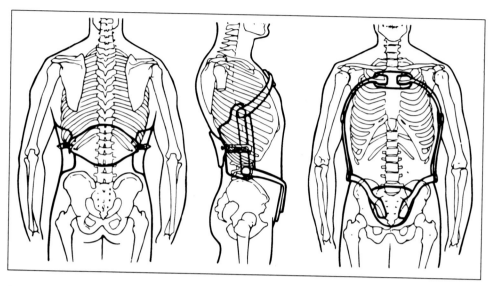

Figure 3–9. Jewett orthosis. (Reproduced with permission from *Spinal Orthotics* [1983]. Sidney Fishman, Ph.D., & Norman Berger [Eds.]. New York: Prosthetic-Orthotic Publications.)

To avoid these complications, the stomach can be decompressed using a nasogastric or orogastric tube.[114, 134, 145]

Stress ulcers may also occur during the acute stage after spinal cord injury. Prophylactic treatment includes the use of antacids to reduce gastric acidity, histamine H_2 receptor antagonists to reduce gastric acid secretion, or sucralfate to enhance gastric mucosal microcirculation and defensive mechanisms.[105, 114, 165] The latter regime for stress ulcer prophylaxis is associated with a lower incidence of pneumonia in patients who are on ventilators.[114, 141, 164]

After spinal cord injury, a bowel program is required to induce bowel movements at regularly scheduled intervals and prevent incontinent episodes between times. Periodic emptying of stool will help prevent constipation, overdistention, and impaction, thus helping to prevent autonomic dysreflexia and other complications. For more information, see Chapter 14 (www.prenhall.com/somers).

Skin care

People with spinal cord injuries are vulnerable to the development of pressure ulcers. This complication can be prevented with proper care.

A critical component of pressure ulcer prevention is the avoidance of prolonged periods of

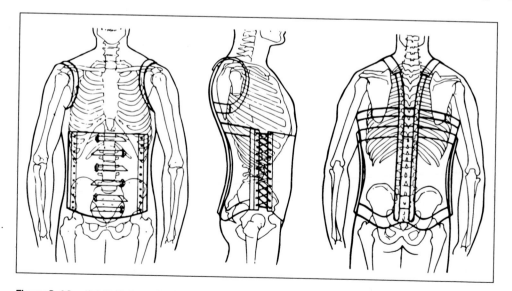

Figure 3–10. Knight-Taylor orthosis. (From Fishman, S.; Berger, N.; Edelstein, J., & Springer, W. [1985]. Spinal orthoses. In: American Academy of Orthopedic Surgeons: *Atlas of Orthotics: Biomechanical Principles and Application* [2nd ed.]. Princeton: C.V. Mosby Company. Reproduced with permission from C.V. Mosby Company.)

unrelieved pressure on the skin, particularly over boney prominences. Prolonged unrelieved pressure is avoided by changing the patient's position periodically when in bed, and by performing pressure-relieving maneuvers (pressure reliefs) when in a wheelchair. Immediately after the injury as the patient is transported to a hospital and undergoes an initial evaluation and emergency interventions, immobilization is necessary. Prolonged periods of immobility during this time, however, can lead to the development of pressure ulcers.[44, 103] To avoid this problem, health professionals should take measures to provide pressure relief to the patient's skin as soon as it is possible to do so without compromising the patient's vertebral stability. Strategies to prevent skin damage during emergency care include insertion of pressure-distributing gel pads under the patient's boney prominences while the patient remains immobilized;[58] minimizing the time involved in transportation, waiting in the emergency room, and x-ray procedures; and admission to the nursing unit as soon as possible.[103]

In addition to the avoidance of prolonged unrelieved pressure, pressure sore prevention involves protecting the skin from shearing forces and friction, providing appropriate equipment, optimizing the patient's health and nutritional status, maintaining clean and dry skin, and educating the patient and family about skin care. Chapter 6 addresses the prevention and treatment of pressure ulcers.

Respiratory care

When spinal cord injury disrupts the functioning of the diaphragm, intercostals, or abdominals, the resulting impaired ability to breathe and cough can lead to atelectasis, pneumonia, and death. The clinical picture is further complicated if the person sustained trauma to the thorax during the initial accident or if she has a history of respiratory disease, aspiration, or smoking.[30, 80, 110]

A high cervical lesion or other injuries that result in seriously impaired breathing ability may make it necessary to initiate mechanical ventilation during the emergency or acute phases of management. Even if unassisted ventilation is adequate initially, respiratory ability can deteriorate in the first few days after spinal cord injury. For this reason, respiratory function should be monitored closely during the initial phase following injury.[13, 114]

Respiratory care should be initiated soon after spinal cord injury and continue throughout acute and postacute rehabilitation. It should include measures to mobilize secretions, enhance breathing and coughing ability, and provide the person with the knowledge and skills required to avoid complications after discharge. Chapter 7 presents respiratory management in detail.

Cardiovascular care

When spinal cord injury interrupts communication between the brain and the sympathetic preganglionic neurons in the spinal cord, peripheral vasodilation and bradycardia result. These effects are usually significant only in people with lesions above T6, and they resolve within a few weeks of injury. During the initial days following spinal cord injury, however, continuous cardiac monitoring is advisable for all patients.[30, 114, 120] Placement of a temporary pacemaker or treatment with atropine (parasympatholytic agent) or inotropic medication may be indicated for severe bradycardia.[30, 64, 80, 128, 134, 163] Vasopressor medication or intravenous (IV) fluids may be indicated to maintain an adequate blood pressure.[114, 120, 163] IV fluids should be administered judiciously; pulmonary edema is likely to result if large volumes are given.[80, 115, 134]

Vasovagal response. Acutely after spinal cord injury, tracheal suctioning or endotracheal intubation can cause a precipitous fall in heart rate and cardiac arrest. This problem may be avoided by administration of oxygen prior to and after these procedures. Atropine may be given prophylactically or to correct the problem if it develops.[15, 80, 115]

Orthostatic hypotension. People with recent spinal cord injuries frequently exhibit orthostatic hypotension when upright activities are first initiated. Strategies for developing tolerance to upright sitting are presented in Chapter 12.

Autonomic dysreflexia. Autonomic dysreflexia is a potentially life-threatening exaggerated sympathetic response to noxious stimulation below the lesion. This complication occurs almost exclusively among people with cervical and high thoracic lesions, usually first appearing 6 or more months after the injury.

Because autonomic dysreflexia can develop rapidly and is potentially life-threatening, immediate response is necessary when it occurs. The signs and symptoms of autonomic dysreflexia include systolic and diastolic blood pressure elevated 20 mm Hg or more above the individual's post-injury normal level; a pounding headache; profuse sweating or skin flushing above the lesion, particularly in the face, neck, and shoulders; piloerection above the level of the lesion; paresthesias in the head, neck, and upper chest; visual deficits; nasal congestion; anxiety; and cardiac arrhythmias.[38, 128, 137, 170] When patients exhibit signs and symptoms of autonomic dysreflexia, their blood pressure should be assessed. During the episode, blood pressure and heart rate should be monitored frequently.[38, 137, 170] If the individual's blood pressure is above her post-injury normal, she should be positioned with her head and torso elevated and the lower extremities lowered. This positioning may lower the blood pressure and promote cerebral venous return.[38, 111, 163] Clothing and other devices that may be constricting should be loosened.[24, 38, 137, 170]

The underlying source of the noxious sensation causing the dysreflexia should be investigated and eliminated as quickly as possible. Since bladder distention is the most common stimulus for autonomic crisis, draining the bladder may stop the crisis. If the blood pressure remains elevated, it may be brought under control using a short-acting antihypertensive medication. A rectal examination can then be performed, and fecal impaction removed if present. Topical anesthetics should be used during both bladder draining and rectal examination and evacuation, to avoid exacerbating the dysreflexic response.[38, 137, 170]

If bladder and rectal emptying do not stop the dysreflexic response, other possible sources of the dysreflexia should be investigated. If the patient's blood pressure remains elevated after the underlying cause has been removed, it can be controlled using antihypertensive medication.[15, 24, 38, 111, 115, 163, 170] If the source of the autonomic dysreflexia cannot be removed immediately (if it is caused by a pressure sore, for example), the patient may be treated with local anesthesia, oral analgesics, or antihypertensive medication.[181]

The underlying cause of an individual's dysreflexic episode should be noted. To some degree, future episodes can be prevented by avoiding the development of the precipitating condition. For example, better urinary management practices may prevent the development of bladder distension and resulting autonomic dysreflexia.[o] Individuals who experience recurrent episodes of autonomic dysreflexia may benefit from prophylactic medication.[170]

Prevention of deep venous thrombosis and thromboembolism.

Deep venous thrombi (DVTs) are common in the early weeks after spinal cord injury and can lead to pulmonary emboli and death. A variety of measures are typically taken during the acute phase after injury to prevent this potentially lethal complication. Thromboprophylaxis is initiated soon after injury and continues for 8 weeks or more, depending on the individual. After the acute phase of injury, an event such as surgery or a period of prolonged bed rest may necessitate the reinstitution of thromboprophylaxis.[39] Table 3–1 presents interventions used for the prevention of thromboembolism following spinal cord injury.

In addition to providing thromboprophylactic interventions, clinicians should monitor patients for signs of DVT. Swelling in one calf or thigh, discoloration, pain, local or systemic temperature elevation, and dilation of the superficial veins are indications of possible deep vein thrombosis.[39, 166, 180] These symptoms are often present without DVT, however, and thrombus formation often occurs without clinically recognizable symptoms.[166] Because DVTs are both common and relatively difficult to detect in people with spinal cord injuries, the index of suspicion for DVTs should be high.[114, 145, 181]

The diagnosis of DVT requires procedures such as venography, impedance plethysmography, Doppler ultrasound, and I-fibrinogen scans.[30, 64, 115, 145, 166, 180] When venous thrombosis is detected, anticoagulant therapy is indicated.[64, 128, 180] Out-of-bed activity and lower extremity exercise should be suspended.[137]

Patients with recent spinal cord injuries should be monitored for signs of pulmonary embolus: chest pain, shortness of breath, tachycardia, sweating, apprehension, fever, and cough.[39, 114, 128, 180] As is true with DVTs, pulmonary embolism can be difficult to detect in people with spinal cord injuries. Diagnostic tests for pulmonary embolism include ventilation/perfusion scans and pulmonary angiography.[114, 145] Treatment involves anticoagulation therapy and placement of a vena cava filter.[114]

Prevention of cardiovascular disease.

People with spinal cord injuries are living longer, thanks to advances in medical and rehabilitative management. Cardiovascular disease, typically a disease of aging, has become one of the leading

---

[o] Trans-urethral sphincterotomy may be indicated when detrusor-sphincter dyssynergia causes repeated bouts of autonomic dysreflexia.[170]

TABLE 3–1.   THROMBOEMBOLISM PROPHYLAXIS FOLLOWING
SPINAL CORD INJURY

Interventions	Indications	Precautions and Contraindications	Timing
Anticoagulant prophylaxis with low molecular weight heparin or adjusted dose unfractionated heparin	• All patients acutely after injury unless contraindicated	Contraindications • Active or potential bleeding that cannot be controlled • Head injury • Coagulopathy Precautions • May be withheld for 24 to 48 hours postinjury due to potential for bleeding and for neurological deterioration • Withheld on day of surgery	Initiated within 72 hours of injury. Duration varies with completeness of lesion, presence of additional risk factors for thromboembolism, access to medical care.
Compression hose or pneumatic compression devices	• All patients acutely after injury unless contraindicated	Precautions • Proper placement of hose and compression devices, and frequent skin inspections • When thromboprophylaxis is delayed more than 72 hours after injury, testing for leg thrombi should precede initiation of compression	First 2 weeks after injury.
Vena cava filter placement	Indicated for patients who have • Failed anticoagulant prophylaxis • A contraindication to anticoagulation Should be considered for patients who have: • C2 or C3 complete motor paralysis • Poor cardiopulmonary reserve • Thrombosis in the inferior vena cava despite anticoagulant prophylaxis	Precaution • May become dislodged during assisted coughing with abdominal compression	Upon detection of failure of anticoagulation prophylaxis.
Mobilization and active or passive extremity exercises	• All patients unless contraindicated	Contraindications • Any orthopedic or medical condition that would make mobilization and passive exercise potentially harmful • Presence of DVT: suspend activity and passive exercise during first 48 to 72 hours of anticoagulation therapy Precautions • Avoid motions or activities that will cause movement in unstable area(s) of spine • Protect skin from damaging forces	Range-of-motion exercise, out-of-bed activities, and active use of functioning musculature should be initiated as soon as is medically and orthopedically feasible. Should continue indefinitely.

Sources: references 39, 64, 114, 128, 180, 181.

PROBLEM-SOLVING EXERCISE 3-1

Your patient, who has C8 tetraplegia, has been practicing rolling from supine to prone on a mat. She states that she has a pounding headache, and you notice that her face is flushed and damp with perspiration.

- What do you suspect as a likely cause of the patient's signs and symptoms?
- How should you respond?

causes of death in this population.[11, 48, 49, 137, 157] Because of this, long-term cardiovascular wellness has become a focus of rehabilitation.

Cardiovascular disease prevention in people with spinal cord injuries includes many of the same elements as it does in the general population: smoking cessation, low-fat diet, weight control, and aerobic exercise.[128] Cardiovascular conditioning through exercise, a critical component of cardiovascular wellness programs, can be problematic following spinal cord injury. Both altered autonomic control of the cardiovascular system and limited skeletal muscle mass available for exercise make it difficult to stress the heart enough to effect adaptive changes.[34, 89, 137] The following activities and interventions, however, have been found to enhance cardiovascular fitness in people with spinal cord injuries: electrically stimulated leg cycling or ambulation, arm ergometry training, combined arm ergometry and electrically stimulated leg cycling, wheelchair ergometry training, wheelchair propulsion, walking with crutches, and participation in wheelchair sports.[9, 42, 51, 72, 87–89, 91, 127, 137, 157, 179]

Cardiovascular fitness training during inpatient or outpatient rehabilitation can enhance patients' exercise tolerance, allowing them to be more physically active. Unfortunately, these fitness gains will not last if the exercise program is discontinued.[42] To achieve a more lasting benefit to the patient's health, the rehabilitation team should focus on the development of a physically active lifestyle that can continue long after rehabilitation is over. The exercise regime most suited to the individual will depend on her preferences, physical abilities, financial resources, support systems, and access to exercise facilities, equipment, and organized sports. Compliance is likely to be higher if the activities are practical and enjoyable.[34, 157]

In designing fitness programs, clinicians should keep in mind the risk of overuse injuries and pain in the upper extremities.[34, 173] Cardiovascular conditioning activities that involve movement patterns that are both biomechanically normal[85] and different from those used during daily activities[157] may help with this problem. An exercise program that develops appropriate flexibility and balanced strength in the shoulders[p] will also help prevent overuse injuries.[85]

In addition to preventing cardiovascular disease, fitness programs may enhance quality of life. Physical deconditioning can lead to an escalating cycle of functional limitation and disability. Fitness programs, by increasing tolerance for physical activity, can make more independent functioning and integration into the community possible.[34, 99]

Management of Musculoskeletal Problems

Osteoporosis. Osteoporosis develops after spinal cord injury in the extremities innervated caudal to the lesion, leading to increased vulnerability to fractures. Ambulation, prolonged standing, and electrical stimulation have been investigated for their effectiveness in reducing or reversing the development of osteoporosis. None of these interventions have been shown to be effective in the lower extremities[10, 12, 16, 98, 101, 130] with the possible exception of *early* weight-bearing through the lower extremities.[46]

Heterotopic ossification. Following spinal cord injury, heterotopic ossification (HO) occurs most frequently in the hips, knees, and elbows.[64] The signs and symptoms of HO include pain, swelling, erythema, warmth, and restricted range of motion in the affected area.[63, 64] Heterotopic ossification may be seen on x-ray, but it can be detected earlier using a bone scan.[6]

Interventions for heterotopic ossification include range of motion exercises to preserve joint range of motion, and treatment with either diphosphonate or nonsteroidal antiinflammatory agents to minimize ossification.[6, 63, 64] Despite these interventions, heterotopic ossification can progress to the point where it significantly impairs the individual's ability to function. When this occurs, the patient may undergo resection of

---

[p] Chapter 12 presents additional strategies for avoiding chronic shoulder pain.

the ectopic bone, often followed by radiation therapy and pharmacologic treatment.[63, 119]

Pain. Pain is a common problem both during the acute phase after spinal cord injury and in the years that follow. This pain can result from a variety of neurologic (examples: nerve root impingement, central neuropathic pain), orthopedic (examples: heterotopic ossification, chronic overuse injuries), or even medical (examples: deep vein thrombosis, visceral disorders) causes.[55, 69, 85, 95, 104, 113, 136, 147, 151, 152] The first step in pain management is an examination and evaluation to determine the pain's source. Once the cause of the pain has been identified, appropriate medical, surgical, or physical therapy interventions can be implemented.[q]

Spasticity and spasms. Spasticity and spasms[r] occur frequently in people with spinal cord injuries, particularly in those who have lesions in the cervical or upper thoracic cord. Elevated muscle tone is not always problematic. In fact, some individuals are able to use it to assist in certain functional activities such as standing and walking. On the other hand, many people have spasticity and spasms that cause pain, interfere with sleep, and lead to increased vulnerability to the development of range-of-motion limitations. Elevated muscle tone can also interfere with independent functioning, and can make it difficult for others to provide assistance.

Spasticity management is highly individualized. Some people find that passive range-of-motion exercises (prolonged stretching) and positioning are adequate to preserve range of motion, keep spasticity-related discomfort within acceptable levels, and prevent spasticity from interfering with independent functioning or dependent handling.[156] When these measures fail and spasticity causes significant discomfort or interferes with sleep or safe functioning (independent or assisted), pharmacotherapy should be considered. Baclofen, clonidine, dantrolene sodium, diazepam, ketazolam, or tizanidine can be taken orally. Each of these medications has potential side effects, ranging in severity from drowsiness to liver toxicity.[70, 77, 125, 156] Intrathecally administered baclofen, an alternative to oral medication, is delivered by a surgically implanted pump. Because the medication is delivered directly into the subarachnoid space surrounding the spinal cord, spasticity and spasms can be controlled with fewer systemic effects. Potential side effects include withdrawal or potentially lethal[5, 156] overdose that can occur when the pump does not function properly.[77]

Both orally and intrathecally administered medications require careful dosage titration. Pharmacotherapy is generally started with low doses, which are increased gradually until the desired clinical outcome is achieved.[53, 77, 156] Optimal dosing reduces the patient's muscle tone enough to decrease discomfort and permit safe functioning, with minimal side effects.

Following spinal cord injury, muscle tone can fluctuate. A variety of conditions such as bladder infections, fractures, pressure ulcers, or hangnails can cause temporary increases in spasticity and spasms. Such sources of increased muscle tone should be investigated and treated before medications are initiated or adjusted.[70, 76, 77]

When problematic spasticity exists in a limited number of muscles, alternative locally acting agents may be utilized. These agents include botulinum toxin, which is injected into muscles, and phenol or ethyl alcohol, which are injected into peripheral nerves or the motor points of muscles. These interventions cause temporary[s] reductions in spasticity.[76, 125, 156] In rare cases when problematic spasticity cannot be controlled using other measures, surgical ablation of nerves (neurectomy), nerve roots (rhizotomy), or the spinal cord (myelotomy) may be considered. These surgeries are irreversible, not always effective in decreasing spasticity, and can cause additional neurological impairments.[70] As pharmacologic management of spasticity has improved, these procedures have become less common.[156]

EDUCATION

Education is a critical component of any rehabilitation program. After spinal cord injury, people need to learn about the altered functioning of their bodies, what they can expect in terms of future motor and sensory functioning, the complications

---

[q] A complete discussion of pain management is beyond the scope of this text. Chapter 12 addresses strategies for preventing chronic shoulder pain from overuse injury.

[r] Spasticity is a velocity-dependent increase in muscle tone in response to passive movement.[62, 112] Spasms are involuntary muscle contractions that occur spontaneously or are elicited by stimuli such as tactile stimulation.[140]

[s] Three to 6 months for botulinum toxin, 2 to 36 months for ethyl alcohol or phenol.[76]

that can occur, and the avoidance and management of these complications. Those who require orthotic stabilization of their spines at the time of discharge must also learn about the proper use of their orthoses.

Although education has always been important in rehabilitation, it has become even more critical as hospital stays have shortened. People are leaving rehabilitation centers earlier, before they have had time for full physiological, functional, and psychosocial adaptation to their injuries. Before patients return home, they must gain the knowledge and skills needed to enable them to stay healthy.

Many people with spinal cord injuries require assistance when they leave rehabilitation, either because they have not yet reached their full functional potential or because their impairments are such that independent functioning is not possible. When individuals are likely to require assistance after discharge, their education programs should include the people who will provide this assistance. This group may include family members, friends, attendants, or other caregivers.

Unfortunately, it is not possible to provide education and training to everyone who will give assistance in the months and years to come. The task of training future caregivers is likely to fall on patients and their families. For this reason, the education program should include instruction and practice in training and directing others in the safe performance of the tasks that will require assistance.

Neurological Return

People with spinal cord injuries should be instructed about their potential for neurological return. Although definitive predictions are often not possible, patients can be apprised of the range of possibilities for neurological return, and the likely time course of any return that may occur. They should also be informed about the rehabilitation team's best estimate of their ultimate outcomes. People with incomplete lesions should be encouraged to monitor themselves for return and to inform the rehabilitation team if significant change occurs.

Prevention and Treatment of Complications

Following spinal cord injury, the threats of pressure ulcers, respiratory complications, bowel and urinary tract complications, and autonomic dysre-

---

PROBLEM-SOLVING EXERCISE 3–2

Your patient wears a thermoplastic body jacket to stabilize his lower thoracic spine. He is on a mat in therapy when you notice that the anterior portion of his orthosis is on upside-down. (You are familiar with these orthoses and are certain that this one has been put on wrong.)

- What should you do about this?
- How can you prevent this problem from reoccurring?

flexia never go away. These complications can be avoided, but only with meticulous care. Cardiovascular disease, although it is not a direct complication of spinal cord injury, also poses a serious threat. Lifestyle changes may help prevent this problem.

During rehabilitation, people with spinal cord injuries must acquire the knowledge and skills needed to stay healthy. Patients should learn about how their bodies function, the complications that can result, how to avoid these complications, and what to do if they occur. They should also gain the self-reliance and communication skills required to take control of their care. Unfortunately, many members of the general medical community are ignorant about the special health needs of people with spinal cord injuries. As a result, someone who places total trust in the system may not get adequate care. People with spinal cord injuries need to learn to manage their own care if they are to stay healthy through the years.

> Our people are really obnoxious when they leave here. Our goal is that when these people leave here, since they have to live with their injury all their lives, is for them to know more about their body than most doctors know. Indeed, most doctors don't know much about spinal cord injury. We want our patients to recognize when they need a urine culture, when they should take antibiotics, when they should not, when they should call a doctor, and what they should tell the doctor they need. We want them to be able to take charge of their own care.
>
> Julie Botvin Madorski[107]

Orthotic Use

Orthoses are effective only if they are worn. A patient who requires orthotic stabilization should be educated about (and *convinced* of) the importance of wearing the device. Otherwise, the orthosis may not be worn. Even a halo, which is attached directly to the skull, can be removed by its wearer.[74]

When orthotic stabilization is required, an orthosis must not only be worn, but worn correctly. Other than halo devices, most orthoses can be removed, reapplied, and adjusted easily. Orthotic wearers should know the circumstances under which their orthoses can be removed safely. They must also know how to reapply and adjust their orthoses properly, or be able to direct these tasks if they require assistance.

As is true with all medical and orthopedic interventions, vertebral orthoses can cause a variety of complications. The wearer of a vertebral orthosis should learn about any complications that the orthosis may cause, and how to respond if these complications occur.

FOLLOW-UP

Follow-up is another important component of health care after spinal cord injury. After discharge, periodic checkups make it possible to monitor and respond to changing physical and psychosocial needs, promote health, detect and treat complications early, and gather feedback on the effectiveness of the rehabilitation program. These postdischarge evaluations should continue indefinitely because many of the sequelae and potential complications of spinal cord injury continue for the remainder of the individual's life.

Follow-up has added significance for people who experience neurological return. As lengths of stay in rehabilitation diminish, the chance of motor return occurring after discharge increases. Significant motor return that is evident at follow-up may indicate the need for further rehabilitation to maximize functional gains made possible by the return. This additional rehabilitation can take place in inpatient, outpatient, or in-home settings as appropriate.

SUMMARY

- Following injury of the spinal column, motion of the spine may result in trauma to previously undamaged neural tissue. Appropriate fracture management is required to preserve neurological function.

- Fracture management starts with immobilization of the spine at the scene of the accident. Definitive management involves operative and/or nonoperative restoration of the spine's alignment, decompression of the neural tissue, and stabilization of the injured structures.

- An orthosis may be used to immobilize the injured spinal column, either in lieu of or following surgery. A variety of orthoses are available for each region of the spine.

- Spinal cord injury leaves an individual susceptible to a variety of serious complications. During acute care and rehabilitation, specialized medical management is necessary to avoid these complications.

- In order to stay healthy, a person with a spinal cord injury must learn to prevent complications, as well as to detect them and respond appropriately when they occur. The educational component of rehabilitation addresses these areas with both the patient and those who will be involved in her care.

- Because spinal cord injury causes life-long vulnerability to a variety of problems, postdischarge follow-up is critical.

4

PSYCHOSOCIAL ISSUES

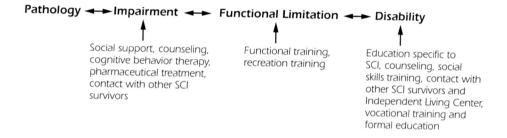

Pathology ←→ Impairment ←→ Functional Limitation ←→ Disability

Social support, counseling, cognitive behavior therapy, pharmaceutical treatment, contact with other SCI survivors

Functional training, recreation training

Education specific to SCI, counseling, social skills training, contact with other SCI survivors and Independent Living Center, vocational training and formal education

Spinal cord injury brings sudden and profound life changes. The person who sustains a cord injury, often an active male in his adolescence or early adulthood, may be swimming, playing football, driving, or earning a living one minute, and the next minute he is incapable of moving his extremities. Over the next days and weeks he finds himself paralyzed, incontinent, immobile, dependent, and isolated. As his rehabilitation progresses and he ventures out from the rehabilitation center, he is faced with a social and physical environment that seems almost hostile in its inaccessibility.

Despite the magnitude and scope of the problems that spinal cord injury can cause, most people who sustain a cord injury are able to adjust. For some people, the injury ultimately results in psychological and spiritual growth. Others never fully recover psychologically from their loss. The outcome depends partly on the individual and partly upon the psychosocial support that he receives. To maximize a person's potential for adaptation and growth following spinal cord injury, the rehabilitation team must address itself to his psychosocial needs.

PSYCHOSOCIAL IMPACT OF SPINAL CORD INJURY

Losses Associated with Spinal Cord Injury

The physical losses engendered by spinal cord injury are perhaps the most obvious. Depending on the completeness and level of the injury, a person can lose control of some or all of his limb and trunk musculature. His physique changes dramatically as his muscles atrophy. Where sensation is affected, he loses the ability to perceive the presence, position, and motion of his limbs or to experience the myriad pleasant and unpleasant sensations from the environment. He is likely to lose bowel and bladder control, and his sexual functioning will be altered.[a]

The person with significant neurological damage from spinal cord injury loses the ability to care for himself and to move from place to

---

[a] Chapter 5 addresses the impact of spinal cord injury on sexuality and sexual functioning and presents strategies for promoting adjustment in this area.

place. Dependent on others to care for him, and placed in an environment where all power and self-direction are taken away, he loses his autonomy. Additionally, he is unable to participate in the recreational, social, educational, and vocational activities that previously filled his days. With rehabilitation, he may regain the capacity to do some of these things, but his manner of doing them will be altered.

Spinal cord injury also threatens financial security and disrupts plans for the future. From 50 percent to 68 percent of people who sustain spinal cord injuries remain unemployed following injury,[25, 29, 51, 73, 119] and those who do work make less money on the average than nondisabled people.[115] Financial difficulties are also created by the expenses of medical care, attendant care, and equipment.[59, 64]

During acute hospitalization and rehabilitation, a person is likely to experience separation from loved ones. Even after discharge, relationships with friends and family members are likely to be different. Roles may be altered, and patterns of communication and levels of intimacy are likely to change.[89, 118] Old friends tend to drift away.[115, 116]

Faced with the changes in his physique, physical functioning, functional capacity, accustomed activities, financial status, relationships, and plans for the future, a person's previous concept of himself no longer fits. Thus, personal identity can be added to the list of losses brought on by spinal cord injury.[75, 115]

Finally, spinal cord injury challenges a person's notions about how the world functions. Each of us has illusions about the world and our place in it. These irrational beliefs, left over from early childhood, may include feelings of invulnerability, immortality, or a sense of total control over one's life.[92, 109] Spinal cord injury can make these and other illusions untenable.

> I think with a spinal cord injury, one realizes that one is not going to live forever, that you are mortal.
>
> Don Rugg[85]

Social Impact of Spinal Cord Injury

People with disabilities are devalued in our society. As a group, they are seen as substantially different from and less desirable than able-bodied people; as a result, they are subject to discrimination.[34, 46, 113, 117]

> Most of us know by now that our physical limitations cut less keenly than the needless limitations placed upon us by an unwittingly hostile society. We should let the world in on that secret.
>
> Barry Corbet[12]

Discrimination against people with disabilities manifests itself in many ways. Architectural and transportation barriers serve to handicap those with mobility impairments. People with disabling conditions encounter discriminatory treatment when seeking education, employment, medical insurance, and housing.[8, 41, 87, 113] Financial disincentives within public assistance programs can make it extremely difficult to break out of a cycle of unemployment and poverty; in some cases, employment can result in a loss of medical insurance[b] and funding for attendant care, meaning that some people with disabilities simply cannot afford to work.[23, 115]

People with disabilities are also subject to discrimination in their interpersonal relationships. When meeting someone with a disability, an able-bodied person's perception of the individual is likely to be dominated by the disability; people focus on the disabling characteristics rather than on the person's other qualities. Likewise, the media tends to focus on a person's disability rather than other, usually more relevant, characteristics. For example, a few years ago a woman was in the local news. Although her disability had no bearing on why she was in the news, it was *always* mentioned when she was discussed. The wording progressed (deteriorated) from "Lucy Jones,[c] the wheelchair athlete," to "Lucy Jones, the woman in a wheelchair," and finally to "Lucy Jones, a 33-year-old wheelchair."

People with disabilities are viewed as fundamentally different from "normal" people and are afforded less esteem and status.[125] They are often perceived as dependent and helpless,[35, 79] tragic victims who remain bitter about their misfortune.[120]

Because of the devaluation and stereotyping of people with disabilities, able-bodied people are

---

b Upon losing Medicare coverage, private insurance may be prohibitively expensive. In addition, policies are likely to exclude any conditions related to the disabling condition. With spinal cord injury, this could result in exclusion of coverage of medical problems associated with the skin, urinary, pulmonary, and musculoskeletal systems.

c Fictitious name.

likely to be uncomfortable talking with them and tend to avoid contact.[35, 54] This discomfort, in combination with architectural barriers in the community, creates a formidable obstacle to community integration. As a result, social isolation is common following spinal cord injury.[53, 115]

After sustaining a spinal cord injury, a person soon discovers that he is a member of a disadvantaged minority, "the disabled." The demoralizing effects of the stereotyping and discrimination that he inevitably experiences are likely to be compounded by his own preexisting prejudices regarding people with disabilities.[117]

> I have never felt despised for being in a wheelchair. I have felt pitied; I have despised myself.
>
> Barry Corbet[13]

Additional Factors Affecting Behavior

Immediately after sustaining a spinal cord injury, a person is likely to be whisked away in an ambulance to an emergency room from which he will proceed to an intensive care unit. Once in the unit, he will be bombarded by a constant stream of monotonous noises from monitors and other equipment. He will have few meaningful sights or sounds to attend to, despite the constant noise, and at the same time he will have an absence of tactile and proprioceptive sensations as a result of his injury. Health care workers will come and go to minister to his physical needs, but he will not have prolonged periods of social contact. Because the activity, sounds, and lighting remain fairly constant through the day and night, his sleep will be disrupted, and he will have few cues to orient him to the passage of time.

> It is too easy to lie in bed just counting spots on the ceiling and allowing the mind to wander and sleep. I know. That's exactly what I did for months; but in my case, as I lay, being turned from side to side, it was the colorful parrots printed on the material covering the screens. I counted them so many times they eventually started flying.
>
> Michael Rogers[104]

During the acute phase following spinal cord injury, a person is likely to experience sensory deprivation, social isolation, lack of time cues, sleep deprivation, and pain. He is likely to be on medications that have psychoactive effects, and may undergo surgery with general anesthesia. He may have sustained a head injury at the time of the accident. Any of these conditions *alone* can have a profound impact on cognitive functioning, emotions, and behavior.[6, 18, 103, 115, 116] When faced with a recently injured person, it is difficult, if not impossible, for the health professional to determine which behaviors are the result of psychological reaction to spinal cord injury and which are due to other circumstances and physical variables.

Many of the conditions just described, particularly medication and sleep deprivation, can persist throughout and beyond rehabilitation. Additionally, during inpatient rehabilitation the person may be bored[38] and may find himself in an environment that encourages complacency and inactivity.

Cautionary note. Many health professionals are quick to interpret any of a variety of behaviors as psychological reaction to spinal cord injury. Before making this judgment, health professionals should keep in mind the multiple factors that can impact on a recently injured person's cognitive functioning, emotions, and behavior. If someone who has recently sustained a spinal cord injury seems confused, is it the result of a psychological response to overwhelming loss? Is it a result of pain, medication, social isolation, or sensory deprivation? If he expresses anger, is this a manifestation of inner turmoil brought on by the injury, or could it be a reaction to demeaning treatment? Before dismissing behavior as "denial," "anger," "depression," or other psychological response to a spinal cord injury, health professionals should consider other possible explanations for the behavior. Most importantly, they should attempt to discern whether anything in the physical or social environment could be contributing to the behavior in question.

Health professionals should also keep in mind the following humbling fact: research has demonstrated that as a group, we are not very good at determining our patients' moods. There is a strong tendency to view patients with spinal cord injuries as more depressed than they actually are.[42, 62, 78] Many people with spinal cord injuries report that they do not view their injuries as tragic or even as the worst thing that ever happened to them.[13, 116] Health professionals who view spinal cord injury in an overly catastrophic light are more likely to convey a defeatist and pitying attitude. This attitude could in turn affect the adjustment of their patients.

PSYCHOLOGICAL ADJUSTMENT AND ADAPTATION FOLLOWING INJURY

Spinal cord injury causes significant losses in many areas: physical, functional, social, financial, personal identity, and world view. In general, the process of adjustment to these losses takes years.[72, 89, 109, 115] As evidence of continuing adjustment over the years, both life satisfaction and quality of life increase with time after injury.[2, 26, 67, 122]

Until relatively recently, it was believed that people who sustained spinal cord injuries went through a specific series of mood states as they adjusted. Typically, each patient was expected to experience shock, denial, depression, anger, dependency, and, finally, adjustment.[76, 116] Although various theorists described slightly different stages of adjustment, it was generally agreed that adjustment required progression through these stages. Anyone who did not fit the pattern was not "doing it right."

Research in recent years has shown the stage theory of adjustment to be inaccurate.[23, 24, 32, 115, 116] People do not progress through a neat series of mood states in a lock-step fashion as they adapt to life following spinal cord injury. Each adapts in his own way.

If people do not pass through a predictable and universal series of stages, what do they do? After spinal cord injury, as after any significant loss, people grieve. Each grieves, however, in his own way and at his own pace. A variety of factors influence the manner in which an individual responds and adjusts to the losses engendered by spinal cord injury. These include personal characteristics such as personality; cognitive style; coping style; values, attitudes, and psychological health prior to the injury; prior loss experiences; and age.[1, 3, 7, 32, 37, 47, 50, 67, 70, 74, 108, 111, 115] The nature of the social support provided by loved ones and health professionals also has a strong influence on adaptation following cord injury.[1, 32, 50, 88, 115] Finally, factors such as financial security,[d] education, and access to transportation impact on adjustment.[5, 26, 50, 115]

Contrary to common assumptions, level of injury is not a significant factor; people with tetraplegia adjust as successfully as those with paraplegia.[19, 20, 39, 44, 48, 49, 50, 83, 86, 100, 108, 110] Moreover, individuals with less profound neurological damage can have greater adjustment problems[e] than those with more severe injuries.[56] Although people with relatively good motor function (Frankel D and E) are likely to function with a high degree of independence, they can also experience many of the same difficulties as those with more complete lesions: orthopedic problems, bowel and bladder dysfunction, pain, medical complications, sexual problems, neurological deterioration, spasticity, depression, and unemployability.[43] Unfortunately, these difficulties may be overlooked or minimized by health professionals, family members, friends, other patients, and others in the community. As a result, individuals with minimal residual neurological deficits may not receive the "permission" and support that they need to grieve their losses and adjust to their injuries.[56]

Tasks of Grieving

Grieving involves more than a passive acceptance, "getting used to" a loss. It is an active process by which a person lets go of what has been lost and formulates a life without it.

Following spinal cord injury, a person may feel that he has literally lost everything. It may seem that all aspects of his life, his relationships, himself, and his future have been destroyed. But in grieving, he gradually gains perspective on his loss. One task of grieving involves sorting through his losses, identifying what aspects of his life and himself he has truly lost, and what remains. He can then let go of what he has lost and reclaim what remains.[111]

In response to the loss of his old self-image, a person with a spinal cord injury forges a new identity.[46, 117] This identity is "an amalgamation of all of the 'I am's' from pre-injury that are still relevant with the new 'I am's' that are consonant with the physical disability."[115]

In addition to finding a new identity, the individual discovers and develops a new lifestyle, with new goals and sources of satisfaction.[30] By creating a new existence rather than holding onto the old, the person with a spinal cord injury can feel good about himself and his life.

---

d Research has provided conflicting information on financial security. Green, Pratt, and Grigsby[50] found that income and employment had no relation to self-concept following cord injury.

e People with injuries classified as Frankel E have higher suicide rates than do individuals with more complete injuries.[56]

Early Reactions to Spinal Cord Injury

After spinal cord injury, people commonly go through a period of confusion and forgetfulness. Often, a newly injured person appears to have difficulty processing information. For example, he may ask a question that he has already asked on several occasions and seem to have no memory of discussing the topic.[f] A newly injured health professional may ask questions or express beliefs that are inconsistent with his medical expertise.

In the past, the period of confusion that often follows spinal cord injury was assumed to be a sign of denial. Lately, however, this assumption has been challenged. Sensory deprivation, social isolation, lack of time cues, sleep deprivation, pain, and medications are other possible explanations.[6, 18, 103, 115, 116]

Research has not demonstrated that denial is the cause of the confused behavior commonly seen after injury. By the same token, research has not *ruled out* the occurrence of denial following spinal cord injury. If people do, in fact, grieve after sustaining spinal cord injuries, denial remains a possibility. Certainly, the losses associated with spinal cord injury are on the magnitude of the loss of a loved one. When grieving such a loss, denial serves a purpose: it allows a person to rally his psychological and social resources and prepare himself for the loss. Denial is *not* a sign of pathology. It is a normal, healthy psychological response that makes it possible for the reality of a loss to sink in gradually as the person becomes able to cope.[75, 79, 92, 109] Whether the confusion commonly seen following spinal cord injury is due to denial, other factors, or a combination remains to be determined. Whatever the source of the confused behavior, health professionals should recognize that recently injured people process information and deal with their losses as best they can. There is no benefit in attempting to force them to face reality.[21]

Grief

After an initial period of confusion, whatever the source, people tend to grieve following spinal cord injury. Grief is a natural, healthy process by which a person adapts to a significant loss. It is not a linear process, with the person plodding through a series of stages one by one. People vary widely in the emotions that they experience after spinal cord injuries, as well as in the order, intensity, and length of time experiencing the various emotions associated with grieving. An individual may alternate rapidly between moods or "move past" a particular mood state, only to return[g] at a later time.[109]

A variety of emotions and behaviors are associated with grief. During normal grief following spinal cord injury, a person *may* experience any of the following: sadness, anger, hostility, anxiety, panic, and feelings of inadequacy, shame, helplessness, and vulnerability.[3, 30] He may have periods of regression and self-neglect.[30, 82] Many consider suicide, although few actually attempt it.[56, 99, 117] In normal grief after the death of a loved one, which is analogous to grief following spinal cord injury,[111] a person may experience hallucinations, changes in sleep and appetite, forgetfulness, and social withdrawal.[126]

It is important to make the distinction between grief, which is a normal and healthy response to loss, and clinical depression, which is pathological. True depression involves a specific, fairly global, and persistent pattern of emotions and behaviors.[h] Whereas most grieve after spinal cord injury, the majority do not exhibit true depression.[32, 62, 67, 86, 110, 115, 116] Among those who become depressed, the depression is usually brief and mild and tends to occur within the first few months of injury.[62, 102, 115, 116]

Outcomes

Most people adapt well following spinal cord injury. After a period of adjustment, they tend to have positive self-concepts[50, 51] and, in general, are satisfied with life,[2, 19, 51] neither more anxious[7, 108] nor more depressed[64, 102, 108] than noninjured people.

We are the living demonstration that even if life circumstances become tough, life satis-

---

[f] At one time, this author was incensed by the apparent fact that nobody was explaining to newly injured people anything about their injuries or prognoses. People who had been injured for months would ask, "Why can't I move my legs? Nobody has explained this to me." Eventually, however, I began hearing the same question from people to whom *I* had provided careful explanations in the early weeks following injury.

[g] This is true for denial, as well as for the various mood states of grieving.[92]

[h] The diagnosis of Major Depressive Disorder requires that the individual exhibits at least five of the following almost every day for at least 2 weeks: (1) significant weight loss or gain, (2) increase or decrease in appetite, (3) insomnia or hypersomnia, (4) psychomotor retardation or agitation, (5) fatigue or energy loss, (6) feelings of worthlessness, (7) excessive or inappropriate guilt, (8) diminished ability to think or concentrate, (9) indecisiveness, or (10) recurrent thoughts of death or suicide.[32]

faction can remain high. We're proof that things can be Hard, but Good. People need to know that.

Barry Corbet[12]

Spinal cord injury is not a devastating catastrophe that creates *victims* who are forever bitter and psychologically impaired. In fact, for many it is a powerful stimulus for growth. Because it brings such profound losses, a spinal cord injury can shatter a person's identity and basic assumptions about himself and his world. In the aftermath of this disruption, it is possible for him to examine and alter his self-image and world view. Thus, he has an opportunity to grow in ways in which he may otherwise never have grown, as these assumptions are rarely questioned except during times of crisis.[96]

> It really changes your perspective. The one thing I really come back to is that I've gained an incredible sense of perspective—different people's realities, how relative the whole bit is. For that, I'm grateful.
>
> John Galland[13]

People often report that they have grown as a result of spinal cord injury.[17] Some even state that they would not opt for a cure if it were available.

> I'm happier now than I was before I broke my neck. I love my wife and my family more. I

have a better rapport with people. I wasn't exactly a jerk when I was still walking, but I'm a better person now than I was before my disability. . . . If nothing else, this experience we have come to call disability has caused me to take a closer look at myself—at the nature of my existence.

> I realize that it's not the physical impressions we make in life that endure, but the mental ones. I roll away knowing that I don't need a cure. I survived. And I'm proud of who I've become.
>
> Ed Hooper[60]

> It was a rebirth—a new beginning. If I could have "the Cure" but I'd have to give up who and what I am, I'd decline.
>
> Anonymous[17]

Although most adapt well after spinal cord injury and many grow from the experience, some do not fare so well. Depression, though not universal, is more prevalent[i] among people with spinal cord injuries than in the general population,[67, 69, 81] as are anxiety and feelings of helplessness.[15] A small percentage exhibits self-neglect, even years after injury.[82] A few find themselves unable to adapt to their disability and never regain a sense of happiness and satisfaction with their lives. The suicide rate among people with spinal cord injuries is 3.3 to 5 times higher than that of the general population.[29, 56] Most of these suicides occur within the first 5 years of injury.[29]

COMMUNITY REINTEGRATION

Humans are social beings. Our relationships with families, friends, neighbors, coworkers, and members of the community at large are important aspects of our lives. Through these relationships, we can gain a sense of belonging and well-being. The roles that we play within these social groups help to define us and give us a sense of purpose.

Spinal cord injury can interfere with relationships and the performance of social roles. This interference has a variety of causes, includ-

---

PROBLEM-SOLVING EXERCISE 4–1

Try to imagine what your life would be like if you had a spinal cord injury. A few years down the road, would you feel that the quality of your life is good? Would you feel like a person of worth?

- If you could not breathe on your own, would you want to be placed on a ventilator or would you rather die than live with high tetraplegia?
- What do your answers tell you about your perceptions about life after a spinal cord injury?

---

i The estimated frequency of true depression following spinal cord injury is 10 percent to 30 percent.[115] Interestingly, this frequency is comparable to the estimated incidence (10 percent to 20 percent) of clinical depression among widows 1 year following their husbands' deaths.[97]

ing the individual's physical capabilities and behaviors, the responses of others, and architectural barriers.

One important focus of rehabilitation is community reintegration, the return to full participation in all aspects of the life of the community. In this context, "community" refers to social groups in a variety of settings: home, neighborhood, work or school, place of worship, and geographic region. Community reintegration includes the performance of age-, gender-, and culture-appropriate roles and activities in natural settings,[j] with normative status, rights, and responsibilities.[27] A high degree of community integration is associated with greater levels of life satisfaction.[55]

STRATEGIES FOR GROWTH AND REINTEGRATION

The purpose of rehabilitation after spinal cord injury is to minimize disability and enable the person to return to a lifestyle as near normal as possible. Teaching the physical skills needed to function independently is not enough to meet this end; living is more than getting in and out of bed and regulating bowels. These activities are not life—they are things that we do to live. To prepare a person to *live* with the sequelae of his spinal cord injury, the rehabilitation team must focus beyond mere functional training and promote psychological and social adaptation as well. This involves providing the needed support as the individual grieves his losses and develops a new identity, lifestyle, future, and world view. It also involves preparing him to function in a society that views him as less than he used to be.

The development of self-advocacy skills is a critical task of social adjustment after spinal cord injury. People with disabilities are protected by law against discrimination in housing, transportation, access to businesses and public facilities, and employment. Unfortunately, these laws are not always enforced. If he is to function in society, a person with a spinal cord injury must be aware of his rights and know how to ensure that they are not violated.

Social adaptation after spinal cord injury involves more than the injured individual; the members of his family have significant adjustments of their own to make. When someone becomes disabled, there is disruption of his fam-

ily's usual mode of functioning.[k] Major changes are likely to occur in lifestyles, roles, communication patterns, and finances. The rehabilitation team can support the family as they learn to cope with these changes. In turn, the family will be better able to provide needed social support to the injured person as he adjusts to the injury and its consequences.

Destructive Practices in Rehabilitation

Most, if not all, rehabilitation professionals would agree that they should (and do) work to prepare people with physical impairments to live as independently as possible and to develop positive attitudes toward themselves and their lives. In practice, however, this is all too often not the case. While we teach the physical skills needed for independent functioning, we can also teach people that they are second-class citizens, incapable or unworthy of self-direction or independence.

Dependence. From the moment a person sustains a spinal cord injury, he loses control of his life. He is handled, poked, prodded, examined, treated, and "done to" by an endless stream of health professionals as they care for his physical needs. Even once he reaches a rehabilitation unit, he is not likely to be treated in ways that enable him to regain control of his life. He is not given any real choices, being expected to conform to the goals and practices of the rehabilitation team. If his desires do not coincide with those of the team, and if he asserts himself, he is likely to be labeled "noncompliant" and a "difficult patient." Passive, compliant behavior is expected and rewarded.[79, 115, 117]

Another harmful practice involves assisting people who are capable of performing an activity independently. This is often done for the sake of expedience. ("Yes, you worked hard in OT to learn how to dress yourself, but I'm going to dress you so that you won't be late for your appointment.") The underlying message is that the person can do the activity in therapy, but in *real life,* he needs others to help him. In addition to receiving this negative message, the person is deprived of practice of the activity. His skill, then, does not develop as it should. Ultimately, he cannot per-

---

[j] An example of a natural setting is a standard workplace rather than a sheltered workshop.

[k] This may be particularly true when spouses take on the role of caregiver. Caregiving spouses of people with spinal cord injuries exhibit higher levels of stress and depression than both their injured partners and the noncaregiving spouses of people with cord injuries.[121]

form the task as well or as quickly as he should, and he in fact ends up needing assistance.

Negative attitudes.   Many health professionals, being products of society at large, have negative attitudes about people with disabilities.[42, 106, 127] These attitudes influence their behavior as they interact with patients. Negative perceptions regarding the potential for adjustment and quality of life after spinal cord injury can influence medical decisions such as whether to initiate or terminate life support.[42] Moreover, health professionals who are overly pessimistic or defeatist can convey these attitudes to patients and their families.[42]

Negative attitudes can also cause health professionals to treat their patients as second-class citizens. By talking to an adult with a spinal cord injury as though he is a child, or by talking about him in his presence as though he cannot hear, the health professional dehumanizes and infantalizes him. We also dehumanize patients by labeling them by their disabling conditions. This practice is so accepted and widespread among health professionals that for many, it is hard to comprehend that there could be any harm in it. But language is very powerful. Anyone who has ever cringed at hearing racist or sexist language knows this. The words that we use express and perpetuate our values and attitudes. When we call a person "patient" even when he is no longer a patient, we communicate the notion that he remains dependent on health professionals. When we label someone by his disabling condition, we focus attention on the disability rather than on the person. It then becomes easier to lose sight of the person himself.

> Many of us insist labels are unimportant. Wrong! Exploitation and oppression are given power through language. In our hierarchical society, it is the social implications of words that do us the greatest damage.
>
> Marta Russell[107]

Medical model.   The practices just described are symptomatic of the medical model of health care. In systems operating according to this model, there is a rigid hierarchy of power with physicians at the top, other health professionals in the middle, and patients and family members at the bottom. The job of the staff is to "fix" patients, and the patients are expected to accept that treatment passively.[8, 22, 95, 115] Health professionals are firmly in control. Even the clothes that they wear,

laboratory coats and uniforms, express their authority.[46] Rounds are likely to be conducted either in the patient's absence or at bedside, with the patient lying down.[52] Clearly, a unit functioning according to the medical model does not provide an atmosphere that encourages those undergoing rehabilitation to exercise their autonomy.

Inherent in the medical model is the inferior, powerless status of the patient. Health professionals dominate all interactions. These practices and values are so ingrained in the medical community that the demeaning domination and subjugation inherent in these interactions is seen by many as appropriate professional–patient relations.

> The submissive and devaluing aspects of the role of patient are so frequently accepted by both patient and staff that some curious phenomena become apparent only when a person in a wheelchair enters a medical institution as a professional. On countless occasions, I have been wheeling along in treatment settings in various parts of the country, attending to my business as a teacher, researcher, or clinical psychologist, when an attendant or nurse would hustle alongside and challengingly or sarcastically say, "Hey, where do you think you're going?" or sometimes "You're not supposed to be out here—go to your room." On one occasion, solely on the basis of my occupancy of a wheelchair, a nurse tried physically to put me in bed! More than once my wheelchair has been hijacked by an attendant who, without comment, wheeled me to the dining room of his institution.
>
> Although I have no objection to consuming a free meal, in general, following one of the "You can't come here" comments or "You must go there" actions, I tactfully explain my business. Invariably the response is, "Oh, I'm sorry, I thought you were a patient!" There is immediate recognition by the staff member that his behavior toward me was inappropriate. But there does not seem to be the slightest trace of awareness that the same ordering, grabbing, and shoving would be inappropriate even if I were a patient.
>
> Nancy Kerr[68]

A facility operating according to the medical model, with its emphasis on "treatments," "patients," and hospital attire, conveys the idea that the people receiving services are sick. This use of the medical model "serves the function of differentiating devalued clients from staff and society and imaging clients as diseased, contagious, impaired, incompetent, passive, and so on."[125]

During rehabilitation, people are often exposed to practices and attitudes that convey to them that they are dependent, sick, incapable of running their own lives, and less than fully human. These messages of dependence and dehumanization may be particularly destructive to a newly injured person. At a time when he is piecing together a new identity, he is likely to be more vulnerable to feedback from others about who he is now that he has a disabling condition. This may be especially true when the feedback comes from health professionals, "experts" on people with disabilities.

Constructive Practices in Rehabilitation

Within the social environment of a hospital or rehabilitation center, there is a massive potential for breaking anyone's spirit. There is also great potential for healing and growth. For the latter to occur, the health care team must consciously and consistently pursue this goal. From day one, from the scene of the accident on, the person with a spinal cord injury must be treated as the thinking, feeling, autonomous person that he is. Instead of relentlessly stripping him of his power and dignity, all members of the team must treat him with respect and support his right to self-determination.

Normalization. Normalization (also called social role valorization) is a philosophy of human service delivery that is highly applicable to physical rehabilitation. It is based on the recognition that certain groups of people are devalued in our society, that these groups are subject to discriminatory treatment, and that service delivery systems often perpetuate and reinforce the devaluation of and discrimination against those whom they serve. The normalization movement focuses on rectifying these problems, using "culturally valued means in order to enable, establish, and/or maintain valued social roles for people."[125]

One facet of normalization addresses the characteristics of the individuals receiving services. Assisting a person to attain or maintain socially valued roles includes enhancing both his image and level of competence. If a member of a devalued group (in this case, someone who has a visible physical disability) projects an image and displays skills (social, intellectual, vocational, etc.) that are valued in our society, he will be afforded greater value. Enhancement of image and competencies can create a positive cycle: someone who projects a valued image is likely to be perceived by others as more competent, and someone who exhibits competence is likely to be seen in a more positive light.[125, 129]

Although normalization principles include addressing individuals' characteristics, this is not the main focus of the movement. Normalization is unique among human service philosophies in that it focuses on "fixing" service delivery systems. The manner in which services are delivered, and the characteristics of the service delivery organizations themselves, affect the image of the people receiving those services.[36, 125] For example, a vocational training program for people with disabilities that labels them "patients" and segregates them from able-bodied trainees will have a negative impact on the social value of those being "served" by the program.

As members of a society in which people with physical disabilities are devalued, rehabilitation personnel are likely to have some negative attitudes about people with disabilities. Though

---

PROBLEM-SOLVING EXERCISE 4–2

Often, unconscious motivations can taint services that are well meaning and, on the surface, good.[125] For example, a rehabilitation unit sponsored a race that included both able-bodied runners and disabled athletes using wheelchairs. (So far so good.) At the awards ceremony after the race, the able-bodied runners received such prizes as athletic equipment and gift certificates from athletic stores. The winning athlete in the wheelchair division received a lap blanket.

- What message did the nature of the awards convey about the participants in the wheelchair division of the race?
- Why does that matter?
- How could the organizers of the race convey a more positive message?

these attitudes tend to remain beneath the surface, unconscious motivations can sabotage good intentions. For this reason, careful and honest self-scrutiny is required if we wish to provide services in a manner that will enhance rather than depreciate the social value of those served.[1]

Independence and autonomy.   Perceived control is strongly associated with life satisfaction in people with spinal cord injuries.[39] To adapt successfully after spinal cord injury, a person must gain (or retain) a sense of personal effectiveness and control over his life. For this to occur, he must be provided with the opportunity to make choices throughout his acute care and rehabilitation. He should be given true control, not just the opportunity to choose between compliance and noncompliance. From the day of his injury onward, he should be provided with information about his condition and treatment options and should be given a voice in setting goals, scheduling activities, and making decisions about his care.

To promote independence, the rehabilitation team should include the patient in problem solving. With guidance and encouragement, he can participate in analyzing problems, coming up with possible solutions, and evaluating outcomes. This can be done while learning functional skills, deciding on bowel and bladder management practices, choosing between equipment options, and determining virtually any aspect of his program. By participating in problem solving in this manner, the patient can develop the ability to problem solve on his own. This skill will prove invaluable to independent functioning during and subsequent to rehabilitation.

Independent functioning also requires a sense of personal responsibility. To live independently, a person must know what to do and when to do it, and must take the initiative to get things done. For this sense of responsibility to develop during rehabilitation, the patient should be given as much responsibility as possible for his rehabilitation. He should know his schedule and be accountable for getting to the various therapies and activities, either under his own power or by asking for assistance when needed. Once in therapy, he should be encouraged to initiate exercises or functional practice without waiting to be told

what to do. The same kind of initiative can be encouraged in his personal care practices, such as pressure reliefs, morning hygiene, and bowel and bladder programs. From the time of his initial hospitalization onward, he should be expected to take as much responsibility for himself as he can, with increasing expectations of independent functioning as he progresses in his rehabilitation.

Positive atmosphere.   While a person is adapting to the sequelae of a spinal cord injury, the physical and social environment of the rehabilitation center can have a powerful impact. A prevailing climate of gloom and tragedy conveys a sense of hopelessness and despair to all involved: those undergoing rehabilitation, family members, friends, and health professionals. A more positive atmosphere will encourage the development of a more optimistic outlook.

The physical environment in a rehabilitation setting is important. Dark corridors and institutional decor convey a feel of sickness and debilitation. At the other extreme, a saccharine and childlike atmosphere communicates a sense of dependence and childishness. Upbeat, age-appropriate decor and music will provide a more positive environment for rehabilitation.

Staff attire also contributes to the atmosphere of a rehabilitation center. Uniforms and laboratory coats help create a hospital-like atmosphere, with all of its connotations of illness and power hierarchies. Likewise, the dress of those undergoing rehabilitation is important. Pajamas are appropriate attire for people who are either sick or asleep. Certainly, they are inappropriate for conferences, therapies, or any other activities that take place outside of an individual's room.

Another element in a rehabilitation setting's atmosphere is the activity level of those undergoing rehabilitation. Long, empty hours in the days and evenings can deaden the spirit. Meaningful activity can provide a sense of purpose and personal control.[46] Active participation in therapies and recreational activities can also reduce boredom, promote better sleep at night,[116] and facilitate the grieving process.[109]

In working to create a positive atmosphere, the rehabilitation team should focus on abilities rather than on impairments. Too often, health practitioners concern themselves with the problems while ignoring the strengths of those whom they serve.[127] To convey a greater sense of optimism, the rehabilitation team should emphasize what a person *can* do rather than dwelling on what he *cannot* do. In discussions during conferences, problem-solving sessions, and informal

[1] Normalization-based evaluation tools such as PASS[123] and PASSING[124] can provide guidance for this self-evaluation and for program planning. These manuals and information about training in their use are available from the Syracuse University Training Institute, 230 Euclid Avenue, Syracuse, NY, 13244-5130. Phone: (315) 443-4264.

interactions, the focus can be placed on abilities and accomplishments. During therapies and other activities, the patient should perform meaningful tasks that are structured in such a way that he can experience success and see his accomplishments. Success experiences can go far to improve motivation[46] and develop a sense of mastery and control.[117]

Although success experiences during rehabilitation can have beneficial effects, it does not follow that all experiences of failure will be detrimental. In physical and occupational therapy, for example, people with significant motor impairments learn new ways to move their bodies and perform various tasks. This functional training inevitably involves a certain number of unsuccessful attempts as the individual gradually masters the motor skills involved. These unsuccessful attempts can be positive learning experiences.

People undergoing rehabilitation should be encouraged to take risks.[98] If an individual's goals and activities are limited to those in which he is certain to succeed, functional progress will be limited. Perhaps more importantly, this over-protectiveness communicates to the individual and others that he is not capable of coping with possible failure. A person who is "protected" from risk may never develop the self-confidence and experience the psychological growth that comes from challenging one's limits.

> There is human dignity in risk. There can be dehumanizing indignity in safety.
>
> Irving Zola[130]

Interactions with staff. Interactions with the staff are critical in rehabilitation; the attitudes and behaviors of rehabilitation professionals have a powerful influence on patients and their families at this time.[80] The values and attitudes that health professionals communicate can serve to demean or to support growth. To foster the development of a positive self-image, all members of the rehabilitation team must treat the patient as an equal, worthy of respect.[m] This respect should be evident in interactions with patients and their families in formal settings, such as in conferences, as well as in informal daily communication.

---

[m] In addition to benefitting those undergoing rehabilitation, equal-status interactions can benefit the staff by promoting the development of more positive attitudes. Equal-status contact is necessary for the development of positive attitudes toward those with disabilities.[45]

Demeaning language should be avoided at all times, even when only health professionals are present. Referring to groups or individuals by their diagnoses serves to reinforce a negative attitude among those present.

Finally, it is imperative for rehabilitation personnel to maintain appropriate "professional" relations with people undergoing rehabilitation. This does not mean that interactions should be cold and formal or patterned on the dominance and submission relations inherent in the medical model. Rather, the relationship should have clearly defined and mutually understood boundaries. A newly injured person who becomes too attached to a health professional may grow dependent on that person. Likewise, a health professional who becomes overly involved with someone undergoing rehabilitation may not act in that person's best interests, prolonging rehabilitation unnecessarily and encouraging dependence.[30] In an appropriate professional relationship, mutual respect, caring, and enjoyment can coexist with an understanding of the relationship's limits.

Social support. Social support can enhance a person's capacity to cope and recover following loss.[9, 97, 109] The rehabilitation team can promote emotional recovery and growth after spinal cord injury by providing this support. Health professionals should listen to people as they air their feelings, helping them to clarify their emotions and reassuring them that their feelings are normal. Staff should listen with empathy, not pity, and avoid judging what they hear.[46, 58, 109, 117] This support should be available from all members of the team, not just from the psychiatric or counseling staff.

Each individual should be allowed to grieve and adapt in his own way; staff members must not impose their own notions of how people should feel and act following spinal cord injury. The recently injured person should neither be required to mourn nor be rushed to complete his grieving prematurely.

Hope and truth. Health professionals have conflicting attitudes about hope and truth. On the one hand, expressions of hope may be labeled as "denial" and seen as signs of failure to cope with reality. On the other hand, health professionals are often reluctant to provide newly injured people with information, in the fear that the truth will crush all hope.

Neither hope nor denial are necessarily bad, as long as they do not interfere with an individual's progress in psychosocial and functional adaptation after injury. In fact, hope can help a person cope with his injury.

> Hope is the most potent of medicines, one that can heal and rejuvenate. Referenced in the future, grounded in the past, and experienced in the present, it involves the expectation that life will be a little more meaningful tomorrow. Hope is essential in any struggle with a major disability or catastrophic illness.
>
> Joan Mader[84]

Whereas hope has its benefits, information is critical to adjustment after a spinal cord injury. Knowledge, even if unpleasant, can help a person with an illness or disability regain a sense of control of his life.[4, 94] Anyone who asks a question has the right to get an honest answer; feigned ignorance and vague or inaccurate answers are not helpful responses.

> The truth is better than telling a patient that he will be fine tomorrow. For tomorrow never comes, and the long-term depressive effect will be greater if the truth is withheld.
>
> Michael Rogers[104]

Although health professionals should provide honest information, they should do so in a way that does not destroy all hope.[21, 116] Perhaps it is best to speak in terms of probabilities rather than absolutes. In truth, we rarely have definitive answers anyway. Who can predict with certainty whether a particular individual will experience neurological return, father a child, or walk again?

Educational model. Many of the growth-enhancing practices just described are inherent in an educational model of rehabilitation. Using this model, health professionals and people undergoing rehabilitation work as partners in pursuit of mutually agreed-upon goals. The model relationship is one of teacher–student[n] rather than healer–patient. This nonmedical orientation conveys the attitude that those undergoing rehabilitation are not sick. This understanding is crucial to coping with a disabling condition.[66]

In the educational model, people undergoing rehabilitation are expected to be active partici-

pants in designing, carrying out, and evaluating their programs. Respect for the individual is inherent in this model. Emphasis is placed on consumerism and autonomous functioning rather than on compliance. Clearly, this approach is superior to the medical model in fostering independence and growth.[115, 116]

A rehabilitation team attempting to implement a program structured on the educational model should keep in mind the fact that it is likely to run counter to their natural tendencies. Having grown up in a society in which disabilities are strongly stigmatized, health professionals are likely to hold negative attitudes about people undergoing rehabilitation. In addition, most of their professional training and practice is likely to have been in delivery systems based on the medical model. Thus, many practices inherent in the medical model (and contrary to the educational model) may go unquestioned.

Because the educational model is likely to run counter to the natural tendencies of health professionals, its implementation requires careful scrutiny and vigilance. All members of the team, and the team as a whole, must take a close look at their own behavior and practices. In *all* formal and informal interactions, health professionals must approach the individuals undergoing rehabilitation with an attitude of respect and equality. All aspects of the social and physical environment must be examined for consistency with the educational model.

Formal Strategies

Personal control, a positive atmosphere, and supportive and respectful interaction provide the necessary foundation for rehabilitation. Additional strategies that can be used to promote growth and adaptation after spinal cord injury are presented in the following sections. These include various approaches to dealing with the personal loss and changes in family dynamics, as well as strategies aimed at successful reintegration into society.

Evaluation. Individuals and their families are highly variable in their responses to the life changes brought on by spinal cord injury. Thus, the psychosocial interventions that are most appropriate will vary. For this reason, evaluation is the logical starting point of planning the psychosocial component of a rehabilitation program.[65, 66, 86] An initial evaluation should be performed soon after injury because many may

---

[n] Teacher–*adult* student.

benefit from intervention during their acute hospitalization.[3] Once an evaluation has been completed, a program can be designed that best meets the needs of a particular individual and his family. Subsequent evaluations will make it possible to alter the program as the needs change.

The psychosocial evaluation can address the patient's personality structure and behavioral style; social problem-solving skills; cognitive abilities; coping styles and ability to cope with the cord injury; current level of anxiety, distress and depression; and past history of interpersonal relations, loss, psychiatric illness, and substance abuse. The assessment can also include an investigation of the patient's social support network and its communication patterns, coping styles, and level of distress. Finally, the evaluation should investigate whether there is a family history of depressive disorder[o] or suicide attempts.[11, 33, 57, 65, 66, 86, 128]

The evaluation results can provide the patient, his family, and health professionals with a better understanding of the individual's and family's reactions to the injury and its sequelae. It can also alert them to potential areas of future difficulty. They can then all work together to identify problems, set goals, and develop a plan of action.

Education.   Education provides a critical foundation for psychosocial rehabilitation. To maintain or regain control of his life following spinal cord injury, a person must first have an understanding of his body's altered functioning and of strategies for avoiding complications and promoting health. Without this understanding, the individual will be unable to participate fully in his rehabilitation program planning or to take responsibility for his self-care.

Education regarding the physical sequelae of spinal cord injury is just a start. Instruction (forewarning) regarding what social problems may arise at home or in the community after discharge can better prepare a person and his family for this transition. To function in society, a person with a disability needs to know about his legal rights and available resources in the community. He will also require financial management skills, and the knowledge and skills required to obtain needed funding from insurance companies. Those who require attendant care must know how to obtain and manage attendants.[46, 59, 115]

Education can take the form of lectures, discussions, audiovisual presentations, and printed material. Inclusion of family members can enhance their capacity to provide constructive support to the person with a spinal cord injury during and following rehabilitation.[59, 105]

Counseling.   Recovering, adapting, and growing after spinal cord injury involves coming to terms with a host of losses, developing a new self-concept, and often redefining roles within a family. Social support can facilitate this process. For many, counseling is an important source of this support.

Group counseling provides an arena for people to discuss their experiences with others who have sustained spinal cord injuries. In this exchange, there is opportunity for the expression of emotions, enhancement of self-awareness, mutual encouragement, exchange of information, role modeling, examination and expansion of values and perceptions, feedback, and problem solving. Participation in group work may enhance motivation, normal grief resolution, and overall adjustment to the spinal cord injury.[46, 77, 90, 126]

Family members can be included in group counseling, either in "family groups" with other families or in family or marital therapy. Family adjustment is important not only for the benefit of the family members but also for the adaptation of the injured person himself. In a group setting, families of people with spinal cord injuries can gain information, express and come to grips with their emotions, give and receive support, grow in their attitudes regarding disability, develop more constructive communication patterns, and learn new coping strategies.[46, 65, 89, 90, 117] Group counseling need not be limited to people with disabilities and their families; other members of a disabled person's social support system may be included.[58]

Some people with spinal cord injuries and their family members also benefit from individual counseling. In one-on-one counseling, a person may receive more individualized support and more assistance with grieving, clarification of intrapsychic and interpersonal conflicts, and the development of new coping skills. Individual counseling is especially (but not exclusively) indicated when a person feels overwhelmed by his emotions, exhibits signs of pathology, or has a personal or family history of early or unresolved loss, psychiatric illness, substance abuse, or difficulty with interpersonal relations.[21, 58, 65, 82, 97, 111, 126]

Social skills training.   Reintegration into society is an important aspect of psychosocial adaptation after spinal cord injury. The social devaluation of people with disabilities can

---

[o] Genetic factors can predispose people to depression.[11]

present a formidable barrier to this reintegration. Following spinal cord injury, an individual is likely to find that people are uncomfortable around him. As a result, he may find it difficult to meet people or to maintain old friendships.

Fortunately, there are things that a person can do to lessen the negative impact of his disability on interactions with others. By projecting a positive self-image and putting others at ease, he can enhance the quality of his interactions with nondisabled people and facilitate a positive change in their attitudes.[10, 54, 115, 129] These behaviors can be acquired in social skills training.

Social skills training involves learning stigma management strategies: verbal and nonverbal behaviors that can improve the quality of interactions with others. These communication techniques center primarily around putting others at ease and establishing rapport during initial encounters. Typical strategies include acknowledging the disability, legitimizing curiosity, providing information, answering questions, behaving assertively, and projecting a positive self-image and acceptance of the disabling condition.[10, 35, 61, 115, 129]

A variety of approaches can be used for social skills training. Through videotapes, lectures, and discussions, people can be introduced to the concept of stigma management and can gain some understanding about behaviors that will help or hinder their interactions with others. Actual practice of communication techniques is helpful in the development of these skills. Feedback from others can alert people to behaviors that they display that may impede interactions. This feedback can also help them to hone their communication skills.[34, 115]

Cognitive behavior therapy. Cognitive behavior therapy is a therapeutic approach aimed at developing more adaptive behaviors, feelings, and thinking patterns.[15] This therapy can include relaxation techniques, visualization, self-hypnosis, cognitive restructuring,[p] increasing levels of pleasant events, training in social skills and assertiveness, and education and discussion of sexual issues.[15, 16] Participation in group cognitive behavior therapy during rehabilitation has been shown to result in higher levels of self-

reported adjustment, lower rates of hospital readmissions,[q] and lower rates of drug use for at least 2 years postinjury.[15] It also reduces depressive mood in individuals who have high levels of depressive mood prior to initiation of therapy, and this benefit continues for at least 2 years after treatment.[14, 16]

Functional training. Functional limitations can interfere with the performance of a variety of social roles. For example, a person who cannot negotiate environmental barriers or manipulate objects will have difficulty performing the activities inherent in the roles of breadwinner, homemaker, or student.[101] Functional training can aid in psychosocial adaptation following spinal cord injury by increasing the capacity for independence. Greater independence enables the person to resume or assume a variety of social roles,[101] and is associated with less anxiety and depression[110] and a higher perceived quality of life.[74]

Recreation training. Many people who acquire disabling conditions find themselves unable to participate in the recreational activities to which they were previously accustomed. This represents a significant loss; leisure activities are an important source of pleasure, personal pride, relaxation, physical wellness, and social support. Through recreation training, people can learn ways to resume many of their previous activities, or find alternative leisure activities. Resumption of an active leisure life can promote physical and psychological health and can provide an avenue for reintegration into society.[6, 93] By including spouses in leisure training, the team can assist couples in finding activities that they can enjoy together. This may in turn have a beneficial effect on marital relations.[118]

Pharmaceutical treatment. People exhibit a variety of emotions as they grieve their losses following spinal cord injury. Often, these emotions are unpleasant, both to experience and to witness. For this reason, it can be tempting to medicate people to lessen their (and our) discomfort.[21] Although pharmaceutical treatment can be beneficial in cases of clinical depression or psychosis,[32, 82, 115] it is not indicated for normal grief reactions. Medication aimed at ameliorating emotional pain

---

p Cognitive restructuring involves learning to isolate negative thoughts, mentally eliminate them, and replace them with rational and positive thoughts, as well as learning positive coping statements, attention-distraction, and pain-reinterpretation techniques.[16]

---

q Hospital readmissions frequently occur as a result of preventable secondary conditions such as pressure ulcers. Thus a reduced rate of hospital readmission probably reflects better self-care practices (less self-neglect).

can impede a person's ability to work through his loss.[91, 109]

Postdischarge strategies. When a recently injured person leaves a rehabilitation center, his adjustment has just begun. Although this has probably always been the case, it has become more so in recent years. Due to shorter inpatient stays, "recently injured individuals are usually back in the home and in the community before confronting the full impact of their losses."[11] Moreover, discharge from inpatient rehabilitation brings a new set of challenges and adjustments. Although during rehabilitation people with spinal cord injuries gain some of the knowledge and skills required for living in the community, they typically find that they have more to learn when they leave. In addition, they are faced with the challenging task of applying their new knowledge and skills in daily life at home and in the community.

Because adaptation and growth after spinal cord injury do not end at discharge, people can benefit from continued psychosocial support after completing their initial rehabilitation. Any of the strategies described previously can be used either during inpatient rehabilitation or in alternative settings following discharge. Additional strategies specific to people living in the community are presented in the following paragraphs.

One approach that can be beneficial is to put a recently injured person in contact with an individual who lives in the same community and has adjusted successfully following spinal cord injury. The "veteran" can share information and coping strategies and can provide support to the person and his family.[115]

Self-help groups are another potential source of social support after discharge. These groups can be helpful both for people with spinal cord injuries and for their families. True self-help groups are comprised of *and run by* people with common experiences,[63] in this case, spinal cord injuries. The focus and structure of self-help groups vary, depending on the needs and priorities of the membership. Groups may concern themselves with any or all of the following: education (of members, health professionals, or society at large), fund raising, sharing emotions, mutual social support, recreation, or social action. Individuals participating in self-help groups can gain information, new coping skills, and an increased sense of personal responsibility for their health and social well-being. Self-help groups can also be a source of affirmation, foster a sense of belonging, and provide motivation and reinforcement for successful coping. Perhaps most importantly, self-help groups can be empowering for the participants as individuals and as a group.[8, 58, 63, 97, 112]

> I think the group support lets you be strong together; the group gives you that real sense of strength and optimism and resilience that most people don't have by themselves.
> Judy Heumann[85]

Independent living centers located (sparsely) throughout the United States provide a variety of services to people with disabilities. These services can include provision of information and logistical assistance with equipment repair, home modification, accessible housing, attendant services, and transportation. Independent living centers can also provide legal advocacy, peer counseling, and financial counseling.[22, 40, 115] Many centers engage in disability rights activism.[85] The independent living movement focuses on improving the quality of life of people with disabilities by increasing architectural and transportation accessibility and by obtaining services that enable people to function independently in the community.[22, 40] Self-help and consumer control are important characteristics of the independent living model.[40, 114]

Vocational rehabilitation and formal education can also facilitate psychosocial adjustment after spinal cord injury. Education and vocational training can enhance a person's self-confidence, increase his or her chances of obtaining gainful employment, and promote social interaction.[31, 50, 71] Among people with spinal cord injuries, education and employment are associated with lower levels of psychological distress[110] and higher quality of life.[28, 74] Because education and employment are valued characteristics in our society, they can serve to increase an individual's social status, facilitating his reintegration into society.

Psychological healing and growth and social adaptation can continue for years after a spinal cord injury. In essence, they continue for the remainder of a person's life[72, 115] as new issues and challenges continue to surface through the years. Rehabilitation professionals can aid the process following discharge by including a psychosocial evaluation in routine follow-up visits[53, 65] and by referring people to appropriate services and resources available in the community.

THE BIGGER PICTURE: OUR IMPACT ON THE COMMUNITY

As rehabilitation professionals, our function is to facilitate adjustment and reentry into society after the acquisition of a disabling condition. Traditionally, to reach this end we have placed our focus exclusively on disabled people themselves, teaching them various physical and social skills needed for living with a disability. The other side of the equation, society, has been largely ignored. The assumption underlying this approach is that the problem of disability lies in those who are disabled rather than in society itself. In recent years, however, the disability rights movement has asserted that people are handicapped not by their physical conditions but by negative attitudes and barriers in transportation, architecture, employment, and public assistance programs.[5, 22, 23, 40] When disablement is seen in this light, it follows that we should direct attention to our impact on society rather than solely concerning ourselves with disabled individuals.

One area with which we must concern ourselves is the devalued status of people with disabilities. Our attention in this area is imperative because of the powerful impact that rehabilitation professionals have on society's attitudes. By our actions and inactions, by what we say and do, and by the nature of our service delivery systems, we can strengthen or weaken the stigmatizing attitudes of those around us and of society at large.

As health care professionals, we are seen as experts on people with spinal cord injuries and other disabling conditions. Our communications about people with disabilities can influence others' attitudes. This communication occurs in a variety of situations, from casual social encounters ("You work with cripples? You must be soooo patient.") to interviews with television or newspaper reporters. Any discussion relating to people with disabilities presents an opportunity to either reinforce devaluing attitudes and beliefs or to portray a more positive picture.

Professional responsibility dictates that rehabilitation professionals direct attention to their impact on society's perceptions of people with disabilities. Additionally, some may choose to promote change through political action. Much work is needed in the areas of architectural barriers in the community, accessible housing, accessible transportation, and discriminatory practices and legislation.[34, 115, 127]

SUMMARY

- Anyone who sustains a spinal cord injury is faced with major losses, ranging from changes in his physique and functional ability to disruption of his relationships, financial security, and future plans. His former self-image no longer fits. He has become a member of a devalued and disadvantaged minority, "the disabled."

- Psychosocial adjustment after spinal cord injury involves coming to terms with these losses, formulating a new identity, and learning communication skills needed for returning to life within his family and in the community.

- Most people with spinal cord injuries are able to adjust satisfactorily, and many even grow from the experience. A minority remains unable to adapt.

- Whether an individual grows from or succumbs to his disability can be influenced by the support that he receives during and after rehabilitation. To promote growth and adaptation following spinal cord injury, the rehabilitation team must support the individual as he comes to terms with his injury and its consequences. Attention must also be directed to empowering him; *all* interactions must be based on respect, equality, and mutuality.

- Formal strategies for enhancing psychosocial adaptation include education, counseling, social skills training, cognitive behavior therapy, functional training, recreation training, pharmaceutical treatment, and a variety of postdischarge strategies.

- Because spinal cord injuries impact on family members as well as those who are injured, and because reintegration into family life will require adaptation by all involved, families should be included in the psychosocial component of rehabilitation programs.

- Rehabilitation professionals should strive to have a positive impact on the community at large, working to increase its inclusiveness of people with spinal cord injuries and other disabling conditions.

5

SEXUALITY AND SEXUAL FUNCTIONING

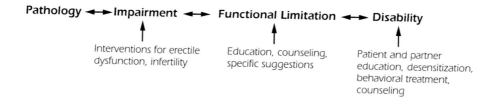

Pathology ◄──► Impairment ◄──► Functional Limitation ◄──► Disability

Interventions for erectile dysfunction, infertility

Education, counseling, specific suggestions

Patient and partner education, desensitization, behavioral treatment, counseling

Sexuality is a central aspect of our lives. From birth on, our gender influences how we define ourselves and how we are seen by others. (Imagine a birth announcement that does not specify the infant's sex!) Because sexuality is such a basic component of our psychological makeup, it is an important ingredient of psychological health. Feelings of sexual inadequacy can impact strongly on a person's sense of identity and self-esteem.[6]

> People treat you differently according to whether you're a boy or a girl; and from the way they react to you, you begin to build your image, your self-esteem. And if somebody or something takes away your sexuality, you don't know who you are or where you fit in.
>
> Ellen Stohl[59]

Sexuality is also important in our social relations. It is used to form and to maintain relationships, to wield power, to communicate with others,[87] and to bolster self-esteem.[50] Feelings of unattractiveness can lead to withdrawal from social and sexual relationships.[65]

We express our sexuality not only, not even mostly, through sexual intercourse. Our attire, interactions with others, the images we present, our flirtations, smiles, and reactions to others are expressions of our sexuality. And yes, we express our sexuality in a wide variety of "sexual acts," ranging from holding hands to more intimate sexual encounters.

The essence of a person's sexual nature is in his or her mind. Spinal cord injury does not alter this. Following cord injury, people continue to be sexual beings, continue to desire sexual expression,[48, 53, 65, 94] and remain sexually active.[13, 55, 71, 94, 115–117] Unfortunately, damage to the spinal cord brings on changes that can interfere with sexual expression and activity. In a recent survey, people with spinal cord injuries reported that decreased sexual function is one of the more difficult sequelae of cord injury to deal with, second only to decreased ability to walk or move.[118]

Perhaps the most obvious way in which a spinal cord injury affects sexuality is in its effect on the person's physical capacity to perform sexual acts. Changes in genital functioning, motor abilities, sensation, range of motion, and muscle tone may interfere with a person's accustomed modes of sexual expression.

Spinal cord injury also brings logistical problems that can get in the way of sexual activity. Altered body language, the potential for bowel and bladder accidents, decreased spontaneity due to managing catheters, and the mechanics of undressing can complicate sexual encounters. In addition, a person with impaired mobility faces architectural and transportation barriers that can impede his or her ability to meet potential partners.

The social consequences of spinal cord injury add to the problem. Paralysis is very visible; a person who uses a wheelchair or orthoses and assistive devices is readily identified as having a disabling condition. As a result, he or she is vulnerable to stigmatization and discrimination. People with disabilities are often viewed by others as sexless, devoid of sexual urges, and undeserving of sexual expression. In a society that places a high premium on physical appearance, people with disabilities are not seen as desirable partners. These societal attitudes can limit the opportunity for sexual expression.[1, 9, 20, 61, 64, 87, 109]

> Although the logistics of lovemaking can be addressed through experimentation and assistance with technique, stereotypic perceptions of people with disabilities as sexually deviant and even dangerous, asexual or sexually incapacitated, either physically or emotionally, are more obdurate obstacles to our sexual fulfillment. These attitudinal barriers can cut off access to intimate partnerships, increase vulnerability to mistreatment, and constrain our choices.
>
> Nancy Eiesland[39]

Attitudinal barriers to sexual expression also come from within. When a person sustains a spinal cord injury, his or her preexisting prejudices do not magically disappear. He or she may see himself or herself, with a now "imperfect" body, as undesirable, undeserving of sexual gratification, even neutered.[87] A great deal of psychological discomfort is likely to result.[50]

The problems brought on by physical changes and internal and external attitudinal barriers are compounded by ignorance. People with spinal cord injuries often do not understand their own sexual potentials. Many find themselves totally in the dark regarding their sexual functioning and ways to go about finding sexual gratification.[87]

In the past the focus of both research and intervention in this area has been on the male, specifically on his genital functioning and fertility.[48, 55, 95, 115, 117] This difference may be due to the higher prevalence of males among people with spinal cord injuries, the fact that male genitals are external and therefore more readily studied, or societal bias.[12, 95] One assumption underlying the predominance of male-oriented research and intervention is that women with spinal cord injuries have an easier adjustment to make because their injuries do not impair their ability to perform in their accustomed role of passive participant in sexual activities.[10, 18] This position, based on outdated notions of sex roles, is no longer defensible. Women now often take the initiative in sexual encounters instead of waiting passively for men to approach them. And many women prefer positions other than the "missionary position" during intercourse. Like her male counterpart, a woman with a spinal cord injury may have difficulty with some of the positions and sexual activities to which she was accustomed prior to her injury. She will have the same potential for problems with bowel and bladder accidents interrupting intimate encounters and will be subject to society's discriminatory attitudes regarding sexuality and disability. She may feel unattractive and undesirable as a result of her injury.[13, 85]

> I used to feel that I really couldn't have real relationships because I thought that, as a disabled woman, I wasn't as desirable. I figured that there was really no reason for anyone to be interested in me if he could have a woman who could walk, totally discounting my whole self and my uniqueness as a person. I didn't feel really good about myself until I started feeling sexually attractive, feeling that I could function, not competitively, but on an equal footing with any other woman.
>
> Susan Schapiro[25]

Some aspects of a woman's sexuality will not be as profoundly affected by cord injury as a man's. Her genital functioning will not be altered as much, and her fertility will not be affected. She may face more social difficulties, however, being more vulnerable than men to being perceived as unattractive and therefore unacceptable as a sexual partner.[7] Health professionals should remember that spinal cord injury significantly affects sexuality whether the person is male or female.

Sexuality and the potential for sexual expression are major concerns for most people who sustain spinal cord injuries.[76] This concern often surfaces very soon after injury.[6, 76] Faced with bodily changes and social stigma, a person with a spinal cord injury may feel less of a man or woman. Depression and lowered self-esteem can result.[22] Because of the psychological and social importance of sexuality, it is critical that this area is addressed during rehabilitation.

PHYSICAL ASPECTS OF SEXUAL FUNCTIONING

Although physical sexual responses are only a part of sexuality, they are certainly a significant part of it. Understandably, physical sexual responses are an area of great concern following spinal cord injury. Sooner or later after injury, people want to know about their capacity to perform various sexual acts, reach orgasm, and have children. Health professionals should be knowledgeable in this area, so that they can educate their patients appropriately.

Neurological Control of Genital Function

Male. The male's genital functions during sexual activity consist of erection, emission, and ejaculation.[a] These functions are controlled by the autonomic and somatic branches of the nervous system.

Erection. Erection is a vascular event, occurring when the erectile bodies of the penis (corpus cavernosa and corpus spongiosum) become distended with blood. This distension occurs when vasodilation of the arteries supplying the penis, combined with relaxation of the smooth muscle of the corpus cavernosum and corpus spongiosum, allows increased blood flow into the erectile bodies. Engorgement of the erectile bodies causes compression of the veins that drain them. The resulting reduction in venous outflow further contributes to the erection by entrapping blood in the erectile bodies.[69, 77, 84, 100]

Both the sympathetic and parasympathetic divisions of the autonomic nervous system are involved in the control of erections. When autonomic input causes the rate of blood flow into the erectile bodies to exceed the rate of flow out, the penis becomes erect.[37, 46, 77, 114] Continuing autonomic stimulation is required to maintain the erection.[86, 114]

Neurological control of erection involves two regions in the spinal cord, as well as higher centers. Efferent pathways from supraspinal centers synapse in the thoracolumbar (sympathetic) and sacral (parasympathetic) erection centers of the spinal cord. The input from higher centers provides both facilitation and inhibition of erection.[30, 32, 84]

Erection can be initiated from two different sources: psychological arousal or sensory stimulation in the genital area or pelvic viscera. *Psychogenic erections* are brought on by psychological arousal. This arousal can be initiated by erotic thoughts or a variety of sensory experiences (smells, sounds, etc.). Erections brought on by sensory stimulation in the genital region or pelvic viscera are called *reflex* or *reflexogenic erections*. Normal functioning involves a combination of psychogenic and reflexogenic erection.[114] In fact, both are needed for an erection to be maintained.[43]

Reflex erections (Figure 5–1) are mediated by the sacral cord. Parasympathetic efferents from S2 through S4 innervate the penile corporal arterioles, causing vasodilation when stimulated. Parasympathetic stimulation also causes relaxation of the smooth muscle fibers in the corpus cavernosum and spongiosum. Erection is initiated when sensory stimulation from the penis, perineal area, rectum, or bladder travels to S2-4. This stimulation causes firing of the parasympathetic efferents, resulting in erection.[43, 46, 84, 100]

The neural control of psychogenic erection (Figure 5–2) is not as well understood as that of reflexive erection. Sympathetic efferents from T11 through L2[27, 28, 30, 37, 44] are known to be involved in psychogenic erections;[b] both humans and experi-

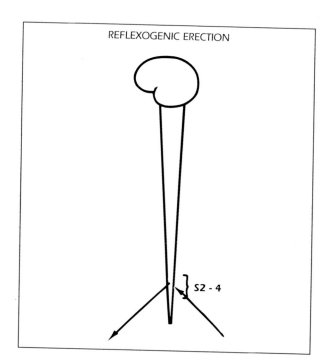

Figure 5–1. *Neurological control of reflexive erection.*

---

[a] Some authors consider emission to be a part of ejaculation. In this chapter, emission and ejaculation will be considered separate entities, as they represent two separate neurologic events.

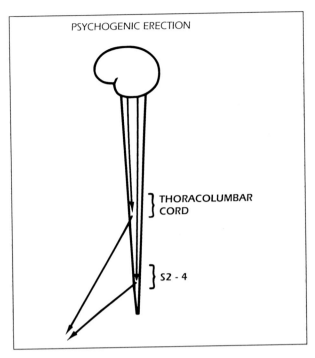

PSYCHOGENIC ERECTION

} THORACOLUMBAR CORD

} S2 - 4

Figure 5–2. Neurological control of psychogenic erection. Thoracolumbar innervation for psychogenic erection is reported by different authors as T11-L2, T10-L2, T10-L3, T11-L3, or T12-L3.

mental animals who lack sacral reflex functioning but have intact thoracolumbar erection centers in communication with their brains exhibit erections in response to psychogenic stimuli.[28, 30, 84] The mechanism by which thoracolumbar-mediated erections occur remains unknown.[84] Psychogenic erections may also be mediated in the sacral cord, occurring when facilitory impulses from higher centers cause the sacral efferents to fire.[77, 114]

Emission. Emission is the process by which semen reaches the posterior urethra in preparation for ejaculation. In emission, peristaltic contraction of the smooth muscle of the vas deferens causes sperm to be transported from the epididymis to the end of the vas deferens (ampulla).[46, 86] Secretions from the seminal vesicles and prostate are added to the sperm to form semen.[41] Contraction of the smooth muscle of the ampulla, seminal vesicles, and prostate, and partial closure of the bladder neck causes the semen to enter the posterior urethra.[43, 46, 86] Figure 5–3 illustrates the structures involved.

Neurological control of emission involves supraspinal centers and both the sacral and thora-

columbar spinal cord (Figure 5–4). Afferents from the genitals enter the second through fourth segments of the sacral cord. From there, they ascend to the brain. Efferents from the brain travel via the anterolateral columns to the thoracolumbar[c] cord. Sympathetic efferents from the thoracolumbar cord innervate the vas deferens, seminal vesicles, prostate, and base of the bladder. The sympathetic outflow to these structures causes emission.[32, 46, 77] Emission can also occur as a result of direct input from the sacral cord to the thoracolumbar cord, without involvement of higher centers. Normally, emission is stimulated by input from both sources.[32]

Ejaculation. Ejaculation is the process by which semen is propelled from the posterior urethra. It involves contraction of striated musculature: the bulbocavernosus, ischiocavernosus, and other pelvic floor musculature.[43, 77] The rhythmic contraction of these muscles, combined with closure of the bladder neck, propels the semen forward[d] and out of the urethra.[46, 86]

Ejaculation occurs as a result of a somatic sacral reflex (Figure 5–5). Sensory afferents are activated when semen enters the posterior urethra as a result of emission. These afferents travel to S2-4, where they synapse with somatic efferents. Reflexive contraction of the bulbocavernosus and ischiocavernosus muscles results,[32, 41, 46] causing propulsion of the semen. The efferents also stimulate reflexive contraction of the vesical sphincter, preventing retrograde ejaculation.[41] During ejaculation, the anal sphincter also contracts rhythmically.[43]

Female. The genital responses exhibited by women during sexual acts include vaginal lubrication; vascular engorgement of erectile tissue in the clitoris, vagina, labia minora, and labia majora; contraction of the smooth muscle of the fallopian tubes, uterus, and paraurethral Skene glands; and rhythmic contraction of the perineal musculature. The genital functioning of females during sexual activity has not been studied as extensively as the functioning of males.

---

b There is disagreement in the literature regarding the exact location of the thoracolumbar erection center. Sympathetic neurons innervating the penis may extend from T10 through L2,[6] T10 to L3,[8] T11 through L3,[77] or T12 through L3.[43, 46]

---

c There is disagreement in the literature regarding the area in the cord that controls emission. It may extend from T10 through L2,[6, 68] T11 through L3,[77] or T12 through L3.[41, 46]

d Normal ejaculation, in which the semen is propelled forward, is called antegrade ejaculation. In retrograde ejaculation, semen is propelled back into the bladder. This occurs when the bladder neck fails to close during ejaculation or when the bladder neck has been resected surgically.[43]

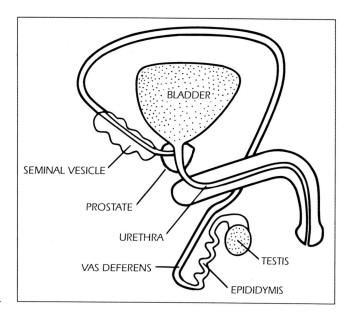

Figure 5–3. Structures involved in emission.

Vaginal lubrication. Vaginal lubrication involves the secretion of mucus from the vaginal epithelium and Bartholin's glands into the vaginal opening. Neurological control of vaginal lubrication is thought to be similar to that of penile erection. Reflexive lubrication occurs as a result of parasympathetic stimulation that arises from S2-4.[6, 49, 51, 100, 111] Both the thoracolumbar and sacral cord are thought to be involved in psychogenic lubrication.[86, 100]

Vascular engorgement. The engorgement of erectile tissue in the corpora cavernosa of the clitoris, vagina, labia minora, and labia majora that occurs during sexual activity is the result of vascular dilation. This dilation is the result of parasympathetic stimulation that arises from S2-4.[6, 51, 108, 111]

Smooth muscle contractions in the fallopian tubes, uterus, and Skene glands. In the female equivalent of emission, the smooth musculature

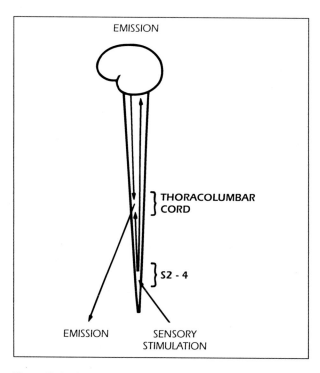

Figure 5–4. Neurological control of emission. Thoracolumbar innervation for emission is reported by different authors as T10-L2, T11-L3, or T12-L3.

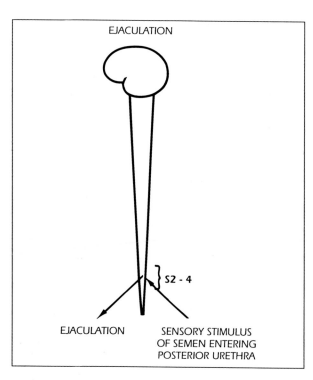

Figure 5–5. Neurological control of ejaculation.

of the fallopian tubes, uterus, and paraurethral Skene glands contracts. The neurological control of these events is similar to the control of emission in the male.[41, 86] These reactions are caused by sympathetic outflow from the thoracolumbar cord.[6, 49, 86, 100]

Striated muscle contractions. As is true with ejaculation in males, the analogous female response involves striated musculature. It consists of rhythmic contraction of the bulbospongiosus (vaginal sphincter) and ischiocavernosus, pelvic floor,[6] and anal sphincter. The neurological control of this response is similar to the control of ejaculation in the male.[41] This muscular response is controlled by a somatic reflex involving S2-4.[6, 49]

Genital Function Following Injury

The impact that a spinal cord injury has on genital functioning is not completely understood. Much of our knowledge is based on studies that have been less than perfect. Much of the data has been gathered using retrospective surveys rather than observation, and there has been inadequate control of variables such as marital status, time since injury, etiology, spasticity, and the influence of medication, surgery, and medical conditions.[48] Moreover, after spinal cord injury in humans, it can be difficult to determine with certainty whether any neurological connections remain between the brain and the centers in the spinal cord that are involved in sexual function.[84]

Despite these limitations, research has shown that the level and completeness of a spinal cord lesion affect its impact on genital functioning. It is not possible, however, to predict *an individual's* potential based on the level and completeness of

the lesion. There are exceptions to any "rule of thumb" that one attempts to impose. It is important to keep this in mind when counseling patients.

Male.   The preservation of erection, emission, and ejaculation capabilities after spinal cord injury varies with the level and completeness of lesion. Additional factors that can influence genital function after cord injury include medication[35] and psychological factors.[28, 77, 105]

In discussions of sexual functioning, cord lesions are sometimes classified as upper motor neuron (UMN) or lower motor neuron (LMN) lesions. So-called UMN lesions leave the functioning of the sacral cord intact. People with these lesions display intact bulbocavernosus reflexes[e] and anal sphincter tone. Most such lesions are above T12.[46] So-called LMN lesions disrupt the functioning of the sacral cord. People with this level of lesion have a lax anal sphincter and absent bulbocavernosus reflex. Usually, the lesion is below T12 in these cases.[46] Table 5–1 presents statistics on male sexual functioning using this classification of lesions.

Erection.   Erection is the most likely of the genital functions to be preserved[f] after spinal cord injury; most men retain the capacity to have erections.[27, 94, 100, 105] This is due to the presence of erectile centers in two areas of the cord; a man with a spinal cord injury is likely to have either his thoracolumbar or sacral erection center functional.

---

[e] Contraction of the bulbocavernosus muscle upon percussion of the dorsum of the penis.
[f] During spinal shock, erections are absent. Resumption of erectile function can occur within a few days, or can be delayed for over a year.[100]

TABLE 5–1.   STATISTICS ON MALE SEXUAL FUNCTIONING FOLLOWING SPINAL CORD INJURY

	UMN Lesions		**LMN Lesions**	
	Complete (%)	Incomplete (%)	Complete (%)	Incomplete (%)
Psychogenic erections	0	25	25–40	80–85
Reflexogenic erections	>90	95–100	0–25	90
Ejaculation[a]	~1	~25	14–35	≤70

[a] These statistics are based on studies that do not distinguish between emission and ejaculation and therefore are inflated.

Sources: references 41, 43, 46, 48, 53, 114.

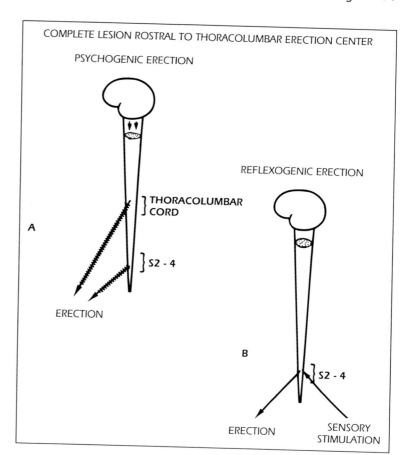

Figure 5–6. Neurological basis of erection capabilities after complete spinal cord injury rostral to thoracolumbar erection center. **(A)** Psychogenic erection impaired due to loss of input from brain to erection centers. **(B)** Reflexogenic erection spared due to preservation of sacral reflex arc.

The neurological basis of the erection capabilities of a person with a complete lesion above the thoracolumbar erection center are illustrated in Figure 5–6. With a complete lesion above T12, the thoracolumbar erection center will no longer be in contact with the brain. As a result, psychogenic erections will not occur.[53] Although men with high lesions do not exhibit psychogenic erections, most retain the capacity for reflex erections.[28, 43, 53, 114] This capacity is due to the fact that the sacral segments of the cord remain functional: the intact sacral reflex arc makes reflex erections possible.[53]

Lesions that lie between the thoracolumbar and sacral erection centers in the cord can spare both psychogenic and reflexive erectile function.[28] Figure 5–7 illustrates the neurological basis of erectile function following lesions that lie below the thoracolumbar center but do not disrupt sacral functioning.

Lower lesions have a more detrimental effect on erections. Figure 5–8 illustrates the effects of complete lesions that extend low enough to disrupt the sacral reflex arc. This disruption of sacral functioning can occur with lesions as high as

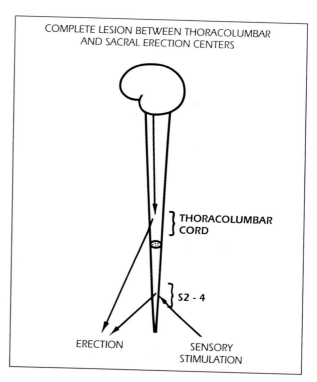

Figure 5–7. Neurological basis of erection capabilities after complete spinal cord injury that is caudal to thoracolumbar erection center but leaves sacral reflex arc intact.

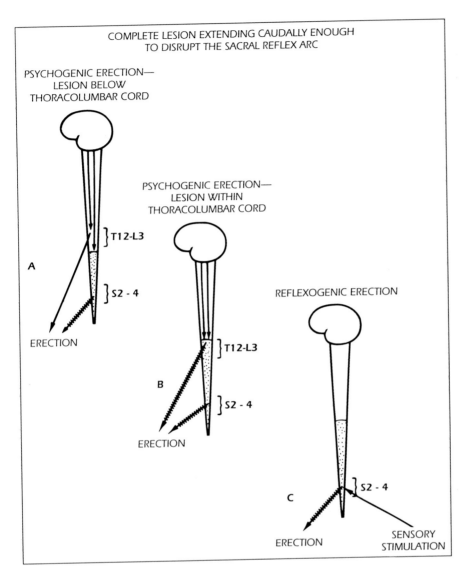

Figure 5–8. Neurological basis of erection capabilities after complete spinal cord injury that extends low enough to disrupt the sacral reflex arc. **(A)** With lesion below thoracolumbar erection center, psychogenic erection may be spared due to preserved input from brain to thoracolumbar erection center. **(B)** With lesion within thoracolumbar erection center, psychogenic erection impaired due to loss of input from brain to both sacral and thoracolumbar erection centers. **(C)** Reflexogenic erection impaired due to disruption of sacral reflex arc.

T12.[28] A complete lesion that falls within the thoracolumbar erection center (between T11 and L2) is likely to lead to the inability to have psychogenic erections.[29, 37] In contrast, a lesion below this level will leave all of the thoracolumbar erection center in communication with the brain. As a result, psychogenic erections will be possible.[29] Reflex erections are not likely to be preserved in people with low lesions, since these lesions are likely to disrupt the functioning of the sacral cord.[30, 46, 53] Men with incomplete lesions are more likely to retain the capacity to have erections.[53]

In summary, most men with spinal cord injuries retain the capacity for penile erection. Men with high lesions are likely to exhibit reflex erections, and those with low lesions may have psychogenic or reflex erections. Incomplete lesions are most likely to result in sparing of erection.

Although most men with spinal cord injuries retain the capacity to have erections, many who have erections are unable to use them in coitus.[32, 41, 48, 100, 103] This makes sense when one recalls that the erections exhibited by neurologically intact men during sexual activity are sustained by input from both the thoracolumbar and sacral erection centers. Loss of input from either center may alter the quality of erection, the ability to sustain an erection, or both.

Emission and ejaculation. The information available on emission and ejaculation following spinal cord injury is not as complete as that on erection. Many studies lump the two functions together, and data are lacking on emission itself. Donovon[37] notes additional limitations of the studies done to date: data are gathered by survey, and there has been poor or no control of conditions that are common in this population and that are known to affect ejaculation (medication, bladder surgery, urinary tract infection).

Emission occurs as a result of sympathetic outflow from the thoracolumbar cord. Because this outflow is caused primarily by input from higher centers,[41, 46] one would expect the effect of spinal cord injury on emission to be similar to its effect on psychogenic erection.

Figure 5–9 illustrates the neurological basis of the effect of a low cord injury on emission. If some or all of the thoracolumbar cord[g] remains in contact with the brain, outflow from this area could cause emission. Higher lesions that interrupt supraspinal input to the thoracolumbar cord would be expected to impair emission (Figure 5–10).

Ejaculation is the most neurologically vulnerable of the genital functions.[h] This vulnerability is due to the fact that two separate spinal cord centers are involved. For ejaculation to occur, semen must be present in the posterior urethra; emission must occur. Emission is brought on by thoracolumbar outflow, in turn stimulated pri-

---

[g] T10-12,[6, 46] T11-L3,[77] or T12-L3.[41, 46]

[h] The following discussion of ejaculatory function following spinal cord injury refers to *ejaculation that occurs during sexual activity*. Ejaculation induced using a vibrator or electrical stimulation is addressed later in the chapter.

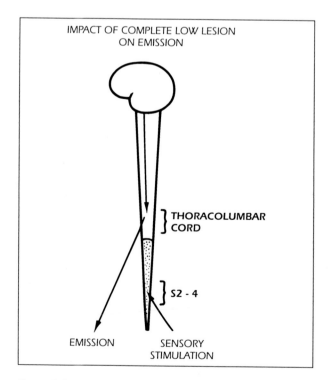

Figure 5–9. Neurological basis of impact of complete low spinal cord injury on emission. Emission may be spared due to preserved input from brain to thoracolumbar cord.

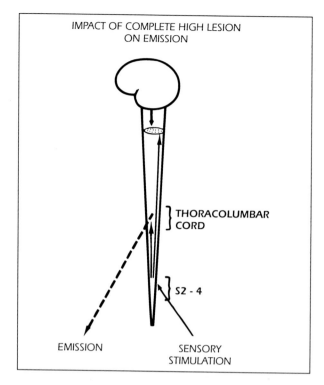

Figure 5–10. Neurological basis of impact of complete high spinal cord injury on emission. Emission impaired due to loss of input from brain to thoracolumbar cord. A small minority of individuals may exhibit emission due to input from the sacral cord to the thoracolumbar cord.

marily by input from higher centers. An intact sacral arc is also required for true ejaculation, since ejaculation occurs as the result of a sacral reflex.

Figure 5–11 illustrates the effect of a complete low lesion on ejaculation. A lesion that is low enough to preserve the thoracolumbar outflow required for emission is likely to interrupt the functioning of the sacral cord. Thus, ejaculation is not likely to occur with a complete low lesion. The incidence of ejaculation is greater with incomplete lesions. Since many studies do not distinguish between emission and true ejaculation, the figures on the incidence of ejaculation (Table 5–1) are inflated. In many instances, what is reported as ejaculation may actually be dribbling of semen due to emission.[i]

A complete lesion that is high enough to allow preservation of the sacral cord is likely to

---

[i] For example, Geiger[43] states that men with cauda equina lesions are more likely to ejaculate than men with higher lesions but that dribbling ejaculation is likely to be associated with flaccid pelvic floor musculature. This description is compatible with a complete LMN lesion and emission, not true ejaculation.

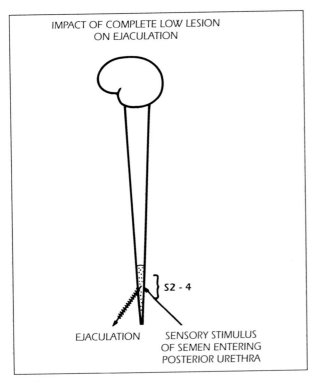

Figure 5–11. Neurological basis of impact of complete low spinal cord injury on ejaculation. Ejaculation impaired due to disruption of sacral reflex arc.

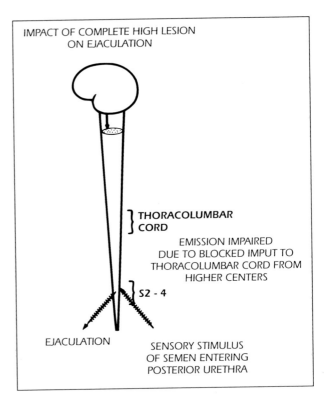

Figure 5–12. Neurological basis of impact of complete high spinal cord injury on ejaculation. Ejaculation impaired due to impaired emission, which results from loss of input from brain to thoracolumbar cord.

interrupt the thoracolumbar cord's communication with higher centers (Figure 5–12). As a result, emission and, therefore, ejaculation are quite uncommon following these lesions.

In summary, few men with spinal cord injuries exhibit true ejaculation. For ejaculation to occur, emission must occur, and ejaculation and emission combined involve supraspinal centers and both the thoracolumbar and sacral areas of the cord. Men with incomplete lesions are more likely to ejaculate than are those with complete lesions. In contrast to erectile capabilities, men with low lesions are more likely to ejaculate than are men with high lesions.[46] Research flaws make the validity of these trends questionable.

Female.   Little is known about the genital functioning of women following spinal cord injury, as few studies have been done in this area.[98] Presumably, one can draw *tentative* conclusions regarding the genital responses of women with spinal cord injuries, based on what is known about the functioning of their male counterparts. Clinical experience often supports this assumption.[43]

The neurological control of vaginal lubrication and vascular engorgement of the genitalia is comparable to the control of penile erection in

men. Based on what is known about the genital functioning of men after spinal cord injury, one would expect most women with spinal cord injuries to retain the capacity for vaginal lubrication and engorgement of the clitoris, labia, and vagina.

If neurological control of genital functioning is comparable in women and men with spinal cord injuries, women with *complete lesions above the thoracolumbar cord* would not be expected to exhibit genital responses as a result of psychogenic excitation but most should exhibit them reflexively (Figure 5–13). A recent study[j] supports these expectations: women with complete spinal cord injuries above T6 exhibited vaginal vasocongestion in response to manual stimulation in the clitoral region, but not in response to audiovisual erotic stimuli.[98]

Lesions that lie below the thoracolumbar portion of the cord but leave the sacral reflex arc intact would be expected to spare both psychogenic and reflexive genital responses. Figure 5–14 illustrates the neurological basis for this presumption.

---

j Additional studies[96, 99] have been inconclusive.

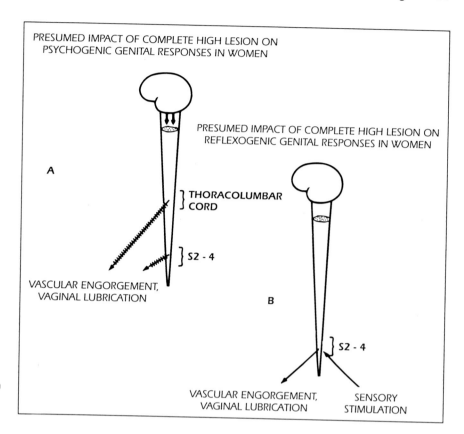

PRESUMED IMPACT OF COMPLETE HIGH LESION ON
PSYCHOGENIC GENITAL RESPONSES IN WOMEN

PRESUMED IMPACT OF COMPLETE HIGH LESION ON
REFLEXOGENIC GENITAL RESPONSES IN WOMEN

A

THORACOLUMBAR
CORD

S2 - 4

VASCULAR ENGORGEMENT,
VAGINAL LUBRICATION

B

S2 - 4

VASCULAR ENGORGEMENT,
VAGINAL LUBRICATION

SENSORY
STIMULATION

Figure 5–13. Presumed impact of complete high spinal cord injury on genital responses in women. **(A)** Psychogenic vascular engorgement and vaginal lubrication impaired due to loss of input from brain to thoracolumbar and sacral cord. **(B)** Reflexogenic vascular engorgement and vaginal lubrication spared due to preservation of sacral reflex arc.

Following *lower complete lesions disrupting sacral cord function*, few should exhibit vaginal lubrication and engorgement of the pelvic structures reflexively. If women have a thoracolumbar center for these responses, some could be expected to exhibit these responses as a result of psychogenic stimuli (Figure 5–15). A small study that gathered information through interviews supported this assumption.[5]

Contraction of smooth musculature in the fallopian tubes, uterus, and paraurethral Skene glands is caused by outflow from the thoracolumbar cord, as is emission in men. Although data is lacking, one can draw *tentative* conclusions about the effects of cord injury based on neuroanatomy. A complete lesion above the thoracolumbar region of the cord would be likely to disrupt these physical responses, and a lesion below this level should leave them intact in most instances.

Rhythmic contraction of striated pelvic musculature, the analogue of ejaculation, is a sacral reflex. If the impact of spinal cord injury is equivalent in both sexes, one would expect few women with spinal cord injuries to exhibit this motor response. The statistics on ejaculation in males following cord injury are highly questionable, however, because studies tend to report emission

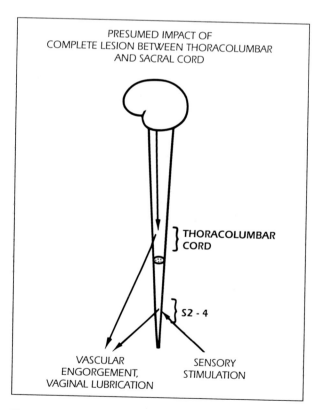

PRESUMED IMPACT OF
COMPLETE LESION BETWEEN THORACOLUMBAR
AND SACRAL CORD

THORACOLUMBAR
CORD

S2 - 4

VASCULAR
ENGORGEMENT,
VAGINAL LUBRICATION

SENSORY
STIMULATION

Figure 5–14. Presumed impact of complete spinal cord injury that is caudal to thoracolumbar erection center but leaves sacral reflex arc intact.

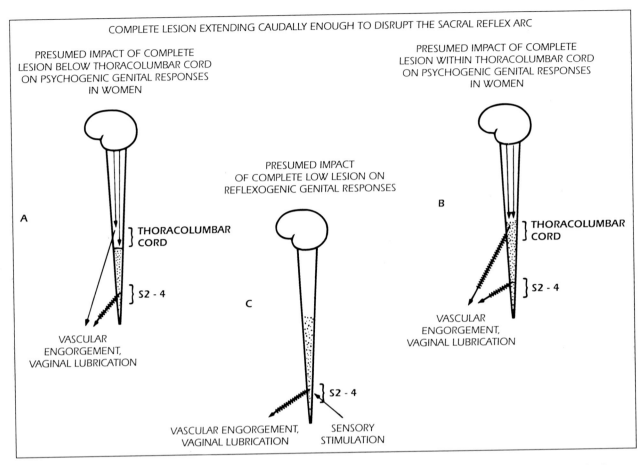

Figure 5–15.   Presumed impact of complete lesion extending low enough to disrupt sacral reflex arc. **(A)** With lesion below thoracolumbar cord, psychogenic vascular engorgement and vaginal lubrication may be spared due to preserved input from brain to thoracolumbar cord. **(B)** With lesion affecting thoracolumbar cord, psychogenic vascular engorgement and vaginal lubrication impaired due to loss of input from brain to sacral and thoracolumbar cord. **(C)** Reflexogenic vascular engorgement and vaginal lubrication impaired due to disruption of sacral reflex arc.

as ejaculation. Thus, it is unknown how many people with spinal cord injuries exhibit the rhythmic contraction of striated pelvic musculature associated with ejaculation in men and its analogue in women.

Present knowledge of male genital responses after spinal cord injury remains imperfect, despite extensive research. The information available needs to be taken with a grain of salt when counseling individuals. Since the extrapolations about female responses presented in the preceding paragraphs are presumptions based on imperfect knowledge, they need to be taken with an even larger grain of salt. Perhaps a whole shakerful.

Extragenital Sexual Responses

Physical responses to sexual excitation are not limited to the genitals. Both males and females exhibit nipple erection, engorgement of breast tissue, a light rash ("sex flush") on the face and upper chest, pupil dilation, and increases in heart rate,

respiration rate, and blood pressure.[43, 50, 108] These responses are controlled by supraspinal centers, and thus are not altered[k] by spinal cord injury.

Orgasm

Orgasm is an intensely pleasurable *subjective* experience. It is usually associated with ejaculation in the male and its physical equivalent in the female. However, orgasm does not have to be associated with these physical responses.[43, 103] It is "essentially a cerebral event."[43]

Because orgasm is a mental event, it is not totally dependent upon genital sensation. Some men and women with complete spinal cord injuries still experience orgasm.[19, 97, 103] In the absence of pelvic innervation, fantasy and erotic imagery can be used to achieve orgasm.[19] Some can achieve orgasm through stimulation of inner-

---

[k] Systolic blood pressure responses are an exception.[98]

vated areas above the level of injury.[5, 13, 18, 49] Others experience orgasm following genital stimulation, despite complete spinal cord injury.[63, 97] The orgasms experienced by people with spinal cord injuries are reported as satisfying, often followed by a resolution of sexual tension similar to that experienced by people without cord injuries.[18, 19, 97]

The incidence of orgasm appears to vary with the level of lesion: it occurs more commonly in people with paraplegia as opposed to tetraplegia.[13, 48, 53] The impact of a lesion's completeness is less clear. People with incomplete injuries may[41] or may not[97] be more likely than people with complete injuries to experience orgasm.

A few people with high lesions report severe spasticity just before and during orgasm.[5, 41] Following orgasm, some individuals (both genders) report that their spasticity is reduced or eliminated for a period of time[5, 49]

Fertility

Spinal cord injury occurs most frequently between the ages of 16 and 30,[45, 78] prime child-bearing years. As a result, fertility is likely to be a significant concern for many who sustain spinal cord injuries.

Male. Few men with spinal cord injuries father children without medical intervention. Most estimates of the incidence of spontaneous paternity following injury are 5 percent or lower.[8, 37, 46, 48, 81]

Impaired erection and ejaculation are obvious sources of infertility after spinal cord injury. Techniques now exist that can be used to elicit ejaculation in men with spinal cord injuries. In one method of harvesting sperm, vibroejaculation, a vibrator is applied to the penis.[8, 77, 81, 83, 91] Ejaculation can be elicited in this manner in 67 percent[89] to over 80 percent of men with lesions above T10,[8, 81, 101] and in 12 percent of men with lesions at or below T10.[81] Vibroejaculation and self-insemination can be performed at home.[8, 33, 79, 89, 101, 103] Autonomic dysreflexia can occur during vibroejaculation,[12, 77, 89] as can bruising and superficial skin damage to the penis.[120]

Electroejaculation, an alternative means of eliciting ejaculation, involves applying electric stimulation using a rectal probe.[8, 11, 18, 33, 77, 91] Successful semen retrieval through electroejaculation is possible in 85 percent to 100 percent of men with spinal cord injury.[8, 33, 74, 101] Electroejaculation must be performed in a hospital or clinic. Potential complications include autonomic dysreflexia, pain, heart arrythmias, and burns.[12, 77, 89, 103] Elec-

troejaculation is most appropriately used in patients for whom vibroejaculation is not successful.[8, 14, 73, 79, 82, 89]

Unfortunately, there is more to the problem of infertility than the inability to place semen in a partner's vagina. Even among men who are able to achieve ejaculation, "naturally" or through technological means, impregnation remains problematic. Men with spinal cord injuries tend to have testicular atrophy. Their sperm tends to have decreased viability, low motility, decreased cervical mucous penetration, and an abnormally high incidence of malformation.[8, 11, 16, 18, 37, 48, 54, 77, 80, 92] Sperm quality does not appear to be related to time since injury.[103]

The cause of inferior sperm quality after spinal cord injury is unknown. Suggested reasons include infection, antibiotic use, elevated scrotal temperature due to prolonged sitting, nondrainage due to impaired ejaculation, a lower state of overall health, abnormal hormone levels, stress, abnormalities in the seminal plasma, antisperm antibodies, and impaired autonomic regulation of semen production.[6, 8, 11, 41, 46, 54, 77, 83, 89, 120] With repeated ejaculations over time, the quality of sperm may[l] improve.[48, 54, 74, 83, 90, 93] Urologic management techniques also have an impact on fertility; men who empty their bladders through intermittent catheterization are more likely to produce motile sperm than are men using other bladder-emptying techniques.[57, 90] Sperm harvested using vibratory stimulation is of higher quality than that harvested using electroejaculation.[8, 33, 73, 77, 82, 103]

In recent years, advances in reproductive technology have benefited people with spinal cord injuries. Sperm can now be harvested using vibroejaculation, electroejaculation, or surgical removal of the sperm directly from the vas deferens, epididymis, or testicle. Fertilization can be achieved through vaginal, cervical, intrauterine, or intrafallopian insemination; in vitro fertilization (IVF); gamete intrafallopian transfer (GIFT); or intracytoplasmic sperm injection[m] combined with IVF or GIFT. Successful impregnation has been reported in a large number of patients using various combinations of these sperm harvesting and fertilization techniques.[8, 15, 33, 73, 77, 79, 83, 89, 91, 101, 106, 113, 119] Unfortunately, any of these approaches can be both financially and emotionally taxing.[17, 77, 89]

Female. Spinal cord injury does not change a woman's fertility.[6, 13, 37, 109] The menstrual cycle

---

[l] Evidence is mixed: some researchers find no improvement of sperm quality with repeated ejaculations.[17, 73, 79]
[m] Injection of a viable sperm into the oocyte.

often stops at the time of injury, but it usually resumes within 5 to 12 months.[3, 13, 18, 37, 41, 77] Women with spinal cord injuries can become pregnant and carry their babies to full term.[18] Most women with spinal cord injuries who become pregnant deliver healthy babies vaginally.[4, 31, 48, 110]

Although a woman remains fertile after spinal cord injury and can deliver normally, pregnancy has its risks. Most women with lesions above T7 exhibit autonomic dysreflexia during labor contractions.[4, 110, 112] Women with lesions above T10[5, 18, 112] can go into labor without realizing it.[n] Other hazards of pregnancy for women with spinal cord injuries include increased risk of anemia, urinary tract infections, pressure ulcers, deep venous thrombosis, respiratory compromise, and constipation.[3, 4, 5, 13, 31, 48, 109, 112] Premature labor and low birth weight are more common than in the general population.[3, 8, 110] Delivery using forceps or cesarean section may occur more frequently.[4, 12, 13]

Because of the complications of pregnancy unique to women with spinal cord injuries, it is advisable for their obstetricians to consult with rehabilitation specialists. With proper management, the increased risks of pregnancy and labor should not pose a major threat to the health of the mother or child. Pressure ulcers, urinary tract infections, respiratory complications, and constipation can be prevented with proper care. A physician aware of the risks of early and undetected labor can monitor the patient closely toward the end of pregnancy and take appropriate precautions when dilation begins. During labor, blood pressure should be monitored continuously. Autonomic dysreflexia can be stopped or prevented with general anesthesia, epidural anesthesia, or various antihypertensive medications.[3, 4, 62, 110, 112]

Since women remain fertile following spinal cord injury, contraceptives are an important concern. The problems posed by the various contraceptive options are different after spinal cord injury. Oral contraceptives further increase the already elevated risk of deep venous thrombosis. An intrauterine device (IUD) can perforate the uterus, and the woman with a spinal cord injury may not detect the problem because of sensory deficits.[18, 37, 109] A woman with impaired hand function would be likely to have difficulty inserting and removing a diaphragm or cervical cap. A diaphragm may be dislodged when a woman performs a Credé maneu-

ver[o] to empty her bladder.[109] The combined use of condom and spermicidal foam is an effective method of birth control,[60] but diminished hand function may complicate the insertion of foam. Assistive devices may make the task easier. Sterilization is an option for women who do not wish to bear children at any time in the future.

Because of the risks and logistical problems associated with the different methods of contraception, the choice may be difficult. The rehabilitation team should address the issue, assisting the patient in finding the solution that is most suitable for her.

THERAPEUTIC INTERVENTION

Spinal cord injury has a significant impact on sexuality and sexual functioning. It can bring about profound changes in genital function, sensation, fertility, and the capacity for bodily movements used in sexual activity. Sexual encounters may be more difficult to orchestrate, and the prospect of incontinence at inopportune moments may always be lurking.

The alterations in physical sexual functioning and the inconvenience that they bring are only a part of the picture. Because a spinal cord injury changes a person from "normal" to "disabled," it places him or her at risk of being perceived as asexual, undesirable, and undeserving of sexual gratification, both by others and by himself or herself. Feelings of sexual inadequacy can undermine a person's self-worth and adaptation to the injury.[85, 107]

Despite the problems that spinal cord injury causes in the area of sexuality, people can adjust. No matter what the level of lesion, what motor abilities, what sensation or genital functioning, people can adapt. They can once again come to see themselves as sexual beings, forming and maintaining relationships, giving and receiving pleasure. But this will not happen automatically; time alone is not enough.[10]

Goals of Intervention

The overall goals of the sexual component of a rehabilitation program after spinal cord injury should be for the person to become comfortable with himself or herself as a sexual being and to learn whatever is needed to make sexual fulfillment possible.

---

[n] Although it is *possible* for labor to go undetected, most women with spinal cord injuries are able to sense the onset of labor. The sensations may be different from those experienced by able-bodied women.[4]

[o] The Credé maneuver is described in Chapter 14 (www.prenhall.com/somers).

The rehabilitation team should affirm the sexuality of the person with a spinal cord injury. The patient and family should receive the message that sexuality and sexual functioning are legitimate concerns and that a fulfilling sex life is a reasonable goal.

People with spinal cord injury also need to gain a basic understanding of how they can function sexually. This understanding should include physical sexual responses before and after injury, fertility, techniques for giving and receiving pleasure, and strategies for dealing with logistical problems such as spasticity or incontinence.

Knowledge in the area of sexuality and sexual functioning is important, but this information will be all but worthless to the person who does not feel worthy of sexual gratification. In a rehabilitation program, a patient should work to regain his or her sense of self-worth, sexuality, and attractiveness as a sexual partner.[85]

Communication is a critical ingredient in all sexual encounters. Perhaps it becomes even more important following spinal cord injury. Patients may need to develop skills in meeting people, putting them at ease, dealing with misunderstandings or misgivings, initiating and refusing sexual activities, communicating likes and dislikes, and letting partners know what they can expect in a sexual encounter.[10, 102, 109]

> I verbalized a lot of things: You know I'm paralyzed, you know I don't have much sensation, or if you don't know this, I'm gonna tell you. And I'm gonna show you. And I'm gonna reach out and touch you, and I'm gonna hold you because that's something I need to do and I want to do. And it's worked.
>
> Mark Johnson[25]

Knowledge, comfort with self, and communication skills are a good start. Ultimately, the goal is for the person to be able to put these things into practice. Patients should be encouraged to explore and experiment, learning how their bodies respond and what is now pleasurable. With their partners,[p] they can try different positions and sexual activities. The rehabilitation team can assist in this process by providing a private room for intimate encounters and providing support when needed.

Strategies

There are a variety of approaches to sexual rehabilitation following spinal cord injury. Several basic strategies are presented in this section. Most programs incorporate more than one of these strategies. Perhaps the perfect program would include elements of all of them.

Psychosexual and physical evaluation. In many centers sexual rehabilitation begins with an evaluation. One or more members of the rehabilitation team assess the patient's sexual functioning in much the same way that they evaluate other areas of function. This evaluation includes obtaining a history and performing a physical examination.

In taking a psychosexual history, a health professional investigates psychosocial issues that can impact on a person's sexual adjustment. Areas of investigation can include the patient's past and present sexual attitudes and behavior, level of understanding of his or her sexual functioning, communication skills, present relationships, feelings about himself or herself as a sexual being, and present sexual desires and concerns.[6, 76] Both the patient's and partner's level of adjustment to the injury should also be addressed.[100]

A sexual evaluation also includes a history of the patient's current and preinjury sexual function and medical status. The health professional investigates the patient's current medications[86, 100] and history of erection or menstruation and pregnancy, urinary tract and bowel functioning and complications, genitourinary surgery, venereal disease, and contraceptive use.[6, 86]

Finally, a thorough sexual evaluation entails an examination that investigates the patient's physical potential for sexual functioning. This examination should address the functioning of both the thoracolumbar and sacral portions of the spinal cord, including genital sensation and responses, sacral reflexes, bladder function,[q] and sensation in the thoracolumbar dermatomes.[28] The evaluation can also include sperm count studies or a pelvic examination, depending on the patient's gender.[6, 40, 76] Finally, the examination can include the patient's strength, range of motion, muscle tone, and functional status, as these areas are relevant to the individual's potential for participating in various sexual activities.[76]

An evaluation of psychosocial and physical sexual functioning is a valuable part of a rehabilitation program. It provides the rehabilitation team

---

[p] Not all patients have sexual partners available. Options in these cases include encouraging patients to explore their bodies on their own and emphasizing strategies for finding partners.

[q] Bladder function can provide insight into the functioning of the sacral and thoracolumbar portions of the spinal cord.[28]

and patient with an understanding of the patient's functioning and enables them to set goals and design a program accordingly. The evaluation itself can also be therapeutic, as it demonstrates to the person that the rehabilitation team considers his or her sexuality and sexual functioning to be an important area of concern.

Education.   In sexual rehabilitation, education is a must and a minimum. Patients should learn about their physical sexual responses and the responses of their partners: how the body responds to sexual stimuli, how and why a spinal cord injury impacts on this function, how these sexual responses can be elicited, and how they can be utilized in sexual encounters. People with spinal cord injuries need to know about their fertility and about options in contraception and assisted reproduction as indicated. They should learn that sexual pleasure and even orgasm are still possible, whether or not they can experience sensations from their genitals. And they should know how to deal with logistical problems such as urinary devices or altered genital functioning. Without this knowledge, a person with a spinal cord injury may be at a loss regarding how to go about pursuing sexual gratification. Worse, he or she may be unaware that sexual gratification is even possible.

The educational component of sexual rehabilitation can take many forms. The information can be presented in lectures, films, slides, group discussions, or question and answer sessions.[40, 88] Romano and Lassiter[88] emphasize that education regarding sexuality should begin with instruction about the physical and emotional aspects of "normal" sexual functioning. The information can be presented as a "review." Like the general public, people with spinal cord injuries are likely to be ignorant in this area but reluctant to admit this ignorance.

People vary in the timing of their readiness to receive information on sexual functioning and fertility after spinal cord injury. Moreover, an individual's needs and priorities may change with time.[75] For this reason, the educational component of a sexual rehabilitation program should include information on resources that will be available in the community after discharge.

Desensitization and attitude.   Sexual activities are emotionally charged and value laden; sexual behavior is immersed in taboos, prescriptions, and proscriptions. People come to rehabilitation with compelling, deep-seated feelings about what they should and should not do in a sexual

encounter, what is desirable, and what is wrong or disgusting. These preexisting attitudes can be a formidable barrier to sexual adjustment after spinal cord injury. They can prevent a person from experimenting comfortably with his or her sexual expression. Attitudes can even inhibit a person's ability to absorb the information presented in an educational program. To achieve sexual fulfillment following spinal cord injury, a person may need to reassess his or her attitudes regarding sexual behavior.

Elements of desensitization and attitude change are incorporated in many sexual rehabilitation programs. Sexual issues can be addressed over time, with the presentations and discussions gradually becoming more explicit. Contact with others who have adapted well sexually after injury can assist with attitude change. In a program described by Steger and Brockway,[102] the process of desensitization is begun in a group setting with participants verbalizing common synonyms of sexual terms.

Behavioral treatment.   Knowledge and attitude change can pave the way for sexual adjustment, but they may not be sufficient. Even armed with an understanding and acceptance of his or her potential for sexual functioning, a person with a spinal cord injury faces social barriers to sexual gratification. The injury may have brought about role changes, conflict, and communication difficulties in preexisting relationships. Meeting people and initiating sexual relations may be problematic; the person with a spinal cord injury is likely to have a strike or two against him or her by virtue of being disabled. Moreover, the person may find that he or she is no longer able to use some tried and true techniques for communicating desires and testing the waters. (The old knee press under the table, for example.)

A variety of communication skills may be helpful to the person with a spinal cord injury (or anyone) in developing and maintaining sexual relations. These skills include verbal and nonverbal expression of affection,[66] desires, and needs; assertiveness; and techniques for meeting and attracting potential partners.[38, 88] Someone who learns to project confidence in himself or herself as a sexual being and knows how to put a partner at ease is more likely to be successful in this arena.

> I'm a little pushy now. Because I lack some of the abilities like hand-holding or flirtatious movements, I take the plunge verbally. I say, 'Well, what now?' or 'I'd like to kiss

you now.' You have nothing to lose, so go for it. If she says no, you're no worse off than you were before.

J. R. Harding[26]

Various approaches can be used to develop communication skills for sexual encounters. Patients can role play, rehearse behaviors, and receive feedback on their communication. They can also practice expressing desires and giving feedback, both verbally and nonverbally.[88, 102] In addition to developing new communication skills, a person with a spinal cord injury needs to learn how his or her body now functions sexually. The partner must also learn and adapt if the relationship is to continue. Couples frequently develop new means of sexual expression after spinal cord injury, and find these alternative sexual activities to be enjoyable and satisfying.[1, 65, 94]

To enhance sexual adjustment, the rehabilitation team should give the couple both the permission and the opportunity to explore their bodies and relearn how to give and receive pleasure. To facilitate this exploration, patients can be instructed in sensory exercises and the use of fantasy. A couple[r] may be given "homework assignments" involving various sexual activities tailored to their needs.[102, 109] In addition to experimenting with giving and receiving pleasure, patients and their partners can practice eliciting genital responses through fantasy or physical stimulation, depending on whether they have retained psychogenic or reflexive genital responses.[28] For inpatients, private rooms can be made available to enable couples or individuals to explore and redevelop their sexual potentials.[76] These rooms may also be used to provide much-needed private time for couples and families.[20]

Counseling. Sexual adjustment following spinal cord injury requires some major adaptations. A person may be faced with altered functioning and loss of sensation in the genitals, a body that no longer looks or works the same as it used to, urinary appliances and the threat of incontinence during sex, loss of fertility, and altered social relations with others. Counseling can help him or her come to terms with these changes.

Group therapy can provide a nonthreatening atmosphere for discussing sexual concerns. Many find it helpful to get together with other people with spinal cord injuries to discuss their feelings and the problems that they anticipate or have already faced. Participants often find comfort in learning that others are facing problems similar to theirs.[40, 88] Group counseling sessions can also provide opportunities for problem solving and mutual support.

More individualized counseling can also be helpful in sexual adjustment after spinal cord injury. One approach involves seeing both the patient and partner, as both have adjustments to make. The two can be seen individually and as a couple. In joint sessions the couple can develop their communication skills and discuss their expectations and emotions with each other.[40, 53]

Specific suggestions. Specific suggestions can be an invaluable aid to sexual adjustment after spinal cord injury. An individual who is simply told to "experiment" and then is turned loose to find his or her own way may have difficulty finding that way. He or she may be reluctant to experiment without at least some initial guidance. Unanswered questions such as "What do I do with this catheter?" or "How exactly can I have intercourse?" may leave the individual reluctant to try sexual activities. Specific suggestions about the logistics of sexual encounters can pave the way for more comfortable and confident exploration.

People with impaired genital sensation may benefit from suggestions for maximizing their pleasure during sexual encounters. They should be encouraged to explore their bodies and find what areas give pleasure when stimulated. People with spinal cord injuries often find that their lowest innervated dermatomes are more sensitive to touch. Many find stimulation of the earlobes, neck, and mouth to be extremely pleasurable. By concentrating on pleasurable sensations, using fantasy, and reassigning pleasurable sensations to the genitals, people with cord injuries can maximize their pleasure, even to the point of orgasm.[18, 49, 102, 109]

Suggestions regarding pleasuring techniques for the partner can also be helpful. Patients can be encouraged to try oral or manual stimulation of the partner's genitals. People with impaired hand function may find that vibrators are useful for stimulating their partners.[102, 109] Vibrators can also be useful for both enhancing pleasure and eliciting genital responses in people with impaired genital innervation.[1]

Another area to address is compensation for dysfunctional vaginal lubrication or penile erection during coitus. Women who do not have functioning sacral cords may not produce adequate vaginal lubrication for intercourse. In these cases, a lubricant can be used. Women who have intact

---

[r] If a partner is not available, the patient can be encouraged to experiment on his or her own.

sacral reflex arcs may require a vibrator or manual stimulation to achieve adequate lubrication.[5, 109]

Erectile dysfunction in men can be more problematic. Men with intact sacral reflexes may be able to elicit or prolong erection by stimulating the penis, scrotum, inner thighs, pubic hair, anus, or lower abdomen. A vibrator or manual stimulation can be used.[42, 53] With or without a functioning sacral reflex arc, a man with erectile dysfunction can use the "stuffing" technique. In this technique the penis is manually "stuffed" into the vagina. This is most easily accomplished with the man on top and the partner's hips flexed.[104] If his partner has adequate voluntary control over her pubococcygeus muscle, she may be able to create a tourniquet effect and cause the penis to become partially erect.[18] If the sacral reflex arc is intact, "stuffing" the penis may elicit a reflex erection.[53] Men with erectile dysfunction may also wish to consider penile prostheses or other physical aids designed to facilitate penile-vaginal intercourse. These physical aids are described in a separate section that follows.

Health professionals can also make suggestions regarding positions for intercourse. A male with a spinal cord injury may prefer the female-superior position, side-lying face to face with his partner, or sitting in a chair or wheelchair with his partner in his lap facing toward or away from him. A woman may prefer the male-superior position or side lying. If she has severe adductor spasticity, a rear approach may be best. Alternatively, she may have intercourse sitting in a wheelchair, sitting at the edge of the seat with her partner kneeling in front of her.[19, 102, 104]

Understandably, people who use indwelling catheters are often concerned about managing this equipment during intercourse. They may fear that they will injure themselves during intercourse or that the catheters will get in the way. Patients should be assured that they can remove catheters prior to sexual intercourse if they prefer, or they can safely leave them in place. A man can fold his urethral catheter back along the side of his penis, either cover it with a condom or leave it uncovered, and lubricate well.[18, 19] A woman who wishes to leave her urethral catheter in place should lubricate it to avoid problems from friction during intercourse,[5] and tape the catheter to her thigh so that it remains out of the way.[18] A suprapubic catheter should be taped to the abdomen, and an ileal conduit bag should be positioned out of the way.[18, 88]

People who manage their bladder incontinence without indwelling catheters may have urinary accidents during sexual activities. This is especially true for people who have reflexively functioning bladders; stimulation of the thighs, genitals, or other pelvic structures may initiate the voiding reflex. This risk can be reduced by emptying the bladder immediately prior to sexual activity[5, 109] and, possibly, by avoiding drinking large amounts of fluid beforehand. In addition, individuals may wish to note which sexual stimuli tend to induce voiding and then avoid these stimuli during sexual encounters. It may also be wise to keep a towel handy and to inform partners of the possibility of bladder accidents.[18, 88] These steps can reduce the embarrassment and inconvenience of any accidents that occur.

Bowel accidents during sexual activity are another area of concern. Patients should be reassured that a regular bowel program can minimize the possibility of having a bowel accident during sex.[109]

A common concern expressed by many patients is that the partner may contract a urinary tract infection during intercourse. Both parties should be assured that this is unlikely[s] if standard hygiene practices are used.[18]

Patients who are subject to autonomic dysreflexia (people with lesions above T6) should be informed that it can be triggered by sexual activity but need not pose a major threat if handled correctly. If a headache occurs during genital stimulation, the couple should stop the stimulation briefly. The headache should then resolve quickly.[t] When it does, the couple can resume their sexual activity, avoiding the particular stimulation that appeared to bring on the headache.[19]

---

[s] Sexually transmitted diseases *should* be a concern, however, just as they are in the general population. Because of the health risks associated with sexual activity, the rehabilitation program should include education on sexually transmitted diseases.

[t] Additional information on autonomic dysreflexia is presented in Chapters 2 and 3.

PROBLEM-SOLVING EXERCISE 5–1

Your patient recently sustained a spinal cord injury classified as T5, ASIA A. He wants to know whether he will ever be able to have sex again. He makes it clear that he is interested in learning about sexual intercourse in particular.

- What should you tell him?

People who require assistance in preparation for sexual activities (undressing, transfers, positioning, management of catheters) may find that having a sexual partner provide this assistance creates problems. Both parties may find it difficult to shift from nurse–patient to lover–lover roles. Moreover, the caretaker/lover may spend so much energy on the preparation that he or she has little left over for the sexual activity. When problems such as these arise, an attendant can be of help.[53]

Suggestions for maximizing pleasure for both partners and suggestions about the mechanics and logistics of sexual activity can be of great assistance to a newly injured person. Ultimately, however, each person still must find his or her own way sexually. He or she will need to experiment, discovering what positions and activities yield the most pleasure and satisfaction.[u]

Interventions for erectile dysfunction. Various physical aids are available for men with erectile dysfunction who wish to include penetration in their sexual activity. Noninvasive options include the use of a firm casing that is worn over the penis or an artificial penis that can either be strapped above the anatomical penis or held in the hand.[40, 52, 104] One option for men who have reflex erections is a constricting band that is placed around the base of the erect penis to trap blood within the erectile bodies and prolong the erection. Alternatively, a vacuum pump may be used to achieve an erection, which is then maintained with a constricting band at the base of the penis.[34, 103, 121] The potential complications that can occur due to the use of vacuum devices and constricting bands include bruises, petechiae, skin irritation or abrasion, edema, erythema, sweating, and leg spasms. To minimize the risk of complications, the user should leave the band in place no longer than 30 minutes.[12, 34]

A man with erectile dysfunction who wishes to have an anatomical erection can undergo surgical implantation of a prosthesis into the erectile tissue of his penis. There are two classes of penile prostheses: inflatable and rod type. Inflatable prostheses include a pump and reservoir and can be inflated or deflated as needed.[104] Rod-type prostheses provide a permanent erection. In addition to providing erection for intercourse, penile prostheses can aid in intermittent catheterization[58] or in the fit of condom catheters.[104]

Penile prostheses have their problems. These include mechanical failure, insufficient rigidity, extrusion of the prosthesis, necrosis, infection, hematoma formation, scarring, and interference with vibroejaculation.[23, 37, 47, 77, 81, 86, 104] Complications occur in approximately 40 percent of cases and usually require revision or removal of the device. Subsequent to removal, reimplantations are likely to fail. Moreover, men who have had penile prostheses removed are often subsequently unable to achieve erections through other techniques such as vacuum erection devices or vasoactive drugs.[47] Because of the problems associated with penile prostheses, all other treatments for erectile dysfunction should be tried before resorting to these devices.[47, 103] Possibly because of the risks associated with prostheses, few men with spinal cord injuries choose to have them inserted.[12]

As an alternative to surgical implantation of penile prostheses, men can achieve erection by injecting vasoactive drugs into their corpus cavernosum. Erection occurs within a few minutes of injection and usually lasts for 1 to 1.5 hours.[12] Complications include liver dysfunction, priapism (erection lasting more than 6 hours),[v] hematoma, mild autonomic dysreflexia, and scarring of the corpora cavernosa with resulting reduction of erectile capabilities.[72, 77, 100, 121]

Sildenafil (Viagra) is a recently developed treatment for erectile dysfunction. This medication is taken orally 20 to 60 minutes prior to intercourse. Sildenafil promotes erection in response to sexual stimulation, increasing the frequency, rigidity, and duration of erections.[69] Studies involving men with spinal cord injuries have demonstrated improved erections in 64 percent of subjects who lack erectile function, and in approximately 75 percent of subjects who have some residual erectile function. Side effects include headaches, flushing, dyspepsia, nasal congestion, shortness of breath, and diarrhea.[36, 69, 77]

A variety of options are available for achieving erections. The rehabilitation team should keep in mind, however, that erection and vaginal penetration are not prerequisites for a satisfying sex life.

> [There's a prevalent belief that] if your neurology is such that you do not get an erection physiologically, then you must have an erection prosthetically. I have no objection to this procedure, but I do object to the proce-

---

[u] The following sources provide additional specific suggestions for sexual activity after spinal cord injury: references 26, 67, 104.

---

[v] Priapism can cause permanent damage to the penis.[86]

dure being offered to newly injured people who have not had an adequate trial at living an integrated life as a para or a quad, who have not learned to *like* themselves again, who still see themselves as some kind of abomination, who think the big thing in sex is genital activity.

George Hohmann[25]

Sexuality as a Part of the Overall Rehabilitation Program

Coming to terms with one's sexuality and sexual functioning is an important component of adjustment after spinal cord injury. Seen in this light, sexual rehabilitation is clearly a key ingredient of rehabilitation after cord injury.

Despite the importance of sexuality, it is often neglected by the rehabilitation team. Because of both poorly defined roles and feelings of discomfort, each team member may avoid the topic, hoping that other team members will deal with it. Individual health professionals or the team as a whole may limit their intervention to discussion of fertility, or even avoid the issue altogether.[19, 24, 75] This problem appears to be more common when the patient is female; women are less likely than men to receive information on sexuality and sexual functioning after spinal cord injury.[55, 115, 117]

When the rehabilitation team does not address sexual functioning, patients are often reluctant to bring up the topic.[6] They may find the subject too embarrassing or may perceive the team's silence as an indication that sex is no longer an appropriate area of concern for them.[21] Even when patients take the initiative to bring up the topic, health professionals may dodge questions and avoid discussions on sexual functioning. This

behavior is likely to increase patients' anxiety about their sexuality and sexual functioning.[50]

To ensure that sexuality is addressed adequately with every patient, sexual rehabilitation (with defined roles and goals) should be an official component of the program. It should not be left to chance, with each team member hoping or assuming that someone else is taking care of it.

Sexuality should be addressed with all patients[w] who have spinal cord injuries, regardless of their gender, age,[2, 70] or sexual orientation. Sexual rehabilitation should be comprehensive, should begin early,[19, 117] and should be tailored to the needs of each individual. If a patient has a sexual partner, that person should be involved in the process, since he or she will also have adjustments to make,[50, 75] and the partner's sexual adjustment can have an impact on the psychosocial well-being of the individual with a spinal cord injury.[66]

Team approach. Successful sexual rehabilitation requires a team approach. The various members of the rehabilitation team should be comfortable affirming patients' sexuality, answering questions about sexual concerns, and supporting the sexual component of the rehabilitation program.[40] Patients will then be able to discuss their concerns with whomever they feel the most comfortable.

Being an effective team member requires more than knowledge in the area of sexual functioning. Values and attitudes are also important. A health professional who is uncomfortable discussing sexual issues, who sees people with disabilities as sexless, or who is repulsed by the sexual options open to people with spinal cord injuries will not be an effective participant in sexual rehabilitation. In fact, he or she is likely to have a detrimental effect on patients. Overtly or covertly, the health professional may convey negative attitudes that undermine the patient's progress.[22, 50]

All members of the rehabilitation team should have the knowledge and attitudes needed to support patients in their sexual rehabilitation. Specialized training may be required to prepare team members for their roles in sexual rehabilitation. Workshops on sexuality and sexual functioning can be valuable experiences for health professionals, increasing their comfort with sexual issues and making them more likely to address these issues with their patients.[21]

PROBLEM-SOLVING EXERCISE 5–2

Your patient has a spinal cord injury classified as T8, ASIA B. After a home visit, she confides that she and her husband "messed around" while she was at home. She then laughs and tells you that she wet the bed "just when things were starting to get interesting."

- How should you respond?

---

[w] Children with spinal cord injuries should receive age-appropriate sexual education that addresses both normal functioning and the impact of spinal cord injury. Their parents should also be provided with education on sexuality, sexual functioning, and fertility after spinal cord injury.[2]

PLISSIT model.   Although the entire rehabilitation team should be able to support the sexual component of the program, not all health professionals must (or even can) provide intensive sexual therapy to their patients. Different professionals will provide different input, depending on their comfort, experience, interest, and expertise.

The PLISSIT model of intervention[x] can be useful for the team approach to sexual rehabilitation. "PLISSIT" is an acronym representing the levels of intervention described in the approach: *Permission, Limited Information, Specific Suggestions,* and *Intensive Therapy.* Using this model, health professionals can supply varying levels of intervention. The level that a given person provides can be determined by both the patient's need and the professional's expertise and comfort.

Permission-giving is the most basic level of intervention in the PLISSIT model. At this level the health professional gives the patient "permission" to be sexual; through verbal or nonverbal behavior, the health professional affirms the patient's sexuality and encourages him or her to explore its expression.[9, 56] This is the minimal level of intervention, which all members of the team should be able to provide. The "permission" from various health professionals will provide much-needed support to the patient.

At the next level of intervention, the health professional provides limited information: the patient is educated about his or her sexual functioning.[9, 53, 56] For patients with spinal cord injury, the education can cover anatomy and physiology, genital functioning following injury, fertility, and birth control.

At the third level of intervention, the health professional provides the patient with specific suggestions.[9] Suggestions can cover the logistics and mechanics of sexual acts, meeting and seducing people, and giving and receiving pleasure. A variety of health professionals may provide this level of intervention, addressing issues most pertinent to their fields. For example, a nurse may discuss options for managing a catheter during sexual encounters, and a physical therapist may make suggestions regarding positioning during intercourse.

Intensive therapy is the highest level of intervention, provided by health professionals with specialized training.[9] Counseling, behavioral treatment, and attitude reassessment fall into this category of intervention.

SUMMARY

- Spinal cord injury has profound effects on sexuality and sexual functioning. Changes in genital functioning, sensation, and musculoskeletal functioning may make a person's accustomed modes of sexual expression difficult or impossible. In addition, the physical and social sequelae of a cord injury are likely to disrupt a person's sense of self, including his or her sense of self as a sexual being. Logistical problems such as incontinence or difficulty in meeting people can further complicate the picture.

- Male genital functions during sexual activity include erection, emission, and ejaculation. Neurological control of these functions involves the sacral and thoracolumbar spinal cord, as well as supraspinal centers. The impact of spinal cord injury on the various genital functions depends on the lesion's level and degree of completeness.

- Female genital functions during sexual activity include vaginal lubrication, vascular engorgement of the genitals, and muscle contractions in both smooth muscles and striated musculature. The impact of spinal cord injury on genital functioning has not been studied as extensively in females as in males; however, tentative conclusions can be drawn based on our understanding of male functioning. The limited research that has been done appears to support these extrapolations.

- Spinal cord injury profoundly impairs male fertility. Recent advances in reproductive technology, however, have made biological fatherhood a reasonable goal.

- Spinal cord injury does not alter a woman's fertility. Because of certain risks involved in pregnancy and childbirth, however, obstetricians caring for women with cord injuries should consult with rehabilitation specialists.

- Sexual rehabilitation is an important component of rehabilitation after spinal cord injury. Different rehabilitation centers take a variety of approaches in addressing sexuality. Some or all of the following elements can be included in a sexual rehabilitation program: psychosexual and physical evaluation, education, desensitization, attitude reassessment, behavioral treatment, counseling, specific suggestions, and interventions for erectile dysfunction.

---

[x] Developed by J. S. Annon.

6

Skin Care

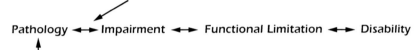

Prevention of pressure ulcers and their sequelae
through medical and nutritional support,
management of tissue loads, skin inspection,
provision of equipment, education and training

Pathology ←→ Impairment ←→ Functional Limitation ←→ Disability

Promotion of pressure ulcer
healing through cleansing and
debridement, application of
dressings, managing bacterial
colonization and infection,
adjunctive therapies, surgery,
medical and nutritional support,
management of tissue loads,
skin inspection, provision of
equipment, education and
training.

Spinal cord injury brings with it a lifelong vulnerability to the development of pressure ulcers. A pressure ulcer is a localized area of tissue necrosis that can occur when soft tissues are subjected to prolonged unrelieved pressure.

Pressure ulcers, also called pressure sores, decubitus ulcers, decubiti, or skin breakdown, are among the most common complications of spinal cord injury.[32, 76, 100, 151, 153] It has been estimated that as many as 85 percent of people with spinal cord injuries develop at least one pressure ulcer at some point after their injuries.[104]

A number of risk factors are associated with the development of pressure ulcers following spinal cord injury (see Table 6–1). Pressure sores are more prevalent among people with complete lesions.[22, 76, 79, 141, 151] Level of injury may or may not be a contributing factor; some studies report a higher incidence of pressure ulcers in people with paraplegia,[22, 141] others report higher rates among people with tetraplegia,[79, 151] and others report no

relation between the incidence of pressure ulcers and level of lesion.[3, 48, 100, 124]

Pressure sores occur almost exclusively over boney prominences. The skin over the sacrum, coccyx, heels, ischium, and greater trochanters are the most common sites of skin breakdown in individuals with spinal cord injury.[32, 61, 69, 133, 141, 151]

ETIOLOGY OF PRESSURE ULCERS

A variety of factors are thought to make people with spinal cord injuries vulnerable to the formation of pressure ulcers. Skin collagen degradation after spinal cord injury may make the skin more prone to breakdown.[120] In addition, the circulatory sequelae of cord injury lead to compromised peripheral blood flow, with resulting reduction in oxygen and nutrient supply to the tissues.[89, 102] The skin and subcutaneous tissues are more vul-

TABLE 6–1. FACTORS ASSOCIATED WITH PRESSURE ULCER OCCURRENCE AND SEVERITY FOLLOWING SPINAL CORD INJURY

	Factors Associated with Higher Risk
Completeness of Injury	Complete injury (ASIA A)
Impairments Resulting from Spinal Cord Injury	Autonomic dysreflexia
	Excessive perspiration
	Fecal or urinary incontinence
	Lower ASIA motor score*
	Muscle tone abnormality: hypotonia or severe spasticity
	Sensory impairment
Emergency Management	Prolonged immobilization after injury
Functional Status	Bed-confined > mobile in wheelchair > ambulatory
	Lower level of independence
Medical Conditions	Cardiovascular disease
	Diabetes
	Hypertension or hypotension
	Urinary tract infections
	Malnutrition (anemia, hypoalbuminemia)
	Previous pressure ulcer
	Pulmonary disease
	Renal disease
Psychological and Social Factors	Impaired cognitive function
	Inadequate social support
	Psychological disorders
Behavioral Factors	Noncompliance with skin care regimen
	Smoking
	Substance abuse
Demographics	Advanced age
	Longer time since injury
	Lower educational level
	Male gender
	Non-white race
	Residence in nursing home or hospital

* The ASIA motor score is presented in Chapter 8.

Sources: references 21, 22, 48, 67, 81, 84, 93, 96, 100, 104, 118, 123, 124, 133, 140, 141, 151.

nerable to trauma; the interruption of skin blood flow caused by external stresses is more pronounced in people with spinal cord injuries than in people with intact nervous systems.[89]

In addition to having skin that is more vulnerable to external stresses, people with spinal cord injuries develop higher interface pressures[a] in sitting than do people without spinal cord injuries.[15, 52, 66] These higher pressures may be due in part to uneven loading on the ischial tuberosities resulting from pelvic obliquity.[66] Atrophy may also contribute to the elevated interface pressures;[66] with muscle atrophy, the soft tissue "padding" over boney prominences is reduced, resulting in an increase in pressure over these areas.

The above-listed problems are compounded by the increased likelihood of trauma to the skin

[a] Interface pressures are the pressures at the interface between the person and the supporting surface.

following spinal cord injury. Combined paralysis and sensory impairment result in areas of the skin being subjected to pressure for prolonged periods. Wherever external pressure on soft tissues is greater than capillary pressure, the capillaries in that region are occluded.[b] This condition exists in tissues compressed between boney prominences and the supporting surface (for example, over the ischial tuberosities when sitting).

Local capillary occlusion does not normally present a problem for people with intact motor and sensory function because these people shift their positions frequently throughout the day. These position changes redistribute pressure long before tissue damage occurs. In contrast, people who have sensory impairments resulting from spinal cord injuries lack the sensation that stimulates protective weight shifts. Moreover, motor paralysis results in more static positioning. The combination of reduced motion and loss of protective sensation results in compression of the tissues between the boney prominences and supporting surfaces or other objects (such as orthoses) for long periods of time. The resulting prolonged ischemia can lead to necrosis of the skin and underlying tissues.[c]

Prolonged unrelieved pressure is the most common cause of pressure ulcers after spinal cord injury.[37] High pressure applied for a short duration can also damage the skin and subcutaneous tissues, causing pressure ulcers.[142, 150] In addition to pressure, shear forces play a significant role in the development of many pressure ulcers.[142, 150] Shearing occurs when tissue is subjected to oppositely directed parallel forces. This shearing causes sliding motion within the tissue. For example, the skin overlying the sacrum is subjected to shear forces when a person lies supine in bed with the head of the bed elevated. In this position, the skin is stabilized against the bed while the deeper tissues slide caudally due to the effects of gravity pulling the person downward toward the foot of the bed.[11, 150] The superficial and deep layers of tissue are pulled in opposite directions, parallel to the shear forces. Shear forces increase the skin's vulnerability to pressure by disrupting the tissues' vascular sup-

ply. In the presence of shear stresses, vascular occlusion can occur at lower pressures.[66]

Several additional conditions can increase the skin's vulnerability to the damaging effects of pressure. Elevation in temperature, locally or systemically, can make the skin and subcutaneous tissue more prone to ischemia because temperature elevation increases the tissues' oxygen requirements.[26, 142] Prolonged exposure to moisture, as can occur with incontinence or excessive sweating, softens the skin and increases its vulnerability to trauma.[102, 109, 142, 150] Both low blood pressure and smoking can reduce peripheral circulation and increase the likelihood of breakdown.[152] Factors that contribute to the development of pressure ulcers are illustrated in Figure 6–1.

SEQUELAE

Pressure ulcers are of major concern because they can lead to osteomyelitis, sepsis, and even death.[35, 39, 151] Additionally, a pressure ulcer that heals leaves a scarred area that remains highly vulnerable to the recurrence of ulcers in the future. Moreover, an extended period of bedrest may be necessary to allow ulcer healing. This prolonged bedrest interferes with vocational and avocational activities, and can lead to the development of a variety of physical problems, including deconditioning, pulmonary complications, joint contractures, additional pressure ulcers, and reduced functional status.

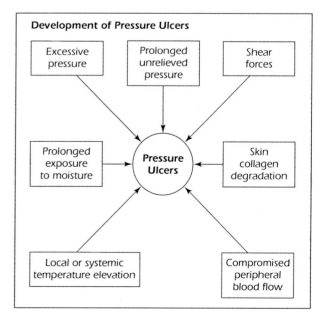

Figure 6–1. *Factors that contribute to the development of pressure ulcers.*

---

[b] Capillary closure is commonly considered to occur at 25 to 32 mm Hg, but a variety of factors can affect capillary closure.[113] Research has demonstrated that tissue blood flow can occur despite significantly higher pressures.[109] Conversely, capillary occlusion can occur at lower pressures.[95]

[c] Ischemia is thought to occur in human skin after it is subjected to 60 mm Hg of pressure for 1 hour.[64] Higher pressures require less time to cause ischemia.

Pressure sores are costly in terms of the expense of hospitalization and surgery, time lost from vocational and avocational activities, and postponement of physical rehabilitation and reintegration into the community.[4, 19, 69, 79, 81, 127, 142] The prevalence of pressure ulcers among people with spinal cord injuries is most tragic when one considers that this complication can be avoided with proper care.

PREVENTION

Pressure ulcers are a serious, common, and preventable complication of spinal cord injury. A lifelong process of skin care beginning at the time of injury is required to prevent pressure sores and their sequelae.[d]

During the initial postinjury phase encompassing acute care and inpatient rehabilitation, meticulous preventive skin care is particularly important because it sets the stage for future care. Pressure ulcer prevention should also be a focus during postacute rehabilitation in outpatient settings and in the home. This continued emphasis on skin care is particularly important in the light of shrinking hospital stays in both acute care and rehabilitation. Postdischarge follow-up care is also critical, as indicated by the fact that pressure ulcers occur with increasing incidence as time passes after injury.[48, 67, 96, 100]

Pressure sore prevention involves avoidance of prolonged unrelieved pressure on the skin, particularly over bony prominences. This is accomplished through periodic repositioning when in bed and by the performance of pressure reliefs when sitting. Specialized equipment (beds, mattresses, mattress overlays, and wheelchair cushions) helps prevent skin breakdown by reducing the pressure on the person's skin when in bed or in a wheelchair.

Periodic relief of pressure is important after spinal cord injury, but it is only one facet of the preventive skin care program. Measures must also be taken to minimize other factors that cause skin breakdown (Figure 6–1 and Table 6–1). The patient and those involved in his care should protect the patient's skin from shear forces, friction, blunt trauma, and exposure to hot objects. Clothes, shoes, and orthoses should fit properly; if too tight, they exert prolonged pressure on the skin. The person's skin should be kept clean and dry,[e] with special attention given to preventing prolonged contact with urine, feces, or excessive perspiration.[11, 55, 56, 75, 87, 91, 102] Skin checks are a necessary component of pressure ulcer prevention. Frequent assessments of the skin's integrity provide feedback on the success of the pressure ulcer prevention program. They also lead to early detection of breakdown or potential breakdown, making it possible to intervene before serious skin damage occurs.

The patient's overall health should also be a focus of the preventive skin care program. Medical conditions that increase the risk of developing pressure ulcers or interfere with wound healing should be brought under control to the extent possible. Additionally, a balanced diet must be ensured, as nutritional deficiencies are important contributors to skin breakdown.[11, 56, 87]

Risk Assessment

All people with spinal cord injuries should be considered to be at risk for developing pressure ulcers, and therefore should be included in pressure ulcer prevention programs. It may be useful, however, to identify those who are at highest risk so that they and the health care team can exercise an even greater level of diligence in pressure ulcer prevention. Figure 6–2 presents a pressure ulcer risk assessment scale that is appropriate for individuals with spinal cord injuries.[f]

Prevention while In Bed

Acutely following spinal cord injury, patients on standard hospital beds must be turned *every 2 hours* around the clock to avoid the development of pressure ulcers.[11, 58, 91, 92, 102, 105, 130] This turning should occur whether or not the spine is stable.[47] Although 2 hours is the standard interval between turning, some patients may require more frequent turning.[87] On the other hand, the time spent in each position may in some cases be increased gradually as skin tolerance allows.

Specially designed beds, mattresses, and mattress overlays can help to maintain the skin's integrity by reducing pressure over bony prominences. These devices should be used in addition

---

[d] The pressure ulcer prevention, assessment, and treatment strategies presented in this chapter are consistent with guidelines published by the U.S. Department of Health and Human Services.[11, 12]

[e] The skin should be dry, but not excessively so. Topical moisturizers may be used if flaking or cracking of the skin occurs.[11]
[f] A self-rating scale, the Pressure Ulcer Risk Assessment Scale for Persons with Paralysis, is more appropriate for people with spinal cord injuries who live in the community.[123]

Risk factor	Coded value		Score
1. Level of activity[a]	0 [ ] ambulatory 2 [ ] wheelchair 4 [ ] bed		
2. Mobility[b]	0 [ ] full 1 [ ] limited 2 [ ] immobile		
3. Complete SCI	0 [ ] no	1 [ ] yes	
4. Urine incontinence or constantly moist[c]	0 [ ] no	1 [ ] yes	
5. Autonomic dysreflexia or severe spasticity	0 [ ] no	1 [ ] yes	
6. Age (years)	0 [ ] ≤ 34 1 [ ] 35-64 2 [ ] ≥ 65		
7. Tobacco use/smoking	0 [ ] never 1 [ ] former 2 [ ] current		
8. Pulmonary disease	0 [ ] no	1 [ ] yes	
9. Cardiac disease or abnormal EKG	0 [ ] no	1 [ ] yes	
10. Diabetes or glucose ≥ 110 mg/dl	0 [ ] no	1 [ ] yes	
11. Renal disease	0 [ ] no	1 [ ] yes	
12. Impaired cognitive function	0 [ ] no	1 [ ] yes	
13. In a nursing home or hospital	0 [ ] no	1 [ ] yes	
14. Albumin < 3.4 or t. protein < 6.4	0 [ ] no	1 [ ] yes	
15. Hematocrit < 36.0% (HGB < 12.0)	0 [ ] no	1 [ ] yes	
Total score			

Risk: Low 0–2, Moderate 3–5, High 6–8, Very high 9–25

[a] **Level of activity**
0 - ambulatory - can walk with/without assistance
2 - wheelchair mobile - sits out of bed only, cannot bear own weight and/or must be assisted into chair or wheelchair
4 - bed mobile - confined to bed during entire 24 hours of the day

[b] **Mobility**
0 - full - independent in moving, no limitations, able to control and move all extremities at will
1 - limited - (slightly to very) requires assistance when moving
2 - immobile - complete immobility, unable to change position. Does not make even slight changes in body or extremity position without assistance, completely dependent on others for movement.

[c] **Minimally controlled urinary bladder** - incontinent of urine at least once a day, absence of control.
Constantly moist - skin is kept moist almost constantly by perspiration, urine, etc. Dampness is detected every time patient is moved or turned

Figure 6–2. Pressure ulcer risk assessment scale for the spinal cord injured. (From Salzberg, C., Byrne, D., Cayten, C., van Niewerburgh, P., Murphy, J., & Viehbeck, M. [1996]. A new pressure ulcer risk assessment scale for individuals with spinal cord injury. *American Journal of Physical Medicine and Rehabilitation*, 75(2), 96–104. Reprinted by permission of Lippincott Williams & Wilkins.)

to, not in place of, regular position changes.[47, 55, 75, 87, 145] Ring-shaped donut cushions are *not* appropriate for either prevention or management of pressure ulcers, as they create ischemia in tissues encircled by the donut.[55]

When people lie in bed, their position will determine which areas of their bodies receive the most pressure and are thus most vulnerable to skin damage. In supine, breakdown is most likely to occur in the skin overlying the occiput, scapulae, sacrum, posterior iliac crests, and heels. In sidelying, breakdown is most common over the greater trochanters and both the medial and lateral aspects of the knees and ankles. In prone, the breasts, anterior iliac spines, knees, and toes are vulnerable. [69, 102, 152]

To prevent the development of pressure ulcers while in a standard bed, a newly injured patient must change positions (turn) at least every 2 hours and the skin should be inspected each time the patient is turned. As skin tolerance improves,[g] the time spent in each position may be increased gradually.[151] When the time between position changes is increased, the skin over the boney prominences should be monitored especially closely for signs of breakdown.

Proper bed positioning after spinal cord injury involves more than turning the patient every 2 hours. In each position, care should be taken to prevent excessive pressure over the boney prominences.[h] Pillows or blocks of foam rubber can be used to relieve pressure on the boney prominences and to prevent skin surfaces from contacting each other.[11, 12, 88, 132] Sidelying with direct pressure on the greater trochanter should be avoided, as this places excessive pressure over this boney prominence.[11] Positioning the patient reclined 30 degrees back from sidelying will provide better pressure distribution.[7, 128]

Proper bed positioning also minimizes shear. To prevent skin damage from shear forces over the sacrum when the patient is supine, the head of the bed should not be elevated above 30 degrees.[73] Time spent with the head of the bed elevated should be kept to a minimum.[11, 12]

In the prone position, pillows are used to bridge areas vulnerable to pressure. One advantage of prone lying is that the hips and knees are extended in this position, preventing the development of flexion contractures. In addition, the time spent in this position can be increased to several hours because bridging with pillows eliminates pressure over the boney prominences. The person can then sleep uninterrupted through the night.[132]

When repositioning patients, health professionals should take care to avoid subjecting the skin to undue shear forces and friction.[11] Draw sheets under patients make it possible to turn them without dragging their skin across the supporting surface.[i]

---

[g] Redness over the boney prominences should disappear within 30 minutes of the position change.[88, 151]

[h] Proper bed positioning also involves positioning the extremities to preserve range of motion. For example, the elbows should be placed in extension and the ankles dorsiflexed to neutral.

[i] Draw sheets have the added benefit of making it easier to turn the patient with less physical strain on the people providing this assistance.

In addition to turning and positioning, pressure ulcer prevention while in bed involves keeping the sheets clean and dry. Sheets should also be free of wrinkles where they come in contact with the patient's skin.[91]

Beds, Mattresses, and Mattress Overlays

Specialty beds, mattresses, and mattress overlays are designed to minimize the risk of skin breakdown while in bed. They can be used to reduce pressure on the skin both to prevent pressure ulcers and to promote healing when skin breakdown has already occurred.

Some authors distinguish between pressure reduction and pressure relief. Surfaces that provide *pressure reduction* distribute pressure more than do standard hospital mattresses, resulting in lower pressures on the skin. The pressure on some areas of the skin remains above capillary closing pressure, however, necessitating a regular turning schedule. In contrast, surfaces that provide *pressure relief* support the body without exceeding capillary closing pressure. On these surfaces, it is possible to prevent breakdown without turning.[113]

Beds. One type of bed designed for pressure relief is a low air-loss bed.[113] This type of bed supports the patient on a number of inflated cushions. Air is pumped into these cushions continually and leaks out of small holes in the cushions. The continual filling/leaking air flow allows the support surface to conform to the patient's body, distributing the supporting forces and, thus, minimizing interface pressures. The flow of air also dries the skin. Low air-loss beds typically have features allowing adjustment of the maximal and minimal pressures in different areas of the bed. Low air-loss mattresses and mattress overlays are also available.[45]

A second type of pressure-relieving bed, an air-fluidized bed,[113] is filled with ceramic microspheres. The patient "floats" on the supporting surface as air is pumped continually through the beads. Air-fluidized beds provide constantly changing supporting forces and distribute pressure by conforming to the patient's body. The constant flow of air has a drying effect on the skin. The air-fluidized feature requires a specialized bed; it is not available in mattresses or mattress overlays.[45]

Low air-loss beds and air-fluidized beds (Figure 6–3) can be used by people with stable spines.[145] A patient with an unstable spine may be placed on a rotating bed (also called an oscillating

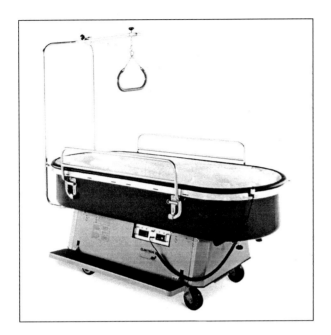

Figure 6–3. Air-fluidized bed. (Photo courtesy of Hill-ROM, 4349 Corporate Rd., Charleston, SC 29405.)

support surface or kinetic treatment table) to prevent pressure ulcers.[j] These beds can be used while the patient is in traction.[91] Rotating beds rock slowly side to side in a continuous motion, constantly redistributing the weight-bearing forces on the patient's skin. A rotating bed must be adjusted properly. Otherwise, it will allow the patient to slide back and forth as the bed rocks. This sliding subjects the skin to shear forces, *causing* skin breakdown instead of preventing it.[145] These beds are most practical for patients who are restricted to bed, as transfers in and out are difficult.

Mattresses and mattress overlays. Pressure-reducing mattresses and mattress overlays are less costly alternatives to specialized beds. They can provide either dynamic or static pressure reduction. These support surfaces can utilize foam, water, gel, or air to reduce pressure on the skin.[113] Each type of mattress or overlay comes in a variety of models made by different manufacturers.

Mattress overlays are placed on top of standard mattresses. Some mattress overlays have been shown to significantly reduce[k] interface

pressures.[40] One disadvantage of mattress overlays is that they can "bottom out," compressing excessively when people are positioned on them. Caregivers should check beneath patients' boney prominences as they lie in the various positions to ensure that bottoming out does not occur[l] on mattress overlays.[12]

Pressure-reducing mattresses are designed to replace standard hospital bed mattresses. A study comparing several brands of pressure-reducing mattresses found large differences in interface pressures over boney prominences.[113]

Most mattresses and mattress overlays provide static pressure distribution. These support surfaces reduce interface pressure by maximizing the contact area between the support surface and the person. The pressure on any given area remains constant until the patient moves.

Alternating pressure mattresses provide dynamic pressure relief. These mattresses are made of air-filled cells that inflate and deflate asynchronously. Because of the cyclic inflation and deflation of the cells, the patient's skin is subjected to fluctuating pressure. Alternating pressure mattress overlays are also available.[45]

Selecting an appropriate support surface. There is a large variety of beds, mattresses, and mattress overlays designed to prevent pressure ulcers and promote healing of existing ulcers. The various support surfaces differ in their effectiveness in reducing pressure over the user's boney prominences. They also differ in the degree to which they reduce shear, cause build-up of moisture and heat, and provide alternating (dynamic) pressure. Each of these factors is relevant to the prevention and treatment of pressure sores. Table 6–2 summarizes the performance characteristics of the different types of support surface. The various brands of similar types of support surface can be very different in the degree to which they reduce interface pressures. Moreover, the performance of a particular support surface can vary. For example, the interface pressures on air-filled mattresses and mattress overlays are determined by their inflation. Under- or over-inflation will result in high interface pressures.[27]

Selection of an appropriate support surface for an individual should be based on consideration of his unique needs. Factors to consider include the presence or absence of pressure ulcers,

---

[j] The Roto-Rest bed provides constant turning. This constant motion reduces the risk of pressure ulcers, enhances pulmonary status, and reduces the risk of pulmonary emboli.[94, 145]

[k] For example, one study found that the RoHo dry flotation mattress overlay significantly reduced interface pressures in patients with spinal cord injuries who had undergone myocutaneous flap surgery. The pressure reduction was slightly less than that provided by air-fluidized beds, but both surfaces prevented flap breakdown.[40]

[l] Bottoming out is detected by placing a hand beneath the mattress overlay while it is underneath the patient. If the support material has compressed to less than an inch at any point, it has bottomed out.

TABLE 6–2.   PERFORMANCE CHARACTERISTICS OF MATTRESSES, MATTRESS OVERLAYS, AND BEDS

	Pressure Reduction or Relief	Shear Reduction	Low Moisture Retention	Reduced Heat Build-up	Dynamic	Requires Power Source	Cost Day	Interferes with Functional Skills
Standard mattress							Low	No
Foam	**Reduction**						Low	Minimally
Static air or water flotation	**Reduction**						Low	Yes
Alternating air mattress or overlay	**Reduction**						Moderate	Yes
Low air-loss bed	**Relief**						High	Yes
Air-fluidized bed	**Relief**						High	Yes
Rotating bed	**Reduction**						High	Yes

Key: ■ = characteristic present.

Sources: references 12, 45, 95, 113.

the skin's tolerance to pressure, feasibility of regular turning with positioning on skin free of breakdown, and the presence of moisture from sources such as excessive perspiration or wound drainage. One consideration unique to the needs of people with spinal cord injury is spinal stability. When the spine is unstable, certain surfaces such as low air-loss beds and alternating pressure mattresses are unsuitable[60] due to the potential for motion at the site of vertebral instability. Another important consideration is the impact of the support surface on function. Many of the pressure-reducing support surfaces increase the difficulty of both independent functioning and dependent handling. Finally, cost should be considered when selecting a bed, mattress, or mattress overlay. The most appropriate support surface will allow prevention of pressure ulcers (and healing if ulcers are present) without unnecessary interference with functioning and with minimal cost per day.

Prevention while Using Wheelchair

The skin overlying the ischial tuberosities, sacrum, and coccyx is susceptible to the development of pressure ulcers in sitting.[102] Proper positioning, an appropriate cushion, periodic relief of pressure on the skin, and a gradual build-up of sitting tolerance can prevent this problem.

Positioning. Appropriate positioning in a wheelchair will reduce the risk of pressure ulcers. During prolonged sitting, the patient's buttocks should be located well back in the chair and the pelvis should be positioned in a slight anterior tilt.[90] In this position, the skin overlying the sacrum and coccyx will not be subjected to excessive pressure.[112] The pelvis should be horizontal, without a right or left lateral tilt. This horizontal orientation will result in equal weight bearing on the right and left ischial tuberosities, reducing the maximal pressure in this area.[66, 77] The patient's buttocks should be centered on the seat. If the pelvis is off-center, the patient is likely to sit with his trunk leaning laterally, resulting in increased pressure on one ischial tuberosity.

Because improper positioning can increase the risk of skin breakdown, health professionals should ensure that patients sit with good posture whenever they are out of bed in a chair. During acute care and early rehabilitation, most patients require assistance to transfer and position themselves in their wheelchairs. Health professionals should take the time to check patients' positions after they transfer, and make adjustments as needed. They should also make adjustments as needed if patients' postures shift during periods of prolonged sitting.

During rehabilitation, patients who have the physical potential to do so should learn how to position themselves optimally in their wheelchairs.[m] Those who are unable to position themselves should learn how to direct others in assisting with this task.

Proper posture in a wheelchair requires that the wheelchair user or those providing assistance place the buttocks and trunk appropriately on the seat. The wheelchair's components, size, and adjustment are also critical for appropriate positioning and pressure distribution in a wheelchair.

Table 6–3 presents wheelchair characteristics that are relevant to positioning and prevention of pressure ulcers.[n]

Wheelchair cushions.   People with spinal cord injuries who utilize wheelchairs require wheelchair cushions[o] to aid in the prevention of pressure ulcers. These cushions are specifically

---

[m] Chapter 11 presents methods for independent positioning in a wheelchair, and therapeutic strategies for teaching these skills.

[n] Chapter 12 provides additional information on wheelchair components, adjustment, and selection.

[o] People with spinal cord injuries should use wheelchair cushions designed specifically for the prevention of pressure ulcers in high-risk populations. Standard foam rubber cushions and donut-type cushions are inappropriate.

TABLE 6–3.   WHEELCHAIR CHARACTERISTICS RELEVANT TO POSITIONING AND PREVENTION OF PRESSURE ULCERS

Wheelchair	Characteristics	Impact on Positioning and Skin
Seat dimensions	Too wide	Promotes the development of a lateral trunk lean, resulting in increased pressure on one ischial tuberosity.
	Too narrow	Skin overlying the greater trochanters may be subjected to pressure from armrests or friction from wheels.
	Too deep (too long from front to back)	Can cause the wheelchair user's buttocks to slide forward on the seat, causing a posterior pelvic tilt with resulting increased pressure on the sacrum and coccyx.
	Too shallow (too short from front to back)	Reduces the area over which sitting forces can be distributed, increasing the pressure on the buttocks.
Footrest height	Too high	Reduces weight bearing on thighs, increasing pressure on buttocks.
	Too low	Does not provide adequate postural support. Allows buttocks to slide out (anteriorly) on wheelchair seat, resulting in a posterior pelvic tilt and increased pressure on the sacrum and coccyx.
Armrests	Present on wheelchair	May reduce risk of developing skin breakdown because of (1) reduced seating pressure due to partial support of body weight; (2) promotion of upright sitting posture; and (3) enhanced stability encouraging the performance of more pressure reliefs.
	Absent from wheelchair	May increase risk of skin breakdown due to absence of above-listed benefits.
	Too low or uneven	Encourage wheelchair user to sit with a lateral lean, increasing pressure on one ischial tuberosity.
Seat and back construction	Upholstered	Stretches over time, reducing postural support. Seat upholstery (sling seat) can also increase shear forces on the buttocks and promote sitting with a pelvic obliquity and posterior pelvic tilt.
	Solid back and solid seat or seat insert	Provides superior postural support, promoting optimal distribution of pressure.

Sources: references 18, 28, 52, 68, 77, 87, 90, 115, 147.

designed for pressure distribution, minimizing the pressure on the skin of the buttocks by spreading the supporting forces over a greater area. Cushions that minimize shear forces on the skin also help to maintain skin integrity.

Selection. Cushions vary in their effectiveness in reducing pressure and shear forces and in providing postural support. They also differ in the degree to which they cause buildup of heat and moisture on the skin, and in their weight, maintenance required, cost, and the amount of difficulty that they cause during transfers. Cushion selection is critical because of the cushion's enormous impact on both skin integrity and the ability to function.

A wheelchair cushion should reduce the pressure on the buttocks enough to enable the wheelchair user to function in a normal day (sitting and performing his accustomed activities all day, *with pressure reliefs*) without skin breakdown. The most critical factor in cushion selection is the cushion's effect on skin integrity. A cushion that is not adequate in this respect is inappropriate for the individual in question.

People with spinal cord injuries are highly variable in the degree to which their skin can tolerate pressure without breaking down. Moreover, people differ in the degree to which cushions distribute pressure on their skin; different people with spinal cord injuries sitting on identical cushions exhibit large variation in the pressure found at their ischial tuberosities.[77] As a result, cushion selection must be individualized.

Because pressure reduction is a critical feature of wheelchair cushions, pressure measuring devices are often used as a part of the cushion selection process. These devices can be used to compare the interface pressures that occur on different cushions. Seating pressures should not, however, be the sole factor considered when selecting a cushion.[20, 108, 147] The only way to determine a given cushion's appropriateness for an individual is to have him use the cushion (or an identical model) for a period of time. If at all possible, he should use a cushion for several days before one is ordered. During the trial period, sitting time on the cushion should be increased progressively and the skin should be checked frequently[20] to determine whether the cushion provides adequate pressure distribution, shear reduction, and heat and moisture dissipation to meet the individual's needs. The patient should participate in activities such as wheelchair propulsion during the trial period, as these activities alter interface pressures.[31, 70] A sec-

ond important consideration in cushion selection is the cushion's impact on posture. A cushion that supports the wheelchair user in a good posture will enhance breathing capacity[p] and functional status, and can help prevent the development of skeletal deformity.[11, 68]

In addition to pressure distribution and posture, the cushion's influence on the patient's functional status must be considered when selecting a cushion.[11] Unfortunately, the cushions that distribute pressure most effectively tend to be heavier and interfere more with transfers. Heavy cushions add to the overall weight that wheelchair users must push when propelling their chairs and can be difficult or impossible for some individuals to take in and out of their chairs independently. Cushions that interfere with transfers can create dependence in people who could otherwise function without assistance. Thus, cushions can have tremendous impact on functional status. Cushion selection involves finding the cushion that provides adequate pressure distribution for the individual in question while creating the least interference with his functioning.

The maintenance required by a cushion should also be considered. Those that need frequent maintenance to retain their effectiveness are appropriate only for people who will take the responsibility to provide or obtain this maintenance.[42]

Expense may also be considered when selecting a cushion. This factor should be of the lowest priority, however, since cushions have such a significant impact on health and function. The cost of even the most expensive cushion is negligible when compared to the potential cost of a single pressure ulcer.

Cushions vary widely in their effect on interface pressures, shear, temperature, and moisture; impact on function; maintenance requirements; durability; and cost. Likewise, people with spinal cord injuries vary widely in their skin tolerance, pressure relief habits and abilities, functional capacity, and willingness or ability to provide regular cushion maintenance. When selecting a cushion, the wheelchair user and the rehabilitation team should work together to determine which cushion will be most suitable to the individual's needs and preferences.

Options. The four classes of commonly used wheelchair cushions are polymer foam, air-filled,

---

p Chapter 7 addresses the impact of posture on breathing.

gel flotation, and honeycomb cushions.q Different brands are available in the various types of cushion, and each brand has a variety of designs.

Foam cushions are made from various types of relatively dense foam.[r] They come in different densities, thicknesses, and seat dimensions. Density and thickness are chosen according to the user's weight and skin tolerance. Options include contoured cushions and cushions composed of two or more layers of different densities. Foam cushions are the least effective type of cushion in distributing pressure, but are adequate for some people with spinal cord injuries. Custom-contoured foam cushions and those made of softer foam provide better pressure distribution than do planar (flat) cushions and those made of stiffer foam.[131] The advantages of foam cushions are that they are light, do not greatly inhibit function, are relatively inexpensive and easily modified, and can absorb moisture. The disadvantages of foam cushions include the following: they cannot be washed, they tend to cause elevated skin temperatures, and they may need to be replaced as often as every 6 months.[42, 49, 68, 90, 106, 129, 147]

Gel cushions are typically made of gel-filled pouches supported on firm, contoured foam bases.[68, 90] Gel cushions provide better pressure distribution than do foam cushions.[137] They can reduce heat buildup[42, 129] and may be the most effective type of cushion in minimizing shear forces on the skin. This characteristic is particularly advantageous for the active person, who is more likely to have skin problems due to shearing. The disadvantages of gel cushions are that they tend to be heavy and can cause moisture buildup on the skin, elevation of local skin temperature after prolonged sitting, reduced sitting stability, and difficulty in transfers.[28, 42, 49, 102, 106]

Air-filled cushions can provide excellent weight distribution. When an air-filled cushion is properly inflated, the person's buttocks are "immersed" in the cushion: the buttocks sink into the cushion as far as they can without bottoming out. This immersion maximizes the area of contact between the person and the cushion, which minimizes the interface pressures.[146] Thus, on properly inflated air-filled cushions, interface pressures are lower than those that occur on either foam or gel cushions.[20, 77, 137] The disadvantages of air-filled cushions include the following: they are heavier than foam cushions, are easily punctured, can reduce sitting stability, and they make transfers *much* more difficult. Some designs can cause buildup of moisture on the skin.[49, 77, 80, 90, 106] Perhaps the greatest disadvantage of air-filled cushions is that they are ineffective in pressure reduction if they are either overinflated or underinflated. To optimize pressure reduction, the inflation pressure should be checked daily.[80]

Honeycomb cushions are made of thermoplastic urethane that is formed into honeycomb-shaped cells. The open cells allow air to circulate, preventing heat and moisture build-up.[68] These cushions are available in contoured or planar designs. They are light in weight, and can be machine washed and dried. Honeycomb cushions are relatively new on the market, and have not been studied as extensively as the other types of cushion. For this reason, it is unknown how their performance in pressure relief and shear reduction compares to other classes of cushion.

Wheelchair cushions are typically used with protective covers. Cushion covers should be selected carefully, as they can influence cushions' effectiveness in pressure distribution. Covers can also increase or decrease moisture and heat buildup on the skin.[26, 42, 147]

Pressure relief. When a person with a spinal cord injury sits for a prolonged period of time, a properly fitting and adjusted wheelchair, a good sitting posture, and an appropriate wheelchair cushion are required to protect the skin over the buttocks and sacrum. These precautions, however, are not sufficient to prevent the development of pressure ulcers. Even an optimal wheelchair and cushion will only reduce interface pressures to a limited degree. When a wheelchair user sits, his skin is subjected to pressures that are high enough to occlude capillary circulation. This is particularly true of the skin overlying the ischial tuberosities. Regardless of the cushion used, periodic relief of pressure is necessary to prevent tissue necrosis.[64]

Starting at the time of injury and continuing through the remainder of their lives, people with spinal cord injuries must perform pressure reliefs whenever they sit for prolonged periods of time. Pressure relief can be accomplished by lifting the buttocks from the seat, or by shifting the trunk forward or to the side. These maneuvers can be performed with assistance or independently,

---

q Dynamic cushions, which provide alternating pressure, are less commonly used because they are cumbersome and require a power source.[49] These cushions may be beneficial for some individuals who are either unable to perform pressure reliefs or are noncompliant with pressure reliefs.[20]

r These foams are *not* to be confused with standard foam rubber, which provides virtually no pressure distribution. The foam rubber cushions that often come with wheelchairs do not provide adequate pressure distribution for people with spinal cord injuries.

depending on the individual's ability. Alternatively, the wheelchair can be tilted or reclined to shift weight off of the ischial tuberosities.[s]

When out-of-bed activities are first initiated, pressure reliefs should be performed every 15 to 20 minutes when sitting.[92, 102, 130] Sitting time should be limited at first, and the skin's status should be monitored closely[t] to determine its tolerance to sitting.[143, 151]

Some individuals are able to tolerate longer times between pressure reliefs without developing pressure ulcers.[109] During rehabilitation, the time between pressure reliefs can be increased gradually *if skin tolerance allows.* When the time between pressure reliefs is increased, frequent skin checks should be performed to determine whether the individual's skin is able to tolerate the longer periods of unrelieved pressure. The skin over the ischial tuberosities, sacrum, and coccyx in particular should be monitored closely for early signs of breakdown or potential breakdown.

Skin inspection.

Following spinal cord injury, insensitive areas of the skin should be inspected at least daily, with particular attention given to the skin overlying boney prominences. More frequent skin checks are indicated in high-risk patients or when there is a change in conditions that could increase the risk of pressure ulcers. For example, the skin should be inspected each time the patient is turned during the early postinjury phase and during periods of bedrest when a patient is ill or has a pressure ulcer. The skin should be checked after each sitting session when sitting is first initiated during the acute hospitalization, when a new cushion is utilized, or when sitting is resumed after a period of prolonged bedrest.

Skin inspection is a critical component of pressure ulcer prevention because the skin's status provides feedback on the effectiveness of the individual's skin care program. Redness[u] that does not resolve within 30 minutes[88, 143, 151] of removal of pressure from the skin may indicate a

problem with the wheelchair cushion, bed support surface, turning or pressure relief schedule, pressure relief techniques, wheelchair components or adjustment, orthotic fit, or any other source of damaging forces on the skin. If skin inspection reveals early signs of skin breakdown or potential breakdown, the patient and health care team should attempt to determine the source of the problem and take measures to eliminate it.

In addition to providing feedback on the pressure ulcer prevention program, skin inspections allow for early detection of imminent or actual breakdown. This early detection makes it possible to intervene before undue damage occurs.

Education and Training

People with spinal cord injuries, particularly those who have significant motor and sensory impairments, are at high risk for developing pressure ulcers. This risk starts at the time of injury and continues through the remainder of their lives. During the initial hospitalization after a spinal cord injury, the health care team bears the responsibility for providing the constant vigilance and meticulous care required to prevent pressure ulcers. By discharge, however, this responsibility must shift to the individual with a spinal cord injury and (if assistance will be required) those who will be involved in his care.

The skin care educational program should provide the patient with information about pressure ulcers: what they are, why they develop, how to prevent them, how to detect them, and how to respond if breakdown occurs. The program should emphasize the severity of pressure ulcers and their sequelae, to underscore the importance of prevention. Individuals who perceive pressure ulcers as being severe may be more likely to comply with their skin care.[114]

The program should also include training in the skills involved in skin care: positioning in bed and in a wheelchair, pressure reliefs, skin inspection, and any equipment maintenance required. If the patient will not achieve independence in his care by the time of discharge from inpatient rehabilitation, those who will be assisting with his care should be included in the education and training program.[v] In addition, individuals who will require assistance should learn how to instruct others in their care. This will enable them

---

[s] Techniques for independent pressure reliefs, strategies for teaching these skills, and power tilt and recline wheelchair features are presented in Chapter 12.

[t] Redness over the boney prominences should disappear within 30 minutes after the end of the sitting session.[88, 151]

[u] People with darkly pigmented skin may not exhibit redness as an early sign of skin breakdown. Early signs of skin damage include discoloration, warmth, edema, induration, or hardness.

---

[v] All members of the health care team should also receive education and training in pressure ulcer prevention.[11, 143]

to continue their skin care programs despite future changes in their support systems.

Table 6–4 summarizes the content of an education and training program for pressure ulcer prevention. For each skin care strategy presented in the program (pressure reliefs, for example), the health care team should provide explanations of the purpose of the action and the hazards of not complying.

In addition to gaining knowledge and skills, the patient needs to develop good skin care habits prior to discharge from inpatient rehabilitation. The health care team cannot assume that education and training will automatically lead to altered behavior. To encourage the development of preventive skin care habits, the staff should involve patients in their care as much as possible. During acute care and early rehabilitation,

TABLE 6–4. CONTENT OF PRESSURE ULCER PREVENTION EDUCATION AND TRAINING PROGRAM

	Program Content
General Information	General information on causes, risk factors and sequelae of pressure ulcers.
Skin Protection in Bed	Positioning: appropriate positions, use of pillows or foam blocks to prevent excessive pressure over boney prominences.
	Turning: turning schedule, techniques for turning.
	Support surface (if specialized support surface is used): operation and maintenance of specialty bed, mattress, or mattress overlay.
	Bed linens: maintain clean, dry, wrinkle free.
Skin Protection in Sitting	Positioning: beneficial sitting posture, methods (independent, assisted, or dependent) of obtaining and maintaining good sitting posture.
	Pressure reliefs: methods, frequency.
	Cushion: maintenance, schedule of use (use whenever sitting!), limitations (will not eliminate the need for pressure reliefs).
Skin Inspection	Frequency: *at least* daily. More frequent under certain conditions, such as during the initial use of new orthoses or shoes, or when medical condition or activity level changes.
	Where to inspect: any surfaces subjected to external loads, with particular attention to boney prominences and weight-bearing surfaces.
	Signs of skin damage or potential breakdown.
	Techniques: visual inspection with mirror where needed, assistance if indicated.
Hygiene	Keep skin clean and dry, especially avoiding prolonged contact with feces or urine.
Response to Signs of Skin Damage	Identify source of skin damage, and take corrective action. Avoid pressure on damaged skin until it has healed.
	Indications for contacting health professional.
General Health Strategies	Maintain good nutritional status. Avoid smoking.
Additional Sources of Skin Trauma	Avoid clothes that exert excessive pressure on the skin, such as pants with heavy seams over the sacrum or coccyx.
	Regularly inspect shoes and orthoses for wear that could result in increased pressure, friction, or shear on the skin.
	During transfers and other functional activities, avoid actions that subject the skin to excessive friction, shear, or high impact forces.

patients' physical capacity to participate in their care may be limited. Health professionals can involve them, however, by explaining pressure ulcer prevention measures as they occur. Patients can also be encouraged to take responsibility for their care. For example, they can be encouraged to remind others to assist them with pressure reliefs at the appropriate intervals. As patients become more physically able, they can gradually increase their participation in skin care activities. They may require frequent reminders at first, but these reminders can decrease as they begin to assume responsibility for their own care.

The rehabilitation team should model appropriate attention to and prioritization of pressure ulcer prevention. Patients' perceptions of the importance of skin care can be influenced by the degree to which health professionals comply with the recommended actions.[5] *All* members of the rehabilitation team should model good pressure ulcer prevention behaviors. Even health professionals who do not normally focus on skin care (speech therapists, for example) should ensure that the patient performs or is assisted with pressure reliefs at the appropriate intervals. If preventive skin care measures are implemented by some team members and not by others, the patient will receive mixed messages about the importance of these measures.

In some cases, poor psychological adjustment leads to self-neglect and noncompliance

with the preventive skin care program. Counseling may help prevent or correct this problem.[w]

One of the greatest challenges of rehabilitation following spinal cord injury involves preparing the patient to prevent pressure ulcers after discharge. With the current trend of shorter hospital stays, this challenge has become greater. Patients may be discharged from inpatient rehabilitation before they have developed the physical skills, knowledge base, and level of psychological adaptation required to assume full responsibility for their skin care. For this reason, education and training in pressure ulcer prevention should extend beyond the traditional inpatient rehabilitation program.[121] Pressure ulcer prevention education and training can continue in day hospital[44] or outpatient settings, as well as in home-based rehabilitation and follow-up visits and phone calls.[38, 72]

PRESSURE ULCER ASSESSMENT

When a pressure ulcer is detected, its management should immediately become a priority. This management should start with an examination of the ulcer and investigation of any factors that may have contributed to its development. A thorough assessment will make it possible to design an appropriate program of interventions, and subsequently to determine the effectiveness of these interventions.

After the initial assessment, pressure ulcers should be examined at least once a week. Examinations should be more frequent if either the patient's medical condition or the ulcer itself deteriorates.[12] Repeat assessments make it possible to evaluate the effectiveness of the interventions, and to alter the program as indicated.

Pressure Ulcer Characteristics

When examining pressure ulcers, health professionals should note their location, size, shape, and stage. (Staging is presented in the section that follows.) They should determine whether the ulcer extends under adjacent tissue in the form of sinus tracts, undermining, or tunneling.[12] Health professionals should also note which of the following are present in the wound bed: exudate, eschar, slough, granulation tissue, or epithelial tissue.[12, 139] Table 6–5 describes the pressure ulcer characteristics that the examination should

---

PROBLEM-SOLVING EXERCISE 6–1

Your patient is a 68-year-old man who has complete T6 paraplegia that resulted from anoxia to his spinal cord during recent surgery (coronary artery bypass graft). He moves his arms independently, but requires assistance to move in bed. He remains in bed on a ventilator, and has developed pneumonia.

- Does this patient have a low, moderate, high, or very high risk of developing a pressure ulcer? (Use the pressure ulcer risk assessment scale in Figure 6–2.)
- What measures would you suggest to prevent the development of pressure ulcers?

TABLE 6-5. PRESSURE ULCER CHARACTERISTICS

Characteristic	Definition	Comments
Location	Anatomic location of ulcer	Can be described in words or by mark on diagram of body.
Size	Length, width, and depth of the lesion	Length can be measured as largest diameter, width can be measured perpendicular to length.
		Alternatively, length can be measured as greatest distance in cephalad to caudal direction, width as greatest distance in line perpendicular to length.
		Depth can be measured at deepest point using sterile probe.
Shape	Configuration of wound's perimeter at the level of the skin surface	Can be documented with drawing or (preferably) photograph.
Stage	Depth of ulcer	Staging system presented in Table 6–6.
Nonblanchable erythema	Redness that persists when pressure is applied with a fingertip	Indicative of Stage I pressure ulcer. Should not be confused with reactive hyperemia, which is a normal response of intact skin. Reactive hyperemia is redness that blanches (turns white or pale) when pressure is applied by a fingertip.
Sinus tract	Cavity or channel underlying a wound that involves an area larger than the visible surface of the wound	Note presence or absence. If present, note location.
Undermining	A closed passageway under the surface of the skin that is open only at the skin surface; generally it appears as an area of skin ulceration at the margins of the ulcer with skin overlying the area	Often develops from shearing forces.
Tunneling	Passageway under the surface of the skin that is generally open at the skin level; however, most of the tunneling is not visible	Note presence or absence. If present, note location.
Exudate	Any fluid that has been extruded from a tissue or its capillaries, more specifically because of injury or inflammation	Note presence or absence. If present, describe amount, color, and opacity.
Eschar	Thick, leathery, necrotic tissue	Appearance: dark brown or black, adherent to ulcer bed.
Slough	Devitalized tissue in the process of separating from viable portions of the body	Appearance: white or yellow, adherent to ulcer bed in clumps or loose strings.
Granulation tissue	Tissue that contains new blood vessels, collagen, fibroblasts, and inflammatory cells, which fills an open, previously deep wound when it starts to heal	Appearance: pink or beefy red, moist, granular, shiny.
Epithelial tissue	Tissue made of epithelial cells that migrate across the surface of a healing wound	Appearance: pink or red. Extends across wound bed in partial thickness wounds, starts at wound periphery, and moves toward center of full-thickness wounds.

Sources: references 12, 73, 139.

address.[x] The condition of the periwound tissue is also relevant; any erythema, induration, or maceration should be noted. Color photographs on grid paper are useful for documenting the ulcer's initial and subsequent condition.[73]

Staging of Pressure Ulcers

The interventions indicated for a pressure ulcer depend on the characteristics of the ulcer. One important feature of pressure ulcers is their depth. Table 6–6 presents a classification system for grading or staging pressure ulcers according to their depth. This system, proposed by the National Pressure Ulcer Advisory Panel,[101] is recommended by the U.S. Department of Health and Human Services.[11, 12] Clinicians should be aware of the following limitations of the staging system: (1) Stage I pressure ulcers are difficult to detect in patients with darkly pigmented skin. (2) Stage I pressure ulcers may be superficial, or they may be evidence of deeper tissue damage. (3) The presence of eschar interferes with accurate staging of a pressure ulcer. Once eschar has been removed, the ulcer can be staged accurately.[10–12, 47]

A pressure ulcer that deteriorates can be assigned a new stage (restaged) to reflect its increased depth. For example, an ulcer that originally appears as a blister or shallow crater extending into the dermis may progress to the point where it presents as a deeper crater extending to the underlying fascia. In this instance, it would be appropriate to change its classification from Stage II to Stage III. In contrast, ulcers should *not* be restaged to reflect healing, since normal tissues are not restored as ulcers heal.[73, 149] Several scales have been developed to assess and document pressure ulcer healing.[8, 43, 78, 135, 138, 149] Figure 6–4 presents the PUSH tool, a scale for healing developed by the National Pressure Ulcer Advisory Panel.[139]

Comprehensive Examination

To treat a pressure ulcer effectively, the health care team must focus on the "whole picture" rather than on the ulcer alone. A variety of factors can contribute to the development of a pressure ulcer and its deterioration or healing, and the assessment must investigate these factors. Relevant areas to evaluate include the individual's medical and nutritional status, psychological and social factors, and possible sources of damaging forces or conditions affecting the skin.

---

[x] If an ulcer is painful, clinicians should also note this fact, as the pain will have to be managed during debriding and other ulcer care. More typically, however, people with spinal cord injuries develop pressure ulcers in areas that are insensitive to pain.

TABLE 6–6.   CLASSIFICATION OF PRESSURE ULCERS[a]

Stage	Characteristics
I	Nonblanchable erythema of intact skin; the heralding lesion of skin ulceration. In individuals with darker skin, discoloration of the skin, warmth, edema, induration, or hardness may also be indicators.[b]
II	Partial thickness skin loss involving epidermis, dermis, or both. The ulcer is superficial and presents clinically as an abrasion, blister, or shallow crater.
III	Full thickness skin loss involving damage or necrosis of subcutaneous tissue that may extend down to, but not through, underlying fascia. The ulcer presents clinically as a deep crater with or without undermining of adjacent tissue.
IV	Full thickness skin loss with extensive destruction, tissue necrosis, or damage to muscle, bone, or supporting structures (for example, tendon or joint capsule). Undermining and sinus tracts may also be associated with Stage IV pressure ulcers.

[a] Proposed by the National Pressure Ulcer Advisory Panel,[101] adapted and recommended by the U.S. Department of Health and Human Services.[12]

[b] Revised version of Stage I definition proposed by the National Pressure Ulcer Advisory Panel:[63] An observable pressure-related alteration of intact skin whose indicators as compared to an adjacent or opposite area on the body may include changes in skin color (red, blue, purple tones), skin temperature (warmth or coolness), skin stiffness, and/or sensation (pain).

PUSH Tool 3.0

Patient Name: _____ Patient ID#: _____

Ulcer Location: _____ Date: _____

DIRECTIONS:
Observe and measure the pressure ulcer. Categorize the ulcer with respect to surface area, exudate, and type of wound tissue. Record a sub-score for each of these ulcer characteristics. Add the sub-scores to obtain the total score. A comparison of total scores measured over time provides an indication of the improvement or deterioration in pressure ulcer healing.

	0 0 cm²	**1** <0.3 cm²	**2** 0.3-0.6 cm²	**3** 0.7-1.0 cm²	**4** 1.1-2.0 cm²	**5** 2.1-3.0 cm²	
Length x Width		**6** 3.1-4.0 cm²	**7** 4.1-8.0 cm²	**8** 8.1-12.0 cm²	**9** 12.1-24.0 cm²	**10** >24.0 cm²	**Sub-score**
Exudate Amount	**0** None	**1** Light	**2** Moderate	**3** Heavy			**Sub-score**
Tissue Type	**0** Closed	**1** Epithelial Tissue	**2** Granulation Tissue	**3** Slough	**4** Necrotic tissue		**Sub-score**
							Total score

Length x Width: Measure the greatest length (head to toe) and the greatest width (side to side) using a centimeter ruler. Multiply these two measurements (length x width) to obtain an estimate of surface area in square centimeters (cm2). Caveat: Do not guess! Always use a centimeter ruler and always use the same method each time the ulcer is measured.

Exudate Amount: Estimate the amount of exudate (drainage) present after removal of the dressing and before applying any topical agent to the ulcer. Estimate the exudate (drainage) as none, light, moderate, or heavy.

Tissue Type: This refers to the types of tissue that are present in the wound (ulcer) bed. Score as a "4" if there is any necrotic tissue present. Score as a "3" if there is any amount of slough present and necrotic tissue is absent. Score as a "2" if the wound is clean and contains granulation tissue. A superficial wound that is reepithelializing is scored as a "1". When the wound is closed, score as a "0".

  4 - Necrotic Tissue (Eschar): black, brown, or tan tissue that adheres firmly to the wound bed or ulcer edges and may be either firmer or softer than surrounding skin.
  3 - Slough: yellow or white tissue that adheres to the ulcer bed in strings or thick clumps, or is mucinous.
  2 - Granulation Tissue: pink or beefy red tissue with a shiny, moist, granular appearance.
  1 - Epithelial Tissue: for superficial ulcers, new pink or shiny tissue (skin) that grows in from the edges or as islands on the ulcer surface.
  0 - Closed/Resurfaced: the wound is completely covered with epithelium (new skin).

Figure 6–4. PUSH Tool (version 3.0) for documenting pressure ulcer healing. (Reproduced with permission of the National Pressure Ulcer Advisory Panel, 11250 Roger Bacon Drive, Suite 8, Reston, VA 20190-5202. Web address: www.NPUAP.org.)

Medical status. The comprehensive examination should investigate the overall health of the patient, with emphasis on determining whether there are any conditions that could affect the healing of the ulcer. Such conditions include cardiovascular disease, diabetes, hypertension or hypotension, urinary tract infection, pulmonary disease, and renal disease.[y]

Nutritional status. The examination should investigate whether the patient's diet is adequate to support healing of the ulcer. The diet should include adequate intake of protein (1.25 to 1.5 g protein/kg/day), calories (30 to 35 calories/kg/day), and vitamins and minerals. Laboratory tests may also be indicated. Serum albumin below 3.5 mg/dL, or a total lymphocyte count of less than 1800/mm^3 indicate clinically significant malnutrition. A drop in body weight of more than 15 percent is also significant.[12]

Psychological and social factors. The assessment should address psychological factors, since they can influence the patient's ability to participate in a skin care program. Impaired mental status, poor learning ability, or depression may limit an individual's capacity to learn or follow through with ulcer care and preventive measures.

Social support is also important. Particularly if the patient is staying at home, the health care team should assess the caregivers' ability to understand and implement the ulcer care and prevention program, as well as the community resources that are available.[12] They should also determine the patient's financial resources, insurance or other, to ensure that the intervention strategies planned are within the individual's means.[73]

Possible sources of skin damage. When a pressure ulcer develops, the source of the problem must be identified: did the skin breakdown occur as the result of trauma to the skin[z] sustained while lying in bed, during functional training, while sitting in a wheelchair, or while wearing an orthosis? Did skin maceration from incontinence or excessive sweating contribute to the problem? Was the skin subjected to friction as a result of repeated

motions caused by spasticity? Identification of the causative factors may make it possible to eliminate or reduce them.

Because pressure ulcers are caused by damaging forces exerted on the skin, it follows that a comprehensive examination of an individual with a pressure ulcer should include an investigation into the source(s) of these damaging forces. Discerning the most likely sources of skin damage is important because it enables the health care team to take corrective action. Eliminating damaging forces and conditions will enhance healing and reduce the likelihood of future breakdown.

One area to investigate is whether the individual's activities have subjected the skin to damaging pressure, shear, or friction. Examples of activities that could cause pressure ulcers include laying in bed with the head of the bed elevated, sliding the buttocks across a transfer board, practicing stair negotiation on the buttocks, sitting for periods of time that are too long for the individual's skin tolerance, allowing too much time to pass between pressure reliefs, and utilizing pressure relief methods that are inadequate. This list is by no means complete—there are virtually limitless ways to traumatize the skin during daily activities.

Faulty or inadequate equipment is another possible source of pressure ulcers. Skin damage can occur as the result of equipment that does not provide adequate pressure distribution to meet the patient's needs. This can be the result of equipment that was improperly selected, incorrectly adjusted or maintained, or has deteriorated over time. The equipment assessment should include the support surface of the individual's bed; the wheelchair cushion; the wheelchair's fit, components, and adjustment; and the fit and alignment of spinal or extremity orthoses. Assessment of equipment is indicated whether the pressure ulcer occurs during the patient's initial hospitalization or at any time later.

In addition to assessing a patient's activities and equipment, the health care team should look for any other possible sources of damaging forces on the skin. Improper positioning in the bed or wheelchair can cause shearing and excessive pressure. Clothes that are too tight or have heavy seams can exert damaging pressure on the skin. Spasticity that causes repeated motions of the extremities can cause friction as the extremities rub against bedclothes or other objects in the environment.

Finally, the health care team should investigate whether any other conditions may have contributed to the development of the pressure ulcer. Prolonged exposure to urine, feces, or perspiration is an example of such a condition.

---

[y] The comprehensive examination should also investigate the presence of complications resulting from the pressure ulcer. These complications include amyloidosis, endocarditis, heterotopic bone formation, maggot infestation, meningitis, perineal-urethral fistula, pseudoaneurysm, septic arthritis, sinus tract or abscess, squamous cell carcinoma in the ulcer, systemic effects of topical treatments, osteomyelitis, bacteremia, sepsis, and advancing cellulitis.[12]

[z] Here, "trauma" can refer to prolonged unrelieved pressure, friction, shear, or blunt force.

Health professionals should assess the individual's activities, equipment, and other potential sources of skin damage in an attempt to discern the most likely causes of the pressure ulcer. The ulcer's location is often a good starting point for this analysis, since it provides a clue about the source of the damaging forces. For example, an ulcer over the ischial tuberosities most likely developed as a result of excessive tissue loads in sitting or during transfers. The individual's wheelchair, cushion, sitting posture, sitting time, pressure relief frequency and technique, and transfer technique are possible problem areas to investigate. In contrast, an ulcer over the posterior heel is likely to result from damaging tissue loads when the patient is supine in bed or when he uses lower extremity orthoses. The patient's position in bed and turning schedule, as well as the bed's support surface, should be evaluated. If the patient wears orthoses, the wearing schedule and the orthoses' fit and alignment should be evaluated.

INTERVENTIONS

A comprehensive ulcer care program addresses both the ulcer itself and any factors that may contribute to its healing or the development of future pressure ulcers. Interventions include prevention of additional pressure ulcers, managing tissue loads, wound cleansing and debridement, use of dressings, managing bacterial colonization and infection, adjunctive therapies to promote wound healing, surgery (if indicated), optimization of the patient's health and nutritional status, and education and training.

Pressure Ulcer Prevention

Anyone with a spinal cord injury who has a pressure ulcer is at risk for developing additional ones. The limitations in activity and positioning necessary for ulcer or surgical flap healing result in greater time spent bearing weight on areas of unaffected skin, increasing the risk of breakdown in these areas. Moreover, once an ulcer heals, it leaves a scarred area that is vulnerable to trauma.

To avoid both the development of new skin breakdown and the recurrence of healed or surgically repaired pressure ulcers, the patient and health care team should develop and institute a pressure ulcer prevention program. Based on the results of their initial assessment, the team should work with the patient to correct any factors that may have contributed to the development of the ulcer or could result in future breakdown.

Managing Tissue Loads

Tissue load management involves protecting both the ulcer and areas of intact skin from damaging pressure, shear, and friction. Minimization of these external forces *on the pressure ulcer* will make it possible for the tissues to heal. Managing the tissue load *on areas of intact skin* will help prevent the development of additional ulcers.

First and foremost, pressure over the affected area must be avoided.[12, 47] A Stage I pressure sore may heal without any intervention other than this relief of pressure.[75] Depending on the source of trauma to the skin, pressure relief may involve adjusting an orthosis or avoiding a certain posture such as supine or sitting.[aa]

When a patient has multiple pressure ulcers, relief of pressure may be problematic: positioning in bed that avoids pressure on one ulcer is likely to involve weight bearing on another one. When this is the case, an air-fluidized or low air-loss bed may promote healing by reducing pressure over boney prominences.[12, 13, 16, 55, 145] Even if a patient has only one ulcer, it may limit the number of positions in which an individual can safely lie in bed. (For example, a sacral ulcer may necessitate the avoidance of supine.) This limitation will effectively increase the time spent in the remaining positions over the course of a day, increasing the risk of developing ulcers while in these positions. A specialized mattress or mattress overlay is indicated to reduce the tissue loads on these areas. Figure 6–5 presents a decision tree for selecting support surfaces to enhance healing and prevent the development of additional ulcers.[bb]

The turning schedule in bed may also have to be adjusted as a part of a pressure ulcer management program.[12] It may be necessary for the patient to turn in bed more frequently in order to keep tissue loads low enough to promote healing and prevent new ulcers from developing.

Cleansing and Debridement

Wound cleansing is a necessary component of any pressure ulcer care program. Ulcers should be cleaned initially and at every dressing change until they have healed. This cleansing reduces the potential for infection and enhances healing by

---

aa People who need to avoid sitting can utilize prone carts for out-of-bed activities. Although these carts are not as comfortable or functional as wheelchairs, they make it possible to be somewhat active and mobile, preventing some of the social and physical sequelae of enforced prolonged bedrest.[103]

bb Additional information on support surfaces and their selection is presented earlier in this chapter.

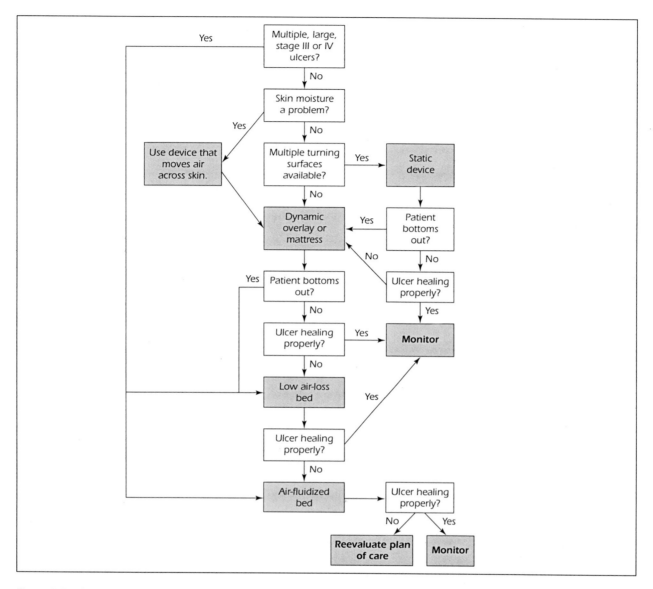

Figure 6–5.   Selection of mattress, mattress overlay, or bed for patient with pressure ulcer. (Adapted from Bergstrom, N., et al. [1994]. *Treatment of Pressure Ulcers*. Clinical Practice Guideline, Number 15. Rockville, MD: U.S. Department of Health and Human Services. Public Health Service, Agency for Health Care Policy and Research. AHCPR Publication No. 95-0652.)

removing nonadherent necrotic tissue, exudate, metabolic wastes, residual topical agents, and dressing residue.[6, 10, 12]

Cleansing is typically accomplished by irrigating the wound. Irrigation pressure should be between 4 and 15 pounds per square inch (psi). Pressures lower than 4 psi do not provide enough force to clean the wound adequately. Pressures higher than 15 psi can traumatize viable tissue and drive bacteria into the wound's tissues. Pressures in the 4 to 15 psi range can be achieved using a 35-mL syringe with a 19-gauge needle or angiocatheter.[12]

Normal saline is the cleansing solution of choice for most pressure ulcers. Irrigation with normal saline provides adequate cleaning in most cases, and this solution does not contain any potentially harmful chemicals. In contrast, many commercially available wound cleansers can be toxic to the wound's viable tissues.[6, 10, 12, 41, 73] Commercial wound cleansers containing surfactant may be indicated for wounds with adherent materials, but clinicians should take care to select solutions that do not contain harmful chemicals.[12]

Many pressure ulcers contain adherent necrotic tissue that cannot be removed by cleansing alone. Necrotic tissue prolongs inflammation, promotes bacterial growth, and interferes with wound healing. For this reason, it should be removed from pressure ulcers to enhance healing and reduce the risk of infection. Debridement of devitalized (necrotic) tissue can be achieved using sharp instruments, wet-to-dry dressings, whirlpool baths, pulsatile lavage, wound irrigation, dextranomers, enzymatic agents, or moisture-

TABLE 6–7. DEBRIDEMENT METHODS

Method	Description	Advantages and Indications	Disadvantages and Contraindications
Sharp debridement	Sharp instruments (scalpel, scissors, forceps) are used to remove devitalized tissue.	Most rapid method of debridement. Indicated for thick, adherent eschar in large ulcers, and when there are signs of advancing cellulitis or sepsis.	Requires skillful clinician. Viable tissue may be debrided.
Wet-to-dry dressings	Ulcer is packed with saline-soaked gauze, which is allowed to dry. Dry gauze adheres to necrotic tissue, so this tissue is removed when dry gauze is removed.	Low-cost materials. Supplies are readily available. Most appropriate for wounds in which wound bed is totally necrotic and those in which both necrotic and granulation or epithelial tissues are present.	Debridement is nonselective: dry gauze removes both viable and necrotic tissue. Granulation and epithelial tissues may be removed from the ulcer bed. Dressings packed too tightly into wound can create pressure within the wound, impeding healing or even causing additional necrosis. If the moist dressing extends beyond the wound margins, skin maceration and candidiasis can result. Wound bed can become desiccated, especially if the patient is on an air-fluidized bed.
Whirlpool	Ulcer is placed in tank of water that is agitated by whirlpool jets. Whirlpool should be followed by irrigation with saline solution.	Can be used to soften eschar and remove thick exudate, slough and loosely adherent necrotic tissue.	Force from whirlpool jets can damage granulation and epithelial tissue. Whirlpool treatments can be physiologically stressful for individuals with cardiovascular or respiratory compromise.
Pulsatile lavage	Wound is cleansed and debrided using device that provides pulsed irrigation (usually with normal saline) and simultaneously uses suction to remove cleaning solution and debris.	Alternative to whirlpool that allows wound cleansing and debridement without physiological challenge of transfers, transport, and immersion in whirlpool. Pressure of pulsatile lavage can be controlled. Can be used to soften, loosen, and remove necrotic tissue and thick exudate.	Units that provide lavage with excessive force may damage granulation and epithelial tissue. May be hazardous if wound is close to major blood vessels, bypass graft sites, or exposed blood vessel, nerve, tendon, or bone.

Method	Description	Indications/Advantages	Disadvantages
Wound irrigation	Wound is washed using syringe or irrigation device.	Can be used to soften eschar and remove unattached eschar and debris.	Inadequate force will not debride effectively. Excessive force can damage granulation and epithelial tissue.
Dextranomers	Small hydrophilic dextran polymer beads placed in wound absorb exudate, bacteria, and other debris. Available in paste formulation.	Indicated for treatment of infected or exudative wounds.	Expensive. Can be difficult to apply.
Enzymatic debridement	Topical debriding agent is applied to necrotic tissue. Enzymes break down devitalized tissue.	Efficacy in removing devitalized tissue and promoting healing has been demonstrated in several studies. Easily applied. Debridement is selective. Alternative to sharp debridement for patients who cannot tolerate it or are in a setting in which sharp debridement may be problematic.	May irritate periwound skin if not contained within the wound.
Autolytic debridement	Wound is covered with moisture-retentive dressing. Endogenous enzymes in wound fluids digest necrotic tissue.	Prevents wound dessication. Debridement is selective. Indicated for patients who cannot tolerate other forms of debridement and who are not likely to develop infections.	Takes longer than other methods of debridement. Not indicated for infected wounds. Improperly applied dressings can cause maceration of periwound skin, promote bacterial and fungal infection.

Sources: references 6, 10, 12, 41, 73, 85, 86, 116, 119, 134.

PROBLEM-SOLVING EXERCISE 6–2

Your patient is undergoing inpatient rehabilitation. She has been using a wheelchair for the past several weeks without exhibiting any problems with her skin. Yesterday, she began using a different wheelchair. All other relevant factors remained unchanged: the patient remained sitting for the same number of hours as usual, participated in her usual activities, continued performing pressure reliefs on the same schedule, and did not change cushions. When she went to bed and inspected her skin at the end of the day, she noticed redness over her ischial tuberosities. This redness blanched when touched with a finger. After 50 minutes, the redness disappeared. In the past, redness over this patient's ischial tuberosities has always resolved within 15 to 20 minutes.

- Does the redness over the patient's ischial tuberosities indicate that she has a pressure ulcer? If so, what stage is the pressure ulcer?
- You suspect that the redness over the patient's ischial tuberosities was caused by the change in wheelchairs. What characteristics of the new wheelchair could have caused this problem?
- What actions should you take to ensure that the patient does not develop a more serious problem in the skin overlying her ischial tuberosities?

retentive dressings.[1, 6, 12, 13, 41, 46, 55, 73, 75, 119, 130] Table 6–7 presents information on the various methods of wound debridement. Different methods of debridement are frequently combined.

Dressings

Dressings are used to protect pressure ulcers and create conditions that are conducive to healing. Conditions that promote healing include a clean and moist ulcer bed, dry surrounding tissues, an absence of unfilled empty space within the wound,[cc] and protection from infection and trauma from external forces.[12, 144]

A large variety of dressings are on the market. These dressings differ in the effects that they have on the wound environment. They also differ in cost per dressing as well as in the frequency with which they should be changed. Table 6–8 presents information on the different types of dressing that are available. Each type of dressing is available from a number of manufacturers. Clinicians should familiarize themselves with the characteristics and manufacturer's usage recommendations of the dressings that they utilize.

Clinicians should select dressings that are most appropriate for their patients. The most important factor in selecting dressings for an individual is the condition of the ulcer: the depth, presence or absence of infection, exudate, and nature of the tissues (necrotic, granulation, or epithelial). Additional considerations include cost,[dd] financial resources, caregiver time required for dressing changes, and (if the patient is at home) access to assistance and health care services.

Adjunctive Therapies to Promote Healing

In recent years, a number of adjunctive therapies have been utilized for the promotion of pressure ulcer healing. Probably the most widely used adjunctive therapy is high voltage electrical stimulation, which has been shown to increase the rate of pressure ulcer healing dramatically.[2, 57, 74] Low intensity direct current can also enhance wound healing.[23, 51] Studies demonstrating enhanced pressure ulcer healing with electrical stimulation have done so using a variety of protocols. For this reason, no one protocol is used universally.[12, 73]

Additional adjunctive therapies include pulsed nonthermal diathermy,[125] ultrasound,[25, 65, 75, 107] hyperbaric oxygen therapy,[25, 65, 73] low-energy laser,[53, 107] ultraviolet,[107] negative pressure therapy,[9, 99] and the application of growth factors.[29] Other than electrical stimulation and pulsed nonthermal diathermy, the efficacy of the various adjunctive therapies in promoting healing in pressure ulcers has yet to be demonstrated in controlled clinical studies.[29]

Managing Bacterial Colonization and Infection

All open (Stage II–IV) pressure ulcers are colonized with bacteria.[12] As long as the number of bacteria remains relatively low, this colonization should

---

[cc] Unfilled empty space within a wound, also called "dead space," can lead to the development of an abscess.[144]

[dd] Cost estimates should reflect the cost per dressing, the frequency of dressing changes, and the cost of nursing care.

not interfere with ulcer healing. When colonization progresses to infection, however, healing is slowed. A wound is considered to be infected (as opposed to colonized) when the bacterial count is greater than 100,000 organisms per gram of tissue.[41]

In addition to slowing healing, infection in a pressure ulcer can spread locally or systemically. Local spread of infection can cause cellulitis, osteomyelitis, infection of involved joints and bursae, and abscess formation.[97] Systemic spread of infection, bacteremia, can be fatal.[98, 126]

One important facet of ulcer care is the prevention of infection. In most cases, this can be accomplished through debridement of necrotic tissue, regular cleansing, dressings, and standard infection control practices.[10, 12] Topical antiseptics should not be used to control bacterial levels within wounds because they are toxic to the wound's viable tissues and can have systemic toxic effects.[10, 12, 151]

Evidence of infection in a pressure ulcer includes purulence, a foul odor, and inflammation in the tissues surrounding the wound. When these signs of local infection are present, the first response should be more frequent cleansing and debridement of any necrotic tissue left within the wound.[ee] If signs of infection continue, or if the wound does not show evidence of healing within 2 to 4 weeks, topical antibiotics should be applied to the wound. If a 2-week course of topical antibiotics does not lead to improved wound healing, the wound should be cultured[ff] and the patient should be evaluated for osteomyelitis in the bone underlying the ulcer.[12]

Although good wound care and topical antibiotics can control infection within a wound, they cannot control an infection once it has spread from the wound. Systemic antibiotics are indicated for anyone who develops advancing cellulitis, osteomyelitis, bacteremia, or sepsis.[12]

Surgery

Surgical closure of pressure ulcers is usually avoided if the wounds can heal satisfactorily with conservative management. One reason for this is that there is a high rate of ulcer recurrence over time after surgery.[gg] Another reason why pressure ulcers are managed conservatively, when possible, is that surgical closure utilizes healthy tissue. This can be problematic in the long run for patients who have recurring breakdown requiring multiple surgeries in the same area. A limited number of surgeries can be performed at a given site, since each surgery takes tissue from nearby areas of the patient's body, and this tissue is in finite supply.[47, 71, 110, 111]

Despite its limitations, surgical closure of pressure ulcers remains an important treatment option for many patients. Although many pressure ulcers can heal with conservative management, this process can take weeks or months when the ulcers are large and deep. Moreover, the healed area will be scarred and, therefore, will remain vulnerable to future breakdown. For these reasons, surgical closure may be considered for Stage III and IV pressure ulcers. For surgical closure of large wounds, a myocutaneous flap procedure has the advantage of filling the wound cavity and creating a well-vascularized and padded area.[13, 36, 40, 71, 130]

When surgery is planned, it is typically preceded by a period of debridement and dressing changes.[126] This period of preoperative management prepares the wound by ridding it of necrotic tissue and reducing the level of bacterial contamination.[126] Moreover, with good wound care during the preoperative period, the ulcer may shrink and as a result require less tissue coverage.[47]

Preoperative care also involves preparing the patient to heal optimally. Nutritional status should be optimized, and any medical conditions that could impede healing should be treated.[73] Smoking cessation during the preoperative period can also enhance healing after surgery.[12] A course of antibiotics is frequently administered pre- and postoperatively,[50, 97, 126] although this practice is not supported by research.[12]

Postoperative care includes a prolonged period of bedrest, with avoidance of pressure on the grafted area through positioning and use of a pressure-reducing support surface.[12, 36, 40] In addition, care should be taken to avoid friction, shearing,[12] or tension on the grafted tissue until adequate healing has occurred. Range-of-motion exercises must be suspended,[13] and antispasmodic medications may be administered to prevent excessive motion caused by spasticity.[130]

Once the surgical site has healed adequately, range-of-motion exercises can resume[54] and the patient can begin bearing weight on the flap. Weight bearing on the surgical site should be undertaken cautiously, with a gradual build-up of weight-bearing time, frequent pressure reliefs, and assessment

---

[ee] As a rule, it is best to use antibiotics only when necessary. Overuse of antibiotics in the past has led to the development of a number of resistant strains of bacteria.

[ff] The culture should be obtained through tissue biopsy or needle aspiration. Swab cultures may not give reliable information on the organisms infecting the ulcer's tissues.[12]

[gg] Reported recurrence rates vary widely.[29] In one study, patients with traumatic paraplegia had a 79 percent recurrence rate within a mean of 10.9 months after surgical repair of their pressure ulcers.[36]

TABLE 6-8. DRESSINGS

Dressing Type	Characteristics	Dressing Changes*	Advantages and Indications	Disadvantages and Contraindications
Alginate	Highly absorptive nonadherent dressing made from seaweed. Calcium alginate fibers become gel as they absorb exudate. Available in sheets or loose packing ribbon. Permeable to oxygen, water, and microorganisms.	Dressing can remain in place up to 7 days in clean wound, 1 day in infected wound.	Absorbs exudate while maintaining moist wound bed. Moist wound bed promotes autolytic debridement. Fills dead space. Indicated for infected or uninfected Stage II to IV ulcers with moderate to large amounts of exudate.	Not indicated for dry or minimally exudative wounds or wounds with black eschar. Can dehydrate wound bed. Should not be packed too tightly into wound. Requires secondary dressing. Does not provide protective barrier from microorganisms or urine.
Collagen	Nonadherent absorptive dressing made with collagen. Available in sheet, pad, gel, or particle form.	Dressing can remain in place up to 4 days in clean wound, 1 day in infected wound.	Absorbs exudate while maintaining moist wound bed. Moist wound bed promotes autolytic debridement. Fills dead space. Indicated for infected or uninfected Stage II to IV ulcers with minimal to moderate amounts of exudate.	Not indicated for highly exudative wounds or wounds with black eschar. Requires secondary dressing.

Continues

116

Type	Description	Duration	Advantages/Uses	Precautions/Contraindications
Film	Clear, adherent, nonabsorptive, polymer-based dressing. Permeable to oxygen and water vapor, not water or microorganisms.	Dressing can remain in place up to 7 days.	Transparency allows easy wound assessment. Protects wound from external forces, chemicals, and microorganisms. Provides moist environment, promotes autolytic debridement. Appropriate for uninfected superficial Stage I to II pressure ulcers. Can be used as primary dressing or secondary dressing over alginates or hydrogels.	Does not absorb exudate. Pooling of exudate under dressing can cause maceration. Contraindicated for deep, exudative, or infected wounds.
Foam	Sponge-like polymer dressing. May or not be adherent. May be impregnated or coated with other materials. Has some absorptive properties. Permeable to oxygen.	Dressing can remain in place 1 to 4 days or until saturated with exudate.	Absorbs exudate while maintaining moist wound bed. Moist wound bed promotes autolytic debridement. Protects wound from external forces. Can be used for mildly to moderately exudative Stage I to IV wounds. Can be used as primary dressing or as secondary dressing over alginates and amorphous hydrogels.	Not indicated for infected or highly exudative wounds. Nonadherent forms require secondary dressing.
Hydro-colloid	Adhesive, moldable wafer made of carbohydrate-based gel-forming material, usually with waterproof backing. Also available in paste or powder form. Most are impermeable to oxygen, water, water vapor, and microorganisms.	Dressing can remain in place up to 3 to 5 days or until exudate reaches dressing edge.	Absorbs exudate while maintaining moist wound bed. Promotes autolytic debridement. Protects wound from microorganisms. Does not require secondary dressing. Cost-effective. Can be used for Stage I to IV pressure ulcers that are mildly to moderately exudative and those that contain necrotic tissue.	Not indicated for wounds that are highly exudative or infected.

TABLE 6–8. DRESSINGS *(Continued)*

Dressing Type	Characteristics	Dressing Changes*	Advantages and Indications	Disadvantages and Contraindications
Hydrogel	Nonadherent, water- and polymer-based dressing. Has some absorptive properties. Available in sheet, impregnated gauze, or amorphous gel form. Permeable to oxygen and water vapor.	Dressing can remain in place 3 to 4 days.	Provides moist environment, promotes autolytic debridement. Protects wound from external forces and microorganisms. Fills dead space. Cost-effective. Indicated for dry or mildly to moderately exudative Stage I to IV wounds, infected or uninfected, with or without necrotic tissue. Can be used for wounds that require packing.	Highly exudative wounds. Hydrogels require secondary dressing.
Continuously moist saline gauze	Cotton or synthetic fabric gauze, moistened with saline and remoistened frequently to prevent drying. Gauze is permeable to water, water vapor, and oxygen.	Dressing remoistened after 4 hours, changed after 8 hours.	Low-cost materials. Supplies are readily available. Can be used for Stage II to IV ulcers.	If allowed to dry out, will desiccate wound bed and will damage healthy tissue when removed. Moist gauze can promote bacterial growth. Time-consuming due to frequent dressing remoistening and change. See additional disadvantages of gauze dressings below.

Dressing	Description	Advantages	Disadvantages/Comments
Wet-to-dry gauze dressing	Cotton or synthetic fabric gauze, moistened with saline and allowed to dry. Removal of dry dressing debrides wound. Gauze is permeable to water, water vapor, and oxygen. Dressing changed after 4 to 5 hours.	Low-cost materials. Supplies are readily available. Can be used to debride Stage II to IV ulcers in which wound bed is totally necrotic.	Dry gauze removes both viable and necrotic tissue. Granulation and epithelial tissues may be removed from the ulcer bed. Dressings packed too tightly into wound can create pressure within the wound, impeding healing or even causing additional necrosis. If the moist dressing extends beyond the wound margins, skin maceration and candidiasis can result. Wound bed can become desiccated, especially if the patient is on an air-fluidized bed. Gauze sheds, contaminating the wound. Time-consuming due to frequent dressing change. Not indicated for shallow pressure ulcers.
Wound fillers	Various forms of beads, gels, granules, strands, pads, pastes, powders. Recommended frequency of dressing change ranges from 2 to 3 per day to 7 days. Frequency depends on the product used, amount of exudate, and presence or absence of infection.	Absorbs exudate while maintaining moist wound bed. Moist wound bed promotes autolytic debridement. Fills dead space. Indicated for moderately to highly exudative deep Stage II to IV wounds, infected or uninfected, with or without necrotic tissue.	

* Clinicians should obtain product information from manufacturers to ensure appropriate use of dressings.

Sources: references 12, 33, 41, 65, 122, 136, 144, 148.

of the skin's status after each sitting session.[12, 36, 47] The physical therapist should assess the patient's wheelchair and cushion to ensure that pressure distribution is adequate. The team should also reinstruct the patient in ulcer prevention strategies.[47]

Nutrition and Health

In addition to treatment of the ulcer itself, optimal pressure ulcer management addresses the patient's general health. Treatment of anemia, hypoalbuminemia, and edema may promote pressure ulcer healing.[75] Systemic antibiotics are indicated for patients who develop abscesses, advancing cellulitis, osteomyelitis, bacteremia, or sepsis.[1, 12, 13, 75, 130]

The patient's nutritional status is also important. Wound healing requires an adequate intake of proteins, carbohydrates, fats, vitamins, minerals, and fluids.[14, 17, 25, 65, 87, 119] Supplemental vitamin C and a high-calorie, high-protein diet may facilitate wound healing. Zinc, iron, magnesium, and vitamin A supplements may be indicated, particularly for people with deficiencies of these nutrients.[1, 25, 55, 75, 130]

Education and Training

Education and training are necessary components of every pressure ulcer care program. This education and training should develop the knowledge and skills required to perform ongoing assessments of the ulcer's status, prevent the development of additional pressure ulcers, and facilitate healing through the management of external forces on the wound, wound cleansing, and dressing changes.

The patient, family, and any others involved in the patient's care should be included in the ulcer care education and training program. The focus of the various participants' education and training will depend on the expected nature of their participation in the ulcer care program. The roles of the different people involved in the wound care program will be determined by the setting (inpatient, outpatient, day hospital, or home). If the patient is at home, the availability of home-health services will influence the degree of responsibility that the patient and family will have for the ulcer care program.

SUMMARY

- Spinal cord injury leads to life-long vulnerability to the development of pressure ulcers, a complication that can have profound medical, functional, and social consequences. Because pressure ulcers are both preventable and serious, skin care is a critical focus of medical management, rehabilitation, and health maintenance following spinal cord injury.

- Preventive skin care after spinal cord injury includes a balanced diet, proper management of bowel and bladder incontinence, avoidance of damaging forces on the skin, and close monitoring of the skin's status. Special attention is given to avoiding prolonged, unrelieved pressure on the skin, particularly over boney prominences.

- Pressure ulcer prevention while in bed involves positioning, regular turning, and the use of a support surface (bed, mattress, or mattress overlay) that is suitable to the individual's needs. Pressure ulcer prevention while in a wheelchair involves positioning, regular pressure reliefs, an appropriate wheelchair cushion, and the use of a wheelchair with dimensions, components, and adjustment that are suitable to the individual's needs.

- Skin inspection is a critical component of pressure ulcer prevention. Regular skin checks give feedback about the effectiveness of the individual's pressure ulcer prevention program, and make it possible to detect early signs of potential breakdown and intervene before it progresses.

- Pressure ulcer care starts with an assessment of the ulcer and a comprehensive examination to identify factors that may have contributed to the development of the ulcer or that may interfere with wound healing.

- Once a comprehensive pressure ulcer assessment has been completed, a wound care program is designed to promote wound healing and prevent the development of additional ulcers. Interventions include correcting any factors that may have contributed to the development of the pressure ulcer, managing tissue loads, cleansing the ulcer, debriding all devitalized tissue, the use of dressings, managing bacterial colonization and infection, adjunctive therapies to promote wound healing, surgery (if indicated), optimization of the patient's health and nutritional status, and education and training.

- People with spinal cord injuries and everyone who will be involved in their care after discharge must learn all aspects of pressure ulcer prevention in order to maintain their skin integrity. Those who have pressure ulcers must also learn ulcer care.

Respiratory Management

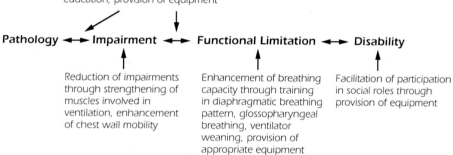

Prevention of secondary conditions through secretion clearance, enhancement of breathing capacity, provision of mechanical ventilation, training in self-cough, education, provision of equipment

Pathology ←→ Impairment ←→ Functional Limitation ←→ Disability

Reduction of impairments through strengthening of muscles involved in ventilation, enhancement of chest wall mobility

Enhancement of breathing capacity through training in diaphragmatic breathing pattern, glossopharyngeal breathing, ventilator weaning, provision of appropriate equipment

Facilitation of participation in social roles through provision of equipment

The respiratory system performs the critical functions of supplying oxygen to and removing carbon dioxide from the body. Spinal cord injury alters this functioning. Depending on the level of lesion, respiratory dysfunction after a spinal cord injury can range in severity from reduced cough effectiveness to a complete inability to breathe.

Respiratory complications are the most prevalent source of morbidity and mortality after spinal cord injury.[28, 30, 31, 55, 56] Many of these complications can be avoided with proper care. Rehabilitation professionals should be familiar with the respiratory sequelae of spinal cord injury, and should work with their patients to develop their ability to breathe and to prevent complications.

Pulmonary function tests are used to examine breathing ability. Table 7–1 presents the various measures and their normal values.

REVIEW OF NORMAL BREATHING

Breathing, or ventilation, is achieved through motions of the ribs and diaphragm. These motions alter the volume of the thoracic cavity, a space bounded by the ribs, sternum, vertebral column, and diaphragm. When the volume within this cavity increases, intrathoracic pressure falls and air is drawn into the lungs. When the space within the thoracic cavity decreases, intrathoracic pressure rises and air moves out of the lungs. The motions involved are illustrated in Figure 7–1.

Motions Involved in Inhalation

Movements that increase the cephalocaudal, anteroposterior, or transverse dimensions of the thoracic cavity cause inhalation.[67, 90, 96] The cephalocaudal dimension of the thoracic cavity increases when the diaphragm descends. The relaxed diaphragm is dome-shaped and extends superiorly into the thorax. When it contracts, it flattens and moves caudally. Because the diaphragm is the caudal boundary of the thoracic cavity, its descent increases the cavity's volume.[16]

Anteroposterior chest expansion occurs when the upper ribs are elevated. At rest, the upper

TABLE 7–1.   PULMONARY FUNCTION TESTS

Measure	Abbreviation	Definition	Normal Values
Tidal volume	TV	The volume of air normally inhaled in one breath during quiet respiration.	~500 mL
Inspiratory reserve volume	IRV	The maximum volume of air that can be inhaled after a normal quiet inspiration.	~3000 mL
Expiratory reserve volume	ERV	The maximum volume of air that can be exhaled after a normal exhalation during quiet breathing.	~1500 mL
Residual volume	RV	The volume of air that remains in the lungs after a maximal exhalation.	~1000 mL
Vital capacity	VC	The maximum volume of air that can be exhaled by forceful exhalation following maximal inhalation. (Equal to the sum of the TV, IRV, and ERV.)	~5000 mL
Total lung capacity	TLC	The volume of air in the lungs at the end of a maximal inhalation. (Equal to the sum of TV, IRV, ERV, and RV.)	~6000 mL
Inspiratory capacity	IC	The maximum volume of air that can be inspired from the end of a normal quiet exhalation. (Equal to the sum of the TV and the IRV.)	~3500 mL
Functional residual capacity	FRC	The volume of air that remains in the lungs at the end of a normal quiet exhalation. (Equal to the sum of ERV and RV.)	~2500 mL
Forced expiratory volume in 1 second	FEV_1	The volume of air that can be expired in 1 second by forceful exhalation following maximal inhalation. (Often expressed as percentage of vital capacity.)	~80% of VC
Maximum positive expiratory pressure	PEP	The maximal positive pressure generated during forced expiration.	Male: 247 cm H_2O Female: 160 cm H_2O
Maximum negative inspiratory pressure	NIP	The maximal negative pressure generated during maximal inhalation.	Male: 132 cm H_2O Female: 94 cm H_2O
Peak expiratory flow	PEF	Maximum rate of air movement during forced expiration.	9.10 liters/second

Normal values vary with age, gender, and height. Most normal values were established in males. Reported normal values also vary between sources.

Sources: references 39, 64b, 67, 73b, 97, 100.

ribs slope downward as they curve forward from the vertebral column to the sternum. When these ribs are elevated, their motion is similar to that of a pump handle: they pivot about an axis located posteriorly where the ribs articulate with the vertebrae. The sternum moves forward and rostrally when this occurs (Figure 7–2A), increasing the anteroposterior dimension of the thoracic cage.[23, 90, 96]

Transverse chest expansion occurs when the lower ribs are elevated. Like the upper ribs, the lower ribs in their resting position slope downward as they extend forward and around the chest

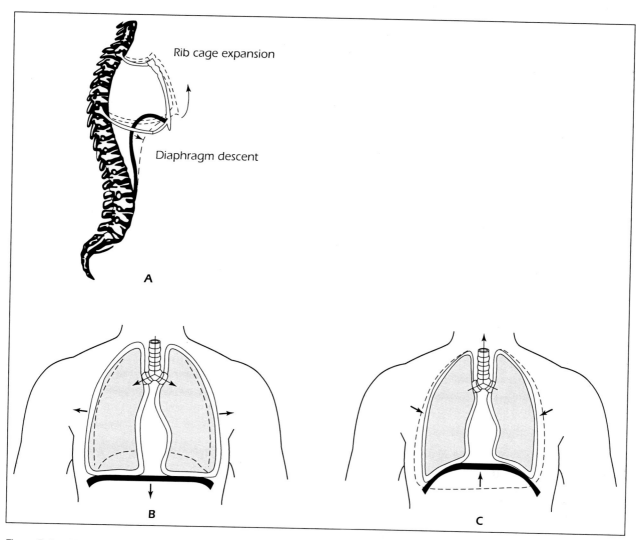

Figure 7–1. *Mechanism of normal breathing.* **(A)** Rib cage expansion and diaphragm descent cause inhalation. **(B)** During inhalation, rib cage expansion and diaphragm descent increase the volume within the thoracic cavity. Intrathoracic pressure falls, and air is drawn into the lungs. **(C)** During exhalation, the rib cage contracts and the diaphragm ascends. Intrathoracic pressure rises, and air is forced out of the lungs. *(Adapted from Fundamentals of Anatomy and Physiology, 4/E by Martini. Reprinted with permission Pearson Education, Inc.)*

from the vertebral column. Their motion during elevation is different, however, because they move about a different axis of rotation. When they elevate, the lower ribs pivot on an axis that runs through both their posterior and anterior attachments. As a result, the motion of the lower ribs during elevation is similar to that of a bucket handle when it is lifted (Figure 7–2B): when the ribs are raised, they swing up and out.[23, 90, 96]

Muscles Involved in Inhalation

During normal breathing, inspiration involves the coordinated action of a number of muscles. These muscles and their actions are illustrated in Figure 7–3A.

Diaphragm. The diaphragm is the principle muscle used in inhalation, contributing most of

the vital capacity[a] during normal breathing. It originates from the lumbar vertebrae, sternum, lower four ribs, and lower six costal cartilages, and inserts into a central tendon.[23, 58, 67] When the diaphragm is relaxed, upward (cephalad) pressure from the abdominal contents pushes it into a dome-shaped resting position. The dome shape and superior position at rest contribute to the efficient functioning of this muscle. Its fibers are elongated in this position, enabling them to generate force more effectively due to the length-tension relationship of muscle contraction.[25, 58] The diaphragm flattens and moves caudally when it contracts, increasing the volume within the thoracic cavity and drawing air into the lungs.

---

[a] Vital capacity and other measures of pulmonary function are defined in Table 7–1.

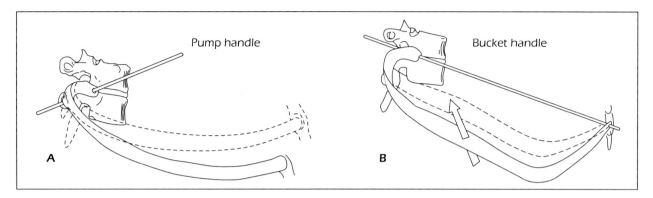

Figure 7–2.   Rib motions during breathing. **(A)** "Pump handle" motions in the upper ribs. **(B)** "Bucket handle" motions in the lower ribs. (From *Hollinshead's Textbook of Anatomy* [5th ed.] by Rosse, C., & Gaddum-Rosse, P. [1997]. Philadelphia, PA: Lippincott-Raven. Reprinted by permission of Lippincott Williams & Wilkins.)

Because the diaphragm lies immediately cephalad to the abdominal cavity, it exerts pressure on the abdominal viscera when it descends. This descent causes the abdominal contents to protrude. When the abdominal contents have protruded as far as the abdominal wall will allow, further descent of the diaphragm is blocked. Continued diaphragmatic contraction then results in elevation of the lower ribs, which in turn causes lateral chest expansion due to the bucket-handle action of the ribs.[23, 24, 77, 96]

Intercostals and accessory muscles. The intercostals and accessory muscles contribute sig-

nificantly to normal breathing through their action on the ribs. These muscles stabilize the rib cage during inhalation, preventing the ribs from being drawn downward when the diaphragm descends. They also elevate the ribs, especially during deep inspiration. By stabilizing and elevating the ribs, the accessory muscles and intercostals contribute to the increase in intrathoracic volume that is required for inhalation.[58]

The intercostal muscles consist of three layers. From most superficial to deepest, they are the external intercostals, the internal intercostals, and the transversus thoracis. Contraction of the intercostals pulls the ribs closer together. If the first rib

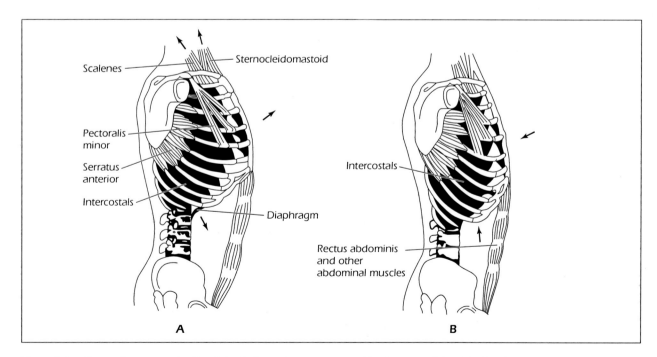

Figure 7–3.   The respiratory muscles. The abdominal muscles are represented by the rectus abdominis. Muscles that stabilize or play a minor role in normal breathing are not shown. **(A)** Inhalation: The sternocleidomastoids, scalenes, pectoralis minor, serratus anterior, intercostals, and diaphragm contract to increase the volume within the thoracic cavity. **(B)** Forced exhalation: The abdominals and intercostals contract to decrease the volume within the thoracic cavity.
(Adapted from *Fundamentals of Anatomy and Physiology, 4/E* by Martini. Reprinted with permission Pearson Education, Inc.)

is stabilized,[b] this opposition of the ribs causes them to elevate.[67, 96] The intercostals also aid in inspiration by preventing the tissues between the ribs from drawing inward when the intrathoracic pressure falls. By making the intercostal spaces more rigid, these muscles make it possible for rib and diaphragm motions to more effectively cause air movement rather than causing distortion of the intercostal tissues.[23, 81, 96]

A variety of accessory muscles aid in inspiration. The scalenes stabilize and may help elevate the rib cage during quiet inhalation.[16] During deep or forced inspiration, additional accessory muscles contract to add force to the inspiratory effort and increase the expansion of the thoracic cage. The scalenes elevate the first two ribs, and the sternocleidomastoids elevate the sternum. The serratus anterior, pectoralis minor, levators costarum, and serratus posterior superior assist in rib elevation. The trapezius, erector spinae, rhomboids major and minor, and levator scapulae stabilize the head, neck, and scapulae so that the accessory muscles listed above can act on the thoracic cage. The pectoralis major can assist in rib elevation when the arms are fixed. Finally, the erector spinae also aid in inspiration by extending the trunk.[16, 23, 67, 81, 96]

Abdominals. The rectus abdominis, internal and external obliques, and transversus abdominis aid in inhalation by providing support to the abdominal viscera, which in turn support the diaphragm in its optimal position for functioning. During inspiration, the abdominals relax to allow the viscera to protrude. This motion makes it possible for the diaphragm to descend.[23, 24, 25, 58]

Motions Involved in Exhalation

Movements that reduce the anteroposterior, transverse, or cephalocaudal dimensions of the thoracic cavity cause exhalation. During quiet breathing, exhalation primarily involves the passive return of the rib cage and diaphragm to their pre-inspiratory positions. During forced expiration, such as occurs in coughing or during heavy exercise, the ribs are drawn downward and the diaphragm is pushed upward to increase the intrathoracic pressure and force air out of the lungs.[16, 23, 67, 96]

Muscles Involved in Exhalation

Exhalation during quiet breathing occurs as a result of passive recoil of the lungs and chest wall as the inspiratory muscles relax. Forced expiration is an active event in which the abdominals and intercostals contract to force air out of the lungs. The muscles involved are illustrated in Figure 7–3B.

Abdominals. The abdominals are the primary muscles of forced expiration. When the external and internal obliques, transversus abdominis, and rectus abdominis contract strongly, they push the abdominal viscera upward against the diaphragm. This upward force moves the diaphragm superiorly into the thoracic cage, pushing air out of the lungs.[16, 23, 58, 67]

The abdominals can also add to the force of exhalation by flexing the trunk.[16, 23] This motion aids in the upward movement of the abdominal viscera and diaphragm. Finally, the abdominals aid in forced expiration through their action on the ribs. The external obliques stabilize the twelfth rib, enabling the intercostals to perform their expiratory function.[96]

Intercostals. Contraction of the intercostals draws the ribs closer together. If the twelfth rib is fixed caudally, intercostal contraction results in depression of the ribs.[96] This rib depression causes a reduction of the anteroposterior and mediolateral dimensions of the thoracic cavity due to the pump-handle and bucket-handle motions of the ribs, described above. Caudal fixation of the ribs is performed by the abdominal obliques, quadratus lumborum, and serratus posterior inferior.[16, 77, 81, 90, 96]

The intercostals also aid in expiration by preventing the intercostal tissues from bulging outward when intrathoracic pressure rises. This reinforcement of the intercostal spaces enables rib and diaphragm motions to more efficiently cause air movement in and out of the lungs rather than bulging of the intercostal tissues.[23, 96]

Diaphragm. Although it is primarily an inspiratory muscle, the diaphragm is also active during expiration. It contracts eccentrically for up to two thirds of expiration, working against the upward (cephalad) force of the abdominal contents. The effect of this eccentric contraction of the diaphragm is to slow the flow of air from the lungs.[25]

Influence of Postural Alignment

Breathing is effected by a variety of muscles working in concert to expand and contract the space

---

[b] Some sources state that the intercostals stabilize the ribs during quiet inhalation and contract more forcefully to elevate them during deep inhalation.[16, 58]

within the thoracic cavity. The muscles of ventilation work optimally when they are in a slightly lengthened position, due to the length-tension relationship of muscle contraction. The alignment of the trunk, neck, and shoulder girdle determines the length of these muscles, and thus influences breathing ability. For example, the scalenes and sternocleidomastoids can work more effectively to expand the upper chest when the cervical spine is extended, as this position places these muscles on a slight stretch.[71]

Trunk and shoulder girdle alignment also influence breathing through their direct impact on movements of the thoracic cage and diaphragm. Postures that limit chest expansion or diaphragm motions make inhalation more difficult. For example, thoracic kyphosis and protracted scapulae make inhalation more difficult by impeding rib elevation.[71] Lumbar flexion, or a posteriorly tilted pelvis, can interfere with inhalation by limiting caudal displacement of the abdominal viscera, which in turn blocks diaphragm descent.

REVIEW OF NORMAL COUGHING

Coughing is an important action by which a person clears her airways when food or other foreign substances enter the trachea from the pharynx, or when respiratory secretions are too thick or copious to be cleared effectively by the normal action of the cilia lining the trachea.[72] During a respiratory tract infection, an inability to cough can lead to atelectasis, pneumonia, and ventilatory failure.[13]

Coughing involves coordinated action of the glottis and the muscles of ventilation. A cough occurs in stages: maximal inhalation, glottis closure, contraction of the muscles of forced exhalation with the glottis closed, and continued forced exhalation with the glottis open.[63, 72, 105] The motions and muscles involved in inhalation and forced exhalation are described in the previous section.

IMPACT OF SPINAL CORD INJURY ON BREATHING AND COUGHING ABILITY

Neurological Level of Injury

After a spinal cord injury, a person's ability to breathe and cough depends largely on the functioning of her ventilatory muscles, which in turn is influenced by the level of her cord lesion.[58, 91, 100] Higher lesions affect breathing and coughing most profoundly because they interrupt innervation to muscles involved in both inhalation and exhalation. Lower lesions leave most of the muscles of inhalation intact, but interfere with the functioning of the muscles used for forced exhalation. Table 7–2 presents the innervation and actions of the muscles involved in breathing.

The following descriptions of ventilatory function after spinal cord injury refer to complete lesions. Breathing and coughing capabilities after an incomplete lesion will depend upon the degree to which motor sparing occurs in the ventilatory muscles innervated below the lesion.

C1 and C2. An individual with a C1 or C2 neurological level of injury[c] retains partial innervation of her sternocleidomastoid, trapezius, and erector spinae, but loses the use of her diaphragm and all other muscles of ventilation. Using the innervated accessory muscles, she may be able to inhale a minimal amount of air.[58] This air movement will be inadequate for survival. Because she lacks a functioning diaphragm, the person with C1 or C2 tetraplegia will require ventilatory support.[d] Additionally, forced expiration will not be possible; exhalation will occur as a result of passive recoil of the lungs and rib cage. The individual will require assistance for airway clearance.

C3. At this level, the diaphragm retains partial innervation. The accessory muscles are more functional, due to full innervation of the sternocleidomastoid and partial innervation of the levator scapulae, scalenes, and rhomboids. The weakly functioning diaphragm and accessory muscles may be able to create sufficient motions of the thoracic cavity to allow for independent breathing. These muscles are likely to fatigue quickly, however, resulting in ventilatory failure.[53, 58] For this reason, the person with C3 tetraplegia will require ventilatory support, at least during the acute stage after injury. Fortunately, ventilator weaning is frequently possible.[87]

Forced expiration will not be possible for a person with C3 tetraplegia; exhalation will occur as a result of passive recoil of the lungs and rib cage, and cephalad pressure from the abdominal contents. The individual will require assistance for airway clearance.

---

[c] Neurological level of injury, as defined by the American Spinal Injury Association, is discussed in Chapter 2.
[d] With training, people can learn to breathe for limited periods of time using their neck accessory musculature (neck breathing) or using mouth, throat, and pharynx musculature (glossopharyngeal breathing).[42]

C4. A person with C4 tetraplegia retains almost full innervation of her diaphragm, the primary muscle of inspiration. Paralysis of her abdominal muscles, however, interferes with the diaphragm's functioning. Because her abdominal muscles are unable to support her viscera, her diaphragm will descend and flatten when she sits with her torso elevated above horizontal. This mechanically disadvantageous diaphragm position will compromise her ability to inhale. Inhalation will be further impaired due to a lack of functioning in the intercostals.

Soon after an injury at this level, the average vital capacity is approximately 24 percent of normal. Although many people with C4 tetraplegia require mechanical ventilation during the acute phase following injury, most are able to develop the capacity for independent breathing without mechanical support.[59]

Although a person with C4 tetraplegia is likely to retain or develop the ability to breathe independently, she will be unable to cough effectively. Because she lacks innervation of her abdominals and intercostals, she will be unable to perform the forceful exhalation involved in coughing. As a result, she will require assistance for airway clearance.

C5 through C8. People with neurological levels of injury from C5 through C8 retain full use of their diaphragms and nearly full innervation in their accessory muscles. For this reason, their capacity for independent breathing is stronger than that exhibited by people with higher lesions. Ventilatory failure occurs less frequently and resolves more rapidly than it does in patients with higher lesions.[50] Because innervation in the intercostal and abdominal musculature is lacking, however, inhalation and forced exhalation remain impaired.[58] Vital capacity soon after the onset of C5 or lower tetraplegia averages approximately 30 percent of normal.[59]

Forced exhalation is impaired at these levels of tetraplegia, due to the absence of intercostal and abdominal motor function. Some capacity for cough is retained, however, through substitution using the clavicular portion of the pectoralis major. This muscle, which receives C5 and C6 innervation, can depress the sternum and upper ribs during coughing.[37, 65]

T1 through T5. Spinal cord injuries with T1 through T5 neurological level of injury differ from higher injuries in that intercostal function is preserved at and above the neurological level of injury. This preserved motor function may slightly enhance a person's capacity for both inhalation and forced exhalation. This enhancement will be limited, however, as the abdominals and the majority of the intercostals remain nonfunctional.[58]

T6 through T12. People with T6 through T12 paraplegia retain the use of those abdominal and intercostal muscles that are innervated above their lesions. This additional motor function enhances their ability to perform both inhalation and forced exhalation, including coughing. This enhanced ability to breathe and cough is more evident in people with lower lesions because they have more motor function preserved in these muscles.[82]

Below T12. Spinal cord damage with a neurological level of injury below T12 leaves intact the vast majority of muscles involved in ventilation,[e] and thus does not have a significant effect on a person's ability to breathe or cough. Respiratory dysfunction may occur, however, as a result of other problems such as prolonged bed rest.

Postural Influences

Following spinal cord injury, a person who lacks innervation of her abdominal musculature typically breathes most easily in supine. In upright postures, her abdominal viscera are allowed to descend and protrude due to a lack of muscular support from the abdominal wall. As a result, her diaphragm descends and flattens to a lower resting position, which places it in a mechanically disadvantageous position and thus impairs inspiration. In contrast, in the supine position gravity exerts force on the abdominal contents that pushes them inward and rostrally so that they support the diaphragm in its normal resting position.[1, 21, 36]

Paradoxical Breathing Pattern

When rib stabilization by the intercostals is lacking, as occurs with cervical and high thoracic spinal cord injuries, abnormal rib motions occur during breathing. When the diaphragm contracts and descends during inhalation, the resulting decrease in intrathoracic pressure pulls the unstabilized ribs caudally and inward. Instead of expanding in its anteroposterior and lateral dimensions during inspiration, the chest decreases

---

e The exceptions are the internal obliques (T7-L1) and quadratus lumborum (T12-L4), both of which assist in forced expiration.

TABLE 7–2. INNERVATION AND ACTIONS OF VENTILATORY MUSCLES

Inhalation Muscles	Actions	Supraspinal	C1	C2
Sternocleidomastoid	Elevates the sternum during deep or forced inhalation.	■ (Black)		■ (Black)
Trapezius	Stabilizes the head, neck, and scapula to enable accessory muscles to elevate the ribs during deep or forced inhalation.	▦ (Grey)		▦ (Grey)
Erector spinae	Stabilize the neck to enable accessory muscles to elevate the ribs and extend the trunk to enhance chest expansion during deep or forced inhalation.		■ (Black)	■ (Black)
Levator scapulae	Stabilize the scapula to enable accessory muscles to elevate the ribs during deep or forced inhalation.			
Scalenes	Stabilize and may help elevate ribs 1 and 2 during quiet inhalation. Elevate ribs 1 and 2 during deep or forced inhalation.			
Rhomboid major and minor	Stabilize the scapula to enable accessory muscles to elevate the ribs during deep or forced inhalation.			
Diaphragm	Descends and moves caudally to increase the cephalocaudal dimension of the thoracic cavity. Elevates the lower ribs when abdominal viscera blocks further descent at the end of inhalation.			
Serratus anterior	Assists in rib elevation during deep or forced inhalation.			
Pectoralis minor	Assists in rib elevation during deep or forced inhalation.			
Pectoralis major, sternal portion	Assists in rib elevation during deep or forced inhalation.			
Intercostals	Elevate the ribs when upper ribs are stabilized, and increase the rigidity of the intercostal spaces.			
Levatores costorum	Assist in rib elevation during deep or forced inhalation.			
Serratus posterior superior	Assists in rib elevation during deep or forced inhalation.			
Abdominals	Provide support to the abdominal viscera, which support the diaphragm in its optimal position for functioning.			
Exhalation				
Pectoralis major, clavicular portion	Can be used to depress the sternum and upper ribs during coughing.			
Intercostals	Depress the ribs when the lower ribs are stabilized, and increase the rigidity of the intercostal spaces.			
Rectus abdominis	Push abdominal viscera rostrally against the diaphragm to increase intrathoracic pressure during forced exhalation and coughing.			
External obliques	Push abdominal viscera rostrally against the diaphragm to increase intrathoracic pressure during forced exhalation and coughing. Stabilize the 12th rib during forced exhalation and coughing, enabling intercostals to draw the ribs caudally.			
Transversus abdominis	Push abdominal viscera rostrally against the diaphragm to increase intrathoracic pressure during forced exhalation and coughing.			
Internal obliques	Push abdominal viscera rostrally against the diaphragm to increase intrathoracic pressure during forced exhalation and coughing.			
Serratus posterior inferior	Depresses the lower ribs during forced exhalation and coughing.			
Quadratus lumborum	Depresses the 12th rib during forced exhalation and coughing.			

This chart presents spinal segment innervation and muscle actions of the muscles involved in breathing and coughing. Because no two sources agree perfectly about either spinal segment innervation or muscle action, this chart contains an amalgamation of the information from several different texts, presenting the points of greatest agreement among the various sources. Key: Black indicates main segmental innervation at that spinal level. Grey indicates additional innervation at that spinal level.

Sources: references 54, 58, 65, 67, 77, 81, 90.

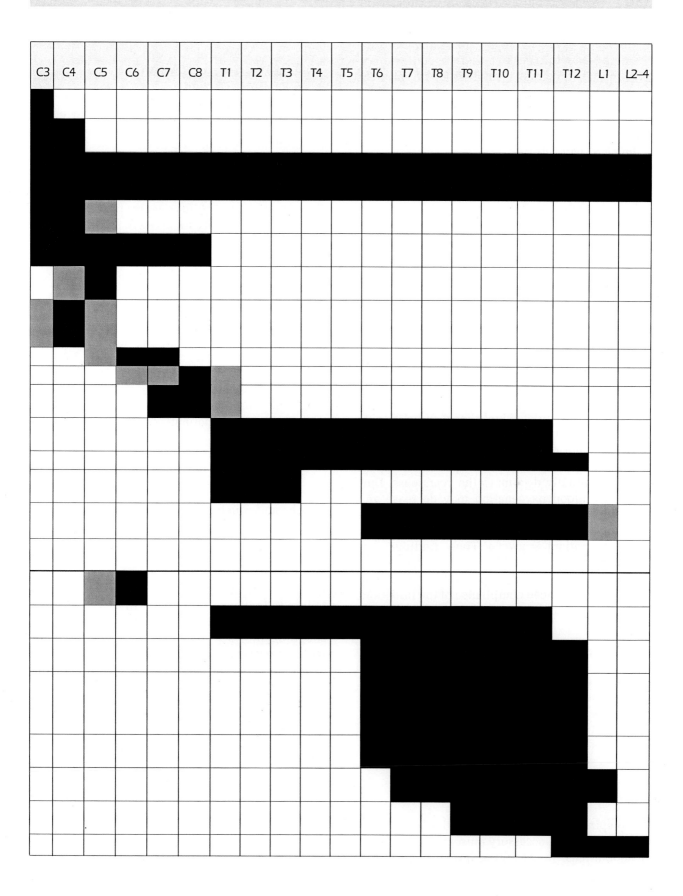

in diameter. This motion, called a paradoxical breathing pattern, causes a reduction in the volume of air inspired.[1] Paradoxical rib motions become less pronounced as time passes, due to increased tone in the intercostal muscles.[46]

Changes over Time

Breathing is most impaired during the early phase after a spinal cord injury. Respiratory function begins to improve within a few weeks of injury, with rapid gains typically seen in the first 5 weeks and continued improvement during the first few months post injury. Vital capacity is likely to double[f] during this time.[58, 59] Additional gains in vital capacity may continue to occur for several years after the injury.[14]

A number of factors may contribute to the improvement of respiratory status during the early months after spinal cord injury. Possible contributing factors include motor return, increasing strength in the accessory muscles and diaphragm, return of tone in the intercostals and abdominals with the resolution of spinal shock, and stiffening of the joints of the rib cage.[46, 58, 59, 82, 94]

Although respiratory function typically improves for a period of time after spinal cord injury, it may eventually decline as the years pass. During sleep, blood oxygenation may decrease and hypercapnia increase despite improvement in vital capacity measurements in sitting and supine when the patient is awake. These findings, evidence of chronic alveolar hypoventilation, may be caused by normal aging, increased obesity and inactivity, or reduced compliance of the lungs and chest wall with chronic spinal cord injury.[14]

Phonation

After spinal cord injury, speech may be impaired due to inadequate breath support. Breath support for speech requires adequate inspiration, followed by controlled exhalation involving eccentric contraction of the muscles of inhalation.[70]

RESPIRATORY COMPLICATIONS

When spinal cord injury disrupts the functioning of the diaphragm, accessory muscles, intercostals, or abdominals, the resulting impaired ability to

---

[f] Other studies have shown that pulmonary function improves as time passes after spinal cord injuries, but have found more variability in the timing and magnitude of these gains.[15]

PROBLEM-SOLVING EXERCISE 7-1

Your patient recently was injured in an automobile accident sustaining a spinal cord injury resulting in complete (ASIA A) C8 tetraplegia.

- List the muscles of inhalation that you would expect to remain fully innervated, partially innervated, and lacking innervation.
- List the muscles used for forced exhalation that you would expect to remain fully innervated, partially innervated, and lacking innervation.
- When the patient lies in a horizontal position, he breathes without any apparent difficulty. When the head of the bed is elevated, his respiratory rate increases and he complains of shortness of breath. Explain the most likely cause of the patient's dyspnea.

---

breathe and cough effectively can lead to a variety of respiratory complications. Inadequate strength in the inspiratory muscles results in reduced ventilation of the lungs, leading to atelectasis. Weakness in these muscles also makes them more likely to fatigue, which can lead to ventilatory failure.[26] Inadequate strength in the expiratory muscles impairs coughing ability. Ineffective coughing allows secretions to build in the lungs, with atelectasis, pneumonia, and respiratory insufficiency resulting.[18, 75, 100, 106] The clinical picture is further complicated if the patient is elderly, sustained trauma to her thorax during the initial accident, or if she has a history of respiratory disease, aspiration, or smoking.[18, 45, 66, 88]

Respiratory complications are extremely common after spinal cord injury. One large study found that the incidence of these complications during the initial acute and rehabilitation hospitalizations was 84 percent among people with neurological levels of injury between C1 and C4, 60 percent among those with levels between C5 and C8, and 65 percent among those with thoracic levels. Pneumonia, ventilatory failure, and atelectasis were the most common respiratory complications among people with neurological levels of injury in the cervical region. Pleural effusion, atelectasis, and pneumothorax or hemothorax were the most prevalent respiratory complications developed by people with thoracic neurological levels of injury.[50]

Although respiratory complications occur most frequently during the initial postinjury phase,[61] they are not limited to the early weeks or months after injury. Both during the acute phase and in subsequent years, respiratory complications are the most common cause of death among people with spinal cord injuries. Pneumonia in particular is the most prevalent cause of death, and causes fatality with greatest frequency when the patient is elderly or has a cervical neurological level of injury.[28–32, 55]

EVALUATION OF RESPIRATORY FUNCTION

A thorough respiratory evaluation should be performed as soon as is feasible after injury. This early evaluation will make it possible to formulate an appropriate plan of care and establish a baseline against which to compare future findings. The evaluation should include assessment of strength in the muscles of ventilation, pattern of chest and abdominal motions during breathing, chest excursion, respiratory rate, coughing ability, ability to move air during breathing (pulmonary function testing), posture, and adequacy of breath support for speech. The evaluation should also investigate the presence of complicating conditions such as chest injury, a history of smoking, or preexisting pulmonary disease. Additional evaluation procedures may be indicated during the acute phase after injury or in patients who are at high risk for pulmonary complications.[17, 75, 82, 84, 89, 101]

Respiratory evaluations should be repeated periodically during the acute and rehabilitation phases of care, and during post-discharge follow-up visits. These evaluations will enable the rehabilitation team to monitor progress or deterioration in respiratory status, and to respond appropriately.

Strength in the Muscles of Ventilation

Innervation of the ventilatory muscles is the most significant determinant of breathing and coughing ability after spinal cord injury. It follows that an assessment of the strength in these muscles is an important component of the respiratory evaluation. The results of muscle testing can be used to prognosticate on the individual's potential for independent breathing and coughing. The findings of the muscle test will also indicate areas of weakness that should be addressed in a strengthening program.

If the patient's spine is stable, the physical therapist can evaluate the strength in her accessory muscles and abdominals using standard muscle testing procedures,[48, 54] adapted as indicated. If the spine is not yet stable, the therapist should avoid muscle test procedures that could cause motion at or create a muscular pull on the affected vertebral area. Chapter 8 presents additional considerations for manual muscle testing of patients with spinal cord injuries.

The respiratory evaluation should include an assessment of diaphragm function. Although diaphragm strength cannot be evaluated using a manual muscle test, the therapist can gain some understanding of this muscle's functioning by observing motions of the patient's abdomen while she breathes.[26] With the patient supine, the therapist should watch for protrusion of her abdomen during inhalation. If the diaphragm contracts through its full excursion, the patient will exhibit a normal amount of epigastric rise. Limited or absent epigastric rise indicate impairment in diaphragm functioning. If the patient is on a ventilator, the therapist can disconnect the ventilator briefly to assess epigastric rise during inhalation.[1]

In addition to testing the muscles of ventilation, the therapist should assess strength in the musculature of the trunk and upper extremities. These muscles provide postural support, and enable the patient to self-cough and perform trunk and shoulder girdle motions to optimize her ventilatory capacity.

Breathing Pattern

Motions of the abdomen and chest, and visible contractions of the neck accessory muscles, provide information on the patient's breathing ability. Normal epigastric motions indicate good diaphragm function. Chest expansion during inhalation gives evidence of intercostal functioning; a paradoxical breathing pattern indicates an absence of intercostal innervation. Visible contraction of the sternocleidomastoids and scalenes during inhalation when the patient is at rest is an indication of diaphragm weakness.[1, 102]

The therapist can assess the patient's breathing pattern by observing and palpating the patient's abdomen, chest, and neck accessory muscles while she breathes. This assessment should be performed both with the patient in supine and in sitting, since upright postures alter diaphragm functioning when the abdominals are not innervated. The therapist should also note any changes in breathing pattern that occur as a result of increased activity.[1, 102]

Chest Excursion

Motions of the rib cage during breathing are a reflection of both ventilatory muscle functioning and chest wall mobility. Chest motions can be assessed using a tape measure with the patient supine. The therapist should measure the chest's diameter at the end of maximal exhalation and at the end of maximal inhalation. The measurements should be taken at the levels of the axilla and the xiphoid process to assess motions of the upper and lower chest, respectively.[1, 102] An increase in chest diameter during inhalation is an indication of functioning intercostals. A decrease in chest diameter during inhalation (paradoxical breathing pattern) indicates that intercostal functioning is absent.

In addition to measuring chest diameter before and after inhalation, the therapist can measure the patient's chest after she performs an air-shift maneuver. In this maneuver, the patient inhales maximally, closes her glottis, and relaxes her diaphragm while maintaining closure of her glottis. This causes a redistribution of air from the lower chest to the upper chest, with upper chest expansion resulting.[1, 89] Using an airshift maneuver, a patient who lacks intercostal innervation can achieve upper chest expansion.

Respiratory Rate

Respiratory rate can be a reflection of the patient's overall respiratory status. In adults, the normal rate of respiration ranges from 12 to 16 breaths per minute.[89, 102] Rapid breathing can be an indication that the individual's ventilatory efforts are not adequate to sustain good oxygenation.

People tend to alter their breathing rate if they realize that it is being observed. For this reason, the therapist should assess respiratory rate without the patient's awareness.[1, 102] One way to do this is to count the patient's breaths while appearing to take her pulse.

Cough

Coughing ability is crucial to survival; a person who cannot cough effectively will be unable to clear her airways of respiratory secretions or foreign substances that she inadvertently inhales. The therapist should observe as the patient attempts to cough, and note the quality of cough that she produces (Table 7–3). If the patient is unable to generate an effective cough, the therapist should note her performance in each of the stages of cough. The patient may have difficulty with any of the following: inhaling an adequate volume of air, exhaling with adequate force, or opening and closing her glottis with appropriate timing during the cough.[72]

TABLE 7–3. QUALITY OF COUGH

Cough Quality	Sound	Number of Coughs Possible per Exhalation	Functional Significance
Functional cough	Loud and forceful	2 or more	Independent in respiratory secretion clearance.
Weak functional cough	Soft, less forceful	1 per exhalation	Independent for clearing throat and small amount of secretions. Assistance needed for clearing large amounts of secretions.
Nonfunctional cough	Sigh or throat clearing	No true coughs; cough attempt has no expulsive force	Assistance needed for airway clearance.

Sources: references 1, 89, 102.

Pulmonary Function Tests

Pulmonary function testing can include a variety of measures of ventilatory ability (Table 7–1). These measurements can provide objective data to assist in both treatment planning and documentation of progress.

Vital capacity, the volume of air that can be exhaled following maximal inhalation, is a particularly useful test. It provides a good measure of ventilatory function in people with spinal cord injuries because it correlates significantly with most[8] other pulmonary function tests.[92] Moreover, vital capacity assessment is a practical means of evaluating ventilatory function in today's health care environment because it can be performed using a hand-held spirometer, which is portable and inexpensive. Measurements should be taken both in supine and in sitting, as breathing ability is likely to differ in these two positions.

Another pulmonary function test that can be useful is negative inspiratory pressure. This measure may be indicated for patients with recent cervical lesions, as it can be predictive of ventilatory failure.[58] Negative inspiratory pressure can also provide information on the potential for ventilator weaning.[52]

Posture

The respiratory evaluation should include a postural assessment. The therapist should note any deformities such as thoracic kyphosis or scoliosis that may interfere with chest motions. The therapist should also assess the patient's sitting posture in a wheelchair, investigating whether her body's alignment will enhance or impede activity in her respiratory muscles and motions of her thorax and abdomen. Any of the following postures can make breathing more difficult: posterior pelvic tilt, thoracic kyphosis, forward shoulders, or forward head.[71]

---

[8] Roth et al[92] performed pulmonary function tests on 52 patients with recent spinal cord injuries (C4 through T6) and found that vital capacity correlated significantly with forced expiratory volume in 1 second, inspiratory capacity, expiratory reserve volume, functional residual capacity, residual volume, total lung capacity, and the residual volume/total lung capacity ratio. Vital capacity did not correlate significantly with the maximal pressures generated during expiration (maximum positive expiratory pressure, or PEP) or inspiration (maximum negative inspiratory pressure, or NIP).

Breath Support for Speech

The respiratory evaluation should include an assessment of the patient's breath support for speech. The therapist can ask the patient to inhale maximally and then either count out loud or say "ah" or "oh" for as long as she can in one breath. The therapist can measure her performance by noting the number that the patient can count to, or by timing the phonation. Patients who have better inspiratory capacity and better eccentric control of their inspiratory muscles will be able to phonate for a longer time with a single breath.[70]

Additional Evaluation Procedures

The respiratory evaluation may include additional assessments, particularly during the acute phase following injury and in patients with severely compromised respiratory systems. Fluoroscopy or chest radiographs can be used to evaluate diaphragm function. Arterial blood gasses can be measured to detect levels of oxygen and carbon dioxide in the blood. Noninvasive pulse oximetry can provide ongoing information on the oxygenation of the patient's blood, both at rest and during activity.[26, 40, 58, 78, 102] End-tidal P_{CO_2} monitoring, also noninvasive, can be used to detect hypercapnia, an elevation in the carbon dioxide level in the blood.[14]

THERAPEUTIC INTERVENTIONS

Respiratory function is a critical focus of medical and rehabilitative care after spinal cord injury, due to the prevalence and severity of complications in this system. This focus should begin soon after injury and continue throughout acute and postacute rehabilitation and post-discharge follow-up.

The respiratory component of a comprehensive rehabilitation program is directed toward the maximization of ventilatory ability and the prevention of pulmonary complications. It includes interventions to ensure adequate ventilation, enhance breathing and coughing ability, mobilize secretions, and provide the patient with the knowledge and skills that she will require to avoid complications after discharge. The specific focus and design of each individual's program will depend upon the results of her respiratory evaluation.

Ensuring Adequate Ventilation

The most basic focus of respiratory care after spinal cord injury is ensuring that the patient has adequate motion of air in and out of her lungs. A person who is unable to breathe, or whose breathing ability is inadequate to maintain alveolar ventilation and meet her metabolic needs, will require assistance in ventilation.

A high cervical lesion that results in seriously impaired breathing ability may make it necessary to initiate mechanical ventilation during the emergency phase of management. Mechanical ventilation may also be required in the presence of lower lesions, particularly if concomitant injuries, preexisting respiratory conditions, or advanced age compromise the patient's pulmonary function.

Even if unassisted ventilation is adequate initially, ventilatory ability can deteriorate in the first few days after a spinal cord injury. This decline in ventilatory function can occur as a result of an ascending lesion, accumulation of pulmonary secretions, or fatigue in the muscles of ventilation.[74, 103] Because of the potential for deterioration, respiratory status should be monitored closely during the initial phase following injury. Repeated checks of arterial blood gasses, vital capacity, and chest radiographs will provide information on the patient's status and will allow prompt response if needed. Mechanical ventilation may be necessary if vital capacity falls too low,[h] oxygen levels in the blood fall too low, or if carbon dioxide levels in the blood rise too high.[6, 45, 58, 75, 79] Warning signs of impending ventilatory failure include rapid shallow breathing, a drop in vital capacity to less than 15 milliliters per kilogram of ideal body weight, or a drop in maximal negative inspiratory pressure to under 20 centimeters of water.[58]

Some individuals with spinal cord injury develop ventilatory insufficiency after years of breathing without mechanical assistance. Late-onset chronic alveolar hypoventilation (CAH) may be due to a decline in vital capacity as a result of aging, obesity, inactivity, or reduced compliance of the lungs and chest walls. Individuals with CAH may exhibit hypersomnolence, frequent sleep arousals, dyspnea, fatigue, sleep-disordered breathing, morning headache, and an increase in respiratory infections. Acute respiratory failure can result.[4, 14]

Positive pressure ventilators. Most assisted breathing is achieved using intermittent positive pressure ventilators (IPPV). This type of ventilator causes inhalation either by delivering a set volume of air (volume-regulated ventilation) or by delivering a set pressure (pressure-regulated ventilation) during inspiration.[41, 53] Exhalation occurs as a result of passive recoil of the lungs and chest wall.

Positive pressure ventilators can work through a variety of modes. These modes differ in the manner in which they support ventilation, and in the degree to which they allow for spontaneous breathing by the patient (Table 7–4).

Positive pressure ventilators are available in both stationary and portable models. With a portable ventilator, the person can be mobile at home and in the community using a power wheelchair.

Both portable and stationary positive pressure ventilators typically interface with the patient through a tracheostomy tube.[86] Over the past few years, there has been increasing focus on alternatives to ventilation using tracheostomies. This is in part due to the high incidence of complications associated with tracheostomies.[i] Alternatives include oral, nasal, and oral-nasal interfaces. Oral interfaces have better cosmesis than do nasal or oral-nasal interfaces. During the day, a mouthpiece can be placed close to the user's face so that she can access it for assisted inspirations as needed. At night, a mouthpiece with a lip seal retention system reduces leakage from the mouth and makes it possible for the ventilator to deliver breaths while the user sleeps.[9, 11, 12] In general, people who have utilized both intermittent positive ventilation via tracheostomy and noninvasive alternatives find the noninvasive methods of ventilation to be preferable in terms of comfort, convenience, appearance, and impact on speaking, swallowing, and glossopharyngeal breathing.[3]

Alternative means of providing assistance to ventilation. There are several alternatives to standard positive pressure ventilators. These alternatives include intermittent abdominal pressure ventilators, negative pressure body ventilators, and phrenic nerve stimulators.

---

[h] There is no generalized agreement regarding the vital capacity values that may necessitate the initiation of mechanical ventilation. The cut-off values range from 500 to 600 mL[45] to 1000 to 1200 mL.[75]

[i] Numerous severe complications are associated with tracheostomies. These complications result from infections, trauma to the trachea, and impairment of swallowing and airway clearance.[6, 10, 12]

TABLE 7–4.   MODES OF MECHANICAL VENTILATION

Mode	Description	Patient's Involvement in Ventilation
Control	The rate and tidal volume are set to deliver a given minute ventilation.	The patient's spontaneous breathing efforts are ignored.
Assist control	The rate and tidal volume are set to deliver a minimum minute ventilation. If the patient has any spontaneous breathing efforts, these efforts trigger the ventilator to deliver the set tidal volume.	The patient can increase the respiratory rate and minute ventilation by triggering more than the set minimum number of breaths. If the patient has no spontaneous breaths, the ventilator will deliver the preset minimum minute ventilation.
Synchronized intermittent mandatory ventilation (SIMV)	The rate and tidal volume are set to deliver a minimum minute ventilation.	The patient can breathe spontaneously between the breaths delivered by the ventilator.
Pressure control	The rate and pressure to be delivered during inspiration are set. If the patient has any spontaneous breathing efforts, these efforts trigger the ventilator to deliver the set pressure for inhalation.	The patient can increase the respiratory rate and minute ventilation by triggering more than the set minimum number of breaths. If the patient has no spontaneous breaths, the ventilator will deliver the preset number of breaths.
Pressure support	The ventilator delivers a set pressure only when triggered by the patient's spontaneous breathing effort.	The patient controls the respiratory rate, tidal volume, timing of inhalation and exhalation, and minute ventilation.
Continuous positive airway pressure (CPAP)	The ventilator delivers positive pressure at the end of exhalation to prevent alveolar collapse.	The patient breathes spontaneously, performing the work of ventilation without assistance from the ventilator.

Source: reference 41.

Intermittent abdominal pressure ventilators (IAPV) work by applying intermittent pressure externally to the abdomen. This type of ventilator interfaces with the patient through an inflatable bladder that is built into an abdominal corset or belt. The corset or belt is worn with the inflatable bladder positioned against the wearer's abdomen. When the positive pressure ventilator inflates the bladder, it compresses the abdominal contents. This compression causes the abdominal contents to push up against the diaphragm, resulting in exhalation. When the ventilator releases the pressure in the inflatable bladder, gravity pulls the abdominal contents caudally. The diaphragm descends and inhalation results. Because inhalation occurs as a result of gravity pulling the abdominal contents caudally, an intermittent abdominal pressure ventilator is effective only when the wearer sits with her trunk elevated *at least* 30 degrees above horizontal.[j] These ventilators are portable, and do not require the presence of artificial airways. They can be used to provide ventilation to people who have no measurable vital capacity, or can be used to supplement the breathing efforts of people who are able to breathe to a limited degree on their own.[6, 9, 11, 80]

Negative pressure body ventilators encompass the torso and cause inhalation by creating a negative pressure on the thorax and abdomen. This negative pressure results in expansion of the thoracic cavity, causing air to be drawn into the lungs. Examples of this type of ventilator include iron lungs, chest shell ventilators, and wrap-style ventilators.[6, 9] Negative pressure body ventilators are cumbersome and restrict activity more than the alternative types of ventilators. As a result, they are used less frequently than other types of

---

[j] Intermittent abdominal pressure ventilators work *optimally* when the trunk is 70 to 80 degrees above horizontal.[9]

ventilatory supports, and tend to be used at night only.[6, 11]

Phrenic nerve stimulators, also called phrenic nerve pacers, diaphragmatic pacemakers, or electrophrenic stimulators, are an alternative to mechanical ventilation for people who have permanently paralyzed diaphragms. With phrenic nerve stimulators, breathing is accomplished through the use of surgically implanted electrodes that stimulate the phrenic nerves. The system includes an external stimulus controller, a transmitter, a subcutaneous receptor, and electrodes. Ventilation using a diaphragmatic pacemaker requires the presence of intact phrenic nerves, diaphragm, lungs, and airway. Diaphragmatic pacing frees the individual from a mechanical ventilator, can achieve superior oxygenation, and allows for more normal speech and breathing patterns.[34, 98, 104] Disadvantages include expense, the need for continued use of a tracheostomy in most cases, and either ineffective or less than optimally effective ventilation in the majority of cases.[6, 9] Because of the potential for failure of the system, a back-up ventilator is generally recommended for the home.[104]

Enhancing Breathing Ability

One of the most important outcomes of respiratory rehabilitation following spinal cord injury is the maximization of the patient's ability to breathe. This task is accomplished by teaching the patient an efficient breathing pattern, strengthening her ventilatory musculature, preserving the mobility of her thoracic cage, optimizing posture, and providing abdominal support when needed.

Breathing pattern. The patient should be encouraged to use a diaphragmatic breathing pattern during quiet breathing, as this pattern is more normal and efficient than an upper chest breathing pattern. To encourage diaphragmatic breathing, the therapist can use verbal and visual cues. If the patient is supine, visual feedback can be provided by placing a large light object, such as a box of tissues, on the abdomen so that the patient can observe its motions as she breathes.

In addition to providing verbal and visual cues, the therapist can provide a quick stretch to facilitate diaphragm contraction. Quick stretch to the diaphragm is performed by pushing the epigastric area[k] in and rostrally immediately prior to asking for the inspiratory effort. Instructing the patient to sniff may also elicit a diaphragmatic response.[73a]

Upper chest breathing occurs when the neck accessory muscles are used for ventilation. Upper chest expansion can be used to increase the volume of inspired air to enhance coughing, improve breath support for speech, or to meet the ventilatory requirements of increased activity.[73a] To develop upper chest expansion, the therapist can place her hands against the patient's upper chest and ask her to push against her hands as she breathes in deeply. To facilitate this motion, the therapist can provide a quick stretch to the neck accessory muscles by pushing the upper chest in and caudally just before asking for the patient's inspiratory effort.

Strength and endurance. Soon after injury, the patient should begin resisted exercises of her muscles of ventilation. These exercises can increase the strength and endurance of innervated respiratory musculature, improve performance on pulmonary function tests, and reduce the perceived difficulty of breathing.[27, 44, 93] Cough ability may also be improved, through the development of a greater inspiratory capacity[82] and increased strength of the abdominals if they are innervated.

Because the diaphragm is the principal muscle of normal inspiration, and because diaphragmatic breathing is more efficient than breathing with the neck muscles,[1] diaphragmatic strengthening is an important component of the exercise program. During initial exercises, the therapist should work with the patient to develop a diaphragmatic breathing pattern. Strategies for teaching diaphragmatic breathing are presented above.

The patient can practice breathing deeply while the therapist applies manual resistance to her epigastric area, and progress to breathing with weights placed on this area. The weights should allow full epigastric rise during inspiration; a reduced rise during inhalation with the weights in place indicates that the resistance is excessive for the patient at that time. To avoid over-fatiguing the diaphragm, the therapist should observe the patient's breathing pattern, and stop the exercises or reduce the resistance if the patient begins using her neck accessory muscles for inspiration.[1, 89, 101, 102]

Resistive inspiratory muscle trainers can be a useful alternative to abdominal weight training. Using one of these devices, the patient inhales against resistance. The resistance can be adjusted to accommodate the individual's inspiratory ability, with increasing resistance provided as her ability improves. Use of inspiratory muscle trainers can result in improved strength and endurance

---

[k] The epigastric area is a triangular area located just caudal to the xiphoid process, between the ribs.[1]

in the muscles of ventilation, improved performance on pulmonary function tests,[27, 44, 93] slower and deeper breathing both during the training sessions and at rest,[64a] reduced use of the neck accessory muscles for inhalation, and increased tolerance for physical activity.[44] Because resistive inspiratory muscle trainers are small and can be self-administered, they can be useful tools for continued respiratory exercise after discharge.

In addition to a strengthening program for the inspiratory muscles, the patient may benefit from exercises that develop strength in her trunk and upper extremities. These muscles provide postural support, and enable the patient to perform trunk and shoulder girdle motions to optimize her ventilatory capacity.

Aerobic training may be another beneficial component of the respiratory rehabilitation program, once the patient is medically able to participate in aerobic activities. Arm cranking exercises have been shown to improve ventilatory muscle endurance in subjects with long-standing thoracic spinal cord injuries.[95]

Eccentric control of exhalation. In addition to addressing inhalation, the therapeutic program should include exercises directed at developing eccentric control of exhalation. This control is required for normal speech production.

To develop eccentric control of exhalation, the patient can practice inhaling maximally and counting or saying "ah" or "oh" for as long as possible before taking another breath. If she can develop the ability to phonate for 10 to 12 seconds, she may be better able to speak normally.[70]

Glossopharyngeal breathing. Many people who have severely limited inspiratory capacity can learn to use glossopharyngeal breathing to increase the volume of air that they can inhale. This technique involves using the tongue and pharyngeal musculature to force air into the lungs in a series of "gulps." This added volume of inspired air can assist with breath support for speech or coughing, improved oxygenation to allow more physical activity, and expansion of the lungs to enhance chest mobility. Glossopharyngeal breathing can also make it possible for people with high cervical lesions and no diaphragm function to breathe on their own for limited periods of time[l] in the event that their ventilators are disconnected or cease to function.[6, 9, 102]

Teaching glossopharyngeal breathing is a highly specialized skill. Therapists who have not undergone training in this area should refer appropriate patients to therapists who are capable of teaching glossopharyngeal breathing.

Chest wall mobility. Chest wall mobility is an important focus of respiratory rehabilitation following spinal cord injury. When the muscles of inhalation are impaired, the rib cage does not move through its normal excursions as the individual breathes, and the chest wall stiffens as a result. Lung compliance is also reduced.[m] Both of these factors increase the work of breathing.[44] Range of motion in the chest wall can be preserved or improved through deep-breathing exercises, passive stretching, joint mobilization, intermittent positive pressure breathing, glossopharyngeal breathing, and airshift maneuvers.[1, 22, 89, 101, 102]

Posture. The alignment of a person's spine, shoulder girdle, and pelvis has a strong impact on her ability to breathe effectively. Sitting posture is particularly important after spinal cord injury because of the amount of time that the individual is likely to spend in sitting. Sitting with an anteriorly tilted pelvis, erect trunk, adducted scapulae, and neutral head and neck alignment will enhance breathing by placing the ribs and accessory muscles in mechanically advantageous positions.[68] During rehabilitation after spinal cord injury, posture should be optimized through exercise, functional training, and the acquisition of appropriate seating equipment.[89]

Abdominal support. When spinal cord injury causes paralysis of the abdominal musculature, inspiration is more difficult in upright positions. This is due to the fact that the paralyzed abdominal musculature allows the abdominal contents to protrude and descend when the patient is upright. This descent of the abdominal contents results in a loss of the cephalad force that they usually exert on the diaphragm. Without the support that it normally receives from the viscera, the diaphragm descends to a lower resting position. In this position, it is not able to contract as effectively. During early out-of-bed activities, an abdominal binder or corset can improve vital capacity, tidal volume, and blood oxygenation by containing the abdominal contents and, thus, placing the diaphragm in a more efficient position for inspiration.[17, 22, 59, 76, 89, 101, 102]

---

[l] In some cases, individuals with no measurable vital capacity may use glossopharyngeal breathing for hours.[6, 10]

[m] When compliance is reduced, higher pressures are required to inflate the lungs.

PROBLEM-SOLVING EXERCISE 7-2

Your patient with complete (ASIA A) C4 tetraplegia exhibits visible contraction of her neck accessory muscles during quiet breathing. Design a treatment program that will decrease her reliance on her accessory muscles for breathing.

In most cases, abdominal binders or corsets can be used as a temporary measure to ease the transition to upright activities. As a person's breathing capacity improves, the binder or corset can be loosened gradually over a period of days and finally, discontinued as the patient accommodates to breathing without it. Alternatively, the patient can gradually accommodate to upright postures without abdominal support by spending time sitting with her trunk in gradually more vertical positions without the support of a binder or corset.[102]

Ventilator weaning. Many people with spinal cord injuries, particularly those who have cervical lesions, require mechanical ventilators during the acute phase after injury. Most who have a neurological level of injury at C3 or lower are able to regain the capacity to breathe independently. Factors that can reduce a person's potential to wean from a ventilator include respiratory or other medical complications, preexisting respiratory conditions, age over 50 years, a vital capacity under 1000, maximal negative inspiratory pressure less than 30 centimeters of water, and a history of smoking.[52, 65, 87, 103]

When a ventilator is used during the acute or rehabilitation phase of hospitalization after injury, the therapeutic program should work toward developing the capacity to breathe without this mechanical assistance. Even when a patient lacks the potential to develop complete independence from mechanical ventilation, a ventilator weaning program may enable her to gain the capacity to breathe independently for brief periods of time. This ability may enhance her survival potential in the event of ventilator failure or accidental disconnection.[87, 103]

Ventilator weaning involves gradually reducing the patient's dependence on a ventilator. Although there are several approaches to ventilator weaning, one method has been used most successfully for people with spinal cord injuries and others who have difficulty developing independence from a ventilator. This approach to weaning, progressive ventilator-free breathing, involves disconnecting the patient from the ventilator for increasing periods of time. This process can start with the patient breathing independently for as little as 1 or 2 minutes at a time. Between sessions she continues to use a ventilator. As her breathing ability develops, the duration and frequency of ventilator-free breathing sessions can be increased.[35, 52, 58, 86, 87] Initial independent breathing sessions should take place with the patient supine, as unassisted breathing will be easier in this position.[65, 86, 103]

The patient is more likely to develop ventilator independence if the respiratory program includes inspiratory muscle training[2, 65] and other measures to enhance breathing capacity, described earlier in this chapter. Secretion management is also critical for ventilator weaning,[52] as accumulation of secretions will increase the work of breathing and lead to the development of respiratory complications.

Clearing Secretions

An inability to cough effectively leads to the accumulation of secretions within the lungs. Enforced recumbency after spinal cord injury compounds the problem. Retention of secretions can lead to atelectasis, infection, and respiratory insufficiency. These complications can be avoided with appropriate management. Acutely following injury, patients with impaired respiratory ability are treated prophylactically with postural drainage and percussion and vibration of the chest.[45, 58, 74, 75, 84, 89] Intermittent positive pressure breathing (IPPB) may also be used prophylactically or as an adjunct to these treatments when patients exhibit retention of secretions and atelectasis.[17, 58] Tracheal and bronchial suctioning may be required to clear secretions, especially when the patient has a tracheostomy or a respiratory tract infection.

Postural drainage, percussion, vibration, IPPB, and suctioning are standard techniques used by respiratory and physical therapists. These techniques can be adapted as indicated to accommodate each individual's medical and orthopedic needs. Additional strategies that are utilized to enhance secretion clearance following spinal cord injury include manually assisted coughing, mechanical insufflation-exsufflation, self-coughing, position changes, and muscle strengthening.

Manually assisted coughing. Manually assisted coughing is an effective means of helping people who lack abdominal musculature clear their respiratory secretions by achieving forceful expiration while coughing.[5, 51, 107] To assist in a cough, the person providing the assistance applies force to the patient's abdomen or chest to push air out of the lungs. This maneuver should be coordinated with the patient's voluntary efforts at coughing after maximal inhalation.

There are several different approaches to providing a manually assisted cough.[1, 69, 102] Probably the simplest technique involves a Heimlich-like maneuver (abdominal thrust). Using this technique, the helper pushes up and in on the patient's epigastric area, taking care to avoid applying force over the xiphoid process (Figure 7–4). An alternative technique involves applying inward and caudally directed forces to the lower lateral ribs. Either of these cough-assist techniques can be administered with the patient in supine, sidelying, or sitting in a wheelchair. In a third technique, which can be applied in supine, semisupine, or sidelying, the therapist applies force to the patient's upper chest and lower chest or abdomen. A final technique, which involves applying rotational forces to the patient's trunk, is provided in sidelying only. The appropriate choice of assisted coughing technique will depend on such factors as medical or orthopedic restrictions,[n] the position of the patient when she needs to cough, effectiveness of cough production with each method, and the preferences of both the person coughing and the person providing assistance.

Regardless of the technique employed for cough assistance, the patient can enhance the cough's effectiveness by participating in all phases of the cough. Instruction in cough assistance should include the steps of cough and the actions that the patient and her helper will perform during the assisted cough (Table 7–5). Both the patient and the helper are likely to require practice to develop optimal timing.

Mechanical insufflation-exsufflation. In some cases, medical or orthopedic conditions preclude the use of manually assisted coughing. In other cases, manually assisted coughing can be provided but is not adequate to clear a patient's respiratory secretions. In either of these situations, a good alternative may be the use of a mechanical

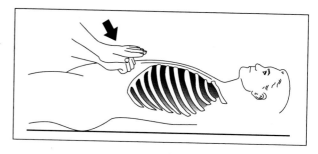

Figure 7–4. Assisted cough, using a Heimlich-like maneuver. (Adapted with permission from K. Johnson, T. Grant, & P. Peterson [1997]. Ventilator weaning for the patient with high-level tetraplegia. *Topics in Spinal Cord Injury Rehabilitation*, 2(3), 19. © 1997 Aspen Publishers.)

insufflation-exsufflation (MI-E) device.[o] This device provides a deep breath to the patient through positive pressure, followed by forced exsufflation created by negative pressure. The treatment can be administered through a face mask or through an endotracheal or tracheostomy tube. An MI-E may be used in combination with an abdominal thrust when there are no contraindications to this maneuver.[5, 7, 8, 13]

Self-cough. One disadvantage of both manually assisted coughing and mechanical insufflation-exsufflation is that they require the presence of a helper. A person who cannot cough effectively without assistance may not cough as frequently as she should, since a helper will not always be available. As a result, she will be more likely to develop respiratory complications.[51, 100]

Most people with C5 or lower spinal cord injuries are able to learn self-cough techniques to "assist" their own coughs.[69] This capability is an important survival skill, as it makes it possible to clear secretions independently.[p]

Self-coughing can be performed using a Heimlich-like maneuver by pushing up and in on the epigastric area while coughing. The strategies presented in Table 7–5 for maximizing cough effectiveness can be utilized during a self-cough.

---

[n] Precautions include any conditions that could make application of force to the thorax or abdomen hazardous. Examples are abdominal surgery, the presence of a Greenfield filter, and osteoporosis or fractures of the ribs.[5]

[o] Mechanical insufflation-exsufflation should be used with caution for patients with recent cervical spinal cord injuries who remain in spinal shock, as it may result in severe bradyarrhythmias in these cases.[7]

[p] In recent years, there has been preliminary research on the effectiveness of electrical stimulation as a method of providing independent cough ability to people with cervical spinal cord injuries. This research has shown that electrical stimulation of the abdominals can enhance the force of cough in some patients, but is less effective than manually assisted coughing.[51, 63, 105, 107] Similar results were found using functional magnetic stimulation to elicit contraction of the abdominal musculature during cough attempts.[62] Both methods of stimulating cough remain experimental, and their effectiveness in mobilizing secretions has yet to be demonstrated.

TABLE 7–5.   PATIENT INSTRUCTIONS FOR MANUALLY ASSISTED COUGHING

Instructions to the Patient	Strategies to Enhance Performance	Purpose
1. Instruct the patient to breathe in as deeply as he can.	• If possible, combine inhalation with trunk and neck extension, and shoulder flexion or scapular adduction.	• The positional changes listed will help maximize the volume of inspired air, which in turn will make it possible to generate a more effective cough.
	• If needed, the patient can use glossopharyngeal breathing to augment his inhalation. If the patient is unable to inhale adequately unassisted, the helper may provide a deep breath using a ventilator, manual ventilation bag, positive pressure blower, or IPPB machine.	• The patient must inhale an adequate volume of air in order to cough effectively.
2. Have the patient hold his breath briefly.	• Allow adequate time for inspiration prior to the "hold" phase of the cough.	• Closure of the glottis is required to allow a build-up of intrathoracic pressure for the expulsion phase of the cough.
3. Instruct the patient to cough.	• If possible, combine forced exhalation with trunk and neck flexion, and shoulder extension or scapular abduction.	• The positional changes listed will help maximize the force and velocity of the exhalation, which in turn will make it possible to generate a more effective cough.
	• The helper should apply the cough-assist forces just prior to the opening of the patient's glottis, and continue applying force as the patient coughs.	• Application of force prior to and after opening of the glottis will maximize the velocity and force of the expired air.

Sources: references 1, 12, 63, 68, 69, 102.

For example, a person who cannot generate adequate cough force using her upper extremities may be able to enhance her cough by falling forward from a sitting position while she coughs. By flexing her trunk and neck as she falls forward and pushes on her epigastric area, she may be able to expel air more forcefully.[69, 102]

Position changes. Frequent changes in position are also helpful in mobilizing secretions.[103] When a person lies in bed in one position for prolonged periods of time, fluid accumulates in the dependent portions of her lungs. Regular changes in position help alleviate this problem by preventing each area of the lung from being dependent for too long.[17, 82, 89] As an alternative to regular turning on standard hospital beds, patients can be placed on rotating beds that keep them in constant motion (Figure 7–5). These beds may prevent the build-up of secretions within the

lungs and reduce the incidence of pulmonary complications.[58, 61] Additionally, early activity out of bed can help mobilize secretions. As soon as it is medically and orthopedically feasible, patients should begin participating in out-of-bed activities.

Strengthening. Strengthening the muscles of exhalation may result in improved cough ability. Patients with innervated abdominal musculature can perform standard strengthening exercises of these muscles, adapted as needed to accommodate profound weakness or orthopedic restrictions. People who lack abdominal musculature but have function in the clavicular portions of their pectoralis majors (C5 and 6 innervation) can use these muscles for forced exhalation. Strengthening of these muscles can lead to an improved capacity for forced exhalation, as evidenced by an increase in expiratory reserve volume.[37]

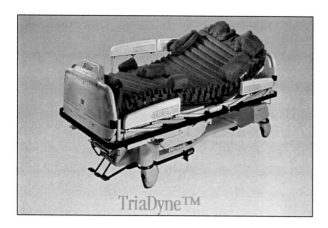

Figure 7–5. TriaDyne® Bed. (Photo courtesy of KCI, San Antonio, TX. TriaDyne is a registered trademark of KCI and is subject to patent and/or pending patent.)

Strengthening the inspiratory muscles can also enhance cough ability, since efficient coughing requires inhalation of an adequate volume of air. Finally, the patient may benefit from exercises that develop strength in innervated muscles in her back, shoulder girdle, and upper extremities. These muscles provide postural support and enable the patient to perform trunk and shoulder girdle motions to optimize her capacity for inhalation and forced exhalation.

Education

Respiratory complications pose a very real threat to the health and survival of a person with a spinal cord injury. Before a patient is discharged from the inpatient phase of her rehabilitation program, she should obtain the knowledge and skills that will be necessary to avoid these complications. If family members or others will be assisting in her care after discharge, they should be included in the education and training. Areas of knowledge to develop include potential respiratory complications, their prevention and early signs, and appropriate measures to take if complications occur. Skills to develop include techniques for secretion clearance and a home program of respiratory exercises for strength, endurance, and chest wall mobility. If a mechanical ventilator or electrophrenic stimulator is used, the individual and anyone who may be involved in her care must learn how to operate the device.[q] They must also learn techniques for providing adequate ventilation in the event of mechanical failure.

Most people with high tetraplegia return to home environments after discharge, and most utilize attendant care. This attendant care is most frequently provided by aides rather than nurses, and the patient is likely to be the one who trains the attendant.[47] Although the rehabilitation team may be able to provide education and training to attendants who will be involved in the patient's care immediately after discharge, this task will fall on the patient or her family in the years that follow. For this reason, both patients and their families should learn how to instruct others regarding respiratory care.

SUMMARY

- Breathing is accomplished through cyclic changes of the volume within the thoracic cavity; increases and decreases in the space within this cavity cause inhalation and exhalation, respectively. The motions involved in breathing occur as a result of the coordinated action of the diaphragm, accessory muscles, intercostals, and abdominal musculature.
- Coughing involves the following sequence of actions: maximal inhalation, glottis closure, contraction of the muscles of forced exhalation with the glottis closed, and continued forced exhalation with the glottis open.
- Spinal cord injury that results in paralysis of any of the muscles of ventilation will interfere with normal breathing and coughing. This can occur when the neurological level of injury is T12 or higher. With *complete* lesions, the level of injury determines the extent to which breathing and coughing are impaired. Higher lesions

---

> ### PROBLEM-SOLVING EXERCISE 7–3
>
> Your patient has incomplete C6 tetraplegia, ASIA C. He is unable to cough effectively without assistance.
>
> - What evaluation procedures would you perform?
> - Design a treatment program that would enhance the patient's independence in effective coughing.

---

q Even if the individual using the ventilator lacks the physical capability of operating it, she should be able to instruct others.

result in impairment of both inhalation and exhalation. Lower lesions interfere less with inhalation, but coughing remains impaired. The extent to which *incomplete* lesions interfere with breathing and coughing depends on both the level of injury and the amount of motor sparing below the lesion.

- Because spinal cord injury impairs breathing and coughing, respiratory complications are common and pose a significant threat to the individual's health and survival.

- The respiratory component of a rehabilitation program after spinal cord injury should begin soon after injury and continue through post-discharge follow-up. The program is directed at maximizing breathing and coughing ability and minimizing the potential for respiratory complications.

Physical Therapy Evaluation and Goal-Setting

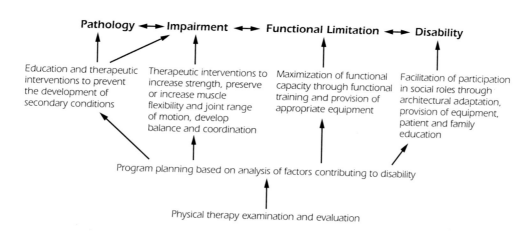

Pathology ⟷ Impairment ⟷ Functional Limitation ⟷ Disability

Education and therapeutic interventions to prevent the development of secondary conditions

Therapeutic interventions to increase strength, preserve or increase muscle flexibility and joint range of motion, develop balance and coordination

Maximization of functional capacity through functional training and provision of appropriate equipment

Facilitation of participation in social roles through architectural adaptation, provision of equipment, patient and family education

Program planning based on analysis of factors contributing to disability

Physical therapy examination and evaluation

The purpose of rehabilitation is the reduction of disability. It follows that appropriate intervention must be based on a careful analysis of the factors contributing to the patient's disability. This analysis starts with an examination of the patient's physical and functional status, as well as other areas relevant to the disablement process. The examination is followed by an evaluation, in which the therapist makes clinical judgments based on the examination results.[38] After identifying the individual's impairments and functional limitations, the therapist makes an estimation of the patient's potential for functional gains. The findings of this assessment are then considered in the context of the patient's priorities, age-appropriate roles, social support systems, physical environment, and resources. Together the patient and therapist establish goals aimed at minimizing disability to the extent possible.

EXAMINATION AND EVALUATION

Examination and evaluation are the foundations of any physical therapy program. The physical therapist requires a thorough and accurate understanding of the patient's status in order to identify areas of strength and weakness, and potential roadblocks to progress. The therapist's evaluation of this data provides the basis for the development of goals and a plan of action tailored to the individual involved.

In addition to providing the information required for setting goals and planning treatment, the therapist's examination establishes a baseline. Documentation of the patient's initial status is needed for later comparison, facilitating the detection of any improvement or deterioration in the patient's condition. This documentation is particularly critical during the early days and weeks after spinal cord injury, when improvement or deterioration in neurological status can occur rapidly. If a good baseline is not available for comparison, these changes are more likely to be missed.

The evaluation process should continue throughout the program. This is not to say that complete, formal evaluations should be performed continually. Rather, the therapist should remain aware of the patient's changing status. By monitoring any significant changes in physical and functional status, the therapist obtains feedback on the program's effectiveness. This feedback allows for adjustments to be made as appropriate.

Periodically, the therapist should perform a more complete reexamination and evaluation. These repeat evaluations provide the opportunity for the therapist and patient to assess progress, reassess goals, and update the program. Reevaluations can also direct attention to areas that may have been neglected inadvertently.

A thorough examination and evaluation at discharge is also important. A complete record of physical and functional status at the end of the program will be useful for health professionals with whom the patient will come in contact in the future. This evaluation is also an important source of feedback for the person with a spinal cord injury, who should be given a clear explanation of his status and potential areas for future progress. Finally, the discharge evaluation provides another opportunity to judge the therapeutic program's effectiveness. With this feedback on the program, the clinician can evaluate the therapeutic strategies employed and alter his approach with future patients when indicated.

After discharge, follow-up examinations are critical. During follow-up examinations, the patient and therapist can identify changes in physical or functional status and determine whether additional services are indicated. They can also identify and address equipment needs during these visits. Perhaps the most efficient and effective approach to follow-up examinations is a clinic in which multiple members of the rehabilitation team are present. Individuals attending the clinic can then undergo a comprehensive multidisciplinary examination that addresses their various medical, orthopedic, psychosocial, and functional needs.

Cooperative Approach

The initial examination often constitutes the first contact between a health professional and a patient, and thus sets the stage for future interactions. Unfortunately, this examination sometimes involves the pokings and proddings of an "expert" who approaches the patient as an object rather than as another person who happens to be a patient at the moment. When this occurs, the health professional dominates the interaction, issuing commands and noting responses. Another unfortunate thing that can occur during evaluations is health professionals being less than forthright. Some health professionals "protect" their

patients from evaluation results, filtering or sugarcoating their findings. This practice may stem from a belief that the information will somehow damage the patient. It may also be due to health professionals' own discomfort regarding communicating bad news to patients.

Whatever the reason behind these approaches to evaluation, they can have a negative impact. By assuming total command of the situation, by treating the person with a spinal cord injury as less than equal, and by withholding information from him, the health professional communicates to the patient that he is helpless and should assume a passive role.

To provide a more constructive experience, the therapist should include the patient as an active participant in the evaluation. (After all, the person being evaluated has a vested interest in the findings!) As an active participant, the person being evaluated is encouraged to express concerns, provide information, and share in any evaluation findings. The evaluation then becomes a positive learning experience in which both parties achieve a better understanding of the patient's status. As importantly, the person undergoing rehabilitation becomes an active participant in his program from the outset. The stage is set for active participation throughout the program.

Precautions

People with spinal cord injuries often have orthopedic or physiological conditions that necessitate care when performing examination procedures. For this reason, health professionals must take appropriate precautions while performing examinations or any other procedures. Precautions for treatment are presented in Chapter 9. These precautions are also appropriate during examinations.

Examination Content

Any complete physical therapy examination includes subjective statements and a history. The examination of someone who has had a spinal cord injury should also include an assessment of the areas of physical functioning that are directly affected by trauma to the cord, as well as the areas in which secondary conditions are likely to occur. The physical therapist should also investigate the patient's functional capabilities, equipment needs, and home environment.

History and subjective statements. Information for the history can be gathered by reading the medical record and interviewing the patient, family members, and others close to the patient. The history should contain any information relevant to the individual's physical or psychosocial status, prognosis, preinjury functional status, and discharge plans. This information will affect goal-setting and the therapeutic strategies employed during rehabilitation.

The therapist should document any relevant statements made by the patient or others that provide information on such matters as the patient's emotional state, concerns, or understanding of the injury. The patient's stated goals should also be included, as they give insight into his priorities.

A history should include the date, level, extent, and etiology of the damage to the spinal cord, any complications or additional injuries sustained at or since the time of the cord injury, and a brief summary of the medical and surgical management received since the injury. It should also note any changes in neurological status that have occurred since the injury. Any preexisting medical conditions that could impact on the person's health or functional status should also be documented. In addition, the history should include a brief summary of any rehabilitation that the patient has undergone since the time of the injury, and a description of his functioning since the injury.

In addition to obtaining information on the patient's medical history, the therapist should investigate social issues, getting a sense of the patient's activities and social roles prior to and since the injury. This information is essential when establishing meaningful goals, as the overall purpose of a rehabilitation program is to enable the person to resume functioning in age-appropriate social roles. Pertinent areas to investigate include vocation and avocations, living arrangements prior to the injury, expected discharge destination, social support available, and the patient's accustomed roles within the various social arenas such as home, work, and school.

Finally, the history should note any medical or orthopedic restrictions that have been placed on the patient's activities. For example, the therapist should document any limitations such as confinement to bed, skeletal traction, fracture precautions, or ventilator dependence.

Voluntary motor function. An accurate examination of voluntary motor function is of vital importance because it will provide a starting point for the therapeutic program. Motor function is one of the most important factors that affects a person's abilities following spinal cord injury; his ultimate potential for physical activities is largely dependent upon the musculature that remains innervated. The results of the manual muscle test are used to prognosticate on the level of functional independence that an individual can expect to achieve. In addition, the findings of the muscle test will indicate areas of weakness that should be addressed in a strengthening program.

Motor function is also significant in that it is a reflection of neurological status. The neurological level of injury is in part defined by the strength that the patient exhibits in the key muscles representative of each cord segment.[a] These key muscles, described by the American Spinal Injury Association,[1] are presented in Figure 8–1. An accurate and complete baseline muscle test will allow comparison to future findings.[b] This is especially important when the cord injury has occurred very recently, because at this stage, it is not unusual for neurological return to occur or for the lesion to progress. Neurological return may manifest itself as return of function in previously paralyzed muscles, and progression of the cord lesion may be shown by loss of motor function.

In addition to providing information on the patient's current neurological status, motor function below the lesion during the acute phase after injury can be an indicator of possible future motor return.[16, 21, 25, 43–45] Thus, the results of early muscle tests are important for patient education, as well as for prognostication about future motor recovery and functional potentials.

Muscles to be tested. A specific manual muscle test is required for accurate assessment of motor function following spinal cord injury. The therapist should test all key muscles on both sides of the body. After testing these muscles, the therapist can calculate the patient's motor score by adding the scores for all of the key muscles (Figure 8–1). This motor score may be useful for documentation of changes in motor function.[42]

When performing a muscle test, the therapist should never assume that all musculature above the diagnosed level of lesion is functioning normally. A therapist who makes this assumption will miss any preexisting weakness or previously undetected signs of neurological damage. To avoid this oversight, all key muscles innervated above the lesion should be tested.

---

[a] Neurological level of injury is explained in Chapter 2.
[b] ASIA publishes a reference manual and series of videotapes that present standardized procedures for performing examination procedures. These resources can be obtained from the American Spinal Injury Association, 2020 Peachtree Road NW, Atlanta, GA 30309.

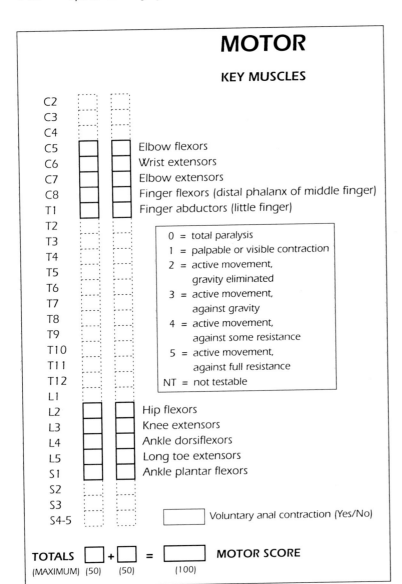

MOTOR

KEY MUSCLES

C2
C3
C4
C5 — Elbow flexors
C6 — Wrist extensors
C7 — Elbow extensors
C8 — Finger flexors (distal phalanx of middle finger)
T1 — Finger abductors (little finger)
T2
T3
T4
T5
T6
T7
T8
T9
T10
T11
T12
L1
L2 — Hip flexors
L3 — Knee extensors
L4 — Ankle dorsiflexors
L5 — Long toe extensors
S1 — Ankle plantar flexors
S2
S3
S4-5

0 = total paralysis
1 = palpable or visible contraction
2 = active movement,
    gravity eliminated
3 = active movement,
    against gravity
4 = active movement,
    against some resistance
5 = active movement,
    against full resistance
NT = not testable

Voluntary anal contraction (Yes/No)

TOTALS ☐ + ☐ = ☐ **MOTOR SCORE**
(MAXIMUM) (50) (50) (100)

Figure 8–1. Motor portion of the scoring form for the International Standards for Neurological and Functional Classification of Spinal Cord Injury. (Reproduced with permission from the American Spinal Injury Association [1996]. Standard Neurological Classification of Spinal Injury Patients.)

Just as the therapist should never assume that motor function is normal above the lesion, he should never assume that it is absent below the lesion. When examining an extremity that appears to lack any motor function, it can be tempting to check only a muscle or two, or even to forgo the muscle test altogether. One reason for this abbreviated examination is that performing a complete muscle test can be time consuming. It can also be discouraging to both the patient and the therapist to run through a long series of unsuccessful attempts at motion. Testing only one or two muscles can lead to inaccurate results, however, with spared motor function going undetected. To avoid this problem, the therapist should test all *key muscles* at and below the neurological level of injury. Doing so will be less time consuming and frustrating than performing a complete muscle test, and will avoid the problem of the therapist overlooking motor sparing that is not immediately apparent.

Certain muscles are functionally relevant but not identified as key muscles. This group includes the deltoids, serratus anterior, latissimus dorsi, trunk musculature, hip abductors and adductors, and hamstrings. In extremities where voluntary motor function is found in the key muscles, the therapist should test the strength in these functionally relevant muscles. Additional musculature can be tested as indicated and as time allows.

Substitution. When performing a muscle test, the therapist should watch for substitution! People with spinal cord injuries quickly learn to use functioning musculature to perform the actions of muscles that are weakened or absent. For example, the anterior deltoid can be used to extend the elbow in the absence of triceps function, and the radial wrist extensors can be used to flex the fingers in the absence of any functioning finger flexors (tenodesis grasp). These compensations can be very deceptive, giving the appearance of normal or partial functioning in musculature that is paralyzed.

Muscle substitution is an important skill for improving functional status, but it can wreak havoc on the evaluation results of an unwary therapist. This is especially true when a long time has passed since the injury, as the person with a spinal cord injury will have become more adept at muscle substitution. To prevent substitution during a muscle test, the therapist should eliminate motions at other joints. In addition, he should carefully palpate the muscle being tested to verify that it is contracting.

Stabilization. Musculature normally used for stabilization during manual muscle testing may be weak or absent. Failure to accommodate for this impaired ability to stabilize can make muscles appear to be weaker than they are. For example, someone with normal (5/5) deltoids and a weak serratus anterior may give the appearance of having weak deltoids during a manual muscle test. He may be able to perform the test motion without resistance, but scapular instability will enable the therapist to "break" the position with less than 5/5 force.

A person's ability to stabilize his entire body must also be taken into account during muscle testing. For example, someone who has recently sustained a cervical or thoracic injury may not have learned how to stabilize his trunk while sitting upright in a wheelchair. During manual muscle testing of his deltoids, he will be unable to maintain the test position against 5/5 force; his inability to stabilize his trunk will make his deltoids appear weak. Thus, if a therapist does not provide the needed trunk stabilization during muscle testing, the test results will be inaccurate.

To obtain accurate results, the therapist must stabilize the patient appropriately. Whenever stabilizing musculature is weak or absent, the therapist must provide the needed stability.

Muscle tone considerations during muscle testing. Elevated muscle tone can also influence muscle test results. Involuntary contraction can occur when a muscle is being tested, making the muscle appear to be stronger than it actually is.

Since abnormal tone can affect muscle test results, its presence should be noted when muscle strength is documented. In addition, the therapist must attempt to distinguish between voluntary and involuntary motor function. To make this distinction, the therapist should ask the patient to contract and relax the muscle on command.

Limiting conditions. Orthoses and orthopedic restrictions often interfere with standard positioning for manual muscle testing. When this is the case, the therapist should simply adapt the tests by performing them in the best positions possible within the limitations. The adaptations in muscle test procedure should be documented.

PROBLEM-SOLVING EXERCISE 8–1

According to the medical record, your patient has complete (ASIA A) C6 tetraplegia. You are performing her initial examination.

- What muscles should you test for strength?

When you are testing for strength in her finger flexors, she is able to flex her fingers through about half of the available range.

- What should you do to determine whether the patient performs this motion by contracting her finger flexors or through muscle substitution?

PROBLEM-SOLVING EXERCISE 8–2

You are performing a manual muscle test on your patient's anterior deltoid while he sits in a wheelchair. He is able to flex his shoulder to 90 degrees, but he is unable to maintain that position when you apply downward force on his arm.

- How can you determine whether he is exhibiting weak deltoids, weak serratus anterior, or both?
- Describe how you could muscle test the anterior deltoid and serratus anterior separately.

Precautions. If the spine is not yet stable, the therapist should exercise caution when testing musculature. Strong contraction of muscles that may exert a pull on the affected vertebral area should be avoided. For example, it is prudent to avoid resistance to the hip flexors if the patient has an unstable lumbar fracture.

Trunk musculature. Testing trunk musculature presents a unique problem. The standard tests for the abdominals and back extensors assume that the musculature is functioning along its entire length. This is often not the case after a spinal cord injury. A given person may have strong contraction of the rectus abdominis from the ribs to the umbilicus and no contraction below this level. What grade can be assigned to this person's rectus? Instead of trying to assign a grade to the musculature in such instances, it may be more meaningful to focus on identifying the approximate myotome levels in which the musculature functions.

The position of the umbilicus during muscle testing can be used as an indicator of function in the abdominal musculature. If it remains central during testing, this indicates that there is a uniform pull in the abdominals; abdominal musculature functions uniformly above, below, and to either side of the umbilicus. For this condition to exist, the abdominals are either absent or functioning uniformly along their entire length; the level of motor paralysis must be either above T5 or below T12. The therapist should palpate to determine which of these is the case. If the umbilicus moves cephalad during testing (Beevor's sign), the muscular pull is greater above the umbilicus than below; the lesion lies between T5 and T12. If the umbilicus moves to the side, the musculature is stronger on the side toward which it moves.

As is true with abdominal musculature, standard manual muscle testing for the back extensors is not appropriate when this musculature is not innervated along its entire length. When testing the back extensors, the therapist should determine the level of motor function by palpating the paraspinals while the patient attempts back extension.

Sensation. Like voluntary motor function, sensation is directly affected by spinal cord injury and is a reflection of neurological status. Pin prick and light touch sensation at key points in each dermatome are used along with motor function to determine the patient's neurological level of injury.[1] Improvement or deterioration in neurological function can be evidenced by a change in sensation. Moreover, spared sensation below the lesion, particularly spared pin prick, during the acute phase after injury can be an indicator of possible future motor return.[21, 44, 45]

Sensation also has an impact on the capacity to perform functional skills, though to a smaller degree than does strength. A person who has intact proprioception and touch sensation in an extremity will find it easier to learn to use that extremity. For example, learning to propel a wheelchair will be easier if some touch sensation is present in the hands, and intact proprioception in the lower extremities will make it easier to control the legs during ambulation.

Pain sensation is particularly important because it serves to protect the skin. The normal reaction to pain is to withdraw from the stimulus, thus avoiding or reducing damage to the skin. Without this protection, an area that lacks pain sensitivity is more vulnerable to trauma. People with spinal cord injuries need to know about this vulnerability and must take measures to avoid trauma to insensate areas.

Sensation to be tested. The therapist should test sensitivity to both pin prick and light touch in all of the key sensory points on both sides of the body.[c] As is true with motor testing, sensory testing should be performed at all key points regardless of whether they fall above, at, or below the level of injury. Figure 8–2 contains the American Spinal Injury Association (ASIA) key sensory points, as well as the ASIA form for recording sensory examination results.[1] After testing sensation in all of the key points bilaterally, the therapist can calculate the patient's pin prick and light touch scores by adding the scores for all of the key sensory points. These scores can be useful for documenting changes in sensory function.

ASIA also recommends testing the patient's awareness of deep pressure/pain and position sense in one joint for each extremity.[1] The therapist may find it useful to test movement and position sense in all major joints of the affected extremities, as this sensation can influence the performance of functional skills.[34, 46]

Sensory substitution. When performing sensory tests, it is important for the therapist to prevent substitution from other senses. In his eagerness to "do well" on the test, a patient may "cheat," possibly without even being aware of it. A variety of senses can be used for this sensory substitution.

---

[c] Because temperature is carried in the same spinal cord tract as is pain, these two sensory modalities are affected equally by cord injuries. For this reason, it is not necessary to test temperature sensitivity.

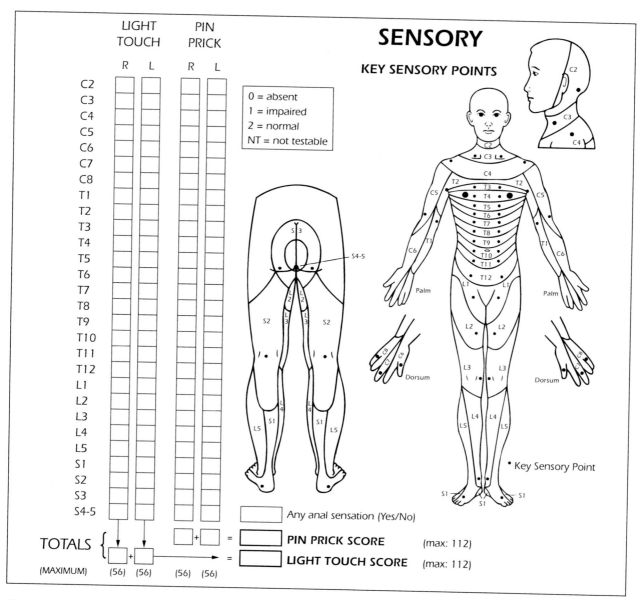

Figure 8–2. Sensory portion of the scoring form for the International Standards for Neurological and Functional Classification of Spinal Cord Injury. (Reproduced with permission from the American Spinal Injury Association [1996]. Standard Neurological Classification of Spinal Injury Patients.)

The patient can watch the therapist performing the test. The therapist's voice intonation and choice of words can also provide hints. A patient who lacks proprioception in a joint can often detect movement through other sensory cues. For example, someone who is lying in bed and has his hip flexed passively may feel his body being pushed toward the head of the bed. To increase the accuracy of sensory testing, the therapist should take measures to eliminate these supplemental sensory cues.

Muscle tone. Abnormal muscle tone[d] is another consequence of spinal cord injury that can play a major role in the disablement process.

Elevated muscle tone can cause pain, joint contractures, and skin breakdown. When severe, it can impair function.[27, 31] Occasionally, people can use abnormal muscle tone to their advantage. For example, some people with incomplete lesions depend upon their elevated muscle tone to augment their voluntary quadriceps function when standing or walking.

A patient's muscle tone can also provide information regarding his medical status. Following spinal cord injury, an increase in muscle tone can be a sign that something is wrong physically, because a noxious stimulus below the lesion can cause an increase in tone. For example, sometimes an increase in spasticity is an early indication of a urinary tract infection.

---

[d] Chapter 2 addresses abnormal muscle tone in greater depth.

When testing muscle tone, the therapist should check for spasticity, which is a velocity-dependent involuntary response to passive stretch.[19, 39] If spasticity is present, the therapist should rate its severity and determine whether it interferes with function. Table 8–1 presents a rating scale for grading spasticity. The patient with elevated muscle tone may exhibit spasms in addition to spasticity. Spasms are involuntary muscle contractions that appear to occur spontaneously or are elicited by stimuli such as tactile stimulation.[35] If the patient exhibits spasms, the therapist should note their frequency and severity, and whether they cause pain or interfere with function.

While examining a patient's spasticity and spasms, the therapist should note whether they are constant or fluctuating, and whether certain conditions, stimuli, or bodily motions influence the patient's muscle tone. This information can be useful to the patient and therapist, who may find ways to utilize these involuntary motor responses to enhance the performance of functional tasks.[18] For example, a patient who exhibits lateral trunk flexion on tactile stimulation of his thigh may be able to use this motor response for righting his trunk in a wheelchair. An understanding of the factors that influence a patient's tone can also be helpful to the patient and therapist as they seek ways to avoid involuntary motor responses that *interfere with function*. For example, a patient who exhibits trunk and extremity spasms when he uses a power recline to perform pressure reliefs in a wheelchair may be able to avoid those spasms by using a power tilt system instead.

Range of motion. Range of motion,[e] like strength and muscle tone, can have a profound impact on functional capabilities after spinal cord injury. Even mild restrictions in motion at crucial joints such as the elbows or shoulders can severely limit a person's functional potential. The therapist should check range of motion of all major joints, starting with a gross test and specifically examining any areas where functionally relevant limitations exist.[f]

The examination should include measurement of hamstring flexibility, due to its impact on functional capabilities. Hamstring flexibility should be tested in supine with the pelvis stabilized. Having a person with a spinal cord injury long-sit and reach for his toes is not an appropriate technique for performing this assessment, as excessive back flexibility can mask hamstring tightness. In addition to checking hamstring length, the therapist may examine flexibility of the biceps brachii, pectoralis major, long finger flexors and extensors, rectus femoris, and gastrocnemius if motion restrictions or functional limitations indicate possible problems in these muscles.

When testing the joint range of motion or muscle flexibility of someone with a recent spinal injury, the therapist should avoid stress to areas of vertebral instability. For example, if a patient with an unstable lumbar fracture has limited hip range of motion, the hip should not be forced beyond the point at which resistance to motion occurs. Even when range does not appear to be limited, it may be prudent to avoid hip flexion past 90 degrees or straight leg raising past 60 degrees in the presence of an unstable lumbar fracture. Motion past these points may cause undesirable motion in the lumbar area. In like manner, an unstable cervical spine necessitates caution when moving the shoulders.

Functional abilities. A functional evaluation investigates what a person is capable of doing,

TABLE 8–1. MODIFIED ASHWORTH SCALE FOR GRADING SPASTICITY

0	No increase in muscle tone.
1	Slight increase in muscle tone, manifested by a catch and release or by minimal resistance at the end of the range of motion (ROM) when the affected part(s) is moved in flexion or extension.
1+	Slight increase in muscle tone, manifested by a catch, followed by minimal resistance throughout the remainder (less than half) of the ROM.
2	More marked increase in muscle tone through most of the ROM, but affected part(s) easily moved.
3	Considerable increase in muscle tone, passive movement difficult.
4	Affected part(s) rigid in flexion or extension.

During testing, the clinician asks the patient to relax and moves the patient's extremities passively through the available range of motion.[4]

Source: Bohannon, R., & Smith, M. (1987). Interrator reliability of a modified Ashworth scale of muscle spasticity. *Physical Therapy,* 67 (2), 207. With permission of the American Physical Therapy Association.

---

e The phrase "range of motion" in this section is used to refer to both joint range of motion and the flexibility of two-joint musculature such as the hamstrings or the biceps brachii.

f Table 9–2 in Chapter 9 presents range of motion requirements for function.

how much assistance he needs, and what equipment he requires to perform various activities. Because the major thrust of the physical therapy component of rehabilitation is to increase functional capability, this part of the examination is very important. The initial functional evaluation provides a starting point for goal-setting and program development.

The functional evaluation performed on completion of the therapeutic program is also critical, as it provides a measure of the program's success. A physical rehabilitation program usually results in improvements in other areas such as strength and range of motion, but these gains are significant only if they contribute to an increase in functional abilities. If the patient is no more independent at discharge than he was initially, the functional training program has failed.[g]

Evaluation and documentation of functional skills should be specific enough to provide a complete picture of the patient's abilities. Blanket statements about areas of functioning do not provide adequate information, as these statements can be interpreted differently by various readers. For example, a statement that an individual is "independent in wheelchair propulsion" does not provide enough information. Does this refer to even surfaces only? One hundred feet or 10 miles? How long does it take for him to propel a given distance? Can he negotiate stairs with the wheelchair? Are specific wheelchair accessories such as handrim projections required? To effectively communicate about the patient's functional status, the therapist should specify the environmental conditions under which the various functional skills can be performed,[h] the equipment required, the patient's level of safety, and other measures relevant to each task such as distance negotiated or time required.

The therapist should also be specific when documenting the amount of assistance that the patient needs to perform each task. Merely noting that a person "needs assistance" does not provide adequate information. For example, the statement that a patient "requires assistance in level transfers" could be true with an individual who is

totally dependent (unable to contribute to the process), someone who requires only stand-by guarding, or anyone who falls between the two extremes. The terminology used in the Functional Independence Measure (FIM) can be useful for describing the level of assistance needed. This terminology is presented in Figure 8–3.

In addition to being specific and thorough, documentation of functional abilities must be as accurate as all other areas of the examination. It can be tempting to "give the patient the benefit of the doubt" in the functional evaluation, calling him independent in an activity when he actually falls slightly short of the mark. For example, a therapist may report that an individual is independent in level transfers, even though he requires guarding because he occasionally loses his balance and falls. A patient should not be called independent in an activity unless he is capable of performing the task alone, without anyone in the area to provide setup or supervision.

To ensure accuracy in the functional evaluation, the therapist must observe the patient performing the activity; he should not take the patient's (or anyone else's) word on his capabilities.[i] An inexperienced person may feel that he is safe in a given activity when in fact he is not. For example, the author once had a patient report that he could negotiate ramps safely in a wheelchair. When asked to demonstrate, he careened down the ramp at a breakneck speed, stopping only when he struck a glass door (fortunately, a sturdy one) about 20 feet beyond the bottom of the ramp. Following this hair-raising display, the patient still maintained that his technique was safe.[j]

The areas commonly covered in a functional evaluation following spinal cord injury include mat and bed activities, transfers, wheelchair skills, ambulation, and the ability to instruct others in dependent activities.

Functional skills to examine. *Mat and Bed Skills:* The therapist should evaluate the patient's capabilities in rolling, coming to sitting, gross mobility (moving to the side, forward, or backward), and leg management. For the sake of convenience, these skills are frequently assessed on an exercise mat in a physical therapy gym. Exercise mats are typically firmer than beds, however,

---

[g] This is not meant to imply that functional gains are the only relevant outcomes of a comprehensive rehabilitation program. Certainly gains made in other areas such as breathing ability, skin integrity, psychosocial adaptation, patient and family education, bowel and bladder regulation, equipment procurement, and home modification are also extremely important.
[h] Environmental conditions include the surfaces on which mat skills and transfers are performed (mat vs. bed, for example), as well as the surfaces over which the individual can walk or propel a wheelchair (linoleum vs. sidewalk vs. grass, for example).

---

[i] If direct observation of the skill is not indicated, the documentation should make it clear that it is the patient's judgment of independence, not the clinician's, that is being reported.
[j] This example illustrates both the need to observe a patient's performance of functional activities and the need to *guard* him while doing so!

DESCRIPTION OF THE LEVELS OF FUNCTION AND THEIR SCORES

INDEPENDENT   Another person is not required for the activity (NO HELPER).

7   Complete Independence—All of the tasks described as making up the activity are typically performed safely, without modification, assistive devices, or aids and within a reasonable amount of time.

6   Modified Independence—One or more of the following may be true: the activity requires an assistive device; the activity takes more than reasonable time; or there are safety (risk) considerations.

DEPENDENT   Subject requires another person for either supervision or physical assistance in order for the activity to be performed, or it is not performed (REQUIRES HELPER).

Modified Dependence   The subject expends half (50%) or more of the effort. The levels of assistance required are:

5   Supervision or Setup—Subject requires no more help than standby, cueing or coaxing, without physical contact, or, helper sets up needed items or applies orthoses or assistive/adaptive devices.

4   Minimal Contact Assistance—Subject requires no more help than touching, and expends 75% or more of the effort.

3   Moderate Assistance—Subject requires more help than touching, or expends half (50%) or more (but less than 75%) of the effort.

Complete Dependence   The subject expends less than half (less than 50%) of the effort. Maximal or total assistance is required, or the activity is not performed. The levels of assistance required are:

2   Maximal Assistance—Subject expends less than 50% of the effort, but at least 25%.

1   Total Assistance—Subject expends less than 25% of the effort.

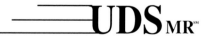

Figure 8–3.   Functional independence measure terminology. (Copyright © 1997 Uniform Data System for Medical Rehabilitation, a division of U B Foundation Activities, Inc. Reprinted with permission of UDS_MR, University at Buffalo, 232 Parker Hall, 3435 Main Street, Buffalo, NY 14214. All of the marks associated with FIM belong to UDS_MR)

and are therefore easier surfaces on which to function. A patient who functions independently on a mat may not perform as well on a bed. For this reason, mat and bed skills should be examined with the patient on a bed before he is judged to be independent.

Transfers: The evaluation should address even and uneven transfers, also called level and unlevel transfers. Even transfers involve moving between the wheelchair and a surface that is level with the wheelchair seat.[k] An uneven transfer involves moving between the wheelchair and a higher or lower surface such as a bathtub, toilet, couch, truck, car, plinth, or the floor. Transfers between a wheelchair and a bed may be even or uneven, depending on the relative heights of the wheelchair and bed.

An independent transfer involves more than merely moving the buttocks from one surface to another. To be independent in a transfer from a wheelchair, a person must be able to set up for the transfer. This includes positioning the wheelchair, locking the brakes, removing or repositioning an armrest, positioning the feet and footrests, and positioning the transfer board, if one is used. The person must be able to move his entire body onto the surface, including his legs. To be independent in a transfer to the wheelchair, he must be able to prepare to leave the area following the transfer. This involves positioning his buttocks appropriately on the wheelchair seat, placing his trunk in an upright position, removing the transfer board (if used), positioning the wheelchair's footrests and armrests, placing his feet on the footrests, and unlocking the brakes.

To transfer safely, a person with a spinal cord injury must move from one surface to another without falling and without traumatizing his skin. Someone who scrapes his buttocks across the wheelchair's tire while transferring has not performed the transfer safely.

Wheelchair Skills: If a patient will require the use of a wheelchair, wheelchair skills should be included in the functional evaluation. The therapist should check the person's capabilities in propulsion over even surfaces, specify the distance that he is able to travel, and note the time required to propel this distance. The evaluation report should note any special equipment that is required for propulsion, such as projections or

surgical tubing on the wheelchair handrims. Obstacle negotiation is also important to address. Evaluation of obstacle negotiation should cover the ability to maneuver over uneven terrain (grass, dirt, gravel, sidewalk), curbs (the therapist should specify the height that can be managed independently), inclined surfaces, doorways, carpet, and stairs. If the patient negotiates obstacles by performing wheelies, the functional assessment should also address his ability to fall safely and right the wheelchair after a fall.

Another important wheelchair skill is the performance of pressure reliefs. A person with a spinal cord injury who cannot perform pressure reliefs independently must have assistance throughout the day in order to prevent the development of pressure ulcers. For this reason, this is an extremely important functional skill to assess. The evaluation should determine both whether the person is capable of performing pressure reliefs and whether he assumes the responsibility to get the relief at appropriate intervals.

Ambulation: If a patient is ambulatory, the therapist should determine how far he can walk, the time required to walk this distance, the gait pattern and equipment used, and the level of assistance required. Capabilities in obstacle negotiation (obstacles listed above in wheelchair skills section) should also be assessed. Additional ambulatory skills that should be addressed include donning and doffing the orthoses (if used), walking backward and to the side, safe falling techniques, coming to stand from the floor, coming to stand from sitting, and returning to sitting from a standing position.

In addition to investigating the patient's ambulatory ability as it relates to level of functional independence, the therapist should perform a gait analysis. This analysis will assist in program planning and equipment selection as the therapist and patient work together to optimize gait.

Instruction of Others: The therapist should determine whether the patient is able to instruct others in safe techniques to assist him with activities in which he is dependent.

Standardized functional assessment tools. Standardized functional assessment tools are frequently utilized as a component of a functional evaluation. These assessment tools provide quantified data that can be useful for communicating with insurance providers about an individual's functional gains. Data gained using a standardized assessment tool can also be used as a measure of a

---

[k] An even transfer is actually between the wheelchair and a surface that is level with the sitting surface. If a wheelchair cushion is used, its top is the sitting surface.

facility's effectiveness, as patients' performance can be compared to the outcomes achieved at other facilities. This information on programmatic effectiveness may be used internally for program development, or externally for accreditation or communication with insurance providers.[13]

The Functional Independence Measure,[l] or FIM instrument (Figures 8–3 and 8–4), is widely used both in the United States and abroad. It is an 18-item instrument that addresses performance in self-care, sphincter control, transfers, locomotion (walking or using a wheelchair), communication, and social cognition. Each item is scored on a scale of 1 to 7, with 1 being total dependence in an activity and 7 being total independence.[12]

The American Spinal Injury Association recommends use of the FIM for functional assessment following spinal cord injury.[1] This assessment tool has been investigated extensively and has been demonstrated to be reliable and valid in general, but may lack the sensitivity to detect some functionally relevant changes among people with spinal cord injury.[1, 26] For example, a person who uses a cane to walk 150 feet would receive the same rating for locomotion as a person who requires a power wheelchair to travel the same distance.

Alternative standardized tools include the Quadriplegic Index of Function,[14, 51] the Barthel Index,[3, 14] and the Spinal Cord Independence Measure.[7] These instruments are not as widely used as the FIM.[26]

Skin integrity. Skin breakdown is a complication of spinal cord injury that can lead to severe medical problems, even death. During the initial examination, the therapist should note any pressure ulcers or early signs of skin breakdown.[m] If a problem is found, pressure over the area must be relieved and the therapeutic program must be modified to avoid any further trauma to the area. The therapist should also notify other members of the team if they are not already aware of the breakdown.

Areas of scarring from healed pressure ulcers should also be noted in the evaluation. Because scar tissue is more susceptible than normal skin to breakdown, care must be taken to minimize trauma to scarred areas. Areas of scarring are also important to note because they provide a history of past skin problems. The presence of healed pressure sores may indicate that the patient has neglected his skin care in the past and needs to learn better habits in this area. These scars may also be the legacy of poor medical care.

Breathing and coughing. Most spinal cord injuries result in at least partial impairment of breathing and coughing ability. As a result, respiratory complications are a significant source of mortality among people with spinal cord injuries. The respiratory evaluation investigates the patient's ability to breathe and clear secretions from his lungs.[n]

Equipment. Equipment has a significant impact upon disability. Someone who lacks needed equipment, or has equipment that is inappropriate or in disrepair, will not be able to function optimally. An equipment check during the initial examination helps to focus attention early on this important area. As soon as a patient's equipment needs have been identified, the process of meeting those needs should be started. If arrangements for equipment purchase or repair are initiated early, the results are likely to be more satisfactory than if equipment procurement is attempted in a rush just prior to discharge.

The therapist should record any orthoses, wheelchairs, or other equipment in the patient's possession and note whether it is rented, on loan, or owned by the patient. The fit, function, and condition of the equipment should be evaluated.[o]

Home environment. One important task during rehabilitation is preparing the person to function in his home. This preparation involves a combination of developing functional skills and adapting the home environment as necessary.

During the initial evaluation, the therapist should find out what environment the patient intends to return to on completion of his rehabilitation. During discharge planning it will be helpful to know, for example, if the patient plans to live alone in an isolated trailer park or with a large family in an apartment building in the city. The therapist should also investigate whether the home has architectural barriers, such as stairs or small bathrooms.

A more detailed assessment of the home should follow. Ideally, a member of the rehabilitation team will visit the home and get a detailed picture of the environment, including door and

---

l The FIM can be obtained from Uniform Data System for Medical Rehabilitation, 232 Parker Hall, 3435 Main Street, Buffalo, New York 14214-3007.

m Skin care and assessment are presented in greater depth in Chapter 6.

n Chapter 7 addresses respiratory evaluation and treatment.

o Evaluation of wheelchairs, cushions, and lower limb orthoses is addressed in Chapters 12 and 13.

FIM™ instrument

	7 Complete Independence (Timely, Safely) **6** Modified Independence (Device)	**NO HELPER**
L E V E L S	**Modified Dependence** **5** Supervision (Subject = 100%+) **4** Minimal Assist (Subject = 75%+) **3** Moderate Assist (Subject = 50%+) **Complete Dependence** **2** Maximal Assist (Subject = 25%+) **1** Total Assist (Subject = less than 25%)	**HELPER**

	ADMISSION	**DISCHARGE**	**FOLLOW-UP**
Self-Care A. Eating B. Grooming C. Bathing D. Dressing - Upper Body E. Dressing - Lower Body F. Toileting			
Sphincter Control G. Bladder Management H. Bowel Management			
Transfers I. Bed, Chair, Wheelchair J. Toilet K. Tub, Shower			
Locomotion L. Walk/Wheelchair M. Stairs	W Walk C Wheelchair B Both	W Walk C Wheelchair B Both	W Walk C Wheelchair B Both
Motor Subtotal Score			
Communication N. Comprehension O. Expression	A Auditory V Visual B Both V Vocal N Nonvocal B Both	A Auditory V Visual B Both V Vocal N Nonvocal B Both	A Auditory V Visual B Both V Vocal N Nonvocal B Both
Social Cognition P. Social Interaction Q. Problem Solving R. Memory			
Cognitive Subtotal Score			
TOTAL FIM Score			

NOTE: Leave no blanks. Enter 1 if patient not testable due to risk.

Figure 8–4.   FIM™ Instrument. (Copyright © 1997 Uniform Data System for Medical Rehabilitation, a division of U B Foundation Activities, Inc. Reprinted with permission of UDS_MR, University at Buffalo, 232 Parker Hall, 3435 Main Street, Buffalo, NY 14214. All of the marks associated with FIM belong to UDS_MR)

hall widths, layout of the bathrooms and kitchen, accessibility of kitchen and bathroom fixtures, accessibility of the entrance to the home, and a variety of other features of the home environment. A family member or the patient can also provide this information if given guidelines for the home evaluation.[p]

Other. The physical therapy examination should cover any other problem areas exhibited by the patient that may require intervention, impact on prognosis, or influence treatment strategies. Possible additional areas of examination that may be indicated include edema, pain, aerobic capacity and endurance, balance, posture, and deep tendon reflexes.[38]

FUNCTIONAL POTENTIALS

After completing the initial examination, the physical therapist makes an informed estimation of the patient's potential for functional gains. This estimation of functional potential, or prognosis, is needed for patient and family education, as well as for goal-setting.[q] Unfortunately, there is no general consensus regarding the functional outcomes that are reasonable to expect following spinal cord injury. Table 8–2 presents functional potentials that are consistent with the guidelines published by the Paralyzed Veterans of America.[r] These descriptions of functional potentials of people with *complete* traumatic spinal cord injuries are meant to assist in goal-setting by providing information about the functional outcomes that are typically achieved by people with various levels of injury. The functional potentials presented here are meant to be used as general "ballpark" guides rather than as rigid guidelines for goal-setting. A given individual may either exceed or fall short of the outcomes presented.

Factors Impacting on Functional Outcomes

Following spinal cord injury, an individual's potential for physical activity is determined largely by his motor function. As a rule, people with more innervated musculature have a greater capacity for independence.[10, 23, 30, 40, 47, 48] The level and extent of a cord lesion determine the motor function that remains after the injury: lower lesions and incomplete lesions leave more of the body's musculature innervated.

If all other factors are equal, a person with a low complete spinal cord lesion can be expected to achieve independence in more advanced activities than are possible for someone with a higher complete lesion. Even the degree of motor sparing within a level can have an impact. For example, someone with only 3/5 strength in the muscles of the myotome at his neurological level of injury may not achieve the same level of independence as another person with the same neurological level of injury who has greater strength in the same musculature. In like manner, preserved motor function in the zone of partial preservation can result in greater functional independence.[s]

Whereas the neurological level of injury is the best predictor of functional gains after a complete injury, it is not a good predictor following incomplete spinal cord injury. When a lesion is incomplete, the degree of completeness and neurological recovery have more relevance to functional potential.[41] People with significant voluntary motor function below their lesions (ASIA D) tend to achieve greater functional independence than do people with more complete (ASIA A, B, or C) lesions.[15]

Although voluntary motor function has a major impact upon a person's functional capacity, it is not the sole determinant. There is no guarantee that someone with a spinal cord injury will be able to master the skills that others with similar injuries have achieved. Research has shown that the following factors are associated with lower functional outcomes: advanced age, pressure ulcers, spasticity, pain, and limitations in range of motion.[10, 22, 27, 33, 37, 49] Clinical experience[2, 20, 29] points to several additional factors that can limit progress in functional training. These factors include obesity, disadvantageous body build (short arms, for example), sensory impairments, impaired mental functioning, inadequate psychological adjustment to the

---

[p] Chapter 15 (www.prenhall.com/somers) addresses architectural design.

[q] The *Guide to Physical Therapist Practice*[38] published by the American Physical Therapy Association distinguishes between goals and outcomes. The term "goals" refers to intended accomplishments related to impairments, and "outcomes" refers to intended accomplishments related to functional limitations and health status. In the portion of that publication that discusses practice patterns, however, both types of intended accomplishments are referred to as "goals." This text will follow that lead: the term "goals" is used in reference to intended accomplishments in all areas rather than being limited to those relating to impairments.

[r] These guidelines, frequently referred to as the "PVA Guidelines," are based on a combination of expert consensus and a review of published research.[8]

---

[s] The zone of partial preservation consists of the myotomes and dermatomes below the neurological level of injury that remain partially innervated after a complete spinal cord injury.[1]

TABLE 8–2. TYPICAL FUNCTIONAL OUTCOMES FOLLOWING COMPLETE SPINAL CORD INJURY

Neurological Level of Injury	Bed Skills	Transfers	Wheelchair (W/C) Skills	Ambulation
C1–3	Total assist	Total assist	**Power W/C:** Independent driving using head, chin, mouth, or breath control. Independent in pressure reliefs using power tilt and/or recline. **Manual W/C:** Total assist.	No functional ambulation
C4	Total assist	Total assist	**Power W/C:** Independent driving using head, chin, mouth, or breath control. Independent in pressure reliefs using power tilt and/or recline. **Manual W/C:** Total assist.	No functional ambulation
C5	Some assist	Total assist	**Power W/C:** Independent driving using hand-control. Independent in pressure reliefs using power tilt and/or recline. **Manual W/C:** Independent to some assist indoors on uncarpeted level floors. Some to total assist outdoors.	No functional ambulation
C6	Some assist	**Even:** Some assist to independent **Uneven:** Some to total assist	**Power W/C:** Independent driving using hand-control. Independent in pressure reliefs either without specialty seating system or using power tilt and/or recline. **Manual W/C:** Independent indoors, some to total assist outdoors.	No functional ambulation
C7–8	Independent to some assist	**Even:** Independent **Uneven:** Independent to some assist	**Manual W/C:** Independent indoors and outdoors on level terrain. Some assist with unlevel terrain.	No functional ambulation
T1–9	Independent	**Even:** Independent **Uneven:** Independent	**Manual W/C:** Independent indoors and outdoors on level and unlevel terrain.	Functional ambulation not typical
T10–L1	Independent	**Even:** Independent **Uneven:** Independent	**Manual W/C:** Independent indoors and outdoors on level and unlevel terrain.	Some assist to independent in functional ambulation using knee-ankle-foot orthoses (KAFOs) and lofstrand crutches or walker
L2–S5	Independent	**Even:** Independent **Uneven:** Independent	**Manual W/C:** Independent indoors and outdoors on level and unlevel terrain.	Some assist to independent in functional ambulation using KAFOs or ankle-foot orthoses (AFOs) and lofstrand crutches or cane

This table is consistent with the outcomes published by the Consortium for Spinal Cord Medicine.[8] More detailed information on functional potentials is presented in Chapters 10–13.

spinal cord injury, poor motivation, fear, medical complications, low endurance, limited equipment options, and poor premorbid athletic ability. Unfortunately, the rehabilitation that is available to an individual can also be a limiting factor. If inadequate time is allotted to rehabilitation, functional gains may be limited. Functional gains can also be constrained if the person undergoes rehabilitation in a setting that is not oriented toward the aggressive pursuit of independence.

Exceptional Cases

Just as some individuals do not achieve the functional outcomes presented in Table 8–2, others achieve greater levels of independence. When youth, health, advantageous body build, a high degree of motivation, good funding, and access to good medical and rehabilitative care combine, the patient may acquire more advanced skills. Table 8–3 presents outcomes that are possible in those exceptional cases.[t]

---

[t] Table 8–3 presents exceptional outcomes for individuals with C8 or higher neurological levels of injury. Functional potentials for people with lower levels "max out" in Table 8–2, as these individuals typically achieve independent functioning.

The information in Tables 8–2 and 8–3 should not be used to set strict upper limits when establishing goals. Therapists who impose inflexible ceilings on patients' goals can limit their functional gains. Greater independence may be achieved if rehabilitation professionals and people with spinal cord injuries attempt to accomplish higher goals, stretching past previous limits.

Incomplete Spinal Cord Injuries

The functional potential of an individual with an incomplete lesion depends largely on the degree of motor sparing or return that he experiences. When voluntary motor function below the lesion is minimal (ASIA B or C), the functional potential is essentially the same as if the individual had a complete lesion (ASIA A) at the same spinal cord level. When significant motor sparing or return occurs in the trunk and extremities (ASIA D and E), a higher degree of functional independence can be achieved.

As is true with complete injuries, voluntary motor function is not the sole determinant of functional outcomes after incomplete spinal cord injuries. Muscle tone is a particularly important consideration when predicting functional potential following incomplete spinal cord injury.

TABLE 8–3. EXCEPTIONAL FUNCTIONAL OUTCOMES FOLLOWING COMPLETE SPINAL CORD INJURY

Neurological Level of Injury	Bed Skills	Transfers	Wheelchair (W/C) Skills
C4	—	—	**Power W/C:** Independent driving using hand control.
C5	Independent; may require equipment	**Even:** Independent; usually require transfer board, may require overhead frame with loops	**Power W/C:** Independent in pressure reliefs without specialty seating system.
C6	Independent	**Uneven:** Independent in slightly uneven transfers; may require transfer board	**Manual W/C:** Independent in negotiation of mild obstacles such as 1:12 grade ramps, slightly uneven (outdoor) terrain, 2- to 4-inch curbs.
C7–8	—	**Uneven:** Independent in uneven transfers, including floor-to-wheelchair	**Manual W/C:** Independent in negotiation of mild obstacles such as ramps with steeper than 1:12 grade, slightly uneven (outdoor) terrain, 4-inch curbs.

Incomplete lesions tend to result in more spasticity than do complete lesions,[24, 36] and severe spasticity can greatly impede progress. Sensory sparing and return can also impact on function after an incomplete spinal cord injury. Because somatosensory feedback is required for normal motor control, sensory impairments can prevent optimal utilization of musculature that remains or returns after a spinal cord injury. Additional factors that impact on functional outcomes are presented above.

Functional Gains after Discharge

Many people with spinal cord injuries experience significant functional gains after they leave rehabilitation.[5, 48, 50] This improvement is at least in part due to the development of skill through practice. In addition, the strength gains that typically occur for an extended period following cord injury[17, 52] may lead to functional improvements.

PROBLEM-SOLVING EXERCISE 8–3

Your patient is a 52-year-old male with complete (ASIA A) C7 tetraplegia. His innervated musculature is strong, his range of motion is normal in all extremities, and he exhibits 1+ spasticity in both lower extremities. He has no medical problems other than the tetraplegia. Prior to his accident he had a sedentary lifestyle. He cooperates in therapy, but does not show a great amount of drive or initiative.

Another patient is a 19-year-old otherwise healthy male with C7 tetraplegia who, remarkably, has identical strength, range of motion, and muscle tone as the 52-year-old. This patient was a star athlete prior to his accident, and shows a very high level of motivation in therapy.

- What functional outcomes might be reasonable to expect for the 52-year-old patient?
- What functional outcomes might be reasonable to expect for the 19-year-old patient?

GOAL-SETTING

Goal-setting is a critical component of a physical therapy evaluation because goals give direction in the development of therapeutic programs. Goals also provide a measure with which the therapist and patient can judge the program's effectiveness.

Setting therapeutic goals involves an analysis of the examination results as they relate to the disablement process. The therapist and patient together consider the impairments, functional limitations, and other factors that could impact on the patient's future health and participation in the various activities that are involved in living. The therapist and patient then set goals that are directed toward minimizing disability, returning the patient to as independent and active a lifestyle as possible.

Patient Involvement

In rehabilitation, people who have experienced a significant loss of bodily function acquire new skills so that they can live more independently. For this process to be successful, patients must be involved in establishing their own goals. A patient's participation in goal-setting ensures that the program is directed toward mastering skills that he values. It also gives him some control over his program, promoting independence.

Setting meaningful goals. Rehabilitation is an active process, requiring patient participation. Functional gains come only after the person with a spinal cord injury has worked long and hard. Setting goals that the patient values may result in better motivation to work in the program, which in turn will enable him to achieve a higher level of independence.

Setting goals that are meaningful to the patient will also increase the likelihood that he will use his newly acquired skills following discharge. A program that focuses on gaining abilities that the patient has no desire to use will only waste time, effort, and money.

The only way to ensure that a program's goals are meaningful to the patient is to involve him in establishing them. The therapist cannot assume that what he wants a patient to achieve will coincide with what that individual wants to learn. A health professional who sets goals without the patient's input runs the risk of establishing goals that he does not value. The therapist may also neglect areas of functioning that the patient wants to address.

Program control. A health professional who dictates a patient's goals places him in a position of dependence. The messages given to the patient are, "We are in control. We know what is best for you. You need us to make these decisions for you. Do as you are told." In contrast, having a patient set his own goals affirms his autonomy, giving him the responsibility of identifying what he wants to achieve. It emphasizes that he is still in control of his life, despite his spinal cord injury.

Placing a patient in control of goal-setting can also improve his motivation in therapy. Having responsibility for the goals may encourage a feeling of greater involvement in his rehabilitation. A person is more likely to feel motivated to achieve goals if he has established them, rather than having had them decreed by a health professional.

The Collaborative Process

Having a patient set his goals does not mean that the therapist cannot provide suggestions and guidance. Goal-setting involves a collaborative process in which the patient and therapist come to an agreement about the intended outcomes of the therapeutic program. The therapist brings to the process an estimation of the patient's functional potential, based on the results of the physical therapy examination. The patient brings to the process his perspective, priorities, and understanding of the social and physical environments in which he is accustomed to living.

Soon after injury. A person who participates in setting his therapeutic goals experiences control in at least one area of his life. This is particularly important for a recently injured person. In the bulk of his experiences since the injury, it is likely that health professionals, family, and even friends have been in charge. By giving the newly injured person some control over his program, the therapist supports his autonomy.

Although it is important to involve patients in setting their goals, a recently injured person cannot be expected to come up with a complete list of rehabilitation goals without any guidance. He is likely to have no idea of his functional potential or of the skills that he will require to function. Yesterday, perhaps a week ago, the recently injured person was probably oriented toward such achievements as paying off a loan, completing college, getting a promotion, or finding a date for the senior prom. The idea of therapeutic goals such as independent transfers or wheelchair mobility is likely to be completely foreign.

To prepare a recently injured person to set his rehabilitation goals, the therapist should share the initial examination results with him and provide an estimation of his functional potential. The therapist should explain what skills are possible to achieve and then ask the patient whether he is interested in learning to perform these activities. The patient should also be given the opportunity to identify any other goals that he wants to pursue.

When discussing goals with an acutely injured person, it is a challenge for the therapist to be forthright and yet tactful. It is important to remember that the patient has not had time to adjust to his injury or even to comprehend its impact. The therapist also needs to understand that the patient may not be overly thrilled with the list of functional skills that are presented as possible goals. Rehabilitation is not an appealing option when compared to recovery.

> Rehabilitation's job is to take your body *as it is* and to maximize your capabilities within recognized limitations. This is a difficult acknowledgment. Rehabilitation seems only second best, which is exactly what it is. To fully accept rehabilitation, for most of us, is to effectively abandon recovery. Rehabilitation can give you strength, reeducation, skills and real improvement, but no cure. Many people find this an easy bridge to cross, and a few find it so upsetting that they temporarily want out of the game.
>
> Barry Corbet[9]

Further down the road. A person who sustained a spinal cord injury months or years ago is likely to have a good understanding of the impact of his injury and should be able to identify specific goals to pursue when he comes for rehabilitation. In these cases, the therapist should start the process of goal-setting by asking the patient what he is interested in achieving in therapy.

The therapist may know of additional functional abilities that the individual has the potential to achieve. These skills may well interest the patient, even though they were not in his list of goals; it may not have occurred to him that these activities were possible. For example, few people would spontaneously come up with the idea of negotiating stairs in a wheelchair. To provide the patient with the opportunity to maximize his functional potential, the therapist should let him know what additional skills he has the potential to achieve and allow him to decide whether he wishes to develop these skills.

Prioritization of Goals

In today's health care environment, funding sources frequently limit the time that a patient can spend in the acute and postacute inpatient phases of rehabilitation.[11, 32] Much rehabilitation now occurs in less expensive alternative settings[6] such as extended care facilities, day rehabilitation programs, outpatient clinics, and patients' homes. Rehabilitation may occur in stages at a series of settings, with the program in each setting building on the patient's prior accomplishments. Because of time constraints, there is typically a limitation in the goals that an individual can achieve during each phase of his rehabilitation.

When the time available in a given phase of rehabilitation is limited, the therapist and patient must identify the goals that are most critical to achieve at that point. Factors to consider when prioritizing goals include discharge destination, assistance available after discharge, availability of therapy following discharge, current medical or orthopedic restrictions on activity, likelihood of significant neurological return, functional potential, financial resources, and the patient's home and community environments.

When funding sources seriously limit the services, equipment, and time in rehabilitation that are available to patients with spinal cord injuries, rehabilitation professionals may have to settle for "adequate outcomes"[u] rather than striving for "optimal outcomes."[32] In these cases, highest priority should be given to goals that are related to basic survival, such as obtaining an appropriate seating system and developing skill in performing pressure reliefs. When setting goals related to functional skills, the therapist and patient may have to accept lower levels of independence, with greater reliance on equipment and assistance. Emphasis must then be placed on education and training of the caregivers, and on teaching the patient how to direct his assistance. The patient and therapist can also establish goals related to activities and a home exercise program that will enable the patient to continue his progress after discharge.

---

[u] This is not to say that the rehabilitation team should "go down without a fight." When faced with funding constraints limiting optimal outcomes, health professionals should utilize the appeals process, seek alternate sources of funding, or both. When these attempts are unsuccessful, the therapist and patient may be forced to settle for adequate rather than optimal outcomes.

Writing the Goals

Emphasis on function. The first step in goal-setting is specifying exactly what functional skills will be pursued in therapy. After the patient and therapist have established a list of purely functional goals, the therapist should determine what impairments need to be addressed in order to accomplish these outcomes. Following spinal cord injury, most new functional skills require an increase in strength, and many require an increase in range of motion. This is because the person with a spinal cord injury now has a limited number of muscles with which to function. Compensation for paralysis requires strength in the muscles left working, and enough flexibility to perform the maneuvers used in functional activities.

The final list of therapeutic goals should include all functional goals plus any goals relating to impairments such as improving strength or flexibility. The goals should also address the equipment procurement, architectural adaptation, and educational outcomes required for optimal functioning and health maintenance after discharge.

Wording of goals. Goals provide direction, focus, and structure for therapeutic programs. Their wording should be specific, with measurable endpoints, because vague goals allow vague therapeutic programs. A program will flounder if the therapist and patient do not have a clear notion of what exactly they are aiming to achieve.

Goals that lack specific endpoints do not identify exactly what is to be accomplished. "Improve wheelchair skills" is an example of such a goal. Technically, if the patient improves even slightly in his wheelchair skills, he has reached the goal as stated. If the objective of the program is for the patient to become independent in a skill, this outcome should be stated clearly.

One way to improve the above goal would be to change it to "independence in wheelchair skills." The patient will have achieved the goal only when he can perform wheelchair skills independently. This wording, however, is still too vague; it does not clarify which wheelchair skills will be addressed in the program. The goal could refer to mastering wheelchair propulsion over even surfaces, learning to negotiate various obstacles, or performing any number of wheelchair-related activities.

A more appropriate wording would be "independence in wheelchair negotiation of 6-inch curbs." This wording communicates a specific skill (negotiation of a particular obstacle) and provides an endpoint (independence).

Goals regarding physical prerequisites (strength, range of motion) should also be specific, with identifiable endpoints. This does not mean that the therapist must state exactly what muscle grade or degree of flexibility will be aimed for. It is not always possible to predict exactly what strength or range of motion a particular individual will need to perform a functional activity, because these requirements vary with body build and ability. For this reason, specifying an exact muscle grade or degree of flexibility is often not appropriate.

How, then, can the therapist write a specific goal? Wording prerequisite goals in terms of function will accomplish this end. For example, "increase strength to the degree required to achieve the above functional goals" provides a verifiable endpoint. When the functional goals have been accomplished, the goal of improving strength has also been accomplished. This wording helps to keep the program's focus on function, preventing it from drifting away from its real purpose.

PROBLEM-SOLVING EXERCISE 8–4

Your patient was in an automobile accident 1 week ago. She sustained an incomplete spinal cord injury with T10 neurological level of injury, plus multiple extremity fractures. She was transferred to your facility today for inpatient rehabilitation. The following orthopedic restrictions are listed in her chart: (1) TLSO (thoracolumbo-sacral orthosis) to be worn at all times. (2) Strict nonweightbearing on the left lower extremity and bilateral upper extremities. You speak with the patient's surgeon about the restrictions and find that the patient should not push or pull with the upper extremities, or bear any weight through either the hands or the forearms. The left lower extremity may be allowed to rest on the floor or on a wheelchair footrest, but the patient is not to bear any additional weight on it.

The TLSO will be worn for approximately 3 months. From your past experience, you do not expect it to hamper her progress in rehabilitation to a large degree. The nonweightbearing restrictions are to be in force for at least 6 weeks. While these restrictions are in place, you do not foresee any significant progress in her functional abilities.

Your facility's case manager informs you that the patient's insurance company will fund 5 weeks of inpatient rehabilitation. From past experience with this company, the case manager feels that the inpatient stay may be extended by a week or two at the most.

- What solution can you think of that would maximize the patient's benefit from therapy? To implement this solution, what will the case manager, nursing staff, and therapies need to do?
- What therapeutic goals would you set at this time?

SUMMARY

- Physical therapy examination and evaluation involve an assessment of the patient's impairments, functional limitations, and other factors that contribute to the disablement process. The data gathered in the examination establishes a baseline and provides the basis for program planning.

- The examination and evaluation should be a collaborative effort between the therapist and patient. Inclusion of the patient as an active participant in the process serves to reinforce his autonomy and ensures that the therapeutic goals established are meaningful to him.

- Following spinal cord injury, a physical therapy examination should include the patient's history and subjective statements, voluntary motor function, sensation, muscle tone, range of motion, functional abilities, skin integrity, ability to breathe and clear secretions, equipment, and home environment.

- After the initial examination is completed, the therapist makes an informed estimation of the patient's potential for functional gains. This estimation is largely influenced by the patient's voluntary motor function. Additional factors to be considered include range of motion, spasticity, age, secondary or preexisting medical conditions, body build, sensation, cognitive and emotional status, and funding for equipment and rehabilitation services.

- Goals are set in a collaborative process in which the patient and therapist come to an agreement about the intended outcomes of the therapeutic program. The patient and therapist must take into account the examination results, the estimated potential for functional gains, the patient's priorities, the social and physical environment in which the patient will function after discharge, and the resources available for rehabilitation.

- When funding sources limit the rehabilitation services available to the patient, goals must be prioritized. Factors to consider when prioritizing goals include discharge destination, assistance available after discharge, availability of therapy following discharge, current medical or orthopedic restrictions on activity, likelihood of significant neurological return, functional potential, financial resources, and the patient's home and community environments.

- Goals are established with an emphasis on increasing functional independence and reducing disability. All goals should be written with specified, measurable endpoints.

9

Strategies for Functional Rehabilitation

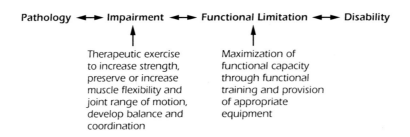

Pathology ◄──► Impairment ◄──► Functional Limitation ◄──► Disability

Therapeutic exercise
to increase strength,
preserve or increase
muscle flexibility and
joint range of motion,
develop balance and
coordination

Maximization of
functional capacity
through functional
training and provision
of appropriate
equipment

The key to designing a successful functional rehabilitation program is understanding the nature of the task: the person with significant motor loss due to spinal cord injury must learn to use her body in a totally different manner after her injury. To sit up, move from one place to another, open a door, or perform any other physical activity, she must use her remaining musculature in unaccustomed ways. Each activity requires adequate strength, joint range of motion, and muscle flexibility to perform the motions involved. In addition to these physical prerequisites, each functional task involves the performance of a set of skills. Functional independence requires the development of all of these physical and skill prerequisites. It also requires the provision of the equipment needed to function optimally. The role of the physical therapist in functional rehabilitation is to work with the patient to identify her relevant impairments and functional limitations, and to address these problems through therapeutic exercise, functional training, and the provision of appropriate equipment.

MOVEMENT STRATEGIES FOLLOWING SPINAL CORD INJURY

Normal movement involves the coordinated action of an array of skeletal muscles; dozens of muscles

function in concert to move the trunk and extremities. Damage to the spinal cord disrupts this normal pattern of motion. The extent of this disruption depends on the completeness and pattern of neurological damage. The manner in which an individual can move after a spinal cord injury will be constrained by the sensory and motor function that returns or is preserved following the injury.

Complete Injuries

After sustaining a complete spinal cord injury, a person who wishes to regain functional independence faces a difficult task. She must learn to use what muscles remain to perform the tasks of now absent musculature. With fewer muscles functioning, she must find new ways to move. Three major tools are available to enable a person with complete spinal cord injury to make the most of what musculature remains functional: muscle substitution, momentum, and the head-hips relationship.

Muscle substitution.   Muscle substitution can be used when the musculature normally causing a motion is weak or absent. In one method of substitution, agonist musculature compensates for a strength deficit. For example, the tensor fascia lata can substitute for a weak or absent gluteus medius in hip abduction. This and other substitutions by agonists should be familiar to all physical therapists, who monitor for them whenever performing manual muscle tests.[9, 11]

Agonists are commonly used to substitute after spinal cord injury. Whenever the agonists of a weak or nonfunctioning muscle remain functional, they work to compensate for the motor deficit. In the paralysis that results from spinal cord injury, however, agonists often are not available for substitution. In these instances, other methods of substitution are used.

The substitutions used following spinal cord injury may seem mysterious to the uninitiated. (Muscles are used to move joints that they do not even cross!) However, a muscle used to substitute does not do anything out of the ordinary. It simply contracts concentrically, eccentrically, or isometrically, pulling in the same direction that it always did. Unless a muscle is moved surgically, it cannot do otherwise. The key to muscle substitution after spinal cord injury is learning to use a muscle's pull differently.

In addition to substitution by agonists, there are three ways in which a muscle can be used to substitute. Muscle action can be combined with the effects of gravity, tension in passive structures, or fixation of the distal extremity to effect a desired motion.

Substitution using gravity. Functioning musculature can be used to reposition a part in such a way that gravity will effect the desired motion. For example, shoulder motion can be used to pronate the forearm. When a person is sitting upright, shoulder abduction and internal rotation can move the forearm to a position in which the palm faces downward slightly. Once the forearm is in this position, the downward pull of gravity will pronate the forearm.

When gravity is used in substitution, the movement's force will be very limited. Any significant resistance will prevent the motion.

Substitution using tension in passive structures. Tension in nonfunctioning musculature can also be used to effect motion. The tenodesis grasp is an example of this method of substitution. When a tenodesis grasp is used, the extensor carpi radialis longus and brevis are used to extend the wrist. The resulting increase in tension in the long finger flexors causes the fingers to flex (Figure 9–1).

This method of substitution can cause a more forceful motion than is possible in substitu-

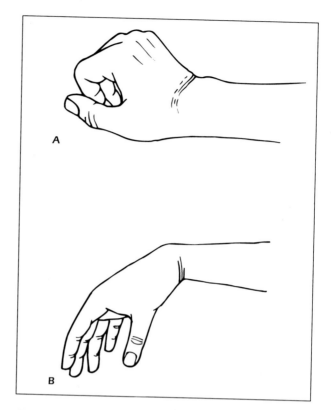

Figure 9–1. *Tenodesis grasp used by people with C6 and C7 tetraplegia.* **(A)** *Fingers close upon wrist extension and* **(B)** *open upon wrist flexion. Gravity provides power for wrist flexion.*

tions using gravity; the motion can be performed against some resistance. For this reason, a tenodesis grasp can be functionally useful in activities such as eating, dressing, and self-catheterization.

Substitution using fixation of the distal extremity. This method of muscle substitution involves fixing the distal end of an extremity by stabilizing it on an object and using proximal musculature to cause motion at an intermediate joint. The anterior deltoid and pectoralis major (clavicular portion) can be used to extend the elbow in this manner.[15] When a person with a spinal cord injury extends her elbow using her proximal musculature, she first stabilizes her hand. In this closed-chain position, she then uses her anterior deltoid and pectoralis major to adduct the humerus. Figure 9–2 illustrates this process. In this example the patient is sitting upright with her hand stabilized beside her on a mat. When the humerus is adducted, the proximal end of the forearm also moves, since it is attached to the humerus. With the hand fixed distally, the forearm moves in an arc (Figure 9–2C). The result is extension of the elbow.

Using this method of substitution, a fair amount of force can be generated. A patient who

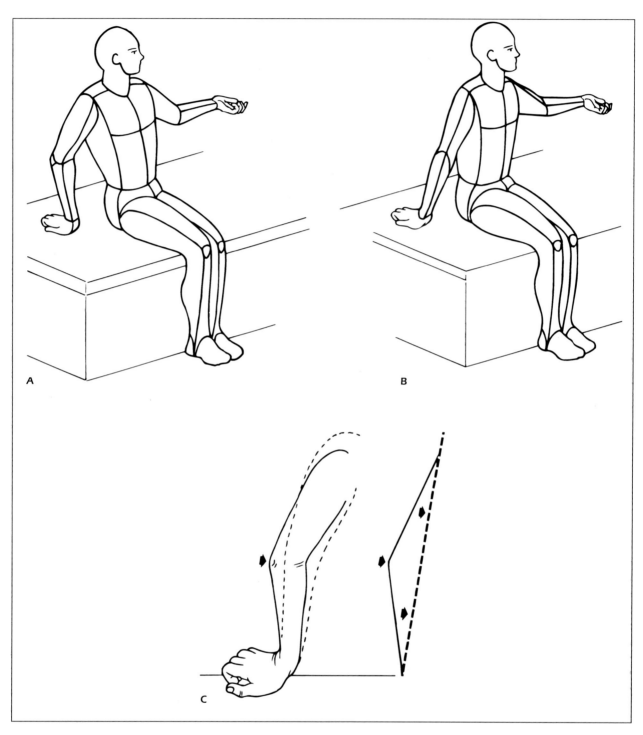

Figure 9–2.   Substitution using fixation of the distal extremity. **(A)** An individual lacking functioning triceps is sitting on a mat, leaning on one arm. The elbow is flexed and the hand is stabilized on the mat. **(B)** The elbow is extended by adducting the shoulder. **(C)** When the humerus is adducted, the proximal forearm also moves medially, resulting in elbow extension.

has adequate strength proximally will be able to extend her elbows forcefully enough to lift her trunk from a forward lean (Figure 9–3).

In a related maneuver, an individual who lacks functioning triceps can "lock" her elbows in extension during weight-bearing activities such as transfers. "Locking" the elbows involves placing the palms on the supporting surface (mat, wheelchair cushion, or bed) and positioning the arms with the shoulders externally rotated, the elbows

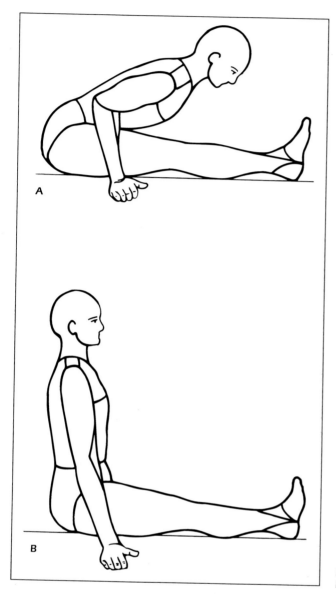

A

B

Figure 9–3. Muscle substitution used to extend the elbows and lift the trunk from a forward lean.

and wrists extended, and the forearms supinated.[a] Elbow extension is maintained during the weight-bearing activity through strong contraction of the anterior deltoids and external rotators.

Angular momentum. Another movement strategy that is used following spinal cord injury involves the use of momentum. Momentum is the tendency of an object to continue moving once it has been set in motion. An object that is rotating about an axis has angular momentum, the tendency to continue its rotation.

Angular momentum can be used to augment motion at a given joint when musculature is weak. A patient who cannot complete an action when she "places" a body part, moving it slowly, may be able to complete the same action if she "throws" the part instead. An example would be someone with weak posterior deltoids who is sitting in a wheelchair and wishes to position her arm behind the wheelchair's push handle. She may find that she is unable to "place" her arm behind the push handle but can move her arm into position by throwing it.

In another use of angular momentum, innervated musculature causes motion, and the momentum of the moving part(s) results in movement in other areas of the body. This use of angular momentum is exemplified by the technique for rolling used by people who lack functioning trunk and lower extremity musculature. To roll, a person lacking

---

[a] The interphalangeal (IP) joints should be flexed to preserve the tenodesis effect. This precaution will be addressed later in this chapter.

trunk and lower extremity musculature throws her head and arms to the side. If the motion is forceful enough and timed correctly, the momentum of the head and arms will carry the trunk from supine.

The angular momentum of a large object (such as a person) is equal to the sum of the angular momenta of all of its parts. Each part's angular momentum is proportional to its velocity, mass, and the moment arm, or distance of the part from its axis of rotation. The effects of these characteristics of angular momentum are important to keep in mind during functional training. They are summarized in Table 9–1.

Head-hips relationship.   The third important movement strategy used to perform functional activities following complete spinal cord injury involves the head-hips relationship. When using this strategy, a person with a spinal cord injury moves her buttocks by moving her head in the opposite direction. To do so, she pivots on her shoulders, which act as a fulcrum in a first class lever (Figure 9–4).

Transfers provide a good example of the use of the head-hips relationship. Someone with a complete injury who wishes to lift her buttocks up and to the left in a transfer does so by moving her head down and to the right while pivoting on her arms.

Incomplete Injuries

The motor and sensory function that remains or returns following incomplete spinal cord injury is highly variable. The movement strategies that an individual with an incomplete injury uses to function will depend upon the extent and pattern of her neurological damage. A person who has sensory sparing but lacks any voluntary motor function below her lesion will utilize the same movement strategies as those used by people with complete spinal cord injuries: muscle substitution, momentum, and the head-hips relationship. Someone with minimal motor sparing is likely to use the same strategies, modified to incorporate the use of functioning musculature. For example, a person who retains some use of her hip flexors could use these muscles while rolling, by combining hip flexion with her head and arm motions.[b] In contrast, a person with significant voluntary motor function remaining below her spinal cord lesion may be

capable of more normal movement patterns; if adequate strength remains in enough musculature below the lesion, she may be able to function without the use of muscle substitution, momentum, or the head-hips relationship. Finally, a person who has an intermediate degree of motor return may utilize these compensatory movement strategies for some activities, and more normal movement patterns for others.

PHYSICAL PREREQUISITES: STRENGTH AND RANGE OF MOTION

Whether an individual learns new movement strategies to compensate for lost musculature, or relearns more normal movement patterns, she requires adequate muscle strength and range of motion to perform the motions involved. During rehabilitation after spinal cord injury, appropriate measures must be taken to ensure that the individual will be prepared for the specific physical activities that she will eventually use to function. To accomplish this end, it is important for clinicians to keep in mind the manner in which the individual will ultimately function. (How will she transfer? How will she grasp objects?)

Muscle Strength

Strengthening is an essential component of any rehabilitation program after spinal cord injury, and should start as soon as therapy is initiated. After spinal cord injury, virtually all innervated musculature is used in various functional activities and thus should be strengthened. The strengthening program should place particular emphasis on musculature that is used in elbow extension, shoulder flexion and horizontal adduction, and scapular protraction and depression, as these muscles are used for most functional activities. Trunk musculature that remains innervated should also be strengthened, so that it can be utilized for upright trunk control and for the performance of mat activities such as rolling and coming to sitting.

Even musculature that exhibits normal (5/5) strength may need to be strengthened because functional activities will place great demands on the patient's musculature. The muscles that remain innervated must compensate for those that have been paralyzed; therefore, innervated muscles are often required to perform actions for which they are not ideally suited. An example is the use of the anterior deltoids to extend the elbows when the triceps are paralyzed. The anterior deltoids, which

---

[b] By flexing her hip while throwing her head and arms, she can add angular momentum in the direction of the roll. This technique is described in more detail in Chapter 10.

TABLE 9-1. PROPERTIES OF ANGULAR MOMENTUM

Property	Impact on Momentum	Application	Clinical Example: Rolling
Summation of momenta	The angular momentum of a large object is equal to the sum of the angular momenta of all of its parts.	Following spinal cord injury, the motions of body parts that remain innervated are used to generate momentum to move parts that are paralyzed. Motions of relatively small body parts (head and upper extremities) are often used to cause larger parts (trunk and lower extremities) to move.	During rolling, momentum from head and arm motions is used to move the trunk and lower extremities. Isolated motions of the head or upper extremities may not create adequate momentum for rolling, but the combined momentum from the head and arms moving synchronously may generate adequate momentum to move the rest of the body.
Velocity	Angular momentum is proportional to the object's (or part's) velocity.	An extremity moving with higher velocity will have greater momentum than the same extremity moving at a slower speed. When a person uses momentum to perform a functional activity, his motions must be performed with adequate speed.	Someone who moves his arms and head too slowly while attempting to roll will not be able to work up enough momentum to move his trunk.
Mass	Angular momentum is proportional to the object's (or part's) mass.	If all other things are equal, an object with greater mass will have greater angular momentum. Because the arms are relatively small, it can be difficult at first to generate adequate momentum using arm motions to cause motion in the pelvis and lower extremities.	Rolling can be made easier by attaching a weight to a patient's forearm. This increases the angular momentum that the arm will have at a given speed, making rolling easier. Although adding a wrist weight to facilitate rolling is not practical as a permanent measure, it can be used to assist rolling during functional training.
Moment arm	Angular momentum is proportional to the object's (or part's) moment arm. A moment arm is the distance of the part from its axis of rotation.	For a given mass and velocity, an object with a longer moment arm will have greater angular momentum. When a person uses momentum from arm motions to move, he will be more successful if he moves his arms in an arc that is as distant as possible from the axis of rotation.	Rolling is easier when the elbows are held in extension and the shoulders are flexed to lift the arms above the trunk. Throwing the arms in this position keeps their mass further from the body, increasing their moment arms. This enables the patient to generate more angular momentum when he throws his arms.

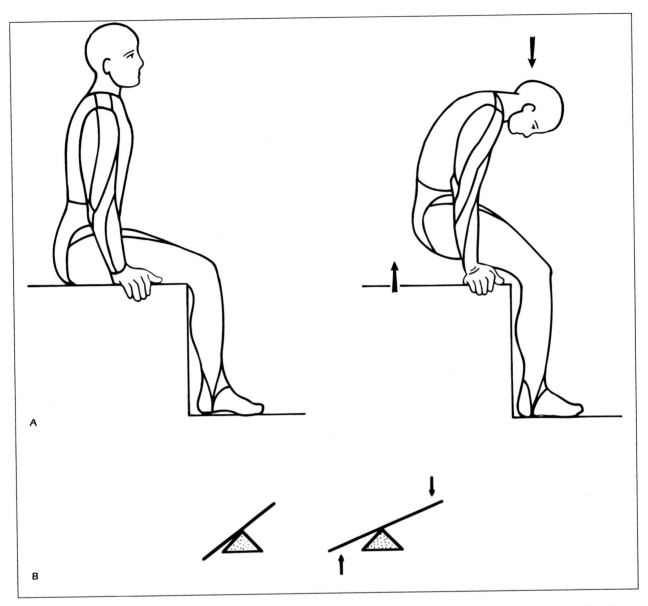

Figure 9–4. The head-hips relationship. **(A)** The person with a spinal cord injury pivots on his arms, moving his head down to lift his buttocks. **(B)** First class lever.

normally flex the glenohumeral joints, must extend the elbows during transfers and maintain this extension while the person supports her weight on her arms. The stronger the anterior deltoids are, the more stable the arms will be during transfers.

Strengthening exercises should consist of active-assisted, active, or resisted motions, depending on the strength of the functioning musculature. To the degree possible within the constraints imposed by orthopedic precautions, the patient can be asked to contract her muscles maximally for short durations. This muscle activity should result in strengthening and hypertrophy of innervated musculature. Lower intensity exercises with longer duration can also be included in the program, to increase resistance to muscle fatigue.[8] The strength-

ening program may include any combination of the following: proprioceptive neuromuscular facilitation (PNF) techniques, isometric exercises, progressive resistive exercises (concentric and eccentric), strengthening through functional activity, isokinetic exercise, and electrical stimulation.[4, 10, 14, 17, 26] During strengthening exercises, care should be taken to avoid placing stress on unstable vertebral areas.[c]

During rehabilitation, the patient with a spinal cord injury should be encouraged to use her functioning musculature as much as possible. While not

---

[c] These precautions are discussed in more detail later in this chapter.

PROBLEM-SOLVING EXERCISE 9-1

Your patient has complete (ASIA A) T5 paraplegia. He is working toward the goal of independent floor-to-wheelchair transfers. He is sitting on the floor in front of his wheelchair, with his right hand on the wheelchair seat and his left hand on the floor.

- In what direction should the patient move his head in order to lift his buttocks up and to the right toward the wheelchair seat?
- Should he throw his head in a rapid motion, or should he place it using a slow and controlled motion?
- Will he need to use muscle substitution to maintain elbow extension on the left?

in therapy, she can maximize her strength by performing isometric exercises, lifting weights, participating in her care, and propelling her wheelchair.

Range of Motion

Maintenance or development of appropriate range of motion is critical during rehabilitation. At best, the development of contractures will slow the rehabilitation process. At worst, contractures will seriously limit the person's ultimate functional potential. To prevent the development of contractures, range-of-motion exercises should be initiated as soon as possible after spinal cord injury. When vertebral instability is present, care should be taken to avoid placing stress on the unstable segments of the spine.[d]

Joint range of motion and muscle flexibility should be increased or maintained (as indicated) through positioning and daily exercises during acute care and rehabilitation. Passive and active range of motion exercises, PNF techniques, joint mobilization, prolonged static stretching, or a combination thereof may be employed.[2, 29] To complement and eventually replace the exercise program provided by health professionals, the family can be

instructed in range-of-motion exercises or the patient can be taught self-range of motion.

When range-of-motion limitations are seriously impeding functional progress, splints or casts may be used to help increase or maintain range between therapy sessions.[2, 21] When these devices are used, however, the health care team must be aware of their potential hazards and take measures to avoid them.[e]

As a rule, normal joint range of motion and muscle flexibility will enhance function. After spinal cord injury, however, greater than normal motion is required in some areas, and mild tightness is desirable in others. Moreover, range and flexibility in some areas will have greater functional significance than in others. For example, limited elbow extension will have greater impact on function than will a comparable limitation in ankle plantar flexion. Table 9–2 summarizes the range of motion requirements of people with spinal cord injuries.

STRATEGIES FOR FUNCTIONAL TRAINING

A program limited to strengthening and range-of-motion exercises will not result in the development of functional skills. The most important component of a functional rehabilitation program is functional training. Through functional training, the individual with significant motor impairments learns the muscle substitutions and acrobatic maneuvers that she will use to move her body, take care of herself, and manipulate her environment. The person with less severe motor deficits relearns more normal movement strategies for performing functional tasks.

The purpose of functional training is the acquisition of certain motor skills that can later be utilized in environments other than the therapy gym. By helping patients acquire functional skills that they can perform at home or in the community, therapists can enhance their capacity to return to their accustomed activities and roles. Theories of motor learning provide some concepts that can be useful in this process.[f] Table 9–3 pre-

---

[d] These precautions are discussed in more detail later in this chapter.

[e] Splints and casts can impair circulation and cause skin breakdown and nerve damage. To avoid these complications, the health care team must ensure that the splints or casts have been fabricated correctly. These devices must also be evaluated regularly to ensure that they continue to fit and function appropriately.

[f] An in-depth discussion of motor learning is beyond the scope of this text. For more information on this topic, the reader is referred to the following references: 19, 22, 23, 24, 27.

TABLE 9–2.   RANGE OF MOTION REQUIREMENTS FOLLOWING SPINAL CORD INJURY

	Ideal Range	Functional Significance
Neck	As normal as possible within orthopedic constraints and precautions.	Mat/bed activities, upper body dressing, self-care, and standing and sitting posture.
Low back	Mild tightness.	Transfers and mat/bed activities.
Shoulders	Normal range in all motions.	Mat/bed activities, upper body dressing.
	In the absence of functioning triceps: greater than normal combined extension/external rotation with elbow extended.	Coming to sitting using certain methods. Note: concerns regarding potential shoulder problems may direct the therapist and patient toward alternate methods of coming to sitting that do not require greater than normal shoulder range.
Elbows	Full extension is essential.	Transfers, mat/bed activities, wheelchair skills, and ambulation.
	Normal or near normal flexion.	Self-care, eating, mat/bed activities, wheelchair skills, and floor-to-wheelchair transfers.
Forearms	Normal supination.	"Locking" elbows in the absence of functioning triceps.
	Normal pronation.	Manipulation of hand-held joystick of power wheelchair.
Wrists	Normal extension.	"Locking" elbows in the absence of functioning triceps. Tenodesis grasp.
	Normal flexion.	Release of tenodesis grasp.
Fingers	In the absence of functioning finger flexors: mild tightness in long finger flexors.	Tenodesis grasp.
Hips	Full extension.	Ambulation.
	At least neutral extension.	Prone lying and prone mat/bed activities.
	Normal or near normal flexion.	Mat/bed activities, dressing, wheelchair skills, and coming to stand from the floor.
	Normal or near normal external rotation.	Dressing.
Knees	Normal extension.	Ambulation.
Hamstrings	110 to 120 degrees of passive straight leg raise.	Long-sitting, dressing, mat mobility, floor-to-wheelchair transfers, and coming to stand from the floor.
Ankles	At least 10 degrees of dorsiflexion.	Ambulation.
	At least neutral dorsiflexion.	Prevention of skin breakdown due to excessive pressure over metatarsal heads and toes while sitting in a wheelchair.

sents some general suggestions for functional training that are consistent with these theories.

Functional training should be initiated as early as possible in the program rather than being postponed until strength and range have been maximized. Early functional training can have tremen-dous psychological benefit, enabling the newly injured person to do things for herself and experience tangible progress toward her goals. As the patient masters and uses more skills, her increased activity level also serves to further develop her strength and flexibility. A balanced program that

TABLE 9–3.   SUGGESTIONS FOR ENHANCING MOTOR LEARNING DURING FUNCTIONAL TRAINING

Suggestion	Reasoning
Plan for successes as much as possible.	It can be frustrating and discouraging to attempt tasks that are too difficult to perform. In contrast, successful accomplishment of a task can be rewarding and motivating. A patient's motivation may be enhanced if her activities in therapy are structured so that she can experience success in many of the tasks that she is asked to perform.
Have the patient practice tasks that are difficult but doable.	If an activity can be performed too easily, practice will not lead to the development of new motor skills. Moreover, practice of a task that is too easy will not engage the patient as effectively in the active learning of the task. Functional training should include tasks that the patient can successfully perform, but with effort.[22] Practice of these tasks will enable the patient to master new skills.
Encourage multiple repetitions of new skills.	Repetition of practice enhances motor learning.[19,23,24] A patient who successfully performs a new skill one time may be unable to repeat the action in the future if she does not practice. If instead she repeats the maneuver multiple times, she is more likely to retain the ability to perform that task in the future.
Once a patient can perform a task, intersperse practice of this task with the practice of other tasks.	Except during early practice of a new motor pattern, retention of learned motor skills is enhanced when the task is interspersed with other tasks (random practice) instead of being practiced repetitively without interruption by practice of other tasks (blocked practice).[19,22,23]
During early practice of a skill, provide physical and verbal guidance to the patient. During subsequent practice, reduce guidance. To the extent possible while ensuring safety, allow the patient to make errors and discover her own solutions to movement problems.	Guidance during early practice can reduce the patient's fear, enhance safety, and guide the patient toward successful performance of the task. During later practice, allowing errors and encouraging the patient to "discover" movement strategies will enhance learning and retention.[19,23,24]
During early practice of a skill, provide frequent feedback regarding the patient's attempts at performing the task. During subsequent practice, reduce the frequency of the verbal feedback.	Feedback on performance (knowledge of results) that is frequent during early practice and diminishes as the person continues to practice may promote the learning and retention of new skills. A possible explanation for this enhanced learning is that with reduced feedback, the person learns to detect errors in performance because she cannot rely so heavily on the feedback.[23]

addresses skill concurrently with strength, muscle flexibility, and joint range of motion will be most efficient in helping the patient progress toward independence.

The task of functional training may seem overwhelming when one is faced with a recently injured person who is unable to roll in bed or even to stay upright in a wheelchair. How on earth will this person achieve the lofty goals that she has identified? The answer is that functional goals can be achieved through the application of a few simple functional training strategies: building a foundation of movement skills, breaking down activities into their component parts, making tasks easier, and learning skills in reverse.

Building a Foundation of Movement Skills

Following spinal cord injury, an individual with significantly impaired or absent voluntary motor function below her level of injury has a limited number of innervated muscles with which to perform tasks that previously involved the coordinated action of the muscles of her entire body. To compensate for lost musculature, she must learn to move in new ways, using muscle substitution, momentum, and the head-hips relationship to function. She must also learn to use her remaining musculature to maintain her balance in the various postures involved in functional activities. Physical therapy involves the development of new motor skills used to move and maintain balance. The emphasis of treatment is on function rather than normalcy.

In contrast, a person who retains or regains adequate motor functioning below her spinal cord lesion may have the potential for more normal movement patterns. Coordinated motor function, however, will not necessarily appear spontaneously as neurological return occurs. For this reason, physical therapy should address the development of normalcy of motion in addition to functional status in instances where significant voluntary motor function remains or returns following spinal cord injury.

Although motor function plays a critical role in movement, sensation is also important. Normal motor control involves input from the visual, vestibular, and somatosensory systems.[1, 3] A person with sensory impairment following spinal cord injury may have limited or absent ability to sense her body's contact with the supporting surface, and may be unable to sense the positions and motions of her body parts relative to each other and relative to the environment. During rehabilitation, a person with significant sensory loss must learn to utilize remaining sensory cues (visual, vestibular, and somatosensory above the lesion) when performing motor tasks.

As a part of building a foundation of movement skills, the person with motor or sensory impairment needs to develop the ability to control her body in the various postures and different environments involved in functional activities. Concepts from theories of motor learning[22–24] as well as proprioceptive neuromuscular facilitation (PNF) techniques[20, 25, 26] can be applied to promote the development of coordinated movement in the trunk, neck, and extremities.

Progression of postures.   Motor control can be developed in a variety of postures. Typically, patients who have profound motor impairments following spinal cord injury first work in basic postures such as sidelying and supine. Coordinated movement may be easier in these positions because of the low center of gravity and large base of support in these postures. Early work can also occur while sitting in a wheelchair. The postural support provided by a wheelchair can provide the postural stabilization that a recently injured person is likely to require in an upright posture.

As a patient's ability to stabilize herself and move within a basic posture develops, she can work in progressively more challenging positions. A more advanced posture is characterized by a higher center of gravity and a smaller base of support. Depending on a patient's muscle function, she may progress to working in a variety of postures such as prone-on-elbows, supine-on-elbows, long- and short-sitting with and without upper extremity support, kneeling, and standing. To develop a foundation of movement skills, the patient can work on the ability to stabilize and move within these and other postures.

"Stages of motor control."   The PNF approach involves progressing the patient from more basic to more advanced motor abilities. The four "stages of motor control" conceptualized in PNF, progressing from most basic to most advanced, are mobility, stability, controlled mobility, and skill.[26] Before one can exhibit a given level of motor control in a particular posture, one must be capable of more basic levels of control in that posture. For example, transferring between a wheelchair and a bed by pivoting on the arms (skill) requires the ability to weight-shift (controlled mobility) when sitting with the hands on the supporting surfaces, which presupposes the ability to maintain a sitting posture (stability) with the hands on the supporting surfaces, which in turn requires adequate range of motion and the ability to initiate motion (mobility). An example in a more basic posture is walking the elbows to the side while in prone on elbows. Walking on the elbows (skill) requires the ability to weight shift (controlled mobility) in prone on elbows, which presupposes the ability to maintain the prone on elbows posture (stability), which in turn requires adequate range of motion and ability to initiate motion (mobility). In therapy, the patient starts by developing basic motor abilities if they are lacking, and then builds on these abilities as her control improves.

Breaking Down the Activity into Its Component Parts

Following spinal cord injury, many functional activities consist of a fairly complex sequence of actions; a "simple" act such as coming to sitting can require a series of five or more separate steps. Each of these steps requires a different set of prerequisite skills. Rather than trying to tackle a complex multistep activity as a whole, it can be more productive to break it down and work toward mastery of each component. Once the patient masters the different steps, she can work on putting them together to perform the functional task.[19, 23, 27]

Making the Task Easier

Certain activities are exceedingly difficult initially, even when broken into separate steps. When working on such a challenging task, functional training may involve practicing an easier version of the task. Using this approach, the patient develops her skill by practicing a maneuver that involves the same technique as the activity in question but is easier to perform. As her skill improves, the maneuver that she practices should increase in difficulty, becoming more similar to the functional skill being addressed.

An example of a task that could be approached using this strategy is the side-approach transfer from the floor to a wheelchair. This activity includes a step in which the person lifts her buttocks all the way from the floor to the wheelchair seat. This maneuver requires great flexibility, strength, and finesse. A patient can develop her technique for floor-to-chair transfers by performing transfers between the floor and successively higher surfaces. She may begin by transferring to and from a surface 1 or 2 inches higher than the floor and gradually increase the surface's height until she can transfer as high as the wheelchair seat.

Another example of this functional training strategy is the practice of bed skills on a mat. A mat, because it is a firmer surface than a bed, provides an environment in which it is easier to perform such tasks as coming to sitting or moving the legs while in a sitting position. It is often beneficial to develop these skills on a more stable surface (mat) during early practice, and progress to practice on a less stable surface (bed).

Learning the Skill in Reverse

Many activities are the most challenging at their starting points. These maneuvers are difficult to initiate and become easier as they approach completion. The task of assuming the prone-on-elbows position is an example of such an activity. It takes a good deal of strength for someone with C5 or C6 tetraplegia to lift her upper trunk off of a mat or bed from a sidelying or prone position. The task becomes easier as her upper trunk rises higher and her arms move into a more vertical position under her shoulders.

Working on the skill in reverse is a useful training strategy for this type of activity. Instead of starting at the beginning of the activity where the task is the most difficult, the patient starts at the endpoint and works backward. Emphasis should be placed on the patient controlling her motion as she works on the skill in reverse. For example, the individual learning to assume the prone-on-elbows position from sidelying can start in prone-on-elbows and practice moving toward sidelying. To develop her skill, she should move slightly toward sidelying in a controlled fashion and then actively return to prone-on-elbows (Figure 9–5). As her ability improves, she should work on moving progressively further from and returning to the prone-on-elbows position in a controlled fashion.

PRECAUTIONS

Strengthening, range-of-motion exercises, and functional training are essential for maximizing functional capabilities following spinal cord injury. These interventions, however, can cause problems if they are applied improperly. Excessive shearing forces or blunt trauma can damage the skin over the buttocks during transfer training. Vigorous strengthening or range-of-motion exercises can place undue stress on an unstable spine and compromise neurological status. Improper techniques in hand and wrist range of motion exercises can overstretch the long finger flexors and compromise the patient's functional grasp. To prevent these and other problems, the health practitioner must take appropriate precautions during all rehabilitative efforts.

Orthopedic Precautions

Following traumatic spinal cord injury, the injured segment of the spinal column is likely to be unstable for a period of time. The duration of spinal instabil-

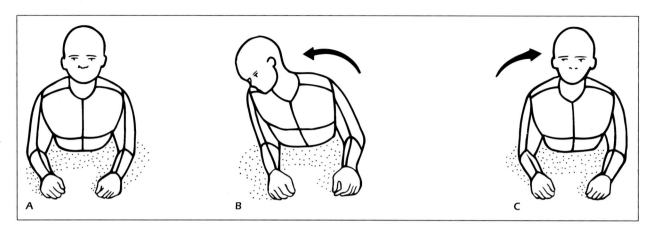

Figure 9–5.   *Learning a skill in reverse: assuming prone-on-elbows. (A) Begin in the end position (prone on elbows in this case). (B) Shift a short distance out of the position. (C) Return to the original position.*

ity will vary with the type and severity of the boney and ligamentous injuries, as well as the surgical and nonsurgical interventions applied. To avoid causing additional neurological injury, health professionals must remain cognizant of the status of the patient's spinal stability, and carefully avoid any activities that could put the unstable spine at risk. Until the patient has been cleared for unrestricted activity, the surgeon should be consulted about the patient's readiness for any new activities that could potentially place stress on the spinal column.

When the cervical spine is unstable, shoulder range-of-motion exercises should be performed cautiously, with the therapist performing the exercises gently to avoid stress to the cervical region. It may be advisable to avoid shoulder flexion or abduction past 90 degrees until the spine has been stabilized.[18] Strong contraction of the shoulder musculature should also be avoided while the cervical spine is unstable, as muscular contraction may place stress on this area of the spine.

When the lumbar spine is unstable, strong muscle contraction of the hip musculature should be avoided because it may cause motion of the lumbar vertebrae. Hip motions should also be restricted; the therapist should perform hip range-of-motion exercises gently, and may need to avoid flexion past 90 degrees. Passive straight-leg raise exercises should be limited to a range in which motions do not cause any tilting of the pelvis. The allowable range will vary, depending on the patient's hamstring flexibility.

Spinal precautions are critical considerations in treatment planning and implementation during the acute and early rehabilitation stages following spinal cord injury. Another orthopedic concern that becomes important as time passes is osteoporosis. Bone mass is rapidly lost after the spinal cord is damaged, resulting in increased risk of fracture.[16] When severe osteoporosis is present, activities that place excessive stresses on the osteoporotic bones should be avoided.

PROBLEM-SOLVING EXERCISE 9–2

Your patient is working toward the goal of rolling from supine to prone. You have instructed her to throw her head and arms (all moving in the same direction) back and forth from side to side in order to roll. From past experience, you know that rolling is most difficult while the patient is supine and the pelvis remains horizontal on the mat. Rolling becomes progressively easier as the pelvis rolls out of this position.

- The patient is unable to roll from supine. What can you do to enable her to practice this skill independently while you work with another patient? (Think of several things you could do to enable her to practice rolling.)
- As her skill develops, how will you progress the program?

Skin Precautions

Pressure ulcers are a common and preventable complication of spinal cord injury that can have serious effects on the person's health and level of disability. During functional training, care must be taken to avoid prolonged pressure, blunt trauma, and excessive shear forces on the skin. The skin should also be monitored regularly for signs of

TABLE 9–4.   SKIN PRECAUTIONS DURING FUNCTIONAL TRAINING

Activities	Vulnerable Areas	Prevention Strategies
Mat/bed skill training	Skin overlying the elbows	Protective elbow pads during prolonged periods of weight-bearing on elbows
Transfer training	Skin overlying the ischial tuberosities, sacrum, and coccyx	Avoidance of blunt trauma or excessive shear forces to the skin through careful instruction and guarding during practice
		Proper clothing (should wear pants rather than hospital gowns; watch for rivets and bulky seams in pants)
Wheelchair skills training	Skills performed in the wheelchair	
	Skin overlying the ischial tuberosities, sacrum, coccyx, and greater trochanters	Properly fit and adjusted wheelchair, appropriate cushion Proper sitting posture Pressure reliefs every 15 to 20 minutes
	Skin overlying the palms (vulnerable during propulsion)	Protective gloves
	Stair negotiation on buttocks	
	Skin overlying the ischial tuberosities, sacrum, and coccyx	Avoidance of blunt trauma or excessive shear forces to the skin through careful instruction and guarding during practice
		Protective padding covering vulnerable areas
Ambulation	Posterior heels, medial malleoli, and any skin in contact with orthoses	Orthoses fit and adjusted to prevent excessive shearing or pressure

breakdown. Special attention should be given to the areas of skin most likely to be damaged, based on the patient's activities and other contributing factors.[g] Table 9–4 specifies areas of skin that can be damaged during functional training, and presents strategies for skin protection during functional training.

Blood Pressure Precautions

Orthostatic hypotension, a drop in blood pressure that occurs when moving toward upright from a horizontal position, commonly occurs when sitting activities are initiated after spinal cord injury. Plac-

ing an abdominal binder and thigh-high elastic stockings on the patient can help prevent dizziness and loss of consciousness during initial upright activities. The patient should also be moved gradually from supine to sitting with the legs placed in increasingly dependent positions.[h] When a patient experiences a drop in blood pressure during upright activities, the therapist can elevate the patient's legs, recline the trunk to a less upright position, or both.

Autonomic dysreflexia is a more serious problem that can occur in people who have cord lesions above T6, usually after 6 or more months have elapsed since the injury. It is caused by

[g] Chapter 6 addresses skin care following spinal cord injury in greater depth.

[h] Chapter 2 presents additional information on orthostatic hypotension. Chapter 12 provides more in-depth information on accommodation to upright sitting.

uncontrolled sympathetic discharge, brought on by a noxious stimulus (such as bladder distension or overly vigorous hamstring stretching) below the lesion. Signs and symptoms include elevated blood pressure, bradycardia, a pounding headache, and sweating and vasodilation above the lesion. When autonomic dysreflexia is suspected, the health professional should place the patient in an upright sitting position with the legs dependent, and should remove the source of the problem.[i]

Preservation of Beneficial Tightness

The precautions just described are required for preventing medical complications and injuries. In contrast, the precautions presented in this section are aimed at preserving the patient's capacity to perform functional skills. Though these precautions may seem to be less important than those described previously, failure to adhere to them can lead to a profoundly diminished capacity for functional independence.

Tenodesis grasp.   People who lack active finger flexion but retain active wrist extension after spinal cord injury can learn to use a tenodesis grasp to perform functional tasks such as writing or self-catheterization. This grasp requires mild tightness in the long finger flexors. With the appropriate degree of tightness in these muscles, the fingers will close upon wrist extension and open fully when the wrist is flexed (Figure 9–1). Overstretching of the long finger flexors results in a loss of the functional tenodesis grasp. At the other extreme, excessive shortening of these muscles will inhibit release.

Whenever the wrists and fingers are extended simultaneously, the long finger flexors are stretched and the tenodesis grasp can be damaged. To ensure the development of appropriate tension in the long finger flexors, range-of-motion exercises should include finger extension to neutral (0 degrees in all joints) with the wrist fully flexed and full finger flexion with the wrist fully extended. Finger extension must be avoided when the wrist is positioned in extension.

The tenodesis grasp is at risk during the performance of functional skills. Simultaneous wrist and finger extension can occur during transfers or functional mat activities when weight is borne on the palms. To avoid stretching the long finger flexors, an individual who uses a tenodesis grasp (or may use this grasp in the future) should keep her interphalangeal joints flexed whenever she bears weight on her palms.

Preservation of mild tightness in the long finger flexors is particularly important because damage to the tenodesis mechanism may be permanent. Once the finger flexors become overstretched, it is difficult to get them to tighten. An overzealous but uninformed therapist can cause lasting problems by overstretching these muscles during the acute stage after injury. In like manner, an uninformed patient or family member may damage the tenodesis grasp mechanism. Many newly injured people and their families are eager to perform exercises on the paralyzed extremities in the hope that these exercises will bring about a return of function. Often, the hands are a focal point of these exercises. For this reason, the patient and her family should be educated regarding the importance of avoiding overstretching the long finger flexors.

Appropriate shortening should be allowed to develop in the long finger flexors of people with C7 or higher tetraplegia, to facilitate tenodesis grasp and release. Although people with C5 and higher tetraplegia do not have the wrist extensors needed for a tenodesis grasp, their long finger flexors should be allowed to tighten. This tightness may make it possible to use the hand as a hook. Moreover, it is common for voluntary motor function to return in one or more levels caudal to the neurologic level of injury during the months and years after injury.[5, 7, 12, 13, 28] Many people with C5, and a few with C4, tetraplegia (motor level) regain function in the C6 myotome during the first 8 months after their injuries.[6] Thus a person who initially lacks wrist extensor function can regain it and may then require finger flexor tightness for a tenodesis grasp.

In addition to requiring mild tightnesss in the long finger flexors, a tenodesis grasp also requires adequate strength in the wrist extensors. During the early stages following spinal cord injury, care should also be taken to prevent overstretching of wrist extensors with less than fair (3/5) strength, as overstretching of weakened musculature can inhibit its functioning. Overstretching can occur when the wrists are allowed to remain positioned in flexion due to the effects of gravity. Positioning the wrists in extension with cock-up splints or hand rolls when at rest can prevent this problem.

---

[i] Chapters 2 and 3 address autonomic dysreflexia in greater depth.

Low back. When spinal cord injury results in significant loss of motor function, many functional skills involve using motions of the arms, head, and upper trunk to move the pelvis and legs. Mild tightness in the low back can enhance the performance of functional skills by allowing head and shoulder motions to be transmitted to the lower body. Excessive flexibility in the low back can interfere with function by allowing disassociation between the upper and lower trunk, permitting the upper trunk to move without any motion occurring in the lower trunk or legs. For example, people with complete spinal cord injuries pivot on their arms and use head and scapular motions to move their buttocks during transfers. A person with an overstretched low back who attempts to lift her buttocks in this manner may find that her back elongates and her buttocks remain on the supporting surface when she attempts to pivot on her arms. To prevent this dissociation between motions of the upper and lower trunk, care should be taken to preserve mild tightness in the low back.

Perhaps the most important precautionary measure that can be taken to preserve beneficial tightness in the low back is the maintenance of proper positioning in a wheelchair. A patient's low back can be overstretched when she sits for

prolonged periods with her buttocks forward on the wheelchair seat, as this position places her lumbar region in a kyphotic posture (Figure 9–6A). When a person with a spinal cord injury sits in a wheelchair, her buttocks should be positioned well back on the seat (Figure 9–6B). This posture will help preserve appropriate tightness in the low back.

Long-sitting can also overstretch the low back if the hamstrings are tight. When the hamstrings are shortened, sitting with the knees extended places stress on the low back. For this reason, long-sitting should be avoided when hamstring tightness prevents passive straight-leg raise to 90 degrees. Additionally, hamstring stretching should be performed in supine rather than in long-sitting.

EQUIPMENT SELECTION

Equipment selection is a critical component of functional rehabilitation following spinal cord injury. Regardless of the level or degree of completeness of an individual's spinal cord lesion, she is likely to require equipment in order to function optimally. The extent and level of the person's neurological damage will influence the type of equipment needed. At one extreme, an individual

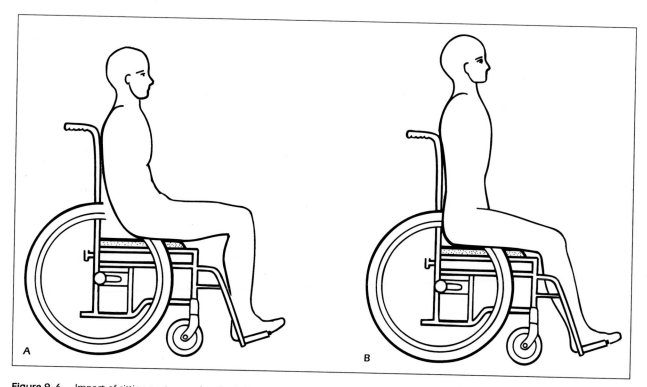

Figure 9–6. *Impact of sitting posture on low back flexibility.* **(A)** *Low back overstretched by sitting with buttocks forward on seat.* **(B)** *Low back protected by positioning buttocks well back on wheelchair seat.*

who has either a very low lesion, or near-normal motor and sensory function below the lesion, may need equipment as simple as a straight cane or an ankle-foot orthosis in order to function safely and independently. At the other extreme, a person who has a high cervical lesion with minimal or no motor function below her injury may require a power tilt and recline wheelchair with computerized controls that interface with environmental control units.

In recent years there has been a virtual explosion in the adaptive equipment market. There is much variability in the quality and usefulness of available products; some are excellent, others have little value. Additionally, a given piece of equipment may be beneficial for some people and useless or even detrimental to others. To maximize functional status, health, and satisfaction, and gain most for their equipment dollar, health professionals and people with disabilities should select equipment carefully.

Establishing Need

The first step in ordering equipment is establishing a need. A person's need for equipment may be functional, medical, or both.

Functional need.   A functional need exists if an individual requires equipment to perform functional activities. Equipment such as wheelchairs, doorknob adaptors, leg orthoses, and vehicular modifications can meet functional needs. Equipment can make the life of a person with physical impairments easier, enable her to do things that she otherwise could not do, and conserve the time and energy used for mundane tasks to free her to do other things. Clinicians should be mindful, however, that equipment is a double-edged sword: it can also create dependence on itself, reducing the user's ability to function without it. A person who is dependent on a piece of equipment has to put up with its drawbacks (bulk, cosmesis, maintenance, etc.). She will also be unable to function in the event that the equipment is lost, broken, misplaced, or left behind.

One challenge in recommending equipment to improve function is determining whether equipment is truly needed. If someone cannot perform an activity satisfactorily without equipment, she may benefit from equipment designed to aid in the task. Judgment regarding the functional need for equipment should take the individual's future potential into consideration. In cases where it is possible that a person could learn to function safely without a particular piece of equipment, the equipment should be purchased only after a thorough rehabilitative effort has failed to enable her to function independently without it. Therapists should be wary of equipment that at first appears to improve function but that the patient could learn to do without. Often, equipment can make a task easier while someone is first learning a skill, like training wheels on a bike. The problem is that therapists often leave these "training wheels" on, thinking that the need remains. The result is that the need does remain and the person is left using unnecessary equipment.

Once it has been determined that someone cannot function well *without* a given piece of equipment, she and the therapist should ascertain whether she can function better *with* it. Through the years much money has been wasted on equipment that turned out to be of limited or no benefit to the intended users. Prior functional training with and "test drives" of equipment prior to purchase could help to eliminate this problem.

Medical need.   A medical need exists if a piece of equipment is required for an individual to maintain or return to a healthy state. Wheelchairs, wheelchair cushions, and vertebral orthoses are examples of equipment that meets medical needs.

Some medical needs are temporary. For example, during the acute phase of rehabilitation, a person with a spinal cord injury may experience orthostatic hypotension as her body readjusts to upright sitting. During this adjustment period, she may require a wheelchair with a reclining back and elevating leg rests. Within a brief period of time, however, she will most likely adjust to upright sitting and will not need these features in a wheelchair. With a temporary medical problem such as this, the needed equipment should be rented or borrowed rather than purchased.[j]

Regardless of whether a piece of equipment meets a temporary or permanent medical need, it should be chosen carefully. Ideally, the equipment will achieve the medically necessary outcome while allowing the patient to function as independently as possible. For example, the vertebral orthosis will stabilize the spine adequately without unnecessarily restricting the patient's extremity motions, or the wheelchair cushion will provide

---

[j] This is not possible with all types of equipment. Vertebral orthoses, for example, must be purchased.

the needed pressure distribution without interfering unnecessarily with transfers.

Choosing Equipment

Once a functional or medical need has been established, the health professional and patient must determine which piece of equipment best meets this need. For most types of equipment, there is a large selection from which to choose. The various brands generally offer different options and vary in quality, price, durability, maintenance required, availability of replacement parts and qualified maintenance facilities, warranty specifications, and other characteristics. With the market constantly expanding, clinicians who are involved in prescribing and advising on equipment must keep current.

When deciding on a piece of equipment, it is best to keep in mind the fact that any equipment has both advantages and disadvantages. For example, pneumatic wheelchair tires are better than solid tires in the following respects: smoother ride and easier propulsion over uneven surfaces, easier negotiation of curbs, and greater traction. Pneumatic tires also have their drawbacks. They go flat if punctured, increase the overall width of the wheelchair, cost more than solid tires, track more dirt into buildings, and must be filled with air periodically. Like pneumatic tires, any equipment or component will have both positive and negative qualities. Clinicians involved in prescribing or advising on equipment should investigate the benefits and drawbacks of the available equipment options.

When possible, equipment (or an identical model) should be used for a trial period before it is purchased. Ideally, several different models will be made available for trials.[k] This practice increases the likelihood that the equipment chosen is really the best match for the individual concerned.

The decision about any piece of equipment should be based on its advantages and disadvantages, considering the needs and priorities of the prospective user. Ultimately, the final choice between equipment options is based on values. When weighing the positives and negatives of different options, should ease of use take priority, or should greatest consideration be given to convenience, durability, maintenance requirements,

price, or aesthetics? Because equipment choice is a value-laden decision with no universal right and wrong answers, the person for whom the equipment is being ordered must be involved in the decision. Otherwise, the piece of equipment chosen by the clinician may not be the one most suitable to the values and priorities of the user. Involving the prospective user in equipment selection also promotes independence, and encourages personal responsibility and consumerism.[l]

SUMMARY

- Functional rehabilitation after spinal cord injury is a challenging task. Depending on the voluntary motor function that an individual retains or regains after injury, she must either learn to use her muscles and move her body in new ways, or relearn to move in a more normal fashion as motor return occurs.

- An individual who has a complete injury learns to use compensatory movement strategies to perform functional tasks. These strategies include muscle substitution, angular momentum, and the head-hips relationship.

- A person who has an incomplete injury will learn to use compensatory movement strategies, more normal movement patterns, or a combination of the two, depending on her motor function.

- The individual with a spinal cord injury who wishes to minimize her level of disability must increase the strength in her innervated musculature and preserve or increase her joint range of motion and muscle flexibility. She must also develop an array of physical skills. The physical therapist assists in this process by working with the patient to develop and implement a program of therapeutic exercise and functional training.

- Four basic strategies can be used in functional training after spinal cord injury: building a foun-

---

[k] Vendors and company representatives are often accommodating when asked to provide equipment for trial.

[l] Involving patients in ordering equipment does not mean ordering them everything that they want or everything that their funding sources are willing to purchase. An individual may want something that is not truly needed or that will be detrimental to her physical or functional status. In an instance such as this, the health professional would be doing the patient a disservice by ordering the requested equipment. The clinician also has a responsibility to third party payers to recommend equipment only when it can be justified as meeting a true need.

dation of movement skills, breaking activities down into their component parts, making tasks easier, and learning skills in reverse.

- During functional training and therapeutic exercise, health professionals must take appropriate precautions. These include a variety of orthopedic and medical precautions, as well as measures to preserve beneficial tightness in the long finger flexors and the low back.

- The patient and therapist also work together to select appropriate equipment that will reduce disability by promoting health and enhancing function.

10

Functional Mat Skills

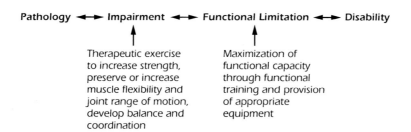

Pathology ←→ Impairment ←→ Functional Limitation ←→ Disability

Therapeutic exercise
to increase strength,
preserve or increase
muscle flexibility and
joint range of motion,
develop balance and
coordination

Maximization of
functional capacity
through functional
training and provision
of appropriate
equipment

Functional mat skills include rolling, coming to sitting, gross mobility on a mat or bed (moving around on a mat or bed), maintenance of an unsupported sitting posture,[a] and leg management. These skills are required for independent mobility; before someone can get out of bed in the morning, he must first be able to sit up and move to the edge of the bed. These skills are also required for independent dressing.

This chapter presents a variety of functional mat techniques,[b] as well as suggestions on how to teach them. It is important for the reader to keep in mind that the motions used to perform any functional task vary between people. This variability is due to differences in body build, skill level, range of motion, muscle tone, and patterns of strength and weakness.

The descriptions of techniques and training presented in this chapter should be used as a guide, not as a set of hard and fast rules. During functional training, the therapist and patient should work together to find the exact techniques that best suit that particular individual.

[a] Unsupported sitting balance is addressed in Chapter 11.
[b] This chapter does not attempt to present all possible functional mat techniques. An individual who is unable to master a skill described in this chapter may fare better with a variation of that technique or with an altogether different method.

PRACTICE ON MAT AND BED

An exercise mat is a good surface on which to learn mat skills. It is firmer than most beds, making it an easier surface on which to practice. At the same time, a mat is soft enough to allow the inevitable tumbles without injury.

Although the skills presented in this chapter are first practiced on a mat, the ultimate goal should be for the patient to function on a bed. This is the surface on which he will most often find himself when he needs to roll over, come to sitting, or get dressed. Since a bed is a more difficult surface on which to function, ability developed on a mat will not automatically transfer to bed function. Thus after an individual has begun to develop some skills on a mat, he should practice them both on a mat and on a bed. This will increase the likelihood that the skills learned in therapy will be utilized outside of therapy.

PRECAUTIONS

Following spinal cord injuries, the activities involved in functional mat training can cause problems if appropriate precautions are not taken. Mat activities can result in excessive motion in unstable segments of the spine, skin damage, and

183

TABLE 10-1. PRECAUTIONS DURING FUNCTIONAL MAT TRAINING

Potential Problems	Mat Activities That Place Patients at Risk	Precautions
Excessive motion at site of vertebral instability, potentially causing additional neurologic and orthopedic damage.	Any activity involving excessive motion or muscular action at or near site of unstable spine. Examples: prone-on-elbows activities while the cervical spine remains unstable, long-sitting while the lumbar spine remains unstable.	• Strictly adhere to orthopedic precautions. • Check fit of vertebral orthoses with patients in the different postures involved in mat training. • When the spine is unstable, avoid activities that may cause motion or strong muscular contraction at site of instability.
Skin abrasions and pressure ulcers.	Any activities creating shearing forces on skin. Examples: dynamic activities while weight-bearing on the elbows, practice moving the buttocks on a mat. Any activities causing prolonged pressure over areas vulnerable to skin damage. Examples: supine activities when there is a pressure ulcer over the sacrum, sidelying activities when there is scarring over the greater trochanters.	• Protective padding over elbows or buttocks during prolonged practice of activities that create shear forces on skin. • Limited time spent in activities that cause shear forces to skin that is not protected by padding. • Bridge vulnerable areas during activities that would expose them to prolonged pressure: have the patient lie on pillows that are positioned proximal and distal to, but not in contact with, the wound or vulnerable skin.
Impaired tenodesis grasp due to overstretching of the long finger flexors.	Any activities involving simultaneous wrist and finger extension. Examples: weight-bearing on palms with fingers extended while coming to sitting or balancing in long-sitting.	• With patients who may utilize tenodesis grasp (people with C7 or higher tetraplegia) avoid simultaneous wrist and finger extension. • When weight-bearing on palms, maintain interphalangeal joints in flexion.
Overstretched low back, resulting in diminished capacity for functional independence.	Any activities involving simultaneous hip flexion with knee extension in patients with hamstring tightness, placing stress on the low back. Example: long-sitting when the hamstrings are tight.	• Avoid long-sitting in patients who lack a minimum of 90 degrees of passive straight-leg raise. • Patients with hamstring tightness may sit safely with their knees flexed and hips externally rotated.

overstretching of the low back and long finger flexors. Table 10–1 presents a summary of precautions for functional mat training.

PHYSICAL AND SKILL PREREQUISITES

Each method of performing a functional activity involves a particular set of skills. Each activity also has strength, joint range of motion, and mus-

cle flexibility requirements. A deficiency in any of these skill or physical prerequisites will impair a person's performance of the activity.

The descriptions of functional techniques presented in this chapter are accompanied by tables that summarize the skill and physical prerequisites. Exact values for the physical prerequisites are not given because the requirements vary among individuals. For example, when coming to sitting using a given method, someone who is strong and coordinated may require less range in shoulder hyperextension than another person who is weaker or less coordinated.

PROGRAM DESIGN

The therapeutic program is designed to enable the patient to achieve all of his functional goals. The steps of program planning follow.

1. Identify the functional goals.[c]
2. Determine the methods that the patient will utilize to perform the activities identified in the goals. This determination will involve choosing the methods that provide the best match between the patient's characteristics and the physical and skill requirements of the activities.
3. Consider the patient's impairments and functional limitations as they compare to the physical and skill requirements of the activities to be achieved.
4. Devise a therapeutic program to develop the needed strength, range of motion, and skills.

For the purposes of program planning, it may be best for the therapist and patient first to consider each goal separately and devise a plan for achieving each goal. The different goals and their plans can then be considered together. Fortunately, there is much overlap of physical and skill prerequisites for the different functional activities. Thus a person working on rolling from supine is potentially progressing toward independence in rolling, assuming prone-on-elbows, and coming to sitting without equipment. Furthermore, work aimed at developing one ability can benefit other, seemingly unrelated, activities. For example, the strengthening and motor learning that results from practicing mat skills may benefit a patient's transfers or basic wheelchair skills.

FUNCTIONAL MAT TECHNIQUES FOLLOWING COMPLETE SPINAL CORD INJURY

After a spinal cord injury, a person's potential for achieving independence in bed skills is determined largely by his voluntary motor function. Table 10–2 presents a summary of the level of independence in bed skills that can be achieved by people who have complete spinal cord injuries at

USING CHAPTER 10 AS A RESOURCE FOR PROGRAM PLANNING

When using this chapter as a resource to assist in designing a program to work toward a functional goal, the therapist should first read the description of that functional activity. These descriptions are located under the headings "Functional Mat Techniques Following Complete Spinal Cord Injury" in the first half of the chapter, and "Functional Mat Techniques and Therapeutic Strategies Following Incomplete Spinal Cord Injury" at the end of the chapter. Based on the description of the functional activity, the corresponding tables, or both, the therapist can determine what physical and skill prerequisites are required to perform the activity. Taking into consideration the patient's evaluation results, the therapist can determine where the patient has deficits relevant to the functional goal. The program should then be designed to address these deficits, developing the needed physical and skill prerequisites.

This chapter presents functional training strategies for each prerequisite skill listed in the tables that accompany the descriptions of mat techniques. These functional training strategies are presented under the headings, "Therapeutic Strategies Following Complete Spinal Cord Injury," and "Functional Mat Techniques and Therapeutic Strategies Following Incomplete Spinal Cord Injury." The therapist can use these suggestions, coupled with his or her own imagination, clinical expertise, and problem solving, to design a functional training program. The program should aim first at developing the most basic prerequisite skills and build to more advanced skills as the patient's abilities develop.

different motor levels (motor component of neurological level of injury). When prognosticating about an individual's capacity to develop bed skills, the clinician should take into consideration the many other factors that also impact on functional gains.[d]

---

[c] Goal-setting is addressed in Chapter 8.

[d] Chapter 8 presents factors that can influence functional outcomes.

TABLE 10–2. FUNCTIONAL POTENTIALS

Motor Level	Significance of Innervated Musculature	Potential for Independence in Bed Skills
C4 and higher	Inadequate voluntary motor function to contribute to bed skills.	Using hospital bed and input through mouth- or voice-control, independent in coming to sitting from supine. Dependent in all other bed skills.
C5	**Partial innervation of the deltoids** makes it possible to extend the elbows using muscle substitution. Deltoid function plus **partial innervation of the infraspinatus and teres minor** make it possible to "lock" the elbows in extension. **Partial innervation of the biceps** brachii, brachialis, and brachioradialis makes it possible to use elbow flexion to pull. Lack of triceps function makes rolling difficult due to flexion of elbows when placing or swinging arms. Minimal serratus anterior function is inadequate to stabilize the scapulae against the thorax.	**Typical Functional Outcomes** **Rolling:** some assist, pulling on bedrail or loops **Coming to sitting:** some assist, either walking on elbows or pulling on loops **Gross mobility in sitting:** dependent to some assist **Leg management:** dependent to some assist **Exceptional Functional Outcomes** Independent in bed skills. Likely to require bedrails or loops.
C6	**Fully innervated deltoids, infraspinatus, teres minor, and clavicular portion of the pectoralis major** allow for stronger elbow extension and "locking" using muscle substitution. **Fully innervated biceps brachii** allows for stronger pull using elbow flexion. **Partial innervation of the serratus anterior** makes it possible to stabilize the scapulae against the thorax. Scapular protraction allows greater lift of the buttocks. **Partial innervation of the latissimus dorsi** enhances shoulder girdle depression, allowing greater lift of the buttocks. Minimal innervation of the triceps brachii is inadequate to contribute significantly to bed skills.	**Typical Functional Outcomes** **Rolling:** some assist to independent, with or without equipment **Coming to sitting:** some assist to independent, with or without loops **Gross mobility in sitting:** some assist **Leg management:** some assist **Exceptional Functional Outcomes** Independent in all bed skills without equipment.
C7	**Partial innervation of the triceps brachii** allows for stronger elbow extension. **Full innervation of the serratus anterior** provides more stable scapula, stronger protraction and upward rotation. **Partial innervation of the latissimus dorsi and sterno-costal portion of pectoralis major** enhances shoulder girdle depression, allowing greater lift of the buttocks.	**Typical Functional Outcomes** Independent to some assist in bed skills without equipment. **Rolling:** independent **Coming to sitting:** independent **Gross mobility in sitting:** independent to some assist **Leg management:** independent to some assist
C8	**Full innervation of the triceps brachii** provides normal strength in elbow extension. **Full innervation of the latissimus dorsi and nearly full innervation of pectoralis major** allow strong shoulder girdle depression. **Nearly full innervation of flexor digitorum superficialis and profundus, and partial innervation of flexor pollicus longus and brevis** provide grasp without muscle substitution, making leg management easier.	**Typical Functional Outcomes** Independent to some assist in bed skills without equipment **Rolling:** independent **Coming to sitting:** independent **Gross mobility in sitting:** independent to some assist **Leg management:** independent to some assist
T1 and below	**Fully innervated upper extremities** make all bed skills more easy to achieve.	**Typical Functional Outcomes** Independent in all bed skills without equipment.

References for innervation: 1, 3, 6, 7, 11. For more complete innervation information, see Appendix B (www.prenhall.com/somers).

Regardless of the level of injury, a person who sustains a complete spinal cord injury has a limited number of muscles with which to perform functional mat skills. To roll, come to sitting, or move about on a bed, he must utilize the muscles innervated above his lesion to move his entire body. During rehabilitation, the patient learns how to perform mat skills using a variety of compensatory strategies, including muscle substitution, momentum, and the head-hips relationship.[e]

Rolling

Rolling is one of the more basic mat skills.[f] It is used to turn in bed and is a prerequisite skill for several methods of coming to sitting. Self-care activities, such as dressing, also involve rolling.

---

[e] These movement strategies are explained in Chapter 9.

[f] "Basic" is not meant to imply that rolling is easy. In fact, learning to roll from supine can be very difficult for people with cervical lesions.

The physical prerequisites for rolling using the three techniques described below are summarized in Table 10–3. Table 10–4 summarizes the prerequisite skills for rolling.

Supine to prone without equipment. To roll from supine to prone without equipment, a person with a complete spinal cord injury turns his body using momentum from head and arm motions.

Some people with complete injuries who are very coordinated, strong, or have low lesions (or any combination thereof) are able to roll in a single maneuver. An individual with this capability simply throws his head and arms forcefully in the direction toward which he wants to roll.

For most people with complete injuries, rolling requires more effort. Momentum for the roll is built by rocking back and forth. To roll in this manner, the person swings his head and arms forcefully to one side and then the other. His trunk rocks from supine with each swing, rolling partially in the direction of the throw. As his trunk falls back toward supine, he adds momentum to

TABLE 10–3. ROLLING—PHYSICAL PREREQUISITES

	Supine to prone without equipment	Supine to prone with equipment	Prone to supine
Strength			
Anterior deltoids	☑	☑	√
Middle deltoids	√	√	√
Posterior deltoids	☑	√	√
Biceps, brachialis, and/or brachioradialis		☑	
Range of Motion			
Shoulder Flexion		√	√
External rotation	☑		
Horizontal adduction	√	√	
Horizontal abduction	√		
Elbow Extension	☑		√
Flexion		√	
Forearm supination	√		√

√: Some strength is needed for this activity, or severe limitations in range will inhibit this activity.

☑: A large amount of strength or normal or greater range is needed for this activity.

TABLE 10-4.   ROLLING—SKILL PREREQUISITES

	Supine to prone without equipment	Supine to prone with equipment	Prone to supine
Supine Skills			
Position elbows in extension (p. 205)	✓	✓	
Maintain elbow extension while flexing shoulders (p. 206)	✓	✓	
Throw arm(s) across body, elbow(s) extended (p. 206)	✓	✓	
Combined arm throw and head swing (p. 206)	✓	✓	
Roll toward prone using momentum (p. 206)	✓		
Position arm to assist in rolling with equipment (p. 207)		✓	
Roll body toward prone by pulling on equipment (p. 207)		✓	
Prone Skill			
Roll from prone by pushing with arm (p. 211)			✓

the motion by throwing his head and arms. By repeatedly throwing his head and arms left and right in coordination with the trunk's rocking motion, the person can build enough momentum to roll (Figure 10–1).

The number of throws that an individual must use to roll will depend on several factors. Someone with greater strength and skill will be able to roll with fewer throws. Body build will also have an impact; obesity or wide hips will make rolling more difficult.

A good deal of momentum is required to move the large mass of the trunk and lower extremities. When using the relatively small mass of the head and upper extremities to roll, their momentum must be maximized. Several things can be done to increase momentum. The elbows should be held in extension to maximize the moment arm. Protracting the scapula at the end of the swing will also increase the moment arm. Arm and head swings should be synchronized and performed forcefully, with maximal velocity.

People with innervated triceps can throw their arms in an arc that is perpendicular to the mat. This is not true for people with C5 or C6 tetraplegia, as they lack functioning triceps. In these cases, the elbows will flex when thrown in this manner, which can result in the person hitting himself in the face. To avoid this problem, an individual who lacks functioning triceps should swing his arms in an arc that is approximately 45 degrees above the plane of his body. (The shoulders are flexed to about 45 degrees.) This position, combined with shoulder external rotation and forearm supination, helps maintain the elbows in extension. It is, however, a less advantageous position for generating momentum for the roll because the arms' mass is positioned closer to the body's axis of rotation.[8] This disadvantageous arm position, combined with absent or minimal pectoralis major innervation, makes rolling difficult for people with C5 or C6 tetraplegia.

Supine to prone with equipment. Weakness, contractures, obesity, spasticity, confusion, low motivation, or inadequate time funded for rehabilitation can keep someone from achieving independence in rolling without equipment. In these instances, many people can learn to roll by pulling on a looped strap, a bedrail, or a wheelchair parked next to the mat or bed. The use of a wheel-

---

[8] The properties of momentum are discussed in Chapter 9.

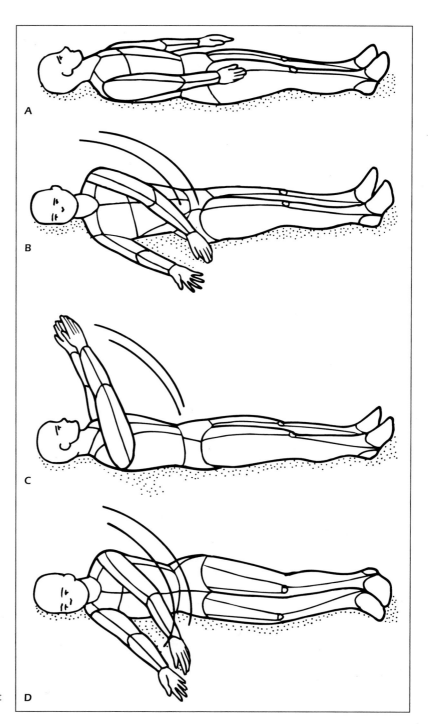

Figure 10–1. *Rolling supine to prone without equipment.*

chair is preferable to a looped strap or bedrail, as it does not require any special equipment.

To prepare to roll using equipment, a person who lacks hand function first positions the arm toward which he plans to roll, stabilizing his arm in the loop, under a bedrail, or under his wheelchair's armrest or wheel rim. The arm should be positioned with the shoulder abducted to about 90 degrees and the antecubital fossa facing the ceiling (Figure 10–2). The forearm should be supinated.

Pulling on the equipment using his biceps and anterior deltoid, the person rolls his trunk toward his stabilized arm. At the same time, he swings his head and free arm in the direction of the roll, adding momentum. In the absence of innervated triceps, the free arm should be swung in an arc that is about 45 degrees above the plane of the body.

The roll can be completed in one of two ways. At the end of the free arm's swing, this arm can be used to pull on the equipment. Alterna-

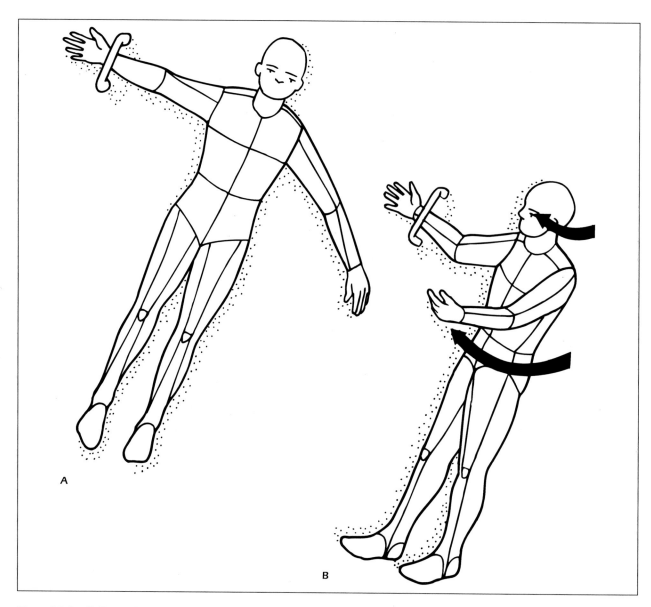

Figure 10–2. Rolling supine to prone with equipment, viewed from above.

tively, the person can reach or punch with his free arm at the end of the swing, protracting his scapula to add momentum to the roll.

Prone to supine. Rolling from prone to supine is far easier than rolling in the opposite direction. A person with a complete spinal cord injury simply pushes on the supporting surface, using the arm away from which he wants to roll. Once he reaches a sidelying position, he can throw his head and arm in the direction of the roll.

Assuming Prone-on-Elbows

Assuming prone-on-elbows is another important basic capability. The prone-on-elbows position

can be used to move in bed, and it is a key position in some methods of coming to sitting.

There are a variety of methods that a person with a complete spinal cord injury can use to get prone-on-elbows. Four methods are presented in this section. The physical and skill prerequisites for these techniques are summarized in Tables 10–5 and 10–6, respectively.

From prone, shoulders abducted. When using this method to get onto his elbows, a person starts in prone with his arms resting on the mat in the position shown in Figure 10–3A. His shoulders are externally rotated and abducted to 90 degrees, and his elbows are flexed to approximately 90 degrees.

TABLE 10–5. ASSUMING PRONE-ON-ELBOWS—PHYSICAL PREREQUISITES

	From prone, shoulders abducted	From prone, shoulders adducted	From sidelying	At the end of a roll from supine
Strength				
Anterior deltoids	☑	☑	√	☑
Middle deltoids			√	√
Posterior deltoids			☑	☑
Biceps, brachialis, and/or brachioradialis			√	
Range of Motion				
Shoulder Flexion	√	√	√	√
Abduction	√	√	√	
External rotation	√		√	☑
Horizontal adduction	√	√	√	√
Elbow Flexion	√	√	√	√

√: Some strength is needed for this activity, or severe limitations in range will inhibit this activity.

☑: A large amount of strength or normal or greater range is needed for this activity.

TABLE 10–6. ASSUMING PRONE ON ELBOWS—SKILL PREREQUISITES

	From prone, shoulders abducted	From prone, shoulders adducted	From sidelying	At the end of a roll from supine
Supine Skills				
Position elbows in extension (p. 205)				√
Maintain elbow extension while flexing shoulders (p. 206)				√
Throw arm(s) across body, elbow(s) extended (p. 206)				√
Roll supine to prone without equipment (p. 206)				√
Prone Skills				
Weight shift in prone-on-elbows (p. 211)	√	√	√	
Walk elbows in from abducted position (p. 212)	√			
Walk elbows forward from adducted position (p. 212)		√		
Sidelying Skill				
Move from sidelying to prone on elbows (p. 214)			√	√

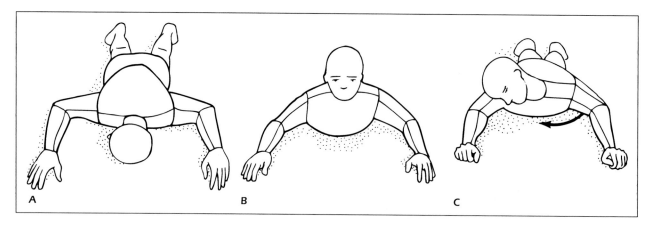

Figure 10–3. Assuming prone-on-elbows from prone, shoulders abducted. **(A)** Starting position. **(B)** Partway up. **(C)** Weight-shifting and moving unweighted arm medially.

From the starting position, the person shifts his weight to one side and horizontally adducts and shrugs the opposite shoulder. He then shifts in the other direction and pulls his other arm medially in the same manner. Each time he performs this maneuver, the unweighted elbow is moved a short distance medially. By repeatedly weight-shifting and repositioning his elbows medially, he gradually "walks" his elbows inward until they are positioned vertically under his shoulders.

From prone, shoulders adducted. An alternate method for getting onto the elbows from prone involves shoulder flexion instead of horizontal adduction. The person starts with his elbows flexed and his shoulders adducted against his sides (Figure 10–4A).

From the starting position, the trunk is lifted slightly, using forceful flexion of the shoulders. Shifting his weight to one side, the person flexes the unweighted shoulder. This maneuver brings the elbow forward slightly, moving it toward a position under the shoulder. The person then shifts to the other side and pulls the opposite elbow forward. By repeatedly weight-shifting to alternate sides and flexing his unweighted shoulders, he "walks" his elbows into position under his shoulders.

From sidelying. When using this method to assume a prone-on-elbows position, the person begins in sidelying with the shoulder and elbow of his lower arm (the arm on which he is lying) flexed. If he does not have fully innervated shoul-

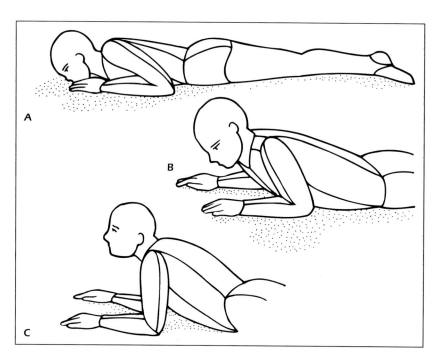

Figure 10–4. Assuming prone-on-elbows from prone, shoulders adducted. **(A)** Starting position. **(B)** Partway up. **(C)** Prone-on-elbows.

der musculature, he may need to stabilize his hand against his head. Stabilizing his hand in this manner enables him to use this arm more effectively as a lever. Figure 10–5 illustrates the starting position with the hand stabilized against the forehead. The hand can be stabilized in other positions, such as against the chin or the side of the head.

Moving to prone-on-elbows from this position involves simultaneous use of leverage by the lower arm and momentum from the free arm.

From the starting position, the person pushes the elbow of his lower arm down into the mat using a strong contraction of his posterior deltoids, lifting his trunk up and forward over his elbow. Once the lift has been initiated, he can tuck his chin to assist in the motion.

While pushing into the mat with his lower arm, the person forcefully swings his free arm forward, adding momentum to help move the trunk. On completion of the arm's swing, he can do one of two things with this arm to help pull his trunk up and over his supporting elbow. He can use momentum by reaching or punching the arm at the end of its swing, protracting the scapula. Alternatively, at the end of the free arm's swing, he can stabilize the hand against his supporting elbow. With his hand stabilized in this manner, he can use this arm to pull the trunk, helping to move it to a position over his supporting elbow.

At the end of a roll from supine. This method for getting prone-on-elbows is possible for someone with C6 or lower tetraplegia who is both strong in his innervated musculature and skillful in rolling without equipment. Using this technique, the person takes advantage of his body's momentum at the end of a roll, using it to get onto his elbows.

This process is started with a forceful roll. As the person rolls past sidelying, he pushes the elbow of his lower arm into the mat. He can use his free arm to assist in the process in either of the two

ways described previously: he can reach or punch at the end of the arm's swing, or he can stabilize the free hand against his supporting elbow and then use this arm to pull. Whichever method is used, these actions must be performed without interrupting the roll from supine. An uninterrupted roll makes it possible for the trunk's momentum to help carry the trunk over the supporting elbow.

Coming to Sitting without Equipment

To dress or transfer out of bed independently, a person needs to be able to get himself into a sitting position. If he can do so without equipment, he will be spared the stigma, expense, and restrictions of special equipment.

With functioning triceps. An individual with intact upper extremity musculature may be able to come to sitting directly from supine by pushing down on the mat with his hands. If he needs to he can rock his trunk side to side slightly as he pushes.

Even without fully intact upper extremities, the presence of functioning triceps makes a large difference in the ability to assume a sitting position. A person with functioning triceps can roll past sidelying, plant his hands on the mat, and push himself into a sitting position.

Assuming a sitting posture is a more involved process when functioning triceps are lacking. The following three methods do not require triceps. Table 10–7 provides a summary of the physical prerequisites for these techniques. Table 10–8 summarizes the skill prerequisites.

Rolling and throwing arms. This method of assuming a sitting position requires very good flexibility. The shoulders must have greater than normal range in extension. The elbows must extend fully with the shoulders positioned in hyperextension and external rotation.

To come to sitting using this method, the person first gets prone-on-elbows using any of the methods just described (Figure 10–6A). He then shifts his weight onto one elbow. With his unweighted arm, he pushes his trunk up and over the supporting elbow, moving to the forearm-supported sidelying position (Figure 10–6B).

From forearm-supported sidelying, the person throws his free arm back in an arc, landing on his palm (Figure 10–6C). To make the next step possible, the hand must land with the shoulder positioned in external rotation and extreme horizontal abduction and hyperextension. The elbow must be fully extended and the forearm supinated.

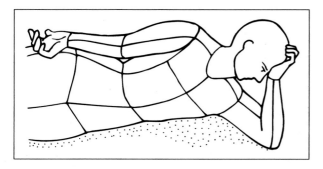

Figure 10–5. *Starting position for assuming prone-on-elbows from sidelying.*

TABLE 10–7.   COMING TO SITTING WITHOUT EQUIPMENT— PHYSICAL PREREQUISITES

		Roll and throw	Straight from supine, hands stabilized	Walking on elbows
Strength				
Anterior deltoids		☑	☑	√
Middle deltoids		√	√	√
Posterior deltoids		☑	√	√
Biceps, brachialis, and/or brachioradialis			☑	√
Internal rotators				√
Range of Motion				
Shoulder	Extension	☑ᵃ	☑ᵃ	
	Flexion	√		√
	Abduction	√	√	√
	External rotation	☑ᵃ	☑ᵃ	
	Internal rotation			☑
	Horizontal abduction	☑ᵃ	☑ᵃ	√
Elbow	Extension	☑ᵃ	☑ᵃ	√
	Flexion	√	√	√
Forearm	Supination	√	√	
Wrist	Extension	√	√	
Hamstring flexibility				☑

√: Some strength is needed for this activity, or severe limitations in range will inhibit this activity.

☑: A large amount of strength or normal or greater range is needed for this activity.

ᵃ These motions (shoulder extension, external rotation, horizontal abduction, and elbow extension) must be present in combination.

From this position, the person shifts his weight onto his extended arm and lifts the other arm (Figure 10–6D).

Balancing on his supporting arm, the person throws his free arm back. When the palm lands on the mat, the elbow of this arm should be extended, the forearm supinated, and the shoulder horizontally abducted, hyperextended, and externally rotated (Figure 10–6E).

From this position, an upright sitting posture is achieved by walking the hands forward. To walk his hands forward, the person shifts first to one side and then to the other, moving the unweighted hand forward by elevating and protracting the scapula.

Straight from supine, hands stabilized. To assume a sitting position using this method, a person with a spinal cord injury must have very strong biceps. Range-of-motion requirements are the same as those for the method described above.

In the supine position, the hands are stabilized by placing them in the pockets, inside the pants, or under the hips. The person then lifts his upper trunk by flexing his elbows forcefully (Figure 10–7B).

Once the person has lifted his upper trunk as high as he can, he moves his elbows posteriorly. Shifting his weight from side to side, he walks his unweighted elbows back until he is in a stable position, supine-on-elbows (Figure 10–7C).

From supine-on-elbows, the individual shifts his weight to one elbow and lifts the unweighted arm (Figure 10–7D). While lifting, he forcefully contracts the anterior deltoid of his supporting arm, turning his upper trunk so that his shoulders are aligned vertically over the supporting elbow.

TABLE 10-8. COMING TO SITTING WITHOUT EQUIPMENT—SKILL PREREQUISITES

	Roll and throw	Straight from supine, hands stabilized	Walking on elbows
Supine Skills			
Weight shift in supine, supported on one elbow and one hand (p. 207)	√	√	
From supine, supported on one elbow and one hand, lift elbow (p. 208)	√	√	
Position elbows in extension (p. 205)	√	√	
Maintain elbow extension while flexing shoulders (p. 206)	√	√	
Stabilize hands in pants or under pelvis (p. 209)		√	
With hands stabilized in pants or under pelvis, lift trunk using elbow flexion (p. 209)		√	
Weight shift in supine-on-elbows (p. 209)		√	
In supine-on-elbows, walk elbows back (p. 209)		√	
Dynamic shoulder control in single forearm-supported supine (p. 210)	√	√	
From supine-on-elbows, lift one elbow (p. 210)	√	√	
From single forearm-supported supine, throw one arm back (p. 210)	√	√	
Prone Skills			
Assume prone-on-elbows position (pp. 212 and 214)	√		√
Weight shift in prone-on-elbows (p. 211)	√		√
Move from prone-on-elbows to forearm-supported sidelying (p. 213)	√		√
In prone-on-elbows, walk elbows to the side (p. 213)			√
Sidelying Skills			
Dynamic shoulder control in forearm-supported sidelying (p. 215)	√		
From forearm-supported sidelying, throw free arm back (p. 216)	√		
In 90-degree forearm-supported sidelying, walk supporting elbow toward legs (p. 217)			√
From forearm-supported sidelying, push-pull into sitting position (p. 217)			√
Sitting Skills			
Extend elbows against resistance[a]			√
Tolerate upright sitting position[b]			√
Dynamic shoulder control in sitting, propped back on one hand (p. 218)	√	√	
From sitting propped back on one hand, throw free arm back (p. 219)	√	√	
Weight shift while sitting, propped back on two hands (p. 219)	√	√	
From sitting, propped back on two hands, walk hands forward (p. 220)	√	√	
Push with arms to lift trunk from forward lean[a]			√

[a] Refer to Chapter 11 for a description of this skill and therapeutic strategies.

[b] Refer to Chapter 12 for a description of this skill and therapeutic strategies.

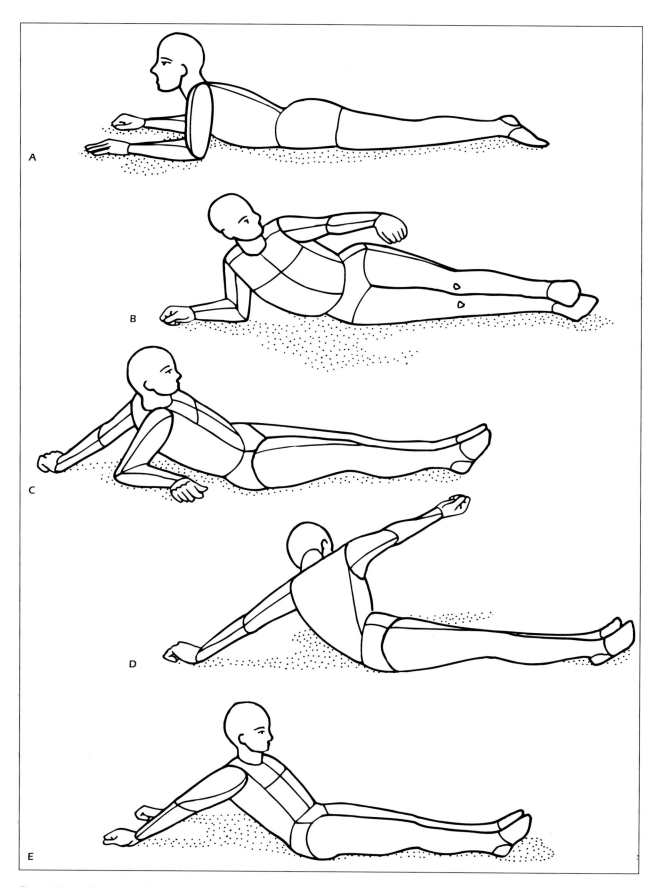

Figure 10–6.   Coming to sitting by rolling and throwing the arms. **(A)** Prone-on-elbows. **(B)** Forearm-supported sidelying. **(C)** Supine supported on one elbow and one hand. **(D)** Supporting elbow lifted. **(E)** Sitting propped back on two hands.

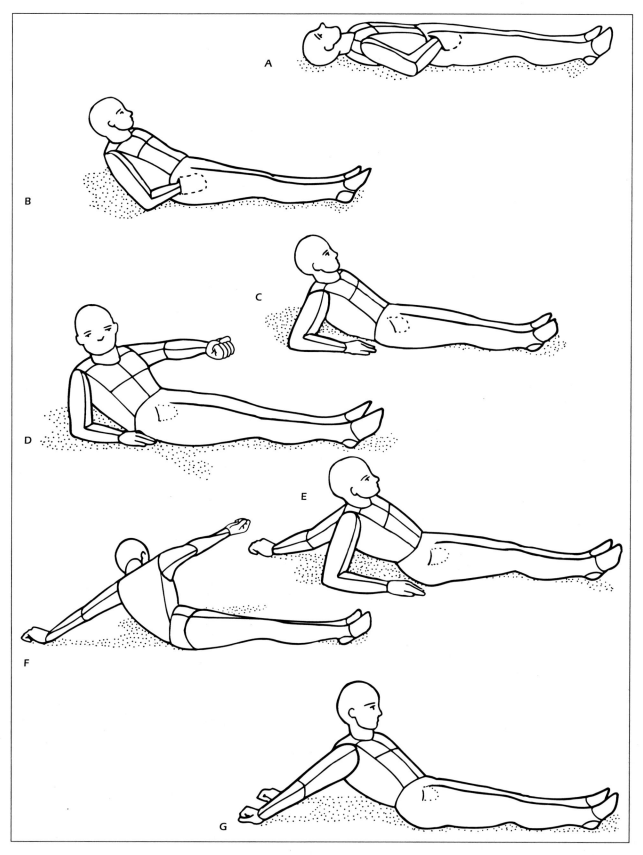

Figure 10–7.   Coming to sitting straight from supine, hands stabilized in pants. **(A)** Starting position: supine with hands stabilized in pants. **(B)** Upper trunk lifted using elbow flexion. **(C)** Elbows walked back to a stable position. **(D)** One arm lifted. **(E)** Free arm thrown back. **(F)** Second arm lifted. **(G)** Second arm thrown back.

From this position, the person comes to sitting in the manner described previously. He throws back first one arm and then the other (Figure 10–7E through G) and walks his hands forward until he reaches an upright sitting posture.

Walking on elbows. This method of assuming the sitting position does not require the range of motion that is needed to perform the methods described previously. Because neither shoulder hyperextension nor full elbow extension is needed, people who have range limitations can use this method to come to sitting. Moreover, because the patient does not position his shoulders in extreme hyperextension while coming to sitting in this manner, he may experience less trauma to his shoulders.

To come to sitting by walking on his elbows, the person first gets prone-on-elbows using any of the methods described above. He then walks his elbows to one side. To do so, he shifts his weight first to one side and then to the other, moving the unweighted elbow each time.

The person continues walking his elbows to the side until he reaches a point where his trunk will not laterally flex any further (Figure 10–8B). In the next step he rotates his pelvis from prone toward sidelying. This involves pushing with the elbows (using shoulder flexion with the elbows stabilized on the mat) to roll his pelvis from prone (Figure 10–8C).

With his pelvis tilted from prone, the person can continue walking on his elbows until his shoulders are close enough to his legs. This position will vary, but it is generally such that the trunk is at a 90-degree or smaller angle to the legs (Figure 10–8D).

Shifting his weight onto the elbow that is furthest from his legs, the person lifts his unweighted arm and hooks the forearm around his thighs (Figure 10–8E). He can then walk the weight-bearing elbow toward his legs, shifting his weight by pulling with the arm that is stabilized on his legs.[h] In this manner, he walks his elbow until it is close enough to his legs for him to perform the next step (Figure 10–8F). The target position for the elbow will vary, depending on the individual's strength and skill.

Shifting his weight off of his supporting elbow, the person internally rotates this shoulder and plants his palm on the mat (Figure 10–8G). Pushing with this arm and pulling with the one sta-

bilized on his legs, he then rocks his body to get his pelvis flat on the mat and his trunk into position over his legs (Figure 10–8H). Once his body is positioned over his legs, he can place both palms on the mat and push his torso to upright (Figure 10–8I).

Coming to Sitting Using Equipment

Weakness, contractures, obesity, spasticity, and inadequate time for full rehabilitation are among the factors that can prevent someone from learning to assume a sitting posture without equipment. In these cases, many can learn to assume a sitting position independently using equipment.

There are various methods that can be used to come to sitting using a loop ladder attached to the foot of the bed or using loops suspended from a bar over the bed. One method for each is presented in this section. Tables 10–9 and 10–10 summarize the physical and skill prerequisites for these methods. A final alternative method of coming to sitting involves the use of a hospital bed. This alternative should be considered for anyone who either does not have the potential to function on a standard bed, or chooses not to pursue this goal.

Loop ladder. A person with a spinal cord injury who is unable to roll or get into prone-on-elbows without equipment may be able to come to sitting using a loop ladder.[i] The ladder is attached to the foot of the bed and lies on the mattress (Figure 10–9A).

The starting position is supine, with the loop ladder lying beside the person. The ladder will be used to pull onto the elbow that is closest to the loops. After placing one or both forearms through the nearest loop, the person drives his elbow into the mat while pulling on the loop, lifting his upper trunk over the elbow (Figure 10–9B).

Balancing on one elbow, he removes his arm(s) from the loop and places the forearm of his free (nonweightbearing) arm through the next loop. Pulling on the loop, he unweights his supporting elbow and inches it toward the foot of the bed (Figure 10–9C). When he has moved as far as he can using that loop, the person moves his free arm to the next loop and repeats the process. In this manner, he walks his supporting elbow around, bending at the hips. This process can be continued until his torso is positioned over his legs.

---

[h] This step may be omitted if strength and skill allow.

---

[i] A loop ladder is a series of loops made of webbing material, sewn end to end. The size and number of loops will vary among individuals.

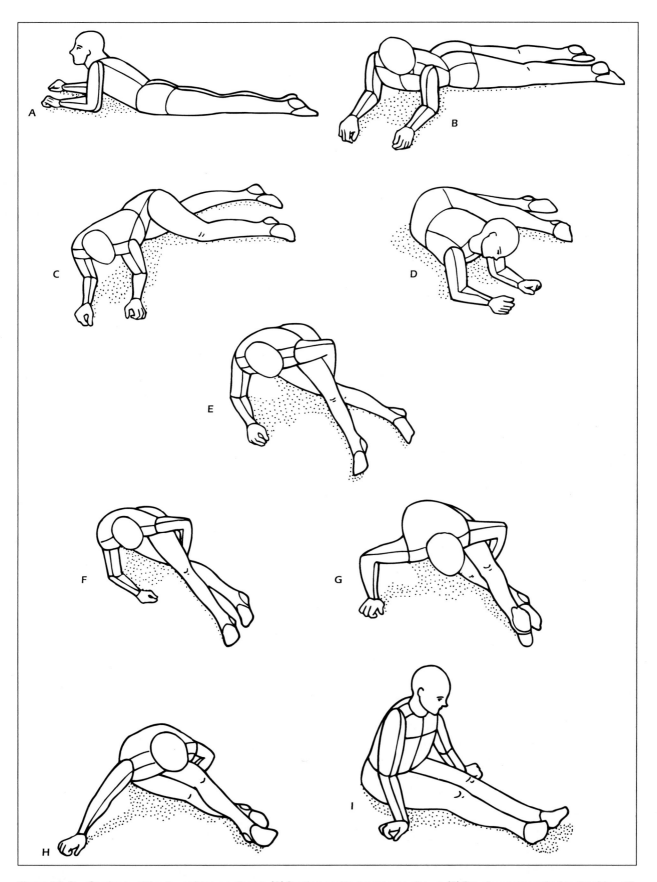

Figure 10–8. Coming to sitting by walking on elbows. **(A)** Starting position: prone-on-elbows. **(B)** The elbows are walked to the side until the trunk will not laterally flex any further. **(C)** The pelvis is rolled from prone toward sidelying. **(D)** The elbows are walked toward the legs. **(E)** An arm is hooked around the thighs. **(F)** The supporting elbow is walked toward the legs. **(G)** The palm is planted on the mat. **(H)** The body is rocked into position over the legs. **(I)** The torso is pushed to upright.

TABLE 10–9. COMING TO SITTING WITH EQUIPMENT—PHYSICAL PREREQUISITES

	Using loop ladder	Using suspended loops
Strength		
Anterior deltoids	☑	☑
Middle deltoids	√	√
Posterior deltoids	√	√
Biceps, brachialis, and/or brachioradialis	☑	☑
Range of Motion		
Shoulder Extension		√
Flexion	√	√
Abduction	√	√
External rotation		√
Horizontal abduction		√
Elbow Extension		☑
Flexion	√	√
Forearm Supination		√
Wrist Extension		√
Combined hip flexion and knee extension	☑	☑

√: Some strength is needed for this activity, or severe limitations in range will inhibit this activity.

☑: A large amount of strength or normal or greater range is needed for this activity.

Someone who routinely uses a loop ladder to come to sitting needs to plan ahead. When he gets into bed at night, he should place the loops where he will be able to reach them the following morning.

Suspended loops. Figure 10–10A shows an overhead frame with loops.[j] This equipment is far bulkier, less esthetic, and more difficult to transport than a loop ladder.

Starting in supine, the person places one or both distal forearms through a suspended loop (Figure 10–10B). Pulling on the loop, he raises his shoulders off of the bed (Figure 10–10C). He then places one elbow on the bed, positioned well under his upper trunk so that he can balance on it (Figure 10–10D).

Balancing on his elbow, the person removes his arm from the first loop and places it through the next one (Figure 10–10E). He then pulls to lift his trunk higher. In doing so, he lifts his supporting elbow off of the bed. While suspended from the loop, he throws his free arm back, ending in the

position shown in Figure 10–10F. The shoulder of the supporting arm must be extended, horizontally abducted, and externally rotated. The elbow is extended fully and the forearm is supinated.

While balancing on his supporting arm, the person moves his other arm to the next loop (Figure 10–10G). Pulling on the loop and throwing his head forward, he unweights his supporting arm and inches the hand forward. When he has moved his hand as far as he can, he balances on his supporting arm and moves his free arm to the next loop. He can then repeat these steps until he reaches an upright sitting posture (Figure 10–10H).

Gross Mobility in Sitting

To get in and out of bed without assistance, a person with a complete spinal cord injury must be able to move his buttocks on the bed while in a sitting posture. This skill can also be used for limited mobility without a wheelchair. This mobility can be useful when the individual is on the floor or the ground, either by choice or after a fall.

Following a complete spinal cord injury, gross mobility in sitting involves pivoting on the

[j] The ideal number, length, and spacing of the loops will vary among individuals.

TABLE 10–10. COMING TO SITTING WITH EQUIPMENT—SKILL PREREQUISITES

	Using loop ladder	Using suspended loops
Supine Skills		
Position elbows in extension (p. 205)	√	√
Maintain elbow extension while flexing shoulders (p. 206)	√	√
Place arm through loop (p. 210)	√	√
Pulling on loop ladder, move from supine to single forearm-supported supine (p. 210)	√	
In single forearm-supported supine, pull on loop ladder and walk supporting elbow toward feet (p. 211)	√	
Lift trunk by pulling on suspended loop (p. 211)		√
Dynamic shoulder control in single forearm-supported supine (p. 210)		√
Sitting Skills		
Tolerate upright sitting position[a]	√	√
With one arm through overhead loop, throw free arm back (p. 220)		√
Dynamic shoulder control in sitting, propped back on one hand (p. 218)		√
In sitting, propped back on one hand, pull on suspended loop and walk supporting hand forward (p. 220)		√
Extend elbows against resistance[b]	√	
Push with arms to lift trunk from forward lean[b]	√	

[a] Refer to Chapter 12 for a description of this skill and therapeutic strategies.

[b] Refer to Chapter 11 for a description of this skill and therapeutic strategies.

arms. The person lifts or unweights his buttocks[k] by leaning onto his arms and tucking his head. If he lacks functioning triceps, he must lock his elbows in extension.[l] If his serratus anterior is functioning, he can increase the lift of his buttocks by protracting his scapulae. While lifting, he swings his head and upper trunk away from the direction in which he wants his buttocks to move.

The physical and skill prerequisites for gross mobility in sitting are summarized in Tables 10–11 and 10–12.

Leg Management

An individual who lacks lower extremity function must position his legs passively. This skill is rela-

[k] An actual lift is preferable, but unweighting will suffice if the individual is unable to lift his buttocks off of the mat.

[l] The procedure for locking the elbows is addressed in Chapter 11.

tively easy; anyone who can come to sitting and move on a mat independently should be able to learn to position his legs.

Figure 10–11 illustrates the technique for positioning the legs passively. Propping on one arm in the sitting position, the person uses his other arm to move one leg at a time. He does so by pulling his leg toward the supporting arm. By forcefully moving his head and torso in the direction of the pull, he can add power to his pull.

Tables 10–11 and 10–12 summarize the physical and skill prerequisites for leg management on a mat or bed.

THERAPEUTIC STRATEGIES FOLLOWING COMPLETE SPINAL CORD INJURY

General Strategies

To perform a functional mat activity, a person with a spinal cord injury must first acquire the

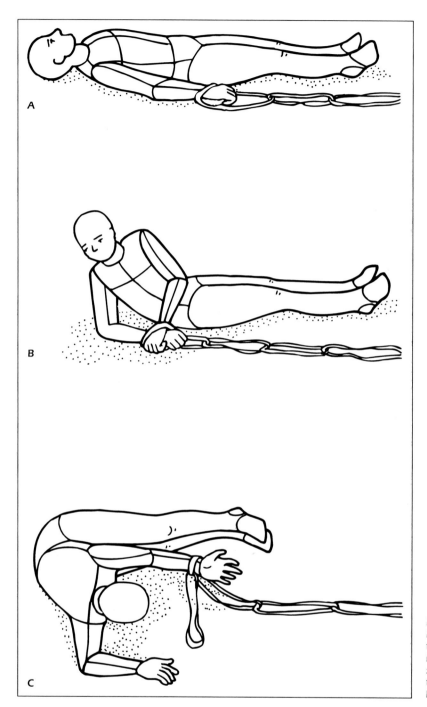

Figure 10–9. Coming to sitting using a loop ladder. **(A)** Starting position. **(B)** The upper trunk is lifted by pulling on the loop and driving the supporting elbow into the mat. **(C)** The supporting elbow is inched toward the foot of the bed. The other arm assists by pulling on the loop ladder.

activity's physical and skill prerequisites. The therapeutic program should work toward developing all of the needed range, strength, and skills.

Rolling, gross mat mobility, and leg management are relatively simple activities, with few skill prerequisites. As a result, planning a functional training program to develop one of these abilities is fairly straightforward. The patient should start by developing the most basic prerequisite skills and then build on these skills until he is able to perform the activity.

In contrast, each method of coming to sitting involves a fair number of steps. Many of the steps are unrelated; the skills required to perform one step are not needed to perform any other steps. As a result, decisions in functional training are less clear-cut. When working toward coming to sitting using the method that involves rolling and throwing the arms, is it best to work first on assuming prone-on-elbows or on balancing on one extended arm? The two steps involve different skills, and neither step is required to practice the other.

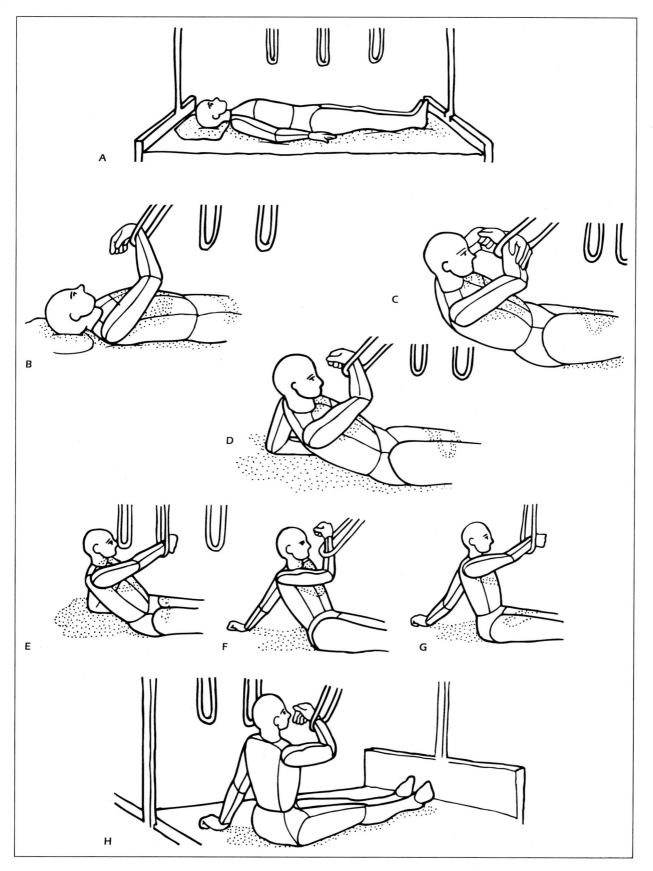

Figure 10–10.   Coming to sitting using suspended loops. **(A)** Starting position. **(B)** One forearm placed through loop. **(C)** Upper trunk lifted from bed. **(D)** Elbow placed on bed. **(E)** Arm placed through second loop. **(F)** Trunk lifted and free arm thrown back. **(G)** Arm placed through third loop. **(H)** Supporting hand walked forward.

TABLE 10–11. GROSS MOBILITY IN SITTING AND LEG MANAGEMENT—PHYSICAL PREREQUISITES

	Gross mobility in sitting	Leg management
Strength		
Anterior deltoids	☑	√
Middle deltoids	√	√
Posterior deltoids	√	√
Biceps, brachialis, and/or brachioradialis	√	☑
Range of Motion		
Shoulder Abduction		√
External rotation	☑	
Elbow Extension	☑	√
Flexion		√
Forearm Supination	☑	√
Wrist Extension	☑	√
Combined hip flexion and knee extension	☑	☑

√: Some strength is needed for this activity, or severe limitations in range will inhibit this activity.

☑: A large amount of strength or normal or greater range is needed for this activity.

TABLE 10–12. GROSS MOBILITY IN SITTING AND LEG MANAGEMENT—SKILL PREREQUISITES

	Gross mobility in sitting	Leg management
Sitting Skills		
Tolerate upright sitting position[a]	√	√
In long-sitting, prop forward on extended arms[b]	√	
In long-sitting, lift or unweight buttocks by leaning forward on extended arms[b]	√	
Control pelvis using head-hips relationship[b]	√	
In long-sitting, lift or unweight buttocks and move laterally[b]	√	
In long-sitting, move buttocks forward and back (p. 221)	√	
In long-sitting, prop to one side on one extended arm (p. 221)		√
Dynamic stability in long-sitting, propped to the side on one extended arm (p. 221)		√
Sitting propped to the side on one extended arm, use free arm to move lower extremity (p. 221)		√

[a] Refer to Chapter 12 for a description of this skill and therapeutic strategies.

[b] Refer to Chapter 11 for a description of this skill and therapeutic strategies.

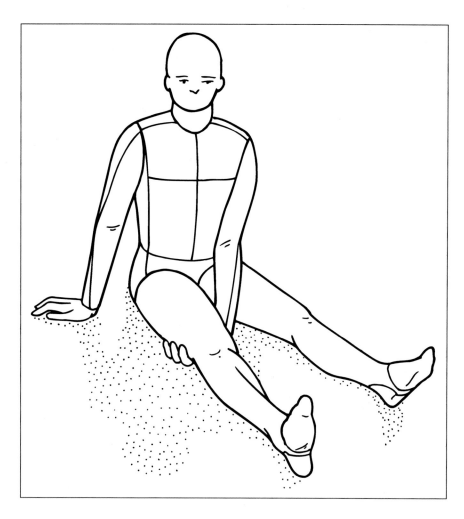

Figure 10–11. Leg management.

In instances in which an individual has a number of unrelated skills to master, it may be best to work on several skills concurrently. Doing so will add variety to the program. This variety may help to keep the patient's interest in the program. It also will make it possible for him to change activities when a group of muscles becomes fatigued, enabling him to work in therapy for longer periods of time by distributing the demands on his musculature.

Before asking a patient to attempt a new skill, the therapist should explain and demonstrate the technique.[m] The demonstration should provide a clear idea of the motions involved, as well as the timing of these motions. The therapist should also demonstrate or explain how the new skill will be used functionally. In addition to observing demonstrations, the patient may find it useful to look at illustrations of the functional technique.

During functional training, the therapist should remember that every individual with a spinal cord injury will perform a particular activity differently. Each person has a unique combination of body build, coordination, strength, and flexibility, and these characteristics influence the manner in which he performs functional tasks. What works for one patient may be a total disaster for the next. The challenge of functional training is finding the timing and maneuvers that best suit the individual involved.

Strategies for developing the various prerequisite skills are presented in this section. The descriptions of skills are grouped according to the patient's position when performing the skills. In instances in which a skill involves moving from one position to another, the skill is defined by its starting position.

Supine Skills

Position elbows in extension. People with complete C5 or C6 tetraplegia have innervated elbow flexors but lack extensors. As a result, a prob-

---

[m] This demonstration can also be provided by another person with a spinal cord injury, if someone is available who has similar impairments but a higher level of functional ability. Alternatively, the patient may watch a videotaped demonstration of the skill.

lem that they often experience when lying supine is that they cannot straighten their elbows once they become flexed. Because these individuals lack functioning triceps, they need to learn an alternate method for extending their elbows. In supine, momentum is used to accomplish this task.[n]

Commonly, an elbow is positioned in flexion with the shoulder internally rotated so that the forearm rests on the trunk. To extend his elbow when his arm is in this position, a patient can flex his shoulder and then slam his elbow into the mat by extending and externally rotating the shoulder abruptly. If he performs this maneuver with enough force, and if he relaxes his elbow flexors while doing so, the forearm's momentum will carry it caudally and the elbow will extend.

The elbow can also be positioned in flexion with the shoulder externally rotated. When this occurs, the elbow can be extended by internally rotating the shoulder while slamming the elbow into the mat. Alternatively, the patient can internally rotate the shoulder to position his forearm across his body and proceed from there as described above.

Many people with spinal cord injuries discover these maneuvers on their own. Others require instruction and practice. Those who have difficulty learning to extend their elbows can practice the techniques starting with their elbows only slightly flexed. (Extending the elbows will be easiest from this position.) As they develop skill, they can practice from increasingly flexed positions.

Maintain elbow extension while flexing shoulders. In the absence of functioning triceps, a person with C5 or C6 tetraplegia must use gravity to hold his elbows in extension when he flexes his shoulders. For gravity to hold the elbows in extension, appropriate positioning is required; the shoulders must be held in external rotation. Internal rotation of the shoulders will result in elbow flexion.

Maintaining elbow extension during shoulder flexion involves more than simply positioning the arms so that gravity extends the elbows. People who lack functioning triceps must also keep their elbow flexors relaxed while they flex their shoulders. After sustaining cervical spinal cord injuries, people often tend to perform shoulder and elbow flexion in combination. (This may be a result of recruitment in response to a partial loss of deltoid innervation.) To use their arms func-

tionally, these individuals must learn to isolate these motions.

Some patients learn without instruction how to maintain their elbows in extension while flexing their shoulders; however, many require instruction and practice. A therapist may assist by giving verbal and tactile cues as the patient learns to contract his shoulder flexors while keeping his elbow flexors relaxed. The patient should first practice flexing his shoulders through only a few degrees of motion and progress through larger arcs as his skill increases.

Throw arm(s) across body, elbow(s) extended. The position of the arms during this maneuver will depend on whether or not the individual's triceps are innervated. People who lack functioning triceps must use positioning to keep their elbows from flexing while they throw their arms across their bodies in supine. The shoulders are held in external rotation and flexed only to about 45 degrees. In this position, the downward force of gravity helps hold the elbows in extension.

A person with a spinal cord injury who wishes to use arm motions to roll must move his arms forcefully. The therapist can help the patient get a feel for the position and force of the arm swings by assisting him through the motions. Once the patient gets a feel for the motion, he can practice on his own.

Some patients are able to throw their arms across their bodies without prior instruction and do not need to practice this skill separately. These patients may proceed directly to practicing combined head and arm motions.

Combined arm throw and head swing. To practice this skill, a patient should be able to maintain his elbows in extension while throwing his arms across his body.

The patient should practice turning his head while throwing his arms across his body, turning his head in the direction of the arm throw. To build enough momentum to roll, he must perform the arm and head motions forcefully and simultaneously. The therapist can give the patient a feel for the force of the arm motions by moving him passively once or twice.

Roll toward prone using momentum. This skill can be practiced from sidelying without the development of any prior skills. For practice rolling from supine, however, the patient must be able to throw his arms across his body while keeping his elbows extended, simultaneously throwing his head in the same direction.

---

[n] Muscle substitution using the anterior deltoid is not generally feasible in supine because it requires the presence of an object on which to stabilize the hand.

It can be very difficult to learn to roll from supine to prone without equipment. To facilitate the acquisition of this skill, the therapist should make the task easier. One way to do so is to cross the patient's legs. During practice rolling to the left, the right leg should be crossed over the left.

Rolling is most difficult from supine and gets progressively easier as the individual approaches sidelying. For this reason, practice should start in sidelying. The therapist should position the patient in sidelying with his legs crossed and instruct him to punch or reach his free arm forward. This motion will move his center of gravity forward, causing him to roll toward prone. Once the patient learns how to rotate his body in this manner, the therapist can assist him to a slightly more supine position and have him practice rolling from there. As the patient's skill increases, he should practice rolling from progressively more supine positions. Throughout the practice, forceful head and arm motions should be encouraged.

A patient who is having difficulty learning to roll may benefit from having wrist weights placed on his arms. The added mass of the wrist weights adds to his arms' momentum, making it easier to roll. As a patient's skill increases, the weights should be removed.

The training strategies just described should be used judiciously. The patient should always start from a position as close to supine as possible and use as little weight as he can. Once he is able to roll from supine, he should practice with his legs uncrossed.

Independent work. To practice this skill independently, the patient should be able to roll back toward supine from prone. The therapist can prepare the patient for rolling practice by crossing his legs, attaching a wrist weight if needed, and placing him in an appropriate position between supine and sidelying. A foam wedge or pillow(s) placed behind the patient's pelvis and lower back will keep him from rolling to a more supine position. These supports should be placed so that they do not restrict arm motions.

Position arm to assist in rolling with equipment. Before practicing this skill, a patient should be able to extend an elbow, using either triceps or momentum. If he can extend his elbow, positioning the arm to assist in rolling should take little practice.

The therapist should begin by showing the patient the appropriate arm position for rolling with equipment: the shoulder is abducted and in neutral rotation so that the antecubital fossa faces the ceiling. The forearm is supinated and stabilized under either the bedrail or the armrest of a wheelchair (Figure 10–2).

Once shown the position, the patient should require little practice to learn this skill. An individual who lacks functioning triceps should first position his elbow in extension, then abduct his shoulder to place the arm.

Roll toward prone by pulling on equipment. Practice of this skill does not require the ability to position the arm. The patient starts with one arm stabilized against a bedrail or wheelchair, positioned as described above. Using elbow flexion and shoulder horizontal adduction of the stabilized arm, he rolls his body toward the equipment. If he is able, he should add momentum to the roll by swinging his head and free arm toward the equipment. Toward the end of the roll, he can use his free arm to assist by reaching or punching in the direction of the roll, by pulling on the equipment, or both.

Rolling can be a difficult skill to master. The therapeutic strategies used to teach rolling with momentum can be used for rolling with equipment. To make the task easier, the therapist can have the patient practice initially from a sidelying position, with the legs crossed. A weight on the free arm may also be helpful during early practice. (A more complete description of strategies for teaching rolling is supplied above.)

Weight shift in supine, supported on one elbow and one hand. For weight shifting in this position to be possible for someone with a complete cervical lesion, the shoulder of the extended arm° must be positioned in extreme hyperextension (Figure 10–12A). If this shoulder is not in enough extension, it will be higher than the other shoulder (Figure 10–12B). This disparity in shoulder height will make it impossible for the patient to shift his weight onto the higher shoulder. The amount of shoulder extension required will vary among people; an individual with greater strength and skill will not require as much range.

This is a difficult position for weight shifts, and thus it is probably best to develop skill in easier positions first. The patient should first learn to shift his weight while sitting upright, propped back on two hands (described in the sitting skills section below). As his skill improves, he can

---

° The arm with the elbow in extension.

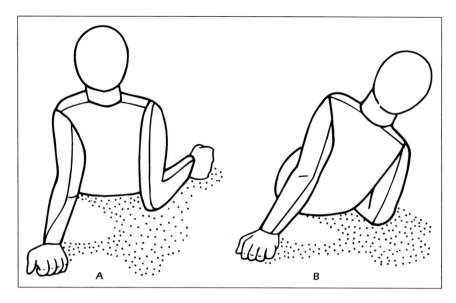

Figure 10–12.   *Supine, supported on one elbow and one hand.* **(A)** *Shoulder of extended arm positioned in extreme hyperextension.* **(B)** *Shoulder of extended arm positioned in inadequate hyperextension. Note the height of this shoulder.*

progress to shifting weight in supine-on-elbows (described in a later section). When he is adept at shifting his weight in these positions, he will be ready to practice while propped back on one elbow and one hand.

The therapist should assist the patient into position and ask him to shift his weight toward the extended arm. If the patient has difficulty shifting his weight, the therapist can place a hand against his shoulder and ask him to push. The patient should shift his weight only as far as he can control the motion and return to his original position. He should increase the arc of motion as his skill develops, gradually working up to the point where he can unweight his elbow completely.

From supine, supported on one elbow and one hand, lift elbow.   In this maneuver the per-

son shifts his weight and lifts the unweighted elbow. As he does so, he pivots his trunk over the shoulder of the supporting arm (Figure 10–13).

Before practicing this skill, the patient must be able to shift his weight while sitting propped back on one elbow and one hand. The weight shift must be large enough to unweight the elbow completely. The patient also should have dynamic shoulder control in sitting, propped back on one hand.

Lifting an arm while in this position is similar to doing so while propped back on two hands or two elbows. The patient should first practice lifting an arm from the easiest position, sitting propped back on two hands. He can then develop skill in supine, supported on two elbows. Once he has learned to lift an arm from these positions, he will be ready to practice from supine, propped on

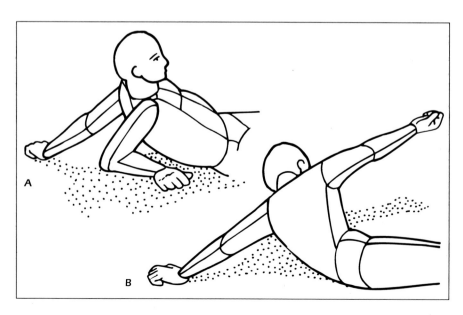

Figure 10–13.   *From supine on one elbow and one hand, lift elbow. Trunk pivots on supporting shoulder.*

one elbow and one hand. The strategies for acquiring these skills will be the same in each position.

Once an individual has developed the necessary prerequisite skills (weight shifts and dynamic shoulder control) in a given position, he can work on lifting an arm. The therapist may start by moving the patient passively to give him a feel for the motion. The patient can then practice shifting his weight and lifting his arm.

A patient who is unable to lift his arm can work on developing the skill in reverse, starting in the end position with his arm lifted. From this position, he can work on lowering his free arm toward the mat and lifting it again. As he does so, he pivots his trunk on the supporting shoulder. He should move in small arcs at first, gradually building to the point where he can lower his elbow or hand to the mat under control and lift it from that position.

Independent work. Once the patient has developed some skill in this maneuver, he can practice on his own. The therapist can assist the patient into position and instruct the patient to practice.

Stabilize hands in pants or under pelvis.
Learning to stabilize the hands in the pants is a relatively easy task. The patient simply needs to practice working his hands into the pants' front pockets or under the waistband. The pants should be made of a nonstretchy material; sweat pants will not adequately stabilize the hands. The pants must be loose enough for the patient to work his hands in without difficulty. This requirement should not present a problem; if the pants are loose enough to allow independent dressing, they should be suitable for this activity also.

Placing the hands under the pelvis can be a more difficult maneuver to accomplish. The patient starts with his arms by his sides with his shoulders internally rotated. Using elbow flexion, he pulls one hand at a time under his pelvis.

With hands stabilized in pants or under pelvis, lift upper trunk using elbow flexion.
During the initial practice of this skill, the therapist can stabilize the patient's distal forearms and have him lift his upper trunk (do "sit-ups") using elbow flexion. Practice can start with the shoulders flexed because this positioning will make the task easier. As the patient gets stronger and more skillful, the therapist can stabilize his arms in progressively lower positions. Once the patient is able to lift his upper trunk with his arms stabilized at his sides, he is ready to practice with his hands stabilized in his pants or under his pelvis.

Weight shift in supine-on-elbows.
This skill involves leaning to the side while propped on two elbows in supine. The patient's elbows should be positioned medial to or in line with (not lateral to) his shoulders.

During initial practice, the therapist can give the patient a feel for the motion by having him push against resistance. To do so, the therapist can place a hand against one of the patient's shoulders and ask him to push against it. Once the patient has shifted slightly, he can return to upright by pushing against a hand placed on the opposite shoulder.

The patient should practice leaning to one side, then the other. He should start with small motions, shifting only as far as he is able to control the motion and return to the starting position. As his skill increases, he can increase the arcs of motion.

Supine-on-elbows is most stable when the elbows are located directly beneath or cephalad to the shoulders. Early practice of weight shifts should be done with the elbows positioned in this manner. As the patient's skill increases, he should practice in less stable positions, with his elbows located caudal to his shoulders. If he plans to learn to come to sitting using the method in which he stabilizes his hands in his pants or under his pelvis, he should build up to the point where he can shift his weight with his hands stabilized in one of these positions.

Independent work. After being placed in supine-on-elbows, the patient can shift his weight to one side and then the other. He should be encouraged to shift as far as he can while maintaining control over the motion; he should shift far enough to make the activity challenging but not so far that he cannot return to upright independently.

In supine-on-elbows, walk elbows back.
In supine-on-elbows, the patient walks his elbows cephalad, moving his shoulders into greater extension. Practice of this skill requires the ability to weight shift in supine-on-elbows.

The patient starts in supine-on-elbows with his elbows medial to or even with his shoulders. From this position he shifts his weight laterally to unweight one arm and extends his unweighted shoulder slightly, moving the elbow a short distance cephalad. He then shifts his weight onto the newly moved elbow and repeats the process with the other arm. In this manner he walks his elbows cephalad.

Walking the elbows back in supine-on-elbows is typically most difficult when the elbows are located caudal to the shoulders. The task becomes easier as the elbows move rostrally into more stable positions. Practice of the skill should start in a relatively easy position, with the elbows only slightly caudal to the shoulders. As a patient's skill increases, he can walk his elbows back from progressively caudal positions.

Independent work. If placed in supine-on-elbows, a patient can work on his own. Frequent assistance may be needed as he either falls or succeeds in walking his elbows and needs to start again.

Dynamic shoulder control in single forearm-supported supine. Dynamic shoulder control in this position is similar to control in sitting, propped back on one hand (described in the sitting skills section that follows). Dynamic shoulder control is easier in the latter position, so it should be developed there first. The training strategies for the two positions are the same.

From supine-on-elbows, lift one elbow. In this maneuver the person in supine-on-elbows shifts his weight and lifts the unweighted elbow. As he does so, he pivots his trunk over the shoulder of the supporting arm (Figure 10–7D).

Before practicing this skill, a patient should have dynamic shoulder control in single forearm-supported supine. In addition, he must be able to weight shift in supine-on-elbows enough to unweight one elbow completely.

Lifting an elbow from this position involves the same techniques as lifting an elbow from supine, supported on one elbow and one hand. The training strategies for developing these skills are presented above.

From single forearm-supported supine, throw one arm back. Before practicing this skill, a patient must have dynamic shoulder control in single forearm-supported supine.

Starting in single forearm-supported supine, the patient throws his free arm back to assume the position of supine supported on one elbow and one hand (Figure 10–7D and E). The free arm must land on the palm with the elbow extended, the shoulder externally rotated and hyperextended, and the scapula adducted. For this to occur, the throw must be forceful and initiated with the shoulder of the swinging arm positioned as high as possible.

Throwing an arm from this position is similar to doing so from forearm-supported sidelying. The reader is referred to the discussion of the latter skill (in the sidelying skills section later in this

chapter) for a more detailed explanation of throwing an arm, and for functional training suggestions.

Place arm through loop. Before working on this skill, an individual should be able to position his elbow in extension. To practice with a hanging loop, he must be able to maintain his elbow in extension while he flexes his shoulder.

It can be difficult to place an arm through a loop that is suspended from above. During early training, the task can be made easier by placing the loop on the mat. With the loop in this position, the patient can practice grabbing it and slipping his hand through.

Once a patient has become adept at placing his arm through a loop that is lying on a mat, he can begin working with a hanging loop.[p] To place his hand through a hanging loop, the patient must first bring his hand to the loop, flexing his shoulder while maintaining his elbow in extension. He then slips his hand through the loop. Once the hand is through and the loop is around his forearm, he can internally rotate his shoulder and flex his elbow to "grasp" the loop with his forearm.

Practice with a hanging loop should begin with a loop that hangs within easy reach. Once the patient becomes adept at placing his arm through the loop, he can practice with loops hung higher.

Independent work. This skill is ideal for independent work. The patient can practice in therapy or in his room in the evenings.

Pulling on loop ladder, move from supine to single forearm-supported supine. In this maneuver, the person uses a loop ladder lying at his side to lift his trunk and get onto an elbow (Figure 10–9A and B). With one or both forearms stabilized in a loop, he pulls by flexing his elbow(s) forcefully. At the same time, he extends the shoulder of the arm closest to the loop ladder, driving the elbow into the mat. With these combined motions, the patient lifts his upper trunk up and over the supporting elbow.

Lifting the trunk is most difficult at the beginning of the lift, when the patient is supine on the mat. The task becomes easier as the supporting shoulder approaches a position vertically over the supporting elbow. Practice of the skill should begin in the easier position: starting in forearm-supported supine with one or both forearms placed through a loop, the patient can practice lowering himself

---

p Of course, this is only necessary if the patient plans to use hanging loops.

slightly and pulling back up. He should be encouraged to lower himself as far as he can while retaining control of the motion and the ability to return to the starting position. As his skill increases, he can move through larger arcs of motion.

Independent work. Once a patient has developed the ability to lower and to raise his trunk slightly when positioned in single forearm-supported supine, he will be able to practice on his own. The therapist can assist the patient into single forearm-supported supine and encourage the patient to practice lowering and raising his trunk by pulling on the loop ladder.

In single forearm-supported supine, pull on loop ladder and walk supporting elbow toward feet. This skill is performed in forearm-supported supine, with the forearm of the free arm placed through a loop ladder. The upper trunk should be rotated toward the supporting arm, so that the free shoulder is higher than the supporting shoulder (Figure 10–9B).

To unweight and reposition his supporting elbow, the person pulls on the loop and throws his head toward his feet. The combined pull and head swing should be forceful and abrupt. As he pulls, the person drags his supporting elbow toward the foot of the bed. This maneuver is repeated until he has walked his elbow as far as he can with that loop.

During initial practice, the therapist can assist the patient with the motions to give him a feel for the maneuver. The therapist should emphasize that the motions need to be abrupt and forceful.

Independent work. Once the patient is able to walk his supporting elbow toward the foot of the bed with at least minimal success, he can practice the skill independently. The therapist can assist him into forearm-supported supine to enable him to practice.

Lift trunk by pulling on suspended loop. This skill is illustrated in Figure 10–10C. If a patient has adequate strength, he should be able to master this skill with minimal practice. With his forearm(s) stabilized in a hanging loop, he simply pulls to lift his trunk. If he is unable to position an arm through the loop, the therapist can place the arm for him. If the patient has inadequate strength to lift his trunk from supine, he may be able to practice with pillows or a wedge positioned under his upper trunk. If he is practicing in a hospital bed, he can practice with the head of the bed ele-

vated slightly. As his strength improves, he should practice with his trunk in progressively more horizontal positions.

Independent work. This skill is ideally suited for independent practice. The therapist should determine the most appropriate position for practice (flat on the mat or with upper trunk propped) and assist the patient into this position. The patient can then practice lifting his trunk.

Prone Skills

Roll from prone by pushing with arm. To practice this skill, a patient must be able to extend his elbow. He can do so using either triceps or muscle substitution with the anterior deltoid.[q]

Rolling from prone to supine is accomplished by pushing with one arm. To roll toward the left, a patient plants his right hand on the mat and pushes with this arm to roll.

Because rolling toward supine is most difficult from prone, practice can start in sidelying. From this position, a small push will rotate the body slightly toward supine. Once the patient has moved out of sidelying, gravity will complete the roll.

Once a patient is able to roll to supine from sidelying, he should practice rolling from a position closer to prone. The therapist can assist him to a position tilted slightly toward prone from sidelying and have him roll back by pushing on the mat. As his skill improves, the patient can practice rolling from positions that are progressively closer to prone.

Independent work. Patients can practice rolling toward sidelying from semiprone positions. (A person practicing independently should not roll past sidelying unless he is capable of returning from supine.) The therapist can place a pillow or bolster in front of the patient's trunk, positioned so that it supports him in semiprone without blocking his arm.

Weight shift in prone-on-elbows. This skill involves leaning to the side while in prone-on-elbows. To do this under control, a person must first be able to stabilize himself in this posture. The therapist can help him develop this ability by placing him in prone-on-elbows and asking him to hold the position. Applying resistance to the patient's

---

[q] The prerequisite skill of extending the elbow using muscle substitution is addressed in Chapter 11.

shoulders in various directions while he holds his posture can help him develop his stability.

Once he has developed the ability to stabilize in prone-on-elbows, the patient will be ready to practice shifting his weight in this posture. During early weight shifting practice, the therapist can give him a feel for the motion by having him push against resistance. To do so, the therapist should place a hand against one of the patient's shoulders and ask him to push against it. After the patient has shifted slightly, he can return to upright by pushing against a hand placed on the opposite shoulder.

The patient should practice leaning alternately to one side, then the other. He should start with small motions, shifting only as far as he is able to control the motion and return to the starting position. As his skill increases, he can increase the arcs of motion.

During early practice of this skill, the elbows should be located directly beneath the shoulders. Weight shifts are easiest to control in this position. As a patient's skill increases, he should practice in less stable positions, with his elbows located rostral or caudal to his shoulders.

Independent work.   After being placed in prone-on-elbows, a patient can shift his weight to one side and then the other. He should be encouraged to shift as far as he can while maintaining control over the motion; he should shift far enough to make the activity challenging but not so far that he cannot return to upright independently.

Walk elbows in from abducted position.
This skill is illustrated in Figure 10–3. To practice, a patient must be able to weight shift in prone-on-elbows.

Walking the elbows in from an abducted position is most difficult at the beginning of the task, when the trunk remains on the mat. The task becomes easier as the arms become more vertical, approaching the stable prone-on-elbows position. Practice of this skill should start from this easier position.

To practice this skill, the patient starts in prone-on-elbows with his elbows directly under his shoulders. From this position, he weight shifts laterally to unweight one elbow. He moves the unweighted elbow a short distance laterally and shifts his weight back onto it. He should then shift the weight off again and move the elbow back in, returning to the starting position. Moving the elbow back in involves a combined motion of shoulder shrug and horizontal adduction. The therapist can help the patient learn this motion

with verbal cueing and by providing resistance at the shoulder and arm.

When the patient has developed the capacity to move an elbow out and back in, he can progress to moving one elbow a short distance laterally, shifting onto it, and moving the other elbow out. He then reverses the steps, walking the elbows back in.

Walking the elbows out from prone-on-elbows is relatively easy; bringing them back in is the difficult task. While practicing, it can be tempting for the patient to walk his elbows out too far, reaching a position from which he is unable to return without assistance. The therapist should encourage the patient to walk his elbows out only as far as he can control the motion and return without assistance.

As his skill develops, the patient should walk his elbows out and back over increasing distances. In this manner, he can build up to the point where he can walk his elbows all the way out laterally and back in. At this point, he will be able to assume prone-on-elbows from prone.

Independent work.   Once an individual has developed the ability to walk his elbows short distances from and return to prone-on-elbows, he can work on the skill independently. The therapist can assist him into the prone-on-elbows position to enable him to practice.

Walk elbows forward from adducted position.
This skill is illustrated in Figure 10–4. Before practicing, a patient should be able to weight shift in prone-on-elbows.

This skill can be developed in reverse, using an approach comparable to that described for developing the skill of walking the elbows in from an abducted position. From a starting position of prone-on-elbows with the elbows directly under the shoulders, the patient practices walking his elbows back toward his pelvis and then returning to the starting position.[r] As his skill develops, he walks his elbows across increasing distances. In this manner, he gradually builds to the point where he is able to walk his elbows back until he is prone on the mat and from that position can walk them forward to return to prone-on-elbows.

Independent work.   Once an individual has developed the ability to walk his elbows back short distances from and return to prone-on-

---

[r] Refer to the section on assuming prone-on-elbows from an abducted position for more detailed functional training suggestions.

elbows, he can work on the skill independently. The therapist can assist him into the prone-on-elbows position to enable him to practice.

Move from prone-on-elbows to forearm-supported sidelying.

This maneuver is illustrated in Figure 10–14. To practice, the patient must be able to weight shift in prone-on-elbows and should have some dynamic shoulder control in sidelying with forearm support. In the absence of functioning triceps, he must also be able to extend one elbow using his anterior deltoid.

In prone-on-elbows, the person shifts his weight to one side and plants the hand of his unweighted arm on the mat (Figure 10–14B). He then pushes to rotate his body up and over the supporting arm, ending in the position of sidelying with forearm support.

The motions of the supporting shoulder are critical to this maneuver. As the patient pushes his torso up and over his arm, the supporting shoulder moves from a position of horizontal adduction to horizontal abduction (Figure 10–14A through C).

Until the patient has developed some skill in this maneuver, he will need assistance to work on it. The therapist can start by demonstrating and passively moving the patient through the maneuver to give him an idea of the motions involved. The therapist can then assist him into a position of sidelying with forearm support, with the "free" hand stabilized against the mat. From this position, the patient can practice rotating his trunk toward prone and back up (Figure 10–15). The power for this motion will come primarily from the "free" arm pushing on the mat. During practice, the patient's motions should be small enough that they remain under his control, yet large enough to be a challenge. As his skill increases, he can increase his arcs of motion.

This skill is easiest when the trunk and lower extremities are in a line, with the hips in approximately neutral extension. The hips remain in this position while a person comes to sitting using the technique that involves rolling and throwing the arms (Figure 10–6). The maneuver is more difficult when the trunk and lower extremities are angled, as when coming to sitting by walking on the elbows (Figure 10–8). Initial practice should be done in the easier position, with the trunk and lower extremities in a line.

Independent work. Once a patient has developed some skill in this maneuver, he can practice on his own. The therapist can assist him into forearm-supported sidelying and instruct him to practice as described above.

In prone-on-elbows, walk elbows to the side.

Before practicing this skill, the patient must be able to weight shift well in prone-on-elbows.

From prone-on-elbows, the person unweights one elbow by leaning laterally. He moves his unweighted elbow medially a short distance and shifts onto it to unweight the other elbow. He can then move the newly unweighted elbow laterally. By performing this sequence repeatedly, he walks his elbows to the side.

While practicing walking on his elbows, the patient must make sure that he does not move

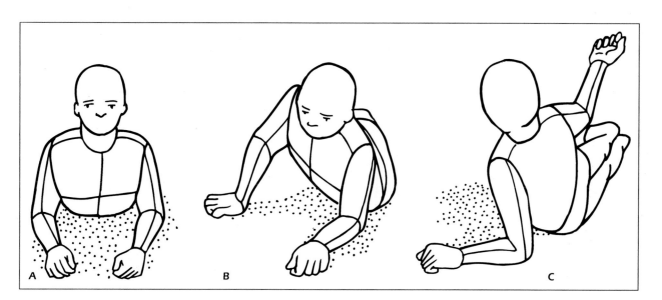

Figure 10–14. Move from prone-on-elbows to forearm-supported sidelying. **(A)** Prone-on-elbows. **(B)** Weight shifted and hand planted. Trunk rotates over shoulder of supporting arm. **(C)** Supporting shoulder has moved from horizontal adduction to horizontal abduction.

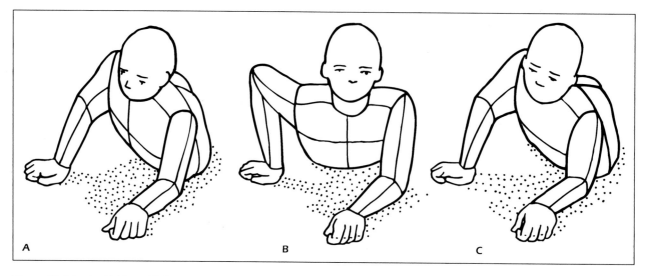

Figure 10–15. In sidelying with forearm support, "free" hand stabilized against the mat. **(A)** Starting position. **(B)** Trunk rotates toward prone. **(C)** Return to starting position.

them too far apart.[s] If he positions his elbows too far apart, he will be unable to shift his weight enough to unweight either elbow. As a result, he will not be able to progress from this position without assistance.

To ensure that his elbows remain close enough together, the patient can make a habit of moving one elbow medially before moving the other one laterally. He should also take small enough "steps" each time he moves an elbow laterally.

Independent work. Once the patient has developed the ability to walk his elbows a short distance while in prone-on-elbows, he can increase

his skill by working independently. The therapist can assist him into the prone-on-elbows position to enable him to practice as described above.

Sidelying Skills

Move from sidelying to prone-on-elbows. This skill is illustrated in Figure 10–16. Before practicing, a patient should be able to weight shift in prone-on-elbows.

When performing this skill, a patient starts in sidelying with his lower shoulder flexed to approximately 90 degrees. He stabilizes the hand of this arm on his chin, forehead, or the side of his head. By positioning his hand in this manner, the patient creates a strut on which he can pivot. Using forceful shoulder horizontal abduction, he

---

[s] The distance that is "too far" will depend upon the individual's strength and skill.

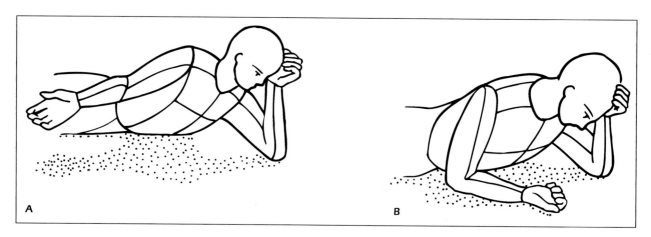

Figure 10–16. Move from sidelying to prone-on-elbows.

pushes his trunk up and over the supporting arm. Toward the end of the maneuver, he can use neck flexion to augment the lift.

This skill is most difficult at the beginning, when the patient lifts his trunk from the mat. It becomes easier as the trunk is lifted higher and the supporting arm becomes more vertical. Practice should start where the task is easiest: in prone-on-elbows, with one hand stabilized on the chin, forehead, or side of the head. From this position, the patient should lean toward the side of the stabilized (supporting) arm, leaning as far as he can without losing control. He then lifts his body back over the supporting arm. To do this, he uses horizontal abduction of the shoulder of the supporting arm. Because the elbow of the supporting arm is stabilized on the mat, shoulder horizontal abduction serves to lift the trunk up and over the arm.

As the patient's skill increases, he can move through larger arcs of motion. As he leans further from vertical, it will become more difficult to return to upright. He may need to use momentum to augment the supporting arm's push. To utilize momentum, he should swing his free arm forward as he pushes his supporting arm into the mat (Figure 10–16A).

The patient should practice leaning and returning to the starting position through larger arcs of motion. In this manner, he can gradually progress to the point where he can lean far enough to touch a shoulder to the mat and return to prone-on-elbows.

Independent work. Once a patient has developed the ability to lean slightly from and return to prone-on-elbows, he can work on the skill independently. The therapist can assist him into the prone-on-elbows position and instruct him to practice as described above.

Dynamic shoulder control in forearm-supported sidelying. In forearm-supported sidelying, the patient maintains his balance while moving the supporting shoulder forward and back. To keep the trunk balanced over the supporting elbow, the patient rotates his trunk in the direction opposite the supporting shoulder's movements; as the shoulder moves forward, his trunk rotates back. (Figure 10–17 illustrates the motions involved.) Motions of the free arm and head can be used to augment balance.

During initial practice, the therapist can assist the patient into forearm-supported sidelying and ask him to maintain the position. At first the patient may just use motions of his head and free arm to maintain his balance.

Once the patient has developed some skill in balancing in forearm-supported sidelying, he can practice moving his supporting shoulder forward and back through small arcs of motion. The therapist may first move the patient passively to give him a feel for the motion involved. The patient should then perform the motions with assistance and guarding.

As the patient's skill develops, he can increase the motions of his shoulder until he is able to move through large arcs. He should always practice moving through an arc that is large enough to be a challenge but small enough to be controlled.

The patient should also practice abducting the scapula of his supporting shoulder when this shoulder is positioned directly over the elbow. This scapular motion raises the trunk, increasing

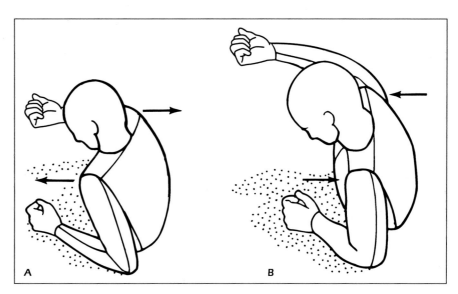

Figure 10–17. *Dynamic shoulder control in forearm-supported sidelying. (A) As the supporting shoulder moves forward, the trunk rotates back. (B) As the supporting shoulder moves back, the trunk rotates forward.*

A   B

the distance between the free shoulder and the mat. This skill is important in coming to sitting using the method that involves rolling and throwing the arms.

Independent work.   Once the patient is able to balance in forearm-supported sidelying while moving his supporting shoulder through small arcs, he should be able to practice independently. The therapist can assist the patient into position and encourage him to practice.

From forearm-supported sidelying, throw free arm back.   This maneuver is illustrated in Figure 10–18. Before practicing this skill, the patient should develop some dynamic shoulder control in forearm-supported sidelying.

Starting in forearm-supported sidelying, the person with a spinal cord injury throws his free arm back to assume the position of supine supported on one elbow and one hand. As he throws his arm, his center of gravity moves from over his base of support, and he falls in the direction of the swinging arm. The palm must land with the arm positioned so that it can accept weight and catch the falling trunk. In the absence of functioning triceps, the final position of the swinging shoulder is key. When the hand hits the mat, this shoulder

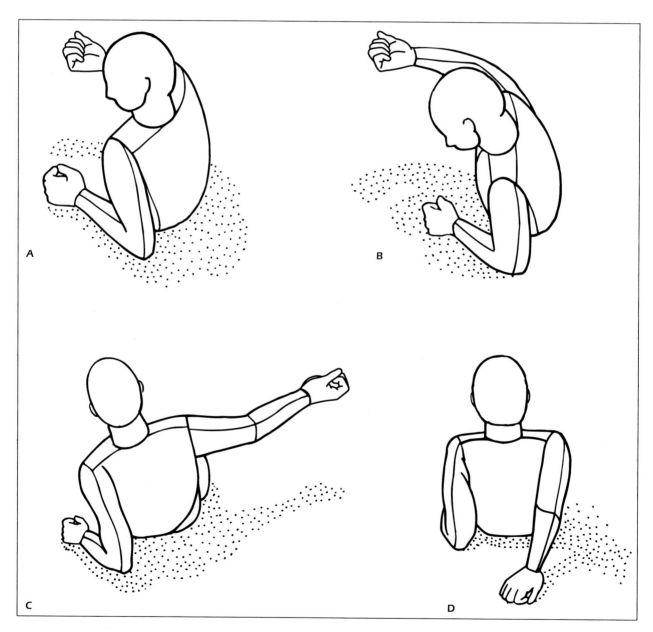

Figure 10–18.   *From forearm-supported sidelying, throw free arm back.* **(A)** *Forearm-supported sidelying.* **(B)** *Ready position to throw: shoulders perpendicular to mat, scapula of supporting arm abducted.* **(C)** *Half-way through throw. Trunk is pivoting on supporting shoulder.* **(D)** *End position.*

must be positioned in extreme horizontal abduction; the hand must land medial to the shoulder. If it lands in a position that is too lateral, the arm will not support the trunk. The elbow will flex, causing the person to fall to the mat.

The thrown arm must land with the hand medial to the shoulder if the arm is to support the trunk. In addition, the shoulder should end in extreme extension. This hyperextension is required for a person lacking functional triceps to come to sitting from this position.

Three factors combine to make it possible for the arm to land with the shoulder positioned appropriately: starting position of the shoulders, velocity of the swinging arm, and direction of the arm's motion.

When the arm throw is initiated, the shoulder of the thrown arm should be as high as possible. Specifically, the shoulders should be aligned perpendicular to the mat (Figure 10–18B) and the scapula of the supporting arm should be abducted. Then, as the patient's center of gravity shifts and the trunk falls, the shoulder of the thrown arm will fall from as high a position as possible. The further it has to fall, the longer the fall will take. A longer fall will allow the free arm to swing further, so the shoulder can end in extreme horizontal abduction.

The swinging arm will also be able to move further if it is thrown forcefully. An arm that travels at a high velocity will travel further as the trunk falls, and as a result will land in a better position.

The patient may find it easiest to throw his arm in the direction of shoulder horizontal abduction rather than extension. If the arm is thrown forcefully in the direction of horizontal abduction, momentum will carry it toward the body's midline at the end of the throw.

The motion of the supporting shoulder is also key to the successful performance of this maneuver. As the patient swings his arm into position, he must pivot his trunk on the supporting shoulder (Figure 10–18C). This pivot will make it possible for the shoulders to end in a stable position when the swing is completed (Figure 10–18D).

It can be quite difficult for a patient to learn to throw an arm back while balancing on the other elbow. For this reason, it is advisable to practice first in an easier position. Throwing an arm back while sitting, propped back on one extended arm, is similar to throwing it from forearm-supported sidelying. Similar initial positioning and motions are involved, but the more upright posture makes the arm throw easier in sitting. By developing this skill in sitting, a patient can prepare himself for practice in forearm-supported sidelying.

Once the patient has some skill throwing an arm in sitting, he can practice from forearm-supported sidelying. During early practice the therapist can place the patient in position, with his free shoulder high. By moving the patient's trunk and free arm passively, the therapist can demonstrate how the supporting shoulder collapses forward as the trunk falls and the free arm swings back. The patient can then practice the technique. He is likely to have many failed attempts as he learns the skill. Verbal feedback from the therapist at this point can help him perfect his technique.

Independent work. Once a patient has developed some ability in this maneuver, he can practice alone. He is likely to need frequent assistance at first, as he will fall periodically.

In 90-degree forearm-supported sidelying, walk supporting elbow toward legs. Before practicing this skill, a patient must be able to weight shift in prone-on-elbows. He should also be able to walk his elbows to the side in prone-on-elbows. From a position of forearm-supported sidelying with the hips flexed to approximately 90 degrees, the patient lifts his nonweightbearing arm and hooks it behind his legs, placing his forearm behind the knees or thighs (Figure 10–8E). Once his arm is stabilized in this manner, the patient is ready to pull his torso toward his legs. To do so, he repeatedly pulls on his legs while throwing his head toward the legs. The combined pull and head swing should be forceful and abrupt, to gain maximal momentum. With each pull, the patient drags his supporting elbow further toward his legs. This step is repeated until the torso has reached the desired position. (The torso's target position will depend on the method that will be used to move the trunk into an upright position.)

During initial practice, the therapist can assist the patient with the motion to give him a feel for the maneuver. The therapist should emphasize that the motions need to be abrupt and forceful. The patient should progress quickly to practicing without assistance.

Independent work. Once an individual is able to walk his supporting elbow toward his trunk with at least minimal success, he can practice the skill independently. The therapist may need to assist him into forearm-supported sidelying with his hips flexed to approximately 90 degrees.

From forearm-supported sidelying, push/ pull into sitting position. Before practicing this skill, a patient must be able to extend one of his elbows, using either his triceps or muscle substitution. This maneuver begins with the person propped on one elbow in sidelying with his hips flexed beyond 90 degrees (Figure 10–8F). The other arm is hooked behind his knees or thighs.

The patient pulls on his legs to unweight the supporting elbow. He then internally rotates the shoulder of the supporting arm, placing his palm on the mat. The shoulder should be internally rotated enough that the elbow points toward the ceiling (Figure 10–8G). Once his hand is planted on the mat, he extends his elbow to push his torso up and over his legs. At the same time, he pulls with the other arm. He can also throw his head toward his legs, using momentum to assist in the motion.

The most difficult part of this maneuver is the beginning, when the person starts pushing and pulling to move his trunk. As the trunk moves up and over the legs, the task becomes easier.

Functional training should begin in the end position, where the skill is easiest. Practice should start with the patient sitting, propped to the side on an arm with its elbow extended. The other arm should be hooked around his legs (Figure 10–19A). From this position, the patient practices lowering his trunk to the side and returning to sitting. He should start with small motions, lowering his trunk slightly and pushing/pulling back up (Figure 10–19B and C). He can lower his trunk further as his skill increases, gradually building to the point where he can raise his trunk

from forearm-supported sidelying. During practice, the motions should be small enough that the patient is able to retain control yet large enough to be a challenge.

Independent work. Once the patient has developed the ability to lean slightly from and return to sitting, he can practice this skill independently. The therapist can assist him into the sitting position and encourage him to practice.

Sitting Skills

Dynamic shoulder control in sitting, propped back on one hand. To perform this activity, a person with a spinal cord injury sits propped on one extended arm and pivots his trunk on the supporting shoulder. He must maintain his balance while moving the supporting shoulder forward and back. To keep his trunk balanced over his base of support, he pivots his trunk in the direction opposite the supporting shoulder's movements: as the shoulder moves forward, his trunk rotates back. (Figure 10–20 illustrates the motions involved.) Motions of the free arm and head are used to augment balance.

The first step in developing this skill is learning to balance while sitting, propped back on one hand. The therapist can assist the patient into position and ask him to maintain the position. The patient uses his head and free arm to balance, using them to keep his center of gravity over his base of

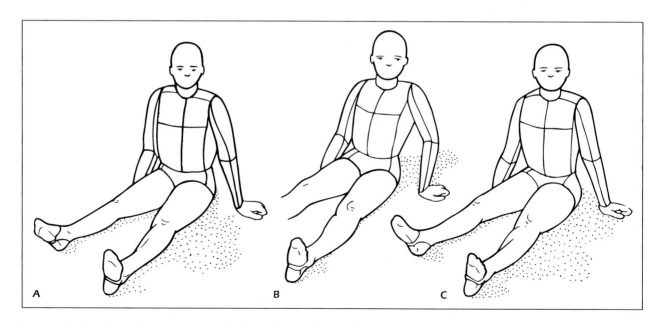

Figure 10–19.   In long-sitting, practice lowering the trunk to the side. **(A)** Starting position: long-sitting, propped to the side on one arm, other arm hooked around legs. **(B)** The patient lowers his trunk to the side. **(C)** Push/pull back to starting position.

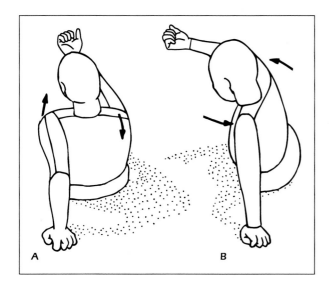

Figure 10–20. *Dynamic shoulder control in sitting, propped back on one hand.* **(A)** *As the supporting shoulder moves forward, the trunk rotates back.* **(B)** *As the supporting shoulder moves back, the trunk rotates forward.*

support: when he starts to fall in one direction, he moves his head and arm in the opposite direction.[t]

Once the patient is able to maintain his balance in this position, he is ready to practice dynamic shoulder control. He should start by moving his shoulder forward and back through small arcs of motion. The therapist may first move him passively to give him a feel for the motion involved. The patient should then perform the motions with assistance and guarding.

As the patient's skill develops, he can increase the forward and back motions of his supporting shoulder until he is able to move through large arcs. He should always practice moving through an arc that is large enough to be a challenge but small enough for him to retain control.

The patient should also practice abducting the scapula of his supporting shoulder when his trunk is rotated to a position vertically over this shoulder. This scapular abduction raises the trunk, increasing the distance between the free shoulder and the mat. This skill is important in the technique of coming to sitting that involves rolling and throwing the arms.

Dynamic shoulder control is most difficult when the supporting shoulder is positioned in extreme hyperextension. Control should be developed first in easier positions with the trunk relatively upright.

---

[t] Prior training in unsupported sitting balance may help prepare the patient for this maneuver. Strategies for developing unsupported sitting balance are presented in Chapter 11.

Independent work. Once a patient is able to balance while moving his supporting shoulder through small arcs, he should be able to practice independently. The therapist can assist the patient into a sitting position and encourage him to practice.

From sitting propped back on one hand, throw free arm back. To practice this skill, a patient must have balance and dynamic shoulder control in this position. He should also have good shoulder range of motion, without any limitations in extension or horizontal abduction.

While sitting propped back on one hand, the patient throws his free arm back. As the arm moves, the trunk pivots on the supporting shoulder and moves past the balance point, falling toward the moving arm. When the hand lands, the swinging arm needs to be positioned so that it can accept weight: the palm should land on the mat medial to the shoulder with the elbow extended, the shoulder externally rotated and hyperextended, and the scapula adducted.

If the hand lands before the upper extremity reaches a stable position, the elbow will flex and the patient will fall to the mat. To increase the likelihood of success, the throw should be forceful and initiated with the shoulder of the swinging arm as high as possible. A more thorough explanation is given above, in the section entitled "From Forearm-Supported Sidelying, Throw Free Arm Back."

During early practice, the therapist can move the patient's trunk and free arm passively. While doing so, the therapist can demonstrate how the supporting shoulder collapses forward as the trunk falls and the free arm swings back. The patient can then practice the technique. He is likely to have many failed attempts as he learns the skill. Verbal feedback from the therapist at this point can help him perfect his technique.

Independent work. Once a patient has developed some ability in this maneuver, he can practice alone. He is likely to need frequent assistance at first.

Weight shift while sitting, propped back on two hands. Before practicing this skill, a patient must be able to tolerate an upright sitting posture. It is not necessary for him to have the skill of extending his elbows because they can be placed by the therapist in a position of passive locking.

In this activity, the patient shifts his weight laterally while sitting propped back on two extended arms. The elbows are "locked" through positioning, with the shoulders extended and externally rotated, elbows extended, and palms on the mat even with or slightly medial to the shoulders. When weight is borne on the arms in this position, the elbows will remain in extension without any muscular effort.

During early training, the therapist can place the patient in position and ask him to shift to the side. He should shift a short distance, return to upright, and shift in the opposite direction. The therapist may help the patient learn to move laterally by placing a hand against his shoulder and having him push laterally against it.

Independent work. Once a patient can shift his weight to the right and left through small arcs while sitting propped back on two extended arms, he can work independently. The therapist can assist him into position and encourage him to practice. As the patient's skill improves, he can increase the distance of his weight shifts. He should work in a range that is challenging, yet within his capabilities.

From sitting propped back on two hands, walk hands forward.

A patient must be able to tolerate an upright sitting position to practice this skill, and must be able to weight shift in this position. To perform this maneuver, a person with a spinal cord injury shifts his weight laterally and moves his unweighted hand forward slightly by elevating and protracting the scapula. He then shifts his weight in the opposite direction and moves the other hand. By repeating these steps, he walks his hands forward toward his buttocks.

The hands must move over short distances and should move straight forward. If a hand is moved too far forward, the trunk can tilt excessively onto the other arm. This makes it difficult to weight shift in the opposite direction. If the person moves his hand laterally instead of forward, this arm will not be in a stable position for accepting weight.

During early practice, the therapist should instruct the patient to lean to one side, then shrug the unweighted shoulder up and forward. If the patient has difficulty moving the unweighted upper extremity, he can add power to the attempt by throwing his head forward and toward the supporting arm.

Independent work. Once a patient can perform this skill with some success, he can practice independently. As an advanced activity for independent work, the patient can walk his hands forward until he reaches an upright sitting position, bal-ance briefly in sitting, throw his arms back, catch himself on his hands, and walk his hands forward again.

With one arm through overhead loop, throw free arm back.

To practice this skill, a patient must be able to tolerate an upright sitting posture.

The endpoint of this maneuver is illustrated in Figure 10–10F. The patient starts in a semireclined position, supporting his trunk with a forearm hooked through a loop that is hanging from overhead. He throws his free arm back, landing with his palm located medial to his shoulder. The thrown arm must land in a position that will enable it to accept weight: elbow extended, shoulder externally rotated and hyperextended, and scapula adducted. To ensure that the arm ends in a proper position, it should be thrown forcefully and in the direction of shoulder horizontal abduction rather than extension.

A patient holding an overhead loop is in a stable position; he does not need to concern himself with maintaining his center of gravity over his base of support. For this reason, throwing an arm while hanging from an overhead loop is not as difficult as doing so while propped on an elbow or hand. Practice should emphasize the force and direction of the throw.

In sitting, propped back on one hand, pull on suspended loop and walk supporting hand forward.

A patient must be able to tolerate an upright sitting posture to practice this skill.

To perform this skill, the patient sits in a semireclined posture with one forearm placed through a suspended loop. The other arm is in a locked position behind him, supporting his trunk (Figure 10–10G). The elbow is "locked" through positioning, with the shoulder extended and externally rotated, elbow extended, and palm on the mat even with or slightly medial to the shoulder.

The patient must unweight his supporting arm to walk the hand forward. To do so, he pulls forcefully on the loop and throws his head forward. At the same time he moves his supporting hand forward toward his buttocks. This maneuver is repeated until the patient has walked his hand as far as he can with that loop.

During initial practice, the therapist can assist the patient with the motions to give him a feel for the maneuver. The therapist should emphasize that the motions need to be forceful.

Independent work. Once the patient is able to walk his supporting hand forward with at least minimal success, he can practice the skill independently. The therapist can assist him into position and encourage him to practice. The patient may be able to alternate practice of this skill with practice lifting the hand from the bed and throwing it back.

In long-sitting, move buttocks forward and back. To perform this skill, a patient must be able to tolerate an upright sitting position, propping on his arms with his elbows extended.[u]

The head-hips relationship is used in these maneuvers. To move his buttocks forward, the person with a spinal cord injury starts in long-sitting, propped forward on his arms. He then pushes into the mat to lift or unweight his buttocks and throws his head back forcefully. To move his buttocks back, he starts with his arms behind and slightly lateral to his buttocks. From this position, he pushes into the mat while throwing his head forward forcefully.

During early practice, the therapist can help the patient get a feel for the maneuvers by assisting him with the motions. Once the patient has a feel for the motion, he can practice with guarding.

Independent work. A patient who has good sitting balance and who has had some initial practice in moving his buttocks on a mat can practice independently. If needed, the therapist can assist him into a sitting position.

In long-sitting, prop to the side on one extended arm. A patient must be able to tolerate upright sitting before practicing this skill. In the absence of functioning triceps, he must be able to lock his elbows.[v] During early practice, the therapist can assist the patient into position and ask him to help hold the elbow of the supporting arm straight. As the patient's ability to support himself improves, the therapist's assistance can be reduced.

Once the patient is able to support his trunk's weight on his arm, he can practice balancing on that arm. The therapist should assist him into position and ask him to stay upright. The patient balances using his head and free arm: when his trunk starts to fall, he moves his head and free arm in the direction opposite the fall.

The patient can work on his balance with guarding at first. To prepare for more advanced

activities, he can practice holding the position as the therapist pushes his shoulders in various directions.

Dynamic stability in long-sitting, propped to the side on one extended arm. To practice this skill, a patient must be able to tolerate upright sitting and prop to the side on one arm with the elbow extended.

While propping to the side in long-sitting, the patient practices maintaining his balance while he rotates his trunk, weight shifts it laterally, and moves his head and free arm in various directions.

Independent work. The activities just described can be performed alone, long-sitting on a mat. The patient should be far enough from the mat's edge to allow him to fall safely.

Sitting propped to the side on one extended arm, use free arm to move lower extremity. Before practicing this skill, a patient should have dynamic stability in long-sitting while propped to the side on one extended arm.

When positioning his legs in long-sitting, a person with a complete spinal cord injury moves one lower extremity at a time. He props to the side on one arm, leaning in the direction toward which he plans to move his leg. He pulls the leg using his free arm, at the same time moving his head and torso forcefully in the direction of the pull.

The therapist should encourage the patient to move his head and trunk forcefully, and to synchronize these motions with the pull. During early practice, the therapist can assist the patient with the maneuver to give him a feel for the motions involved.

Independent work. Once the patient can move a leg with at least minimal success, he can practice the skill independently.

FUNCTIONAL MAT TECHNIQUES AND THERAPEUTIC STRATEGIES FOLLOWING INCOMPLETE SPINAL CORD INJURY

The movement strategies that an individual can use to perform functional tasks after sustaining an incomplete spinal cord injury will depend primarily on his voluntary motor function. A person who retains or regains only sensory function below his injury (ASIA B) will utilize the techniques that are used by people with complete spinal cord injuries, as just described. A person who has minimal motor sparing or return (ASIA

---

[u] Strategies for developing the ability to lock the elbows and to prop forward on extended arms in sitting are presented in Chapter 11.

[v] Strategies for develop the ability to lock the elbows are presented in Chapter 11.

PROBLEM-SOLVING EXERCISE 10–1

Your patient has complete (ASIA A) tetraplegia. She is young, healthy, and highly motivated. She is also dependent in all functional activities. One of her goals is to come to sitting independently in a bed without using equipment.

The patient's muscle test results are as follows.

Muscles	Left	Right
Deltoids (anterior, middle, and posterior)	5/5	4/5
Shoulder internal rotators	5/5	4/5
Elbow flexors	5/5	5/5
Radial wrist extensors	5/5	4/5
Triceps	3/5	2/5
Long finger flexors	0/5	0/5
Abductor digiti minimi	0/5	0/5
Trunk and lower extremity musculature	0/5	0/5

The patient's joint range of motion and muscle flexibility are normal throughout, with the following exceptions.

Motions	Left	Right
Shoulder extension	5 degrees	10 degrees
Elbow extension	–15 degrees	–15 degrees
Passive straight-leg raise	80 degrees	70 degrees
Long finger flexors	mild tightness	mild tightness

- Using the ASIA classification system, what is (are) this patient's motor level(s)?
- What method of coming to sitting without equipment is this individual likely to achieve most readily?
- What are the physical prerequisites for this method of coming to sitting?
- What strength and range should the therapeutic exercise program emphasize to facilitate the attainment of this goal?
- What are the skill prerequisites for this method of coming to sitting?
- Describe a functional training program for this patient.

C) is likely to utilize similar movement strategies, but may be able to add trunk or lower extremity motions to make the tasks easier. In contrast, an individual who has significant motor function below his lesion (ASIA D) will be able to perform mat skills using more normal movement patterns.

Another factor that can have an impact on the performance of mat skills is spasticity. People with incomplete lesions tend to exhibit more spasticity than do people with complete lesions, and spasticity tends to be more severe among those with ASIA B and C lesions.[2, 4, 10] Involuntary muscle contractions can interfere with the functional use of voluntary motor function that is preserved below the lesion. When elevated muscle tone interferes with function, the rehabilitation team can work with the patient to reduce the abnormal tone.[w] In addition, the therapist and patient should note the conditions and bodily motions that tend to elicit involuntary muscle contractions. They can then work together in an effort to find ways in which the patient can move without causing these involuntary contractions. In some cases, they may also find ways in which spasticity can be used to enhance the performance of some activities.

---

[w] Strategies for treating spasticity are presented in Chapter 3.

Perhaps the most challenging aspect of functional mat training after an incomplete spinal cord injury is determining the methods that the individual can utilize to perform the skills. Each patient has a unique pattern of muscle strength and weakness, spasticity, joint range of motion, muscle flexibility, and body build. It is often difficult to predict what methods of performing mat skills will best suit the individual; some physical maneuvers will be within his potential and others will not. Functional training involves problem solving as the therapist works with the patient to help him discover and develop the movement strategies that will enable him to achieve his functional goals.

Rolling

In a neurologically intact person, rolling involves coordinated motions of the entire body. The patterns used to roll vary a good deal between adults. In one commonly used rolling pattern, cervical and trunk rotation and reaching with an upper extremity are combined with lower extremity flexion when rolling from supine to prone. Other rolling patterns found in normal adults include pushing with an arm, pushing with one or both legs, and rolling without trunk rotation.[9]

Regardless of the rolling strategy employed, a neurologically intact adult typically utilizes motions of his head, trunk, upper, and lower extremities. In contrast, a person with a complete spinal cord injury throws his head and upper extremities to roll using momentum. The strategies that a person with an incomplete spinal cord injury can use to roll will depend largely upon the voluntary motor function that is preserved at and below his neurological level of injury.

Minimal motor sparing. When very limited voluntary motor function is present in the trunk and hip musculature, the patient can use head and arm motions to roll using momentum, and can add trunk and hip motions to assist in the maneuver. Preserved function in the abdominal musculature may be used to rotate the trunk partially in the direction of the roll to assist with the motion. Preserved hip musculature can be used to add momentum in the direction of the roll. For example, when rolling from supine to prone toward the right, the individual can flex his left hip as he rocks his body toward the right.

Even musculature that is very weak may be of some benefit. For example, a patient may have hip flexors that are not strong enough to work against gravity, but can flex the hip through partial range when he is sidelying. These hip flexors will not be of benefit at the beginning of the roll, when the person remains supine and gravity resists hip flexion. Toward the end of the roll as he approaches or reaches sidelying, however, he will be able to flex his hip and add the momentum of this motion to assist in the roll.

More extensive motor sparing. A person who retains or regains significant innervation of his trunk and hip musculature may be able to roll using normal patterns of motion. Typical rolling in neurologically intact adults involves segmental motions, with either the upper body (head, upper extremities, and upper trunk) or the lower body (lower extremities and lower trunk) leading.[8] There is, however, a good deal of variability in rolling patterns used by normal adults.[9] A patient who has adequate strength to flex his hips, rotate his trunk, and reach his arms across his body while lying supine may be able to roll from supine to prone with normal or near normal movement patterns. Likewise, an individual who can extend his hips and rotate his trunk from a prone position may be able to learn to roll toward supine with normal or near normal movement patterns.

Therapeutic strategies. The patient should practice rolling, using either momentum or a more normal movement strategy, depending on the therapist's assessment of his potential. Emphasis should be placed on efficient timing and coordination of motions of the head, trunk, and extremities. If needed, the therapist can use demonstration, verbal cueing, tactile cueing, quick stretch, or any combination of these strategies to help the patient learn to perform the motions involved. These inputs should be withdrawn as the patient's rolling ability develops.

Regardless of the rolling strategy used, early practice can begin in sidelying, where the task will be easier. As the patient's skill develops, he can practice rolling from progressively supine positions.

In addition to functional training, the therapeutic program should include strengthening of the muscles involved in rolling. The strengthening program should emphasize shoulder flexion and extension, scapular protraction and retraction, hip flexion and extension, and trunk rotation. The shoulder girdle and hip strengthening exercises that are appropriate will depend on the strength of the musculature. Exercises may be active, active-assisted, or resisted, and may be performed against gravity or with gravity eliminated. Trunk rotation can be strengthened in sidelying or hooklying.[x] In these positions, the patient can rotate his trunk with assistance, independently, or against resistance. As an additional exercise, he may be able to perform sit-ups with rotation. If he does not have adequate strength to perform sit-ups starting with his trunk horizontal, he may be able to do so starting with his trunk in a less challenging position. For example, his trunk can be elevated by placing wedges behind his back to support him in a semireclined position. If necessary, the patient can be supported with his trunk in a nearly vertical position. As his strength improves, he can perform sit-ups with his trunk starting in progressively horizontal positions.[y]

Coming to Sitting

People with intact nervous systems typically use musculature in the trunk and all extremities to come to sitting. The motions involved vary. One supine-to-sit strategy involves flexing the neck and trunk and pushing with the arms to rise straight from supine. The lower extremities are also involved in the task, with the lower extremities serving as an "anchor" as the hip flexors help pull the lower trunk toward sitting. An alternative supine-to-sit strategy involves rolling to the side and pushing to sitting using the arms and trunk musculature. Lower extremity musculature may be used to assist in the roll and to help lift the lower trunk to sitting.

Following a complete spinal cord injury, a variety of methods can be used to come to sitting from supine. The maneuvers involved are performed using motions of the head and upper extremities. The strategies that a person with an incomplete spinal cord injury can use to assume a sitting position will depend on the voluntary motor function that he has below his lesion.

Minimal motor sparing. An individual who retains or regains only minimal voluntary motor function below his lesion will come to sitting using strategies similar to those used by people with complete spinal cord injuries.[z] Spared musculature below the lesion may be used to assist in stabilizing or moving the trunk as the person performs the compensatory motions involved in coming to sitting.

More extensive motor sparing. When adequate voluntary motor function exists below the lesion, a person with an incomplete spinal cord injury may be able to come to sitting using a normal or near-normal movement pattern. The movement strategy that is most effective will depend on the individual's pattern of strength and weakness. If trunk and lower extremity muscles are strong but shoulder girdle musculature is weak, the patient may be able to come to sitting straight from supine by performing a sit-up. If the individual's upper extremity musculature is relatively strong, he may find it easier to roll to his side and then push into a sitting position. A person who has asymmetrical weakness may find it easiest to roll onto his weaker side and use his stronger arm to push to sitting.

Therapeutic strategies. Because there are so many possible strategies for coming to sitting, the therapist and patient should work together to determine which method will be most effective for the individual involved. Together they can analyze the patient's patterns of strength, weakness, abilities and limitations, and find a method of coming to sitting that best utilizes his capabilities.

Regardless of the method of coming to sitting chosen, the patient can develop his skill by practicing the motions involved. If his goal is to come to sitting using a multistep method similar to one used by people with complete injuries, he may benefit from practicing the various steps and then combining them as his skill develops. If the patient's goal is to come to sitting using a more normal movement strategy (sitting up straight from supine, or rolling to the side and pushing to sitting), he may benefit from practicing the task as a whole without prior practice of the skill's components.

One therapeutic strategy that may be particularly beneficial for developing the ability to come to sitting is practice of the skill in reverse. A patient who is unable to assume a sitting position may find it beneficial to start in sitting and practice lowering his trunk into a more horizontal position. He should lower his trunk backward or to the side, depending on the method of coming to sitting that he plans to achieve.[aa]

In addition to functional training, the therapeutic program should include strengthening of

---

[x] The hooklying position is supine with the hips and knees flexed and the feet planted on the mat.

[y] As an alternative to working on a mat, the patient may perform sit-ups with rotation on a tilt table. The section on therapeutic strategies for coming to sitting contains a more detailed description of sit-ups on a tilt table.

[z] These strategies are presented in the first half of this chapter.

[aa] Chapter 9 contains a more complete explanation of the functional training strategy of learning a skill in reverse.

PROBLEM-SOLVING EXERCISE 10-2

Your patient has incomplete tetraplegia. He is dependent in all functional activities. He would like to learn to roll from sidelying toward prone and supine, so that he can sleep more comfortably.

The patient's pin prick and light touch sensation are intact in the C4 and higher key sensory points, and impaired in C5 and below. His muscle test results are as follows.

Muscles	Left	Right
Trapezius (upper, middle, and lower)	4/5	4/5
Deltoids (anterior, middle, and posterior)	2/5	2/5
Elbow flexors	2/5	2/5
Radial wrist extensors	0/5	0/5
Serratus anterior	1/5	1/5
Pectoralis major (clavicular and sternocostal)	1/5	1/5
Triceps	0/5	0/5
Flexor digitorum profundus	0/5	0/5
Abductor digiti minimi	1/5	1/5
Rectus abdominis (palpable from ribs to pubis)	2/5	2/5
External and internal obliques	2/5	2/5
Hip flexors	2/5	2/5
Hip adductors	2/5	2/5
Quadriceps	2/5	3/5
Tibialis anterior	3/5	4/5
Hip abductors	3/5	4/5
Extensor hallucis longus	4/5	4/5
Hamstrings	4/5	4/5
Plantar flexors	4/5	4/5
Gluteus maximus	4/5	4/5

The patient's joint range of motion and muscle flexibility are normal throughout his upper and lower extremities bilaterally. He exhibits elevated muscle tone in all extremities and his trunk: rapid motion (active or passive) of his extremities results in strong involuntary extension of the trunk and all extremities.

- What is this patient's neurological level of injury? What is the lesion's classification, using the ASIA Impairment Scale?
- What movement strategy could this patient use in an attempt to roll from sidelying toward prone?
- What movement strategy could this patient use in an attempt to roll from sidelying toward supine?
- What strength and range should the therapeutic exercise program emphasize to facilitate the attainment of this goal?
- Describe a functional training program for this patient.

the muscles involved in coming to sitting. The movement strategies used and the patient's pattern of strength and weakness will dictate what muscles should be prioritized in the strengthening program. If he plans to use his upper extremities to help push his trunk to upright, he may benefit from closed-chain exercises in which he bears weight on his palms and uses his arms to lower and raise his trunk from upright. Trunk strengthening exercises are also likely to be beneficial, and can emphasize either flexion or lateral flexion, depending on the method that the patient plans to use to come to sitting. To improve his ability to laterally flex his trunk, the patient can practice lowering his trunk laterally from a sitting position, and returning to sitting. He can start with small arcs of motion at first, and increase the excursion of his motions as his strength improves. The trunk flexors can be strengthened through sit-ups on a mat. The patient can start either with his trunk horizontal or supported in a semireclined position, depending on his ability to flex against gravity.[bb] Alternatively, if there are no medical or orthopedic problems preventing upright positioning or weight bearing through his lower extremities, he can perform sit-ups on a tilt table. The patient's legs and pelvis should be secured to the tilt table with straps, and his trunk left free to move. The table should then be tilted enough to enable him to perform sit-ups. As his strength improves, he can work with the tilt table in progressively horizontal positions.

Gross Mobility in Sitting

Gross mobility in sitting (moving the buttocks forward, back, or to the side while in a sitting position) is a skill that is used to position the buttocks on the bed before or after a transfer. This skill can also be used for limited mobility on the floor or ground without a wheelchair. Following a complete spinal cord injury, gross mobility in sitting involves pivoting on the arms and using scapular and head motions to move the buttocks. A patient who has an incomplete cord injury with minimal motor sparing will use essentially the same maneuvers, adding spared trunk or lower extremity musculature to assist in the task.

A person who has an intact nervous system has numerous possible movement strategies for moving his buttocks while in a seated position. Using his trunk and leg musculature, he can move his buttocks with or without using his arms to assist. Moreover, he can move in the bed in a variety of other positions, such as scooting in hooklying or even in sidelying. A person who has an incomplete spinal cord injury with significant motor sparing may move on a mat or bed using normal or near-normal patterns of motion.

To develop the skill of gross mobility in sitting, the therapist and patient should work together to discover the movement strategies that will be most effective for this individual. Therapeutic strategies include practice of the skill and its component skills, and exercises to develop the strength and range needed to perform these actions.

Leg Management

People with intact nervous systems move their legs actively during functional activities, and they frequently combine leg repositioning with other elements of functional tasks. For example, when rising from a bed, people with intact nervous systems typically assume a short-sitting position at the side of the bed without first assuming a long-sitting position. Leg repositioning is performed in concert with trunk motions while rising from supine or sidelying to a sitting position at the side of the bed.[5, 12]

In contrast, leg management following complete spinal cord injury involves positioning the legs passively using the upper extremities. This repositioning is performed as a separate step rather than as an action performed simultaneously with other motions.

The movement strategies used by a person with an incomplete spinal cord injury will depend on his muscle function below his lesion. He may reposition his legs using his arms only, his legs only, or a combination of leg and arm motions. Similarly, he may move his legs while performing other components of the functional task, or he may move them as an isolated step in the process.

To develop the skill of moving the legs during functional activities, the therapist and patient should work together to discover the movement strategies that will be most effective for this individual. Therapeutic strategies include practice of the skill and its component skills, and exercises to develop the strength and range needed to perform these actions. Patients who have significant motor return below their lesions may benefit from practicing positioning their legs in concert with other actions involved in the functional task.

SUMMARY

- Mat skills are functional activities that are typically performed on a mat or bed. These skills are required for independent transfers and dressing.

[bb] Strategies for adapting sit-ups on a mat when the abdominal musculature is weak are presented above, in the section on therapeutic strategies for developing rolling following incomplete injury.

- A person with a complete spinal cord injury who wishes to function independently must learn compensatory strategies for performing mat skills. This chapter presents a variety of techniques that can be used to roll, come to sitting, move the buttocks on a bed, and move the legs during mat activities.

- The movement strategies possible for a person with an incomplete spinal cord injury will depend on the extent of motor sparing or return below his lesion. If he has little or no voluntary motor function below his lesion, he will use movement strategies similar to those used by people with complete injuries. If he has more significant motor function in his trunk and lower extremities, he may be able to use more normal movement strategies to perform mat skills.

- During rehabilitation, the therapist and patient work together to discover the movement strategies that will enable the patient to perform mat skills most effectively. The therapeutic program then consists of activities directed at developing the strength, range of motion, and skill needed to perform these functional tasks. This chapter presents a variety of strategies for developing the skills involved.

- The therapist and patient should take appropriate precautions during functional mat training to prevent motion of unstable vertebrae, skin abrasions and pressure ulcers, and overstretching of the long finger flexors and the low back

11

Transfer Skills

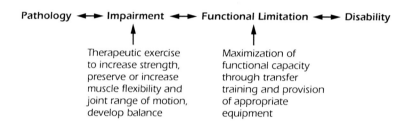

Pathology ◄──► Impairment ◄──► Functional Limitation ◄──► Disability

Therapeutic exercise
to increase strength,
preserve or increase
muscle flexibility and
joint range of motion,
develop balance

Maximization of
functional capacity
through transfer
training and provision
of appropriate
equipment

Transfers are crucial for independent mobility; before a person can go anywhere in her wheelchair, she must first get out of bed. A person who can transfer independently can get out of bed in the morning without waiting for assistance and can leave her wheelchair to sit on a couch, get into a car, or get onto the ground for a picnic. Independent transfer skills also make it possible to get back into the wheelchair after a fall.

This chapter presents a variety of transfer techniques,[a] as well as suggestions on how to teach them. It is important for the reader to keep in mind that the exact motions used to perform any functional task vary among people. This variability is due to differences in body build, skill level, range of motion, muscle tone, and patterns of strength and weakness. Because of these differences, each individual differs slightly in hand placement, starting position, and the degree and force of head and trunk motion used to accomplish the task.

The descriptions of techniques and training presented in this chapter should be used as a guide, not as a set of hard and fast rules. During

functional training, the therapist and patient should work together to find the exact techniques that best suit that particular individual.

PRECAUTIONS

Following spinal cord injuries, the activities involved in transfer training can cause problems if appropriate precautions are not taken. Transfer activities can result in excessive motion in unstable segments of the spine, skin damage, overstretching of the low back and long finger flexors, and injuries from falls. Table 11–1 presents a summary of precautions for transfers and transfer training.

PHYSICAL AND SKILL PREREQUISITES

Each functional activity involves a particular set of skills. Each activity also has strength, joint range of motion, and muscle flexibility requirements. A deficiency in any of these skill or physical prerequisites will impair a person's performance of the activity.

The descriptions of functional techniques presented in this chapter are accompanied by tables that summarize the physical and skill pre-

---

[a] This chapter does not attempt to present all possible transfer techniques. An individual who is unable to master a transfer described in this chapter may fare better with a variation of that transfer or with an altogether different method.

TABLE 11–1. PRECAUTIONS DURING TRANSFERS AND TRANSFER TRAINING

Potential Problems	Transfer Activities That Place Patients at Risk	Precautions
Excessive motion at site of vertebral instability, potentially causing additional neurologic and orthopedic damage.	Any activity involving excessive motion or muscular action at or near site of unstable spine. Examples: upright activities while the spine remains unstable.	• Strictly adhere to orthopedic precautions. • Check fit of vertebral orthosis with patient in the different postures involved in transfer training. • When the spine is unstable, avoid activities that may cause motion or strong muscular contraction at site of instability.
Skin abrasions and pressure ulcers.	Any activities creating shearing forces on the skin. Example: sliding buttocks on transfer board or mat.	• When possible, instruct patient to lift buttocks instead of sliding. • Vary activities to avoid prolonged periods during which shearing forces are placed on skin. • Careful guarding during practice. • Proper clothing during transfer training (pants rather than hospital gowns)
	Any activities in which the patient's buttocks may forcefully contact the wheelchair. Example: transfers between wheelchair and mat (risk of blunt trauma from contact with wheel).	• Emphasize the development of control during transfers, with avoidance of contact between the buttocks and wheelchair components that can cause injury.
Impaired tenodesis grasp due to overstretching of the long finger flexors.	Any activities involving simultaneous wrist and finger extension. Example: weight-bearing on palms with fingers extended while practicing short-sitting propped forward on two arms.	• With patients who may utilize tenodesis grasp (people with C7 or higher tetraplegia), avoid simultaneous wrist and finger extension. • When weight-bearing on palms, maintain interphalangeal joints in flexion.
Overstretched low back, resulting in diminished capacity for functional independence.	Any activities involving simultaneous hip flexion with knee extension in patients with hamstring tightness, placing stress on the low back. Examples: practice lifting legs onto mat, or side-approach floor-to-wheelchair transfers when the hamstrings are tight.	• Avoid long-sitting in patients who lack a minimum of 90 degrees of passive straight-leg raise. • When hamstrings are tight, avoid prolonged practice of activities that involve simultaneous hip flexion and knee extension.
Injury from fall from wheelchair.	Any transfers to or from wheelchair involve some risk of falling.	• Education and training in safe transfer techniques. • Appropriate guarding during functional training.

requisites. Exact values for the physical prerequisites are not given because the requirements vary among individuals. For example, a person who is thin, coordinated, and has relatively long arms will probably require less anterior deltoid strength to perform a particular transfer than someone who is overweight, uncoordinated, and has short arms.

PROGRAM DESIGN

The therapeutic program is designed to enable the patient to achieve all of her functional goals. The steps of program planning follow.

1. Identify the functional goals.[b]
2. Determine the methods that the patient will utilize to perform the activities identified in the goals. This determination will involve choosing the methods that provide the best match between the patient's characteristics and the physical and skill requirements of the activities.
3. Consider the patient's impairments and functional limitations as they compare to the physical and skill requirements of the activities to be achieved.
4. Devise a therapeutic program to develop the needed strength, range of motion, and skills.

---

[b] Goal-setting is addressed in Chapter 8.

For the purposes of program planning, it may be best for the therapist and patient first to consider each goal separately and devise a plan for achieving each goal. The different goals and their plans can then be considered together. Fortunately, there is much overlap of physical and skill prerequisites for the different functional activities. Thus a person working on propping forward on two extended arms is potentially progressing toward independence in a variety of transfers. Furthermore, work aimed at developing one ability can benefit other, seemingly unrelated, activities. For example, the strengthening and motor learning that results from practicing transfers may benefit an individual's mat or ambulation skills.

TRANSFER TECHNIQUES FOLLOWING COMPLETE SPINAL CORD INJURY

After a spinal cord injury, an individual's potential for achieving independence in transfers is determined largely by her voluntary motor function. Table 11–2 presents a summary of the level of independence in transfers that can be achieved by people who have complete spinal cord injuries at different motor levels (motor component of neurological level of injury). When prognosticating about an individual's capacity to develop transfer skills, the clinician should take into con-

USING CHAPTER 11 AS A RESOURCE FOR PROGRAM PLANNING

When using this chapter as a resource to assist in designing a program to work toward a functional goal, the therapist should first read the description of that functional activity. These descriptions are located under the headings "Transfer Techniques Following Complete Spinal Cord Injury" in the first half of the chapter, and "Transfer Techniques and Therapeutic Strategies Following Incomplete Spinal Cord Injury" at the end of the chapter. Based on the description of the functional activity, the corresponding tables, or both, the therapist can determmine what physical and skill prerequisites are required to perform the activity. Taking into consideration the patient's evaluation results, the therapist can determine where the patient has deficits relevant to the needed physical and skill prerequisites.

This chapter presents functional training strategies for each prerequisite skill listed in the tables that accompany the descriptions of transfer techniques. These functional training strategies are presented under the headings, "Therapeutic Strategies Following Complete Spinal Cord Injury" and "Transfer Techniques and Therapeutic Strategies Following Incomplete Spinal Cord Injury." The therapist can use these suggestions, coupled with his or her own imagination, clinical expertise, and problem solving, to design a functional training program. The program should aim first at developing the most basic prerequisite skills and build to more advanced skills as the patient's abilities develop.

TABLE 11–2. FUNCTIONAL POTENTIALS

Motor Level	Significance of Innervated Musculature	Potential for Independence in Transfers
C4 and higher	Inadequate voluntary motor function to contribute to transfers.	Dependent in all transfers.
C5	**Partial innervation of the deltoids** makes it possible to extend the elbows using muscle substitution. Deltoid function plus **partial innervation of the infraspinatus and teres minor** make it possible to "lock" the elbows in extension. **Partial innervation of the biceps brachii, brachialis, and brachioradialis** makes it possible to use elbow flexion to pull. Minimal serratus anterior function is inadequate to stabilize the scapulae against the thorax.	**Typical Functional Outcomes** Dependent in all transfers. **Exceptional Outcomes** Even: independent; those who transfer independently are likely to require transfer boards, and some use boards plus overhead loops
C6	**Fully innervated deltoids, infraspinatus, teres minor, and clavicular portion of the pectoralis major** allow for stronger elbow extension and "locking" using muscle substitution. **Full innervation of the biceps brachii** allows for stronger pull using elbow flexion. **Partial innervation of the serratus anterior** makes it possible to stabilize the scapulae against the thorax. Scapular protraction allows greater lift of the buttocks. **Partial innervation of the latissimus dorsi** enhances shoulder girdle depression, allowing greater lift of the buttocks. Minimal innervation of the triceps brachii is inadequate to contribute significantly to transfers.	**Typical Functional Outcomes** Even: some assist to independent in even transfers with or without transfer board Uneven: some to total assist **Exceptional Outcomes** Even: independent without equipment. Uneven: independent in transfers between the wheelchair and surfaces a few inches above or below the level of the sitting surface; may require transfer board
C7	**Partial innervation of the triceps brachii** allows for stronger elbow extension. **Full innervation of the serratus anterior** provides more stable scapulae, stronger protraction and upward rotation. **Partial innervation of the latissimus dorsi and sternocostal portion of pectoralis major** enhance shoulder girdle depression, allowing greater lift of the buttocks.	**Typical Functional Outcomes** Even: independent in even transfers without equipment Uneven: independent to some assist in transfers between the wheelchair and surfaces a few inches above or below the level of the sitting surface **Exceptional Outcomes** Uneven: independent in uneven transfers, including transfers between the wheelchair and the floor, using a side-approach transfer

(Cont.)

TABLE 11–2. *(Continued)*

Motor Level	Significance of Innervated Musculature	Potential for Independence in Transfers
C8	**Full innervation of the triceps brachii** provides normal strength in elbow extension. **Full innervation of the latissimus dorsi and nearly full innervation of pectoralis major** allow strong shoulder girdle depression. **Nearly full innervation of flexor digitorum superficialis and profundus, and partial innervation of flexor pollicus longus and brevis** provide grasp without muscle substitution, making leg management easier.	**Typical Functional Outcomes** **Even:** independent in even transfers without equipment **Uneven:** independent in transfers between the wheelchair and surfaces a few inches above or below the level of the sitting surface **Exceptional Outcomes** **Uneven:** independent in uneven transfers, including transfers between the wheelchair and the floor, using a side-approach transfer
T1-9	**Fully innervated upper extremities** make all transfers more easy to achieve. Trunk musculature inadequate to assist in transfers.	**Typical Functional Outcomes** **Even:** independent in even transfers without equipment **Uneven:** most achieve independence in transfers between the wheelchair and surfaces a few inches above or below the level of the sitting surface; many achieve independence in transfers between the wheelchair and the floor; a side, front, or back approach may be used to transfer from the floor to the wheelchair
T10 and below	**Partial to full innervation of trunk musculature (T6-L1)** enhances transfer ability.	**Typical Functional Outcomes** **Even:** independent in even transfers without equipment **Uneven:** independent in all uneven transfers, including between the wheelchair and the floor; a side, front, or back approach may be used to transfer from the floor to the wheelchair

References for innervation: 6, 9, 11, 12, 16. For more complete innervation information, see Appendix B (www.prenhall.com/somers).

sideration the many other factors that also impact on functional gains.[c]

Regardless of the level of injury, a person who sustains a complete spinal cord injury has a limited number of muscles with which to move her body. To transfer from one surface to another, she must utilize the muscles innervated above her lesion to move her entire body. During rehabilitation, she learns how to transfer between her wheelchair and various surfaces by using a variety of compensatory strategies, including muscle substitution, momentum, and the head-hips relationship.[d]

Accessory Skills

When most of us think of transfers, we consider only the leap from one surface to another. In fact, a great deal more is involved. To move from a wheelchair to a bed, for example, an individual must be able to position the wheelchair, lock the

---

[c] Chapter 8 presents factors that can influence functional outcomes.

[d] These movement strategies are explained in Chapter 9.

wheel locks, reposition or remove an armrest (if armrests are used), and position the footrests. She must also position her legs, buttocks, and torso in preparation for the transfer and pull her legs onto the bed following the transfer. If a transfer board is used, it must be placed before the transfer and removed afterwards. These accessory skills are an integral part of every transfer. Each technique is used in a variety of transfers. To avoid repetition, the accessory skills will be described separately here.

The physical and skill prerequisites required to perform these accessory skills are summarized in Tables 11–3 and 11–4.

Stabilizing the trunk in a wheelchair. While sitting in a wheelchair, someone who lacks functional trunk musculature must use her arms for stability when her trunk is in any position other than resting forward on the legs or resting back on the backrest. She must also stabilize her trunk in any situation in which her trunk is likely to be pulled off balance. An example of such a situation is when she lifts one arm to the side. Even such a minor act can shift a person's center of gravity enough to cause her trunk to fall to the side.

TABLE 11–3. ACCESSORY SKILLS—PHYSICAL PREREQUISITES

	Stabilize trunk in wheelchair	Move trunk in wheelchair	Move buttocks on seat	Position wheelchair	Lock brakes	Position armrests	Manage legs	Position footrests	Manage sliding board
Strength									
Anterior deltoids	√	√	√	√	√	√	√	√	√
Middle deltoids	√	√	√	√		√	√	√	√
Posterior deltoids	√	√	√	√		√	√	√	√
Biceps, brachialis, and/or brachioradialis	√	√	√	√	√	√	√	√	√
Range of motion									
Shoulder Extension	√	√	√			√			
Abduction	√	√	√			√			√
Flexion			√		√		√	√	
Elbow Extension	√	√	√	√	√			√	√
Flexion	√	√	√			√	√		

√: Some strength is needed for this activity, or severe limitations in range will inhibit this activity.

TABLE 11–4.   ACCESSORY SKILLS—SKILL PREREQUISITES

	Stabilize trunk in wheelchair	Move trunk in wheelchair	Move buttocks on seat	Position wheelchair	Lock brakes	Position armrests	Manage legs	Position footrests	Manage sliding board
Tolerate upright sitting position (p. 318)			√		√	√	√	√	√
Place arm behind push handle (p. 257)	√	√	√		√	√			
Hold push handle to stabilize trunk (p. 257)	√	√	√		√	√			
Move trunk in wheelchair by pulling with arms (p. 257)		√	√		√	√	√	√	√
Move trunk in wheelchair using momentum (p. 258)		√	√		√		√	√	
Move trunk in wheelchair by pushing with arms (p. 256)		√	√		√		√	√	
Manipulate armrests (p. 258)						√			
Slide buttocks on wheelchair seat (p. 259)			√						
Extend elbows using muscle substitution[a] (p. 255)	√	√	√		√				
Prop forward on extended arms (p. 259)	√								
Lift buttocks by pushing on armrests (p. 260)			√						
Lift on armrests and move buttocks (p. 261)			√						
Propel wheelchair[b]				√					

[a] In the absence of functioning triceps.

[b] Skill addressed in Chapter 12.

To stabilize her trunk in an upright position, a person with a spinal cord injury can simply hook one arm behind a push handle. Alternatively, someone who can extend her elbow using her triceps or muscle substitution can push on her thigh or on an armrest to hold herself upright.

Stabilizing the trunk while leaning forward involves similar strategies: the individual can either lean on her arm(s) or hook one arm behind a push handle. When using the latter strategy, the arm's position is determined by the angle of the trunk's forward lean. Figure 11–1 shows different arm positions that can be used.

Trunk stabilization when leaning to the side can be accomplished by hooking an arm behind a push handle. Alternatively, the individual can hold the armrest away from which she is leaning, using her hand, wrist, or forearm.

Moving the trunk in a wheelchair. In the absence of functioning trunk musculature, a person with a spinal cord injury uses her arms and head to move her trunk. She can push or pull on the wheelchair or use momentum from arm and head motions to move her trunk.

One way to lean the trunk forward while sitting in a wheelchair is to pull on an anterior part of the chair such as the front of the armrest or seat. The person who leans forward in this manner can return to upright by pushing on her thighs, the front of the chair, or the armrests. This push to upright can be accomplished using either the triceps or muscle substitution to extend the elbows.

Momentum can also be used to lean the trunk forward. If the individual throws her head and an arm forward forcefully enough, her body will fall forward. One arm should remain hooked

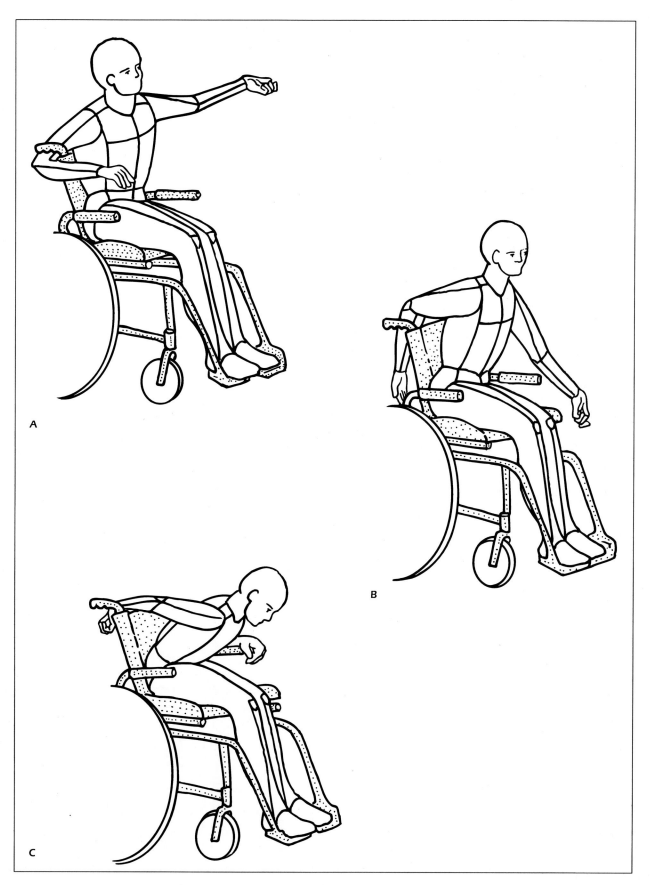

Figure 11–1.   Arm positions for stabilizing the trunk in a wheelchair. **(A)** Sitting upright. **(B)** Slight forward lean. **(C)** Pronounced forward lean.

behind the wheelchair's backrest or push handle to provide stability once the trunk has moved forward. This arm should remain relaxed until the trunk has leaned far enough forward; holding too tight will prevent the trunk's forward motion. The arm that remains hooked behind the chair can be used to pull the trunk back into an upright position. The other arm can assist by pushing on a thigh, the front of the chair, or an armrest.

The trunk can also be brought forward by pushing on the wheelchair's tires, behind the seat. The person using this technique should hook one arm behind a push handle for stability and to return to upright.

Any of the methods just described can be combined to bring the trunk forward. For example, an individual may push on a tire with one hand while throwing her head and the other arm forward.

To lean to the side, a person lacking trunk musculature can either pull sideways on an armrest or throw her head and an arm to the side and allow their momentum to move her trunk. To return to upright, she can pull on the opposite armrest or push handle.

Moving the buttocks in a wheelchair. A person with a complete spinal cord injury uses the head-hips relationship to move her buttocks in the wheelchair: to move her buttocks in one direction, she moves her head and upper torso in the opposite direction. Someone who has intact upper extremity musculature can move on a wheelchair's seat with relative ease. She can simply lift her buttocks by pushing on the armrests or wheelchair seat and throw her head in the direction opposite to where she wants to move.

In the absence of functioning triceps, the exact methods used to move the buttocks on a wheelchair are as varied as the people performing them. What works for one person may not work for the next. The descriptions that follow are some examples.

To move her buttocks forward on the seat, a person with a complete spinal cord injury can throw her head back repeatedly and forcefully. She may be able to improve her performance by pushing on the wheelchair's backrest with her elbows while throwing her head.

Another technique that a person can use to move her buttocks out on the wheelchair seat is to lean her head and upper torso back and shimmy, twisting her trunk right and left repeatedly. This shimmying motion is accomplished by throwing the head and arms right and left.

A third method for moving the buttocks out on the wheelchair seat involves larger twisting motions. Using this approach, a person moves her buttocks out and to one side by twisting her head and upper torso in the opposite direction. To twist out and to the left, she hooks her right shoulder behind the wheelchair's right push handle and hooks her left hand on the right armrest. Pulling with her arms, she twists her head and upper trunk to the right and back (Figure 11–2). This motion will cause the buttocks to slide to the left and forward. The distance that the buttocks will move depends on the magnitude of the head and upper trunk motion. Someone who is unable to move far enough by twisting to one side can repeat the twist in the opposite direction.

To move her buttocks straight to the side for a short distance, a person with a spinal cord injury can lean in the opposite direction. For example, someone who desires to move to the right can hook her right arm around the chair's right push handle and lean to the left.

To move her buttocks laterally over larger distances, an individual can lean her torso forward and to the side, pushing her buttocks back and to the other side. If she is already sitting with her buttocks well back on the seat, the buttocks will move laterally only. (The backrest prevents any further motion toward the back.) To move her buttocks back and to the left, the person stabilizes her trunk by holding the right push handle with her right forearm or wrist and twists forward and

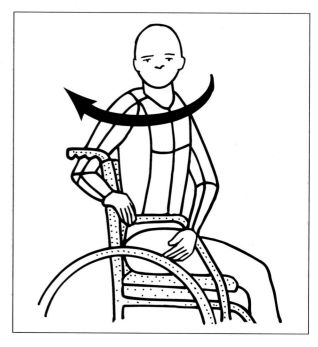

Figure 11–2. *Moving the buttocks out in the wheelchair seat. The person twists his head and upper torso to the right and back to move his buttocks forward and to the left.*

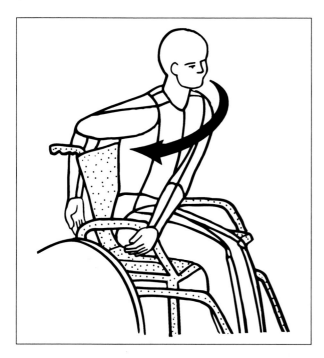

Figure 11–3. *Moving the buttocks back and to the left by leaning forward and twisting the head and upper torso to the right.*

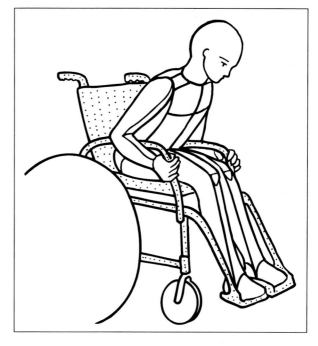

Figure 11–4. *Moving the buttocks back in the seat.*

to the right by pulling on the right armrest with her left forearm (Figure 11–3).

This method of twisting forward and to the side can also be used to move the buttocks back on the seat. The person should twist first to one side and then to the other while leaning forward. Doing so will ensure that her buttocks are centered instead of being lodged to one side when she has completed the backward motion.

Another method for moving back on the seat involves leaning forward and shimmying. The person leans her body well forward and stabilizes her hands against the front of the armrests, as shown in Figure 11–4. She then shimmies her head and shoulders right and left while pushing her hands forward. The result is a backward motion of the buttocks.

Positioning the wheelchair. During a transfer from a wheelchair to a surface such as a mat, bed, or couch, the wheelchair should be positioned as close to the other surface as possible. The chair should be parked at about a 30-degree angle to the object, with the rear wheel and caster as close as they can get to the other surface. Positioning the wheelchair in this manner will minimize the gap between the surfaces, making the transfer easier and safer.

Someone who has difficulty angling her wheelchair as described above should start by positioning the chair parallel to the object, close

enough for the rear wheel to touch it. She should then lock the brake closest to the object and push forward on the other wheel to angle the chair.

When a person plans to transfer from the floor to her wheelchair after a fall, she may first have to move the chair into an upright position. To do so she should lock the brakes and then pull down on the front of the chair to place the chair upright (Figure 11–5).

Engaging the wheel locks. To engage a wheelchair's wheel locks (lock the brakes) while sitting in the chair, the person either pushes or pulls on the lock's lever, depending upon its construction. To reach the wheel lock, she may have to lean forward and to the side.

Positioning the armrests. Armrest styles vary. Some can be rotated out of the way, either up and back or to the side and back. With these armrest styles, a person can prepare for a transfer by pulling up on the armrest and pushing it out of the way. Other armrests must be removed prior to a transfer. Removing the latter type of armrest involves unlocking it (if locked) and lifting it out of its channels. The lift should be straight upward. Any lateral, forward, or backward pull can jam the armrest in its channels.

It can be tempting to place (or even throw) an armrest on the floor or bed after removing it

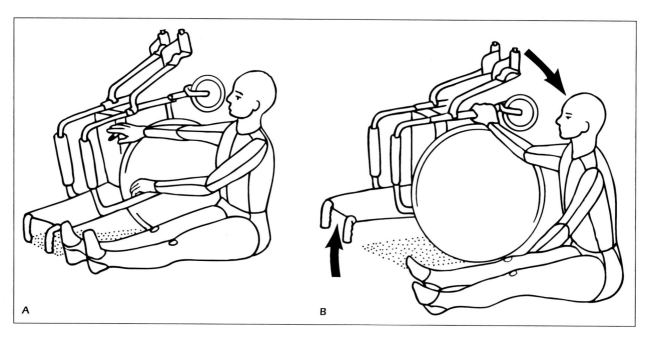

Figure 11–5. *Righting the wheelchair prior to transfer.* **(A)** *Locking the brakes.* **(B)** *Righting the wheelchair by pulling down on the front of the chair.*

from the wheelchair. The problems with this practice are twofold: the armrest may be damaged, and it is likely to be in the wrong place when needed. (It gets kicked under the bed, moved to the other side of the bed, etc.) To preserve her equipment and to save herself the trouble of hunting down misplaced armrests, it is a good idea for someone who uses a wheelchair to get into the habit of storing the armrest on the wheelchair, out of the way but still accessible. An armrest can be hung on one of the wheelchair's push handles, but it is likely to fall off from this position. The rear armrest channel will provide more stable storage. Figure 11–6 shows the position of the armrest for storage.

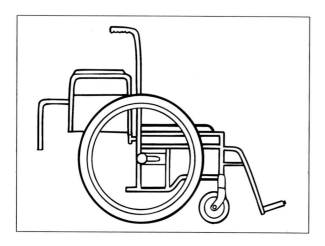

Figure 11–6. *Position of armrest for storage.*

Placing an armrest in this position can be more of a bother than putting it onto the floor or hanging it on a push handle. It will, however, be less bothersome than having the armrest repaired or locating it after it has fallen off of the chair.

Managing the legs.   Legs play an important role in transfers, even in the absence of any motor function. If they are positioned correctly, the legs will bear weight during a transfer. This makes the transfer easier by reducing the weight that the person must lift on her arms. The legs can also help to stabilize the trunk during the transfer, making it easier to pivot on the arms.

Lifting the feet on and off of the footrests.   A person who has intact upper extremity motor function is likely to find it easy to lift her feet on and off of her chair's footrests. To perform this task, she can move one leg at a time by grasping it with one hand and lifting. She can use her other arm to stabilize her trunk.

In the absence of functioning finger flexors, leg management is slightly more involved. To remove her foot from a footrest, a person leans forward while stabilizing her trunk with one arm.[e] She can use her free arm to lift either the ipsilateral or contralateral leg. If lifting the ipsilateral leg, she places her forearm under the thigh and

---

[e] Techniques for stabilizing the trunk are described above.

lifts. If lifting the contralateral leg, she reaches between her legs, places her forearm under the contralateral thigh, and lifts. Power can be added to the lift by stabilizing the proximal forearm on top of the other thigh, using this leg as a fulcrum.

Whether the ipsilateral or contralateral leg is lifted, the foot will slide back off of the footrest as the thigh lifts. If the shoe gets snagged on the heel loop of the footrest, the person can push the leg back with her hand.

Before performing an even transfer, a person with a spinal cord injury should place her feet flat on the floor with the legs vertical. This can be done by pushing or pulling on the legs to move the feet into position, or by lifting one thigh at a time and letting the unweighted foot swing into position.

To place her foot back on the footrest, the person can use the lifting techniques just described. As her foot gets high enough, she pushes it forward with her forearm and places the foot over the footrest.

Lifting the feet on and off of the mat. To be independent in transfers between a wheelchair and a mat (or bed), a person must be able to get her legs onto and off of the mat. When lifting her legs onto a mat following a transfer, the individual balances on one arm and lifts with the other arm. She starts by propping on one extended arm, leaning away from the wheelchair. She then places her free arm under the thigh of the leg furthest from the wheelchair (Figure 11–7A). Balancing on the extended arm, she pulls the thigh onto the mat (Figure 11–7B). She can add power to the lift by leaning away from the leg. Once her foot is well onto the mat, she straightens her knee by pushing her foot and leg with her hand (Figure 11–7C). She then repeats the process to lift the other leg. Getting the feet back onto the floor involves the same process, done in reverse.

Positioning the footrests. If the wheelchair's front rigging is movable, it should be repositioned during transfers so that it does not cause injury or interfere with the transfers. Repositioning the front rigging involves either folding the footplates or swinging the entire footrest mechanism out of the way.

Folding the footplates provides adequate clearance for many transfers. To fold a footplate, a wheelchair user first places her foot on the floor. If she is stabilizing her trunk by holding on to the back of the wheelchair, she needs to shift her hold more distally on the stabilizing arm so that she can lean forward further. She then can reach down with her free hand and fold the footplate by pulling it up. If she cannot grasp the footplate, she can move it by placing her hand or forearm under the plate and pulling upward on it.

During some transfers, such as those between a wheelchair and the floor, one or both footrests must be swung out of the way rather than merely folded. To reposition a footrest, the person leans forward and operates the footrest release, using the arm on the same side of the chair as the

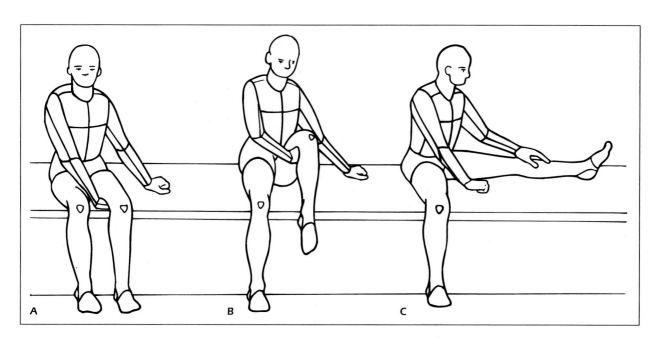

Figure 11–7. Leg management after a transfer. **(A)** Balancing on one arm, the person places his free arm under the thigh of the leg furthest from the wheelchair. **(B)** Pulling the leg onto the mat. **(C)** Straightening the leg on the mat.

footrest. The other arm is used to stabilize the trunk.

Placing and removing the transfer board. To place a transfer board, a person grasps the far end of the board and pulls the near end under her proximal thigh and buttocks. Moving the board back and forth laterally while pulling will help to work the board into position. The board should be angled with the far end higher than the near end, so that it will slide under the thigh instead of being pushed against it. Leaning away from the board will make placement easier.

An individual with impaired grasp can pull on the transfer board using either her forearm or the back of her hand. Nonstandard designs can make board placement and removal easier. For example, a short board or one that has a cut-out for the hand may be easier to manipulate. An "offset sliding board" (Figure 11–8) has a small projection that can be useful: with the projection placed against the anteromedial surface of the chair's wheel, the person can slide the board under her thigh using the wheel as a pivot point for the board. If a patient is unable to learn to place and remove a board with any of these features, a loop of webbing can be added to the board to make it easier to manipulate.

Someone with good hand function can remove a sliding board by grasping it and pulling it out. In the absence of good hand function, she can use her palm to push outward on the board, pushing either on the top surface or on the sides. Leaning away from the board and working it back and forth will make this task easier.

Even Transfers without Equipment

Even transfers, also called level transfers, involve moving between two surfaces of equal height. During even transfers a person with a complete spinal cord injury pivots on her arms, using the head-hips relationship to lift and swing her buttocks.

An even transfer to a mat or bed can be performed with the legs down (feet on the floor) or up (feet on the mat or bed). In the following descriptions, the legs are down. This is due to the author's preference rather than any particular advantage.

Whenever an even transfer is performed with the legs down, the feet should be positioned with the soles flat on the floor and the legs perpendicular to the floor. This positioning will maximize the weight accepted through the legs during the transfer. Tables 11–5 and 11–6 summarize the physical and skill prerequisites for even transfers.

In the absence of functioning triceps. In the absence of functioning triceps, a person must lock her elbows whenever she bears weight through her arms during transfers. This locking is done

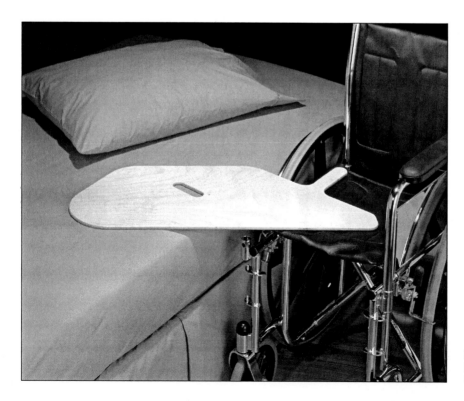

Figure 11–8. *Offset sliding board. (Reproduced with permission from Sammons Preston, Bolingbrook, IL.)*

TABLE 11–5. EVEN TRANSFERS—PHYSICAL PREREQUISITES

	No equipment	Sliding board, upright method	Sliding board, alternate method	Board and loops
Strength				
Anterior deltoids	☑	☑	☑	√
Middle deltoids	√	√		√
Posterior deltoids			☑	√
Biceps, brachialis, and/or brachioradialis			☑	√
Infraspinatus and teres minor	√	√	√	√
Serratus anterior	•	•	•	•
Pectoralis major	•	•	•	•
Latissimus dorsi	•	•		
Triceps brachii	•	•	•	•
Range of motion				
Shoulder Extension				☑
Abduction			√	☑
Flexion	√	√	√	
External rotation	☑	☑		
Internal rotation				☑
Elbow Extension	☑	☑		
Flexion		√		√
Forearm supination	☑	☑		√
Wrist extension	☑	☑		√

√: Some strength is needed for this activity, or severe limitations in range will inhibit this activity.

☑: A large amount of strength or normal or greater range is needed for this activity.

•: Not required, but helpful.

TABLE 11–6. EVEN TRANSFERS—SKILL PREREQUISITES

	No equipment	Sliding board, upright method	Sliding board, alternate method	Board and loops
Tolerate upright sitting position[a]	√	√	√	√
Accessory skills	√	√	√	√
Extend elbows using muscle substitution[b] (p. 255)	√	√		
Lock elbows[b] (p. 256)	√	√		
Prop forward on extended arms[c] (p. 259)	√	√		
Prop forward on one extended arm[c] (p. 259)	√	√		
Unweight buttocks by leaning forward on extended arms[c] (p. 259)	√	√		
Control pelvis using head and shoulders (p. 260)	√	√	√	√
Move buttocks laterally while propping on extended arms[c] (p. 260)		√		
Lift buttocks by pivoting on extended arms[c] (p. 261)	√			
Lift buttocks and move laterally (p. 262)	√			

[a] Skill addressed in Chapter 12.

[b] In the absence of functioning triceps.

[c] Arm(s) with elbow(s) positioned in extension.

through a combination of positioning and muscular contraction. The following is a description of a technique for transferring from a wheelchair to a mat. The same technique is used to transfer to a bed and is performed in reverse to return to the wheelchair.

After moving her buttocks forward in the wheelchair, the person sits upright and positions her hands in preparation for the transfer. Her hands should be anterior to her hips, far enough forward to enable her to lean on them during the transfer. They should not be so far anterior that she cannot pivot on them when leaning forward.

The hand on the wheelchair should be placed next to the person's thigh. The hand on the mat should be positioned far enough away to leave adequate space on the mat for the buttocks at the end of the transfer. This hand should be more anterior than the hand on the wheelchair, to enhance forward stability during the transfer.

The arms should be positioned with the shoulders externally rotated fully, the elbows and wrists extended, and the forearms supinated. This position makes it possible to lock the elbows in extension. The interphalangeal (IP) joints should be flexed to preserve the tenodesis grasp. Figure 11–9A shows the starting position of the transfer. The person maintains her elbows in extension during the transfer through strong contraction of her anterior deltoids, shoulder external rotators,

and clavicular portion of her pectoralis major (if innervated).

To transfer, the person leans forward on her arms, tucks her chin, and rolls her head downward. By pivoting on her arms in this manner, she lifts her buttocks from the wheelchair seat. If any serratus anterior or latissimus dorsi function is present, she should protract and depress her scapulae to increase the height of the lift.

When pivoting on her arms, the person needs to lean forward enough to get adequate clearance of her buttocks. At the same time, she must not pivot so far forward that she moves past her balance point. Doing so will result in a forward fall.

While she pivots on her arms, the person swings her buttocks toward the mat: keeping her head down, she forcefully swings her head and twists her shoulders away from the mat (Figure 11–9B). This twisting motion causes the buttocks to swing toward the mat. It is important for the head to remain down during the transfer to maintain the lift.

The sideways motion of the buttocks during the transfer is *not* accomplished by pushing laterally with the arms; it is achieved by swinging the head and twisting the shoulders. Pushing laterally on the wheelchair will cause the chair to slide. If this problem is to be avoided, the arms must push straight downward throughout the transfer.

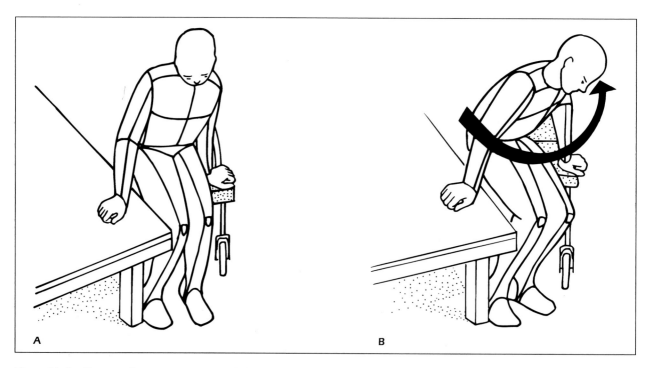

Figure 11–9. *Even transfer without equipment.* **(A)** *Starting position.* **(B)** *Head thrown down and away from the bed to lift the buttocks up and toward the bed.*

In the presence of functioning triceps. Innervated triceps make it easier to support the body's weight on the arms during transfers. If the triceps are strong enough to maintain elbow extension while the individual pivots on her arms, she does not need to lock her elbows with positioning and muscle substitution. The transfer technique just described is used, with the exception that the shoulders may be internally rotated and the elbows do not have to remain fully extended during the transfer.[14]

Even Transfers with Equipment

Weakness, contractures, obesity, spasticity, confusion, or low motivation can keep an individual from achieving independence in even transfers without equipment. In these instances, many people can learn to transfer using a transfer board or using a transfer board and loops.

Even transfers with a transfer board. During a transfer, a board can be used to bridge the gap between the wheelchair and the other surface, making it possible to transfer without lifting the buttocks.

Like any piece of equipment, a transfer board has disadvantages. Although a board may appear to make a transfer easier, it adds an extra step to the process. Worse, it *must be there* for the transfer. Someone who depends upon a transfer board will be out of luck if it is ever misplaced or left behind.

This is not to say that transfer boards are inherently bad or should never be used. Many people who are unable to transfer without equipment can gain independence using a board. If this equipment makes independent transfers possible for someone who would otherwise be dependent, it is certainly indicated. But if an individual has the potential to transfer without equipment, the extra time and effort required for training will be well worth it.

Upright method. This method is similar to an even transfer without equipment. The person first moves her buttocks forward in the chair and positions the transfer board. During the transfer, her hands should be anterior to her hips, far enough forward to enable her to lean on them. The hand on the wheelchair should be placed next to the thigh, and the hand toward which the individual is transferring should be placed on the board. If the transfer is to be done in one motion, the hand on the board should be far enough away to make room for the buttocks to slide across the board. If

the transfer will be performed in several steps, this hand can be placed relatively close to the thigh and repositioned when necessary.

In the absence of functioning triceps, a person uses her anterior deltoids to lock her elbows using the technique described above: her upper extremities are positioned with the shoulders externally rotated, the elbows and wrists extended, and the forearms supinated. If the triceps are functioning with adequate strength to maintain the elbows in extension during the transfer, this positioning is not necessary.

Although the buttocks do not have to be lifted when using a transfer board, the person does need to shift some of her weight off of them to make it possible to slide. To unweight her buttocks, a person with a complete spinal cord injury leans forward onto her arms. While doing so, she twists her head and shoulders away from the mat. This twisting motion causes the buttocks to slide toward the mat. If the individual has sufficient strength and skill, the transfer can be executed in one twist.

An individual who lacks adequate strength or skill to transfer in one motion may have to twist repeatedly during a transfer with a board. The twist of the head and upper torso away from the mat should be forceful, causing the buttocks to slide toward the mat. When moving back into position to prepare for another twist, the motion should not be forceful. A forceful motion toward the mat will cause the buttocks to slide back toward the chair.

Alternative method. Biceps spasticity, poor balance, or contractures can make it impossible to prop and twist on the arms with the elbows in extension. Some people with these limitations who are unable to perform an upright transfer with a board are able to use an alternate method, although finding a method that works for a given individual can be difficult. The therapist and patient will need to be creative in coming up with a solution to the problem.

The following is a description of one alternative method for transferring from a wheelchair to a bed. For clarity, the transfer will be described with the person moving toward the right.

After positioning the transfer board, the person turns away from the bed. To do so, she first hooks her left arm behind the wheelchair's left push handle and hooks her right forearm around the wheelchair's armrest. This position is shown in Figure 11–10A. Some people are more successful performing this maneuver with the left hand stabilized against the chair's left wheel.

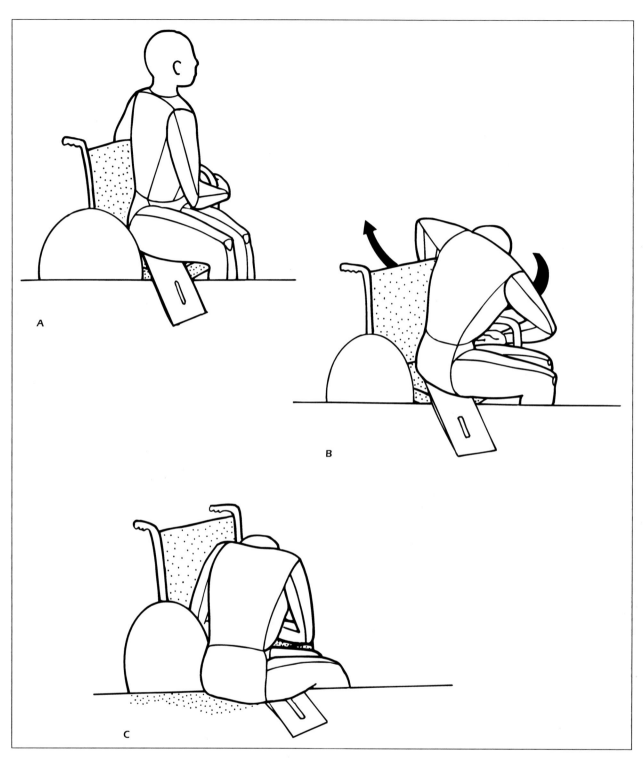

Figure 11–10. Even transfer using sliding board, alternate method. **(A)** Starting position. **(B)** Twisting to slide the buttocks out and toward the bed. **(C)** The transfer is completed with the weight borne on the elbows.

The person twists her head and shoulders back and to the left by pulling on the push handle and the armrest. This twist causes the buttocks to slide forward and to the right toward the bed (Figure 11–10B). Depending on the individual's strength and ability, positioning the buttocks on the right front corner of the seat may take one or several twists.

From the right front corner of the seat, the person pushes her buttocks across the transfer board toward the bed. To do this, she first places her right palm against the inside of the armrest.

Keeping her head low, she pushes on the wheelchair's push handle and armrest and shimmies her head and upper trunk back and forth. This shimmy involves rapid lateral flexion to the right and left alternately.

Once the person has moved her buttocks as far as she can with her arms in the initial position, she needs to move her arms to a position in which weight is borne on the elbows on the left side of the wheelchair seat (Figure 11–10C). Keeping her head low, she moves toward the bed by pushing with her arms and shimmying her head and upper trunk. The push and shimmy are continued until the buttocks and thighs are completely on the bed.

To sit up, the person can push on the wheelchair seat, extending her elbows with her anterior deltoids. In the presence of elbow flexion contractures, she may have to use overhead loops to come to sitting.

Even transfers with board and loops. If an individual does not have adequate strength or range of motion to perform a transfer with just a board, she may be able to achieve independence using a board and loops hanging from an overhead frame. Hanging loops should be used only as a last resort. The loops and frame are bulky, unsightly, and not very portable.

An overhead loop system is shown in Figure 11–11. The exact spacing and length of the different loops will vary between individuals. During transfer training, the therapist and patient should work together to find the optimal configuration of loops for the individual involved.

The following is a description of a chair-to-bed transfer, moving to the left. A transfer in the reverse direction will simply involve reversing the steps.

The person moves her buttocks forward in the chair and places the sliding board. She then positions her hands for the transfer. The left hand should be placed in the nearest loop, palm facing downward. The right hand should be placed on the wheelchair cushion beside the right thigh, well forward on the seat. An alternate position for this arm is over the wheelchair's backrest, with the weight borne above the elbow.

The next step involves positioning the arms and trunk for the transfer. The transfer will be performed with the trunk leaning well forward to unweight the buttocks. The person assumes this position by leaning forward, supporting her weight on both arms. Both elbows should point upward, with the shoulders internally rotated and the elbows flexed. Figure 11–12 shows the starting position for the transfer.

The buttocks are moved toward the bed using the head-hips relationship. While supporting her weight on her hands, the person forcefully throws her head and upper trunk away from the bed. This motion is repeated multiple times. Some are able to perform this transfer using one loop. Others need to reposition their hands to additional loops when they have moved as far as they can from the starting position. An individual repositioning her hands should place her left hand in the next loop and her right hand next to her thigh. She can then resume the twisting motion. The process should continue until the buttocks and thighs are securely on the bed.

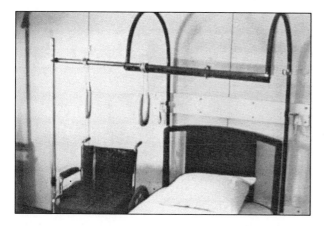

Figure 11–11. Suspended loops for transfers between wheelchair and bed. (*Reproduced with permission from Ford, J., & Duckworth, B. [1987]. Physical Management for the Quadriplegic Patient. Philadelphia, PA: F.A. Davis. [2nd ed.].*)

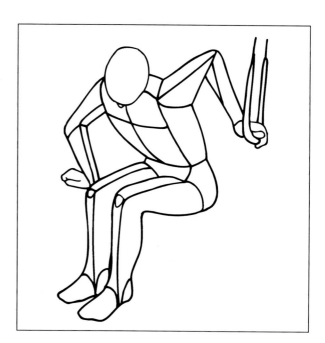

Figure 11–12. Starting position for even transfer from wheelchair to bed using sliding board and overhead loops.

Uneven Transfers

Uneven transfers include any transfers between surfaces of unequal height. These transfers require greater strength and skill than do even transfers.

Able-bodied people live in a multilevel world. They can stand, sit on surfaces of various heights, and get onto and off of the ground. Someone who uses a wheelchair and is unable to perform uneven transfers has few alternatives. She can choose to be in her wheelchair or on a surface (usually a bed) that is exactly as high as the wheelchair seat. She is "confined" to her wheelchair.

A person with a spinal cord injury who can perform uneven transfers has more options open to her. She can leave her wheelchair to sit on a couch or on the floor if she likes and can get back up if she falls. She can get into a car or truck independently, freed from the necessity of a lift. All of these options make for a more flexible lifestyle.

The physical and skill prerequisites required to perform uneven transfers are summarized in Tables 11–7 and 11–8.

Floor transfers.   Transfers between the floor and a wheelchair enable a person to get onto and off of the floor or ground. This ability can be life enriching, enabling a person to get into the water at the beach, take a picnic on the ground, or get onto the floor to play with children or pets. Independent

TABLE 11–7.   UNEVEN TRANSFERS—PHYSICAL PREREQUISITES

	Side approach floor to chair	Front approach floor to chair	Back approach floor to chair	Intermediate levels	Wheelchair to higher surfaces	Toilet	Bathtub
Strength							
Anterior deltoids	☑	☑	☑	☑	☑	☑ᵃ	☑
Middle deltoids	☑	√	√	√	√	√	√
Posterior deltoids	√	√	√	√	√	√	√
Biceps, brachialis, and/or brachioradialis	√						
Infraspinatus and teres minor	√	√	√	√	√	√	√
Serratus anterior	☑	☑	☑	☑	☑	√	☑
Triceps	√	☑	☑	√	☑		√
Pectoralis major		☑	☑		☑		√
Latissimus dorsi		☑	☑				√
Range of motion							
Shoulder Extension	☑	√	☑	√	√		√
Abduction	☑			√	√	√	√
Flexion	☑	√		√	√	√	√
Internal rotation			☑		√		√
Elbow Extension	☑	√	√	√	√	☑ᵃ	√
Flexion		√	√	√	√		√
Wrist extension	√		√		√	☑ᵃ	√
Combined hip flexion and knee extension	☑						

ᵃ In the absence of functioning triceps.

√: Some strength is needed for this activity or severe limitation in range will inhibit this activity.

☑: A large amount of strength or normal or greater range is needed for this activity.

TABLE 11–8.   UNEVEN TRANSFERS—SKILL PREREQUISITES

	Side approach floor to chair	Front approach floor to chair	Back approach floor to chair	Intermediate levels	Wheelchair to higher surfaces	Toilet	Bathtub
Tolerate upright sitting position[a]	✓	✓	✓	✓	✓	✓	✓
Accessory skills	✓	✓	✓	✓	✓	✓	✓
Extend elbows using muscle substitution[b] (p. 255)						✓	
Lock elbows[b] (p. 256)						✓	
Control pelvis using head and shoulders (p. 260)	✓	✓	✓	✓	✓	✓	✓
Lift buttocks by pivoting on extended arms (p. 261)	✓				✓	✓	
Lift buttocks and move laterally (p. 262)	✓				✓	✓	
Lift buttocks to the side from floor to higher surfaces (p. 263)	✓						
Straight lift from floor (p. 264)		✓	✓				✓
Turn body to drop onto wheelchair seat (p. 264)		✓					

[a] Skill addressed in chapter 12.

[b] In the absence of functioning triceps.

floor transfers are also an important survival skill. Even if a patient does not foresee using the skill by choice, it is quite likely that she may find it helpful at some time in the future. Many people who use wheelchairs over a period of time eventually fall. At those times, it is useful to be able to get up from the floor, the street, or the basketball court.

The first step in transferring from the floor to a wheelchair involves ensuring that the chair is upright with the brakes locked. Once the chair is positioned and locked, the individual can transfer using a side, front, or back approach.

Side approach. This technique for transfers between the floor and a wheelchair has the advantage of being fast. Speed is important when a person finds herself on the street in the middle of an intersection or on the floor in the middle of a basketball game.

Using the side approach method, a person utilizes finesse to move her body from the floor to a wheelchair seat. A great deal of strength is not required. For this reason, some people with motor levels as high as C7 can perform this transfer. As can be seen in Figure 11–13, loose hamstrings are necessary.

During the actual lift of the transfer, one hand stays on the floor and one stays on the wheelchair seat. For the purpose of this discussion, the hands will be referred to as the floor hand and the chair hand, respectively.

The starting position for a side-approach floor-to-chair transfer is shown in Figure 11–13A. The person sits in front of the wheelchair with her legs at a 30- to 45-degree angle to the chair. The transfer is likely to be easier if her knees are bent, pointing upward. The buttocks should be slightly in front of the casters, closer to the one behind the person. The hand closer to the wheelchair is placed on the seat, on the furthest front corner. The palm should face down, and the elbow should point upward. The other hand is placed on the floor, a few inches lateral and anterior to the hip.

To lift her buttocks onto the seat, the person swings her head and upper torso down and away from the wheelchair while pushing downward with her arms. The twist must be forceful and the downward motion of the head must be very pronounced to lift the buttocks high enough. To provide extra lift, the person should protract the scapula of the floor arm at the end of the trans-

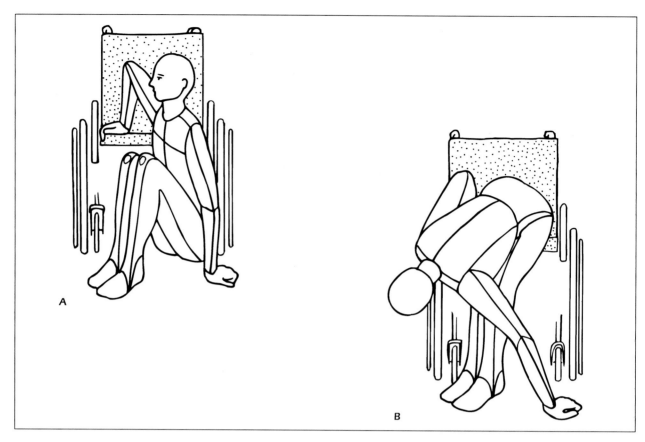

Figure 11–13.   *Side-approach transfer from the floor to a wheelchair.* **(A)** *Starting position.* **(B)** *Buttocks onto seat.*

fer. She ends in the position shown in Figure 11–13B.

The next task is to assume an upright sitting position. This involves placing the floor hand on the legs and walking it up the legs (Figure 11–13C). Once she has placed her hand on her legs, the person unweights the hand by pushing on the leg and throwing her head back and laterally toward the chair. The other arm can be used to assist in this process, pulling on the armrest or on the push handle of the wheelchair. When the hand on the legs is unweighted, the person quickly moves it and catches her weight on a more proximal handhold. This step is repeated until she achieves an upright sitting position (Figure 11–13D).

The same procedure (with minor changes) is used in reverse when transferring down to the floor. After moving her buttocks to the front of the wheelchair seat, the person positions her legs at a 30- to 45-degree angle to the chair. The hand facing out from the chair becomes the "floor hand." To position the floor hand, the individual can either walk her hand down her legs or place it directly on the floor while holding onto the

wheelchair's push handle, backrest, armrest, or seat with the other hand.

The next step involves moving the buttocks onto the floor. The person slides her buttocks off of the seat by twisting her head and upper torso slightly toward the back of the chair. Once the buttocks have moved from the seat, gravity provides the downward force for the transfer. The person's task at this point is to control the motion so that she lands without trauma to her buttocks. To do so, she slows the downward motion by resisting the upward and chairward twist of her head and upper torso. She *should not* swing her head and upper trunk up and toward the chair forcefully during the transfer because that would increase the speed of her descent and result in trauma to her buttocks.

Front approach. This transfer technique requires less skill and hamstring flexibility than does a side-approach transfer, but it requires greater strength. Fully innervated upper extremities are necessary.

The starting position for this transfer is shown in Figure 11–14A. The person is side-sitting with

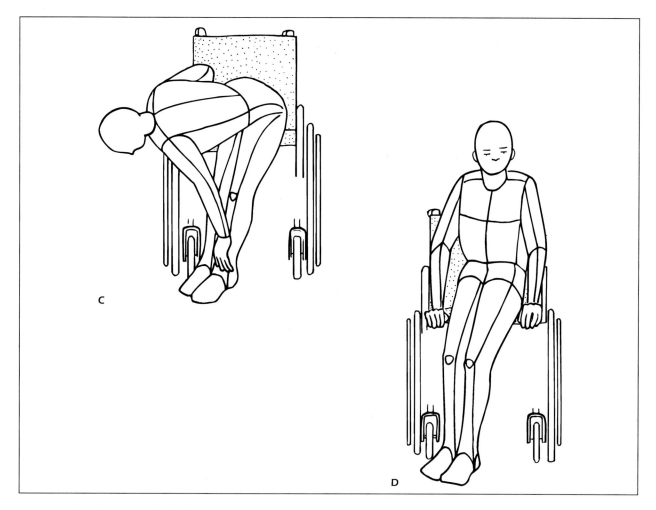

Figure 11–13. *(Continued)* **(C)** Walking hand up legs. **(D)** Sitting upright.

her knees flexed. The knees are located *in front of* the wheelchair's casters, centered between them. One hand is on the wheelchair seat, and one is on the floor.

The person lifts her buttocks off of the floor, using the head-hips relationship to do so. Pushing downward on both hands, she twists her head and upper torso down and away from the chair (Figure 11–14B).

In the next step, the person pushes on the chair and raises her trunk to assume an upright kneeling position in front of the wheelchair (Figure 11–14C). While doing so, she must push downward on the chair, as pulling on it will tip it over.

During the next step of the transfer, a forceful downward push on the armrests or (if there are no armrests) seat is used to lift the body (Figure 11–14D). Again, the person must refrain from pulling on the chair. While pushing on the armrests or seat, she tucks her head, protracts her

scapulae, and raises her buttocks high above the level of the seat. She then releases one hand and twists, turning and landing on the wheelchair seat.

This transfer is not a particularly good method for returning to the floor. The side-approach technique is much faster and easier to perform.[f]

Back approach. The third method for floor-to-wheelchair transfers requires fully innervated upper extremities. The person performing this transfer also needs greater strength and shoulder flexibility than are required to perform a front-approach transfer.

The starting position for this transfer is shown in Figure 11–15A. The person sits on the

---

[f] In contrast to a side-approach transfer from the floor to a wheelchair, a high level of skill is not required when using a side approach to transfer *down* from a wheelchair.

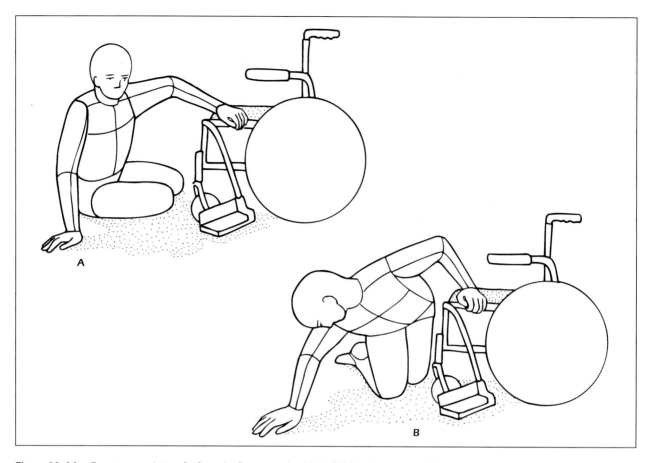

Figure 11–14.   Front-approach transfer from the floor to a wheelchair. **(A)** Starting position. **(B)** Lifting buttocks from floor.

floor in front of the wheelchair, facing directly away from the chair. Her buttocks should be in front of the casters and centered between them. The transfer will be easier if her knees are bent. The person places her palms on the front corners of the wheelchair seat, with the fingers facing forward. This hand position requires a great deal of shoulder flexibility. Many people are not able to perform this transfer because they are unable to assume the starting position.

The person lifts her buttocks from the floor by pushing down hard on the wheelchair seat. This maneuver requires the muscles to function in a position of extreme stretch, making this step prohibitively difficult for most people.[8] As she pushes down, the person should lean back with

---

[8] People who cannot achieve independence in a direct transfer from the floor to a wheelchair may be able to transfer using an indirect approach: they transfer first from the floor to an intermediate-height surface such as a stool, and from the stool to the wheelchair seat. The techniques used are as described for a direct floor-to-chair transfer.

her head and upper torso until her buttocks reach the seat level (Figure 11–15B).

Once the wheelchair seat has been cleared, the person uses the head-hips relationship to lift her buttocks higher and to move back further on the seat. She pivots on her arms, leaning forward and curling her head downward (Figure 11–15C). Additional lift is achieved through strong protraction of the scapulae. As is true for the front approach, this transfer method can be used to return to the floor but is less convenient than the side approach.

Transfers to intermediate levels.   To transfer between a wheelchair and a lower surface such as a couch, a person with a complete spinal cord injury uses a method similar to that used for even transfers without equipment. The difference is that the head and upper torso motions used to lift the buttocks from the lower surface must be more forceful and exaggerated to get an adequate lift. When transferring down from the wheelchair, gravity supplies the power to move the body. The person's task is to control the motion so that she can land without injury.

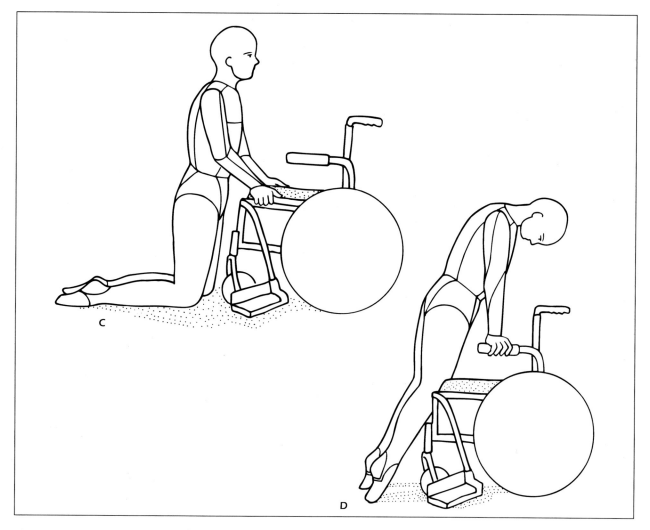

Figure 11–14. (*Continued*) **(C)** Kneeling in front of wheelchair. **(D)** Lifting buttocks by pushing down on armrests.

Wheelchair to higher surfaces.   The ability to transfer from the wheelchair to a higher surface is another useful skill. Many beds are significantly higher than wheelchair seats, as are many "accessible" toilets in public restrooms. An uneven transfer is also required to get into trucks, vans without lifts, or tractors.

The person planning to transfer first locks her brakes with the wheelchair positioned as close as possible to the surface toward which she plans to transfer. If moving toward the right, she places her right hand on the higher surface, several inches in front of the wheelchair seat. The other hand is placed on the wheelchair's seat or armrest, depending on the height of the surface. Placing the hand on the armrest makes a higher transfer possible but increases the risk of the chair sliding to the side during the transfer. Figure 11–16A shows the starting position for the transfer.

While pushing straight down and pivoting on both arms, the person tucks her head and upper torso downward and swings them away from the higher surface. To achieve an adequate lift, the downward motion of the head must be pronounced. To move her buttocks further onto the surface and to gain a more stable position, the person protracts her scapulae strongly.

Once the individual is sitting securely on the higher surface, she leans her torso to a position over the surface (Figure 11–16B). She can then move her hand from the wheelchair to the higher surface and push herself upright.

Bathroom transfers.   Most bathrooms are very small, with little room for maneuvering a wheelchair. The approach that is used for a toilet or tub transfer may be dictated by the bathroom's layout. During transfer training, the therapist and patient should develop a method of transferring

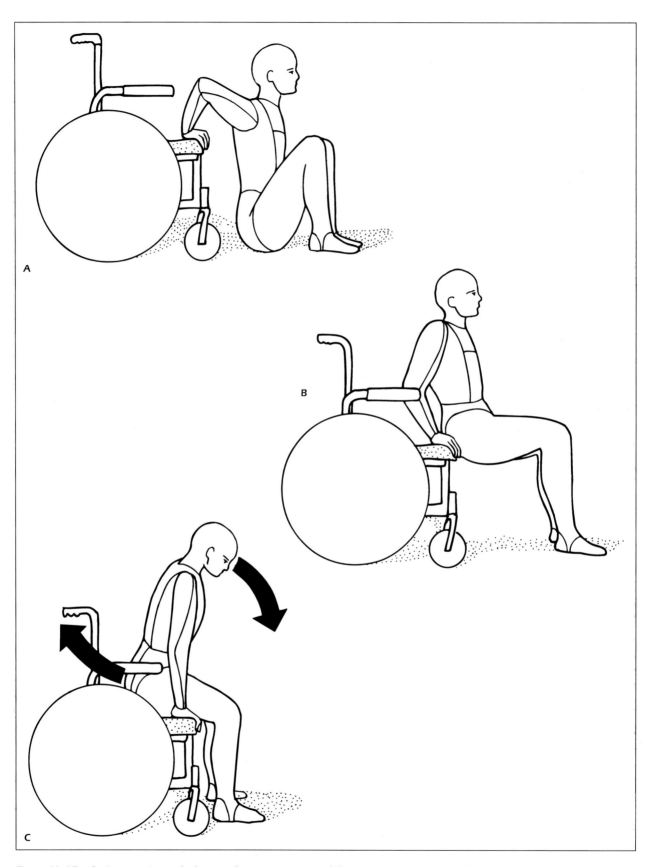

Figure 11–15.   Back-approach transfer from the floor to a wheelchair. **(A)** Starting position. **(B)** Lifting the buttocks from the floor. **(C)** Moving the buttocks back on the seat.

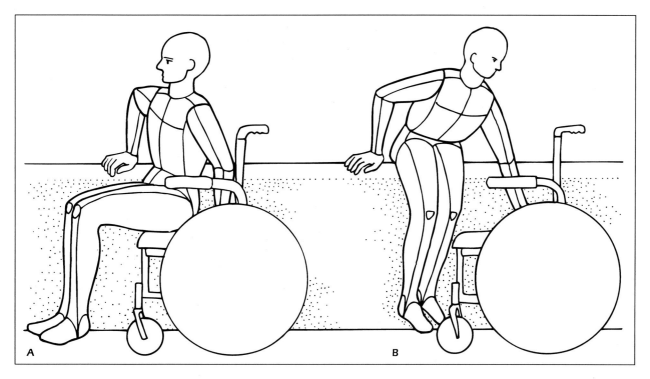

Figure 11–16. *Transfer to higher surface.* **(A)** *Starting position.* **(B)** *Buttocks lifted onto higher surface.*

that will be applicable in the patient's home bathroom.

Toilet. If space permits, a person with a spinal cord injury can transfer to a toilet using a technique that is essentially the same as the even transfer without equipment described previously. The wheelchair is positioned against a front corner of the toilet seat, angled in as with a mat transfer. Using the methods described earlier, the person removes the armrest closest to the toilet, positions her legs, moves the footplates out of the way, and gets into position for the transfer. One hand is placed on the far side of the toilet seat, and the other hand is placed on the wheelchair seat next to the thigh. The person then pivots forward on her arms, twisting her head and upper torso down and away from the toilet. The transfer is likely to be slightly uneven, so a higher lift will be required. This can be accomplished by throwing the head and upper torso into a lower position when pivoting the arms. To return to the chair, the same steps are performed in reverse.

In an alternative method, the person straddles the toilet. To use this technique, she approaches the toilet from the front, facing it directly. The footrests are swung out of the way, and the feet are placed on either side of the toilet. The chair is moved into position against the front of the toilet. After the person moves her buttocks

forward in the chair, she leans forward and props on her arms (elbows extended) with one hand on either side of the toilet seat. She then pushes down hard with her arms and depresses her shoulder girdle while leaning forward. This maneuver lifts her buttocks onto the toilet seat. To return to the chair, the person first places her hands on the wheelchair seat, one on each side. She then moves her buttocks back by pushing down with her arms and depressing her scapulae.

Bathtub. A person who has impaired pain and temperature sensation may sustain serious burns if she transfers into a bathtub full of hot water or fills the tub while sitting in it. To prevent burns, an individual with impaired sensation should fill the bathtub and check the water temperature before transferring into the tub.

To prepare for a tub transfer, the person approaches the tub directly facing its side. The chair should be positioned toward the end opposite the faucet. The person transferring swings her wheelchair's front rigging out of the way, lifts her legs, and places her feet in the tub. After positioning the chair close to the side of the tub, she locks the brakes. She may find the transfer easier with the chair directly against the tub or slightly back from it.

The actual transfer is performed in two steps: from the wheelchair to the side of the tub and from there into the tub. To transfer to the side of the tub, the person places one hand on the near side of the tub and one on the front of the wheelchair's seat or armrest. She then pushes down to lift her body and lower her buttocks onto the side of the tub.

Stabilizing her trunk by balancing on an arm with the hand placed on the far side of the tub, the person uses her free hand to move her feet toward the faucet. She then lowers her body into the tub, with one hand on each side of the tub. To transfer back to the chair, the same steps are performed in reverse.

Transfers in and out of a bathtub without adaptive equipment require fully innervated upper extremities. People who have impaired upper extremity function or other limiting factors, or who simply prefer an easier transfer, can utilize a tub bench. Transfers to and from tub benches are performed using techniques similar to those used for even transfers.

Vehicle transfers. The skills used for the basic even and uneven transfers described earlier can be applied to transfers between a wheelchair and a car, truck, or van. The person angles her wheelchair as close as possible to the vehicle's seat and moves the armrest and footplates out of the way. With one hand on the vehicle's seat and one on the wheelchair seat, she pivots on her arms and transfers. As the therapist and patient work together on the transfer, they can experiment with different hand positions.

After transferring into a car, the person places her feet in the footwells and loads the wheelchair. She can load it either behind or next to herself.[h] If the chair has a folding frame, she turns the chair so that it faces the car (footplates toward the car) and folds the chair. She then lifts the casters through the door and finally pulls the chair into the car. If the chair has a rigid frame, she removes the wheels, folds the backrest, and places the chair and wheels in the car.

THERAPEUTIC STRATEGIES FOLLOWING COMPLETE SPINAL CORD INJURY

To accomplish a functional goal, the patient must acquire both the physical and skill prerequisites for that activity. For example, when working on a

side-approach floor-to-chair transfer, a person with a complete spinal cord injury must develop adequate hamstring flexibility and upper extremity strength as well as the ability to pivot on her arms to lift her buttocks.

When developing skill prerequisites for a functional goal, the patient should start with the most basic prerequisite skills and progress toward more challenging activities. (There is no point in working on lifting the buttocks by pivoting on the extended arms if the individual cannot independently maintain an upright sitting position by propping forward on her arms with the elbows extended.)

It is generally best to work on even transfers first and to progress to uneven transfers. As a person develops the strength, range of motion, flexibility, and skills to perform an even transfer, she lays the foundation for more advanced transfers.

Before asking a patient to attempt a new skill, the therapist should explain and demonstrate the technique. The demonstration should provide a clear idea of the motions involved and the timing of these motions. The patient should also be shown how the new skill will be used functionally.

During functional training, the therapist should remember that every patient will perform a particular activity differently. Each person has a unique combination of body build, coordination, strength, and flexibility, and these characteristics influence the manner in which she performs functional tasks. As a result of these individual variations, each person is unique in the exact placement of her hands; the timing of her pushes, pivots, and twists; and the degree to which she must dip her head to get an adequate lift of her buttocks. What works for one patient may be a total disaster for the next. The challenge of functional training is finding the timing and maneuvers that best suit the individual involved.

As a therapist and patient work together on a skill, they can learn from failed attempts by analyzing the problem. Is the patient strong enough to perform the maneuver? Is she flexible enough? Did she pivot too far forward on her arms, or did she fail to pivot far enough? Were her hands too far anterior or not anterior enough?

Trial and error can be another useful strategy for functional training. For example, the best way to determine whether the hands were too far forward in a failed attempt may be to try the maneuver with the hands positioned further back. The relative success of the attempt may provide an answer.

It is important for the therapist and patient to keep in mind that functional training can take a

---

[h] If loading chair with a folding frame in the front, the driver must perform the initial transfer into the passenger side of the car and slide across the seat to the driver's side.

long time; independence in a given transfer may require an extended period of functional training. It is a mistake to give up on a functional goal after only a few trials. (Assuming that the patient has adequate innervation, of course!) When funding constraints limit the time available for functional training during inpatient rehabilitation, the patient may continue working toward independence in an alternative setting such as an outpatient clinic or in the home.[2]

Strategies to address the various prerequisite skills are presented in the following sections.

Tolerate Upright Sitting Position

When upright activities are first initiated, people with spinal cord injuries may experience orthostatic hypotension. Before an individual can learn to perform any transfers, she must first develop the capacity to tolerate an upright sitting posture. This capacity can be developed through gradual accommodation to progressively upright postures. Strategies for developing upright sitting tolerance are presented in Chapter 12.

Unsupported Sitting Balance

An individual with a spinal cord injury will probably never need to sit with both hands in the air to perform a transfer; however, practicing unsupported sitting balance can be a useful therapeutic activity. Developing the ability to use head and arm motions to maintain upright sitting will make other activities easier.

To sit unsupported, a person must be able to tolerate an upright sitting position. Once she can tolerate an upright sitting posture, a patient's first task in working on unsupported sitting balance is finding her position of balance, the position in which her trunk is balanced over its base of support. In long- or short-sitting, the therapist supports the patient at her shoulders and helps her find her balance point. When the patient's trunk is balanced, the therapist will not feel her pushing forward, backward, or laterally.

The therapist should explain and demonstrate how the patient can maintain an upright position with her hands in the air, using hand and head motions: if her trunk starts to fall, the patient moves her hands and head in the opposite direction.

The patient should practice this skill, getting a feel for how her head and arm motions cause her trunk to move. She will need to experience the loss of balance and learn to regain the balance

point using head and arm motions. Her reactions may be slow at first, and she may tend to overcorrect. The therapist can help the process by giving verbal feedback.

As the patient becomes more adept at maintaining her balance point, the therapist should reduce the support being provided at her shoulders. The patient can progress from practicing with light support, then with the therapist's hands hovering inches away, and finally practice without spotting.

To develop the patient's unsupported sitting balance further, the therapist can disturb her balance or have her catch and throw objects. The patient can also practice maintaining her balance while she reaches her arms in different directions.

Independent work. Once the patient has developed some initial skill in unsupported sitting, she can practice alone while long-sitting on a mat or short-sitting between mats.

Extend Elbows Using Muscle Substitution

When triceps function is absent or inadequate for functional use, the anterior deltoids and clavicular portion of the pectoralis major can be used to extend the elbows.[4, 8] This muscle substitution should be taught early in the program; practice can begin before the patient has been cleared for out-of-bed activities. The therapist can manually stabilize one of the patient's hands with the elbow in a slightly flexed position, and ask her to push. When approached in this manner, many patients will utilize muscle substitution without having to think about it. For an individual who is not able to do so, the therapist can cue her to use her anterior deltoid, reminding her verbally ("use this muscle") and touching or tapping the skin over the muscle.

If a patient cannot extend her elbow while the therapist supplies the verbal and tactile cues just described, the following alternative approach can help her learn the motions involved. The therapist positions the patient's elbow in extension, and stabilizes her hand. She then asks the patient to hold her elbow straight while she (the therapist) applies resistance over the distal humerus or antecubital fossa in the direction that would cause elbow flexion. To hold her elbow against this force, the patient contracts her anterior deltoid. Once the patient learns to stabilize her elbow using her anterior deltoid, the therapist can use the therapeutic strategies described previously to teach her to extend her elbow with this muscle. Alternatively, the therapist may place the patient's elbow in slight flexion, place her (the therapist's) hand against the patient's antecubital fossa, and ask her to push. ("Push against my hand.")

Whichever strategy is employed to teach muscle substitution, the therapist stabilizes the patient's hand during the activity. This stabilization enables the anterior deltoid to work with the arm in a closed-chain position, simulating the muscle's action during a transfer. Once the patient has learned to extend her elbows using muscle substitution, the process can be repeated with the shoulders in a variety of positions.

From a Forward Lean in Sitting, Push Trunk to Upright

To work on this skill, the patient must be able to tolerate upright sitting. She must also be able to extend her elbows against resistance, using either her triceps or muscle substitution.

Probably the best position for working on this activity is short-sitting between two mats, with the mats positioned as shown in Figure 11–17. With her hands stabilized on the mat in front of her, the patient lowers her trunk slightly by allowing her elbows to flex a few degrees and then pushes herself back upright. She should lower her trunk only as far as she can maintain full control of the motion and push back to upright. As the patient's ability improves, she should increase the distance of her pushup.

Some time should also be spent practicing this activity while sitting in a wheelchair. The hands can be placed on or beside the distal thighs.

Independent work. The activities just described are ideal for independent work.

Lock the Elbows

When pivoting on her arms during a transfer, a person who does not have functioning triceps needs to lock her elbows using positioning and muscle substitution. The position for locking is as follows: shoulders externally rotated, elbows and wrists extended, forearms supinated. Weight is borne on the palms. The elbows are held in extension using the anterior deltoids and shoulder external rotators.

After demonstrating the technique for elbow locking, the therapist can help the patient position her arms. The patient then holds the "locked" position while the therapist applies resistance, pushing the elbow toward flexion.

Once the patient has a feel for the position and muscle contraction involved, she can practice locking and unlocking her elbows. If necessary, the therapist can help by supporting the trunk as the patient leans on an arm and practices moving it in and out of position.

Independent work. Sitting in a wheelchair, the patient can stabilize her palms on the wheelchair seat or on a nearby mat and practice locking and unlocking her elbows. This is a good "home-

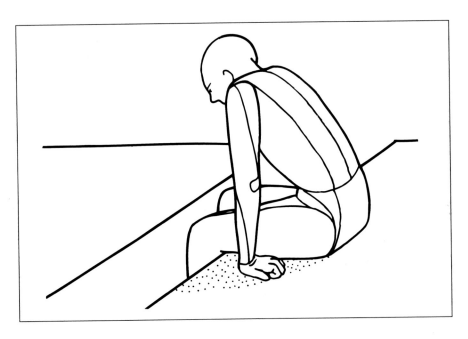

Figure 11–17. Short-sitting on mat with second mat placed in front to allow independent practice of transfer skills.

"work" activity for her to work on when not in therapy.

Place an Arm Behind Wheelchair Push Handle

Before practicing this skill, the patient must be able to tolerate an upright sitting position.

Many people with spinal cord injuries are able to place an arm behind their wheelchair's push handle without any practice. Someone who finds the maneuver more difficult may need to use momentum to get her arm into position. Starting with her arm crossed across her torso, she can throw the arm back and up. The motion should be forceful enough to provide adequate momentum to carry the arm to a position behind the push handle.

The therapist can help at first by assisting with the throw to give the patient a feel for the motion. An individual who continues to have difficulty can practice with a small wrist weight. The weight will add to the arm's momentum, making it easier to throw the arm back.

Practice of this skill should start with the patient sitting upright in a wheelchair. Once she has become proficient in this position, she should work to develop the skill while leaning forward, to the side, or both. As her ability improves, the patient should practice in increasingly tilted positions.

Independent work. This skill can be practiced at any time when the patient is in her wheelchair. It is another good "homework" activity to be performed when not in therapy.

Stabilize Trunk by Holding Wheelchair Push Handle

To work on this skill, a person must be able to tolerate an upright sitting position. It is not necessary for her to be able to place her arm behind the push handle independently.

With her arm hooked behind the wheelchair's push handle, the patient practices holding her body stable. Starting in an upright sitting position, she uses one arm to hold her body upright while she moves the other arm to various positions. This activity can be made more challenging by adding weight to the free arm and by throwing this arm more forcefully.

Once an individual has mastered the skill in upright, she should practice with her trunk leaned in various directions. The degree of lean can increase as she becomes more proficient.

In addition to developing the ability to stabilize her trunk, the patient needs to learn how to adjust her hold on the chair's push handle to allow her trunk to lean. When sitting upright, the trunk is stabilized using the upper arm. When moving from upright, the person must relax her arm enough to allow the hold to slide more distally. The therapist can help with initial practice of this skill by lowering the patient's torso while she adjusts her hold on the chair. As her skill improves, the patient can participate in the control of her trunk's descent, leaning progressively further as she relaxes her hold on the push handle. She should work to the point where she can lower her trunk independently and can stop the descent at any point.

Independent work. Once the patient has developed some initial skill in this activity, she can practice whenever she is in a wheelchair.

Move Trunk in Wheelchair by Pulling with Arms

To work on pulling her trunk forward or returning to upright from a forward lean, a person must be able to tolerate upright sitting. To tilt her trunk forward, a person with a complete spinal cord injury can pull on the wheelchair's armrests. A patient who has adequate upper extremity strength should not have difficulty learning this maneuver. Someone who has difficulty moving in this manner can use momentum from head motions to augment the pull. To return to upright, one hand can be used to push on the legs or the anterior part of the seat while the other hand pulls on the chair's push handle. When the patient first begins practicing these skills, the therapist can provide assistance with the trunk's motions. As the patient's skill develops, this assistance should be reduced.

Practice leaning the trunk laterally in a wheelchair can begin before the patient is able to tolerate upright sitting. Sitting in either a partially reclined or upright position, the patient can practice pulling on her armrest to tip her body to the side and pull back to midline. She should start with small excursions, leaning only as far as she can maintain control and return to midline. As her skill increases, she should move through longer arcs of motion.

Independent work. Once the patient has developed some initial skill in these activities, she can practice whenever she is in a wheelchair.

Move Trunk in Wheelchair Using Momentum

To work on this skill, the patient must be able to tolerate upright sitting.

To move her trunk using momentum, a person with a complete spinal cord injury throws her head and an arm in the direction toward which she wants her trunk to move. The other arm remains behind the wheelchair's push handle for stability.

Initially, patients are often reluctant to throw their heads and arms forcefully. As a result, they are unable to move using momentum. The therapist should encourage the patient to move with abrupt, powerful, and exaggerated motions. It can be helpful for the therapist to give the patient a feel for the motion by moving her arm passively. A wrist weight can also be helpful, adding to the arm's momentum and enabling the person to move her trunk. As her skill improves, she should practice without the weight.

Independent work. Once the patient has developed some initial skill in this activity, she can practice whenever she is in a wheelchair.

Manipulate Armrests

To work on managing her armrests, a patient must be able to stabilize her trunk in the wheelchair.

A person with intact upper extremity function should be able to manipulate her armrests

PROBLEM-SOLVING EXERCISE 11-1

Your patient has C5 tetraplegia, ASIA A. He is practicing the skill of leaning his trunk forward from upright while sitting in a wheelchair. He uses one arm to stabilize himself in the chair while he throws his head and the other arm forward in an attempt to lean forward using momentum. He is unable to lean his trunk forward using this technique.

- What could be causing this problem?
- Describe functional training strategies to develop this patient's ability to lean forward in his wheelchair using momentum.

without difficulty, once she has been shown how they work. People who lack active finger flexors have more difficulty with the task. If the armrest can be repositioned by rotating it up or to the side, the person lacking hand function moves the armrest by pulling/pushing on it with her forearm or the back of her hand (wrist extended). A conventional armrest can be pulled out of and replaced in its channels using either of the holds shown in Figure 11–18. The person can balance the armrest in her lap while turning it around.

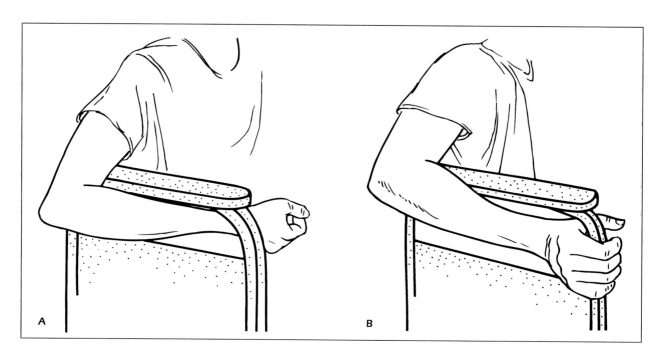

Figure 11–18. *Methods for lifting armrest.* **(A)** *Lifting with forearm.* **(B)** *Lifting using tenodesis grasp.*

Learning to remove and replace armrests is simply a matter of practice. With conventional armrests, the patient needs to spend time lifting the armrests, turning them around, and placing them in the rear channels.

Independent work.   Armrest manipulation can be practiced whenever the patient is in a wheelchair.

Slide Buttocks on Wheelchair Seat

To practice sliding her buttocks on a wheelchair seat, a patient needs to be able to move and stabilize her torso in the wheelchair.

A variety of methods, all involving the head-hips relationship and described above, can be used to slide the buttocks on a wheelchair seat. During early practice of this skill, the therapist can help the patient perform the head and upper torso movements while she tries the maneuvers. This assistance can give the patient a feel for the required force and excursion of the motions.

It is difficult at first for people with spinal cord injuries to move on their wheelchair seats. A therapist can aid the process by pulling on the patient's buttocks or legs to enable her to move. The therapist should time the assistance to coincide with the patient's efforts and should apply just enough force to effect some motion. As the patient's skill improves, the therapist can reduce the assistance given.

Independent work.   Once the patient has developed some initial skill in this activity, she can practice whenever she is in a wheelchair.

Prop Forward on Extended Arms in Sitting

Before someone can learn to prop on extended arms,[i] she must be able to tolerate upright sitting. She must also be able to extend her elbows and hold them in extension against resistance, using either triceps or muscle substitution.

When propping forward on extended arms, a person leans forward slightly and supports her trunk on her arms. Her palms are lateral to her thighs and anterior to her hips.

After assisting the patient into position, the therapist asks her to help hold her elbows straight. As the patient's ability to support herself improves, the therapist's support is reduced.

The patient should also practice placing her arms in position to support her trunk. As the therapist stabilizes her trunk, she can position her hands and extend her elbows. The patient will soon be able to support her trunk independently by propping forward on extended arms. To prepare for more advanced activities, she can hold the position as the therapist applies resistance, pushing her shoulders in various directions.

Independent work.   Once assisted to a position of propping forward on extended arms in sitting, the patient can practice bending and extending her elbows, lowering and raising her trunk. This can be done long-sitting on a mat or short-sitting between two mats (Figure 11–17).

Prop Forward on One Extended Arm in Sitting

Before someone can prop forward on one extended arm in sitting, she should be able to prop forward on two extended arms.

After being assisted into the position of propping forward on two extended arms, the patient should be instructed to shift her trunk laterally. At first, the therapist can facilitate the weight shift by placing a hand on the lateral surface of one of the patient's shoulders and having her push against it.

The patient should shift *under control* through increasing arcs of motion until she is able to lean far enough to support her trunk on one arm. She can then lift the unweighted arm and balance in that position. She should practice this with each arm. To increase her skill, she should practice balancing with the supporting arm in various positions and reaching the free arm in different directions.

Independent work.   The activities just described can be performed alone, long-sitting on a mat, or short-sitting between two mats.

Unweight Buttocks by Leaning Forward on Extended Arms

To develop this skill, a person with a complete spinal cord injury must first be able to prop forward on two extended arms in sitting.

Starting with the patient propped forward on two extended arms in sitting, the therapist should instruct her to lean forward and tuck her chin. The therapist can facilitate the lean by plac-

---

[i] "Extended arms" refers to arms with the elbows positioned in extension.

ing her hands on the anterior surface of the patient's shoulders and having her push against them.

Independent work. Once she has developed some initial practice in this skill, the patient can practice while long-sitting on a mat or short-sitting between two mats.

Control Pelvis Using Head and Shoulders

To perform any transfer independently, a person with a complete spinal cord injury must use the head-hips relationship. By moving her head and upper torso in one direction, she causes her buttocks to move in the opposite direction. Many of the activities described in the sections that follow can help develop this ability; however, the therapist and patient may find it helpful to address head-hips control more directly. In doing so, they develop a basic skill that is crucial to all transfers.

Quadruped is an excellent position for working on this skill. This is true whether or not upper extremity motor function is intact. In the absence of functioning triceps, the patient's elbows must be locked using muscle substitution.

When first working in quadruped, the therapist assists the patient to her hands and knees, and the patient attempts to maintain the position. The therapist helps her maintain her stability at first, and reduces the assistance as the patient's skill improves. The patient can progress to maintaining the position while the therapist applies resistance in various directions.

Once the patient is able to stabilize herself in quadruped, she can progress to moving her buttocks forward and back or side to side using head and shoulder motions. She should move only as far as she can control the motion, increasing the arc as her ability improves.

Someone who has innervated triceps can also practice utilizing the head-hips relationship to assume the quadruped position. Starting in prone, the patient places her palms on the mat next to her shoulders. Simultaneously pushing down and forward (cephalad) with her arms, she pushes her head down to lift her buttocks.

If a patient has elbow flexion contractures or inadequate strength to work in quadruped, she may be able to work on head-hips control while positioned on elbows and knees. This activity may be easier if her elbows are supported on a stack of folding mats so that her trunk is in a horizontal position.

Slide Buttocks Laterally While Propping on Extended Arms

To perform this activity, the patient must be able to unweight her buttocks by leaning forward on her extended arms. During a transfer, a person with a complete spinal cord injury twists her head and upper trunk away from where she wants her buttocks to go. The motion should be forceful and abrupt, to provide enough force to move the buttocks.

The patient starts in sitting, propped forward on extended arms. She then attempts the motion as described above. Initial attempts are often done without adequate force, and as a result the buttocks do not move. Verbal encouragement to increase the force and excursion of the twist may not work. In these cases, the therapist can help the patient to feel the required motion by assisting her during the attempt, applying force at the patient's shoulders.

Once an individual gets a feel for the head and upper torso motions required, the therapist can help with the lateral slide. Timing the assistance to coincide with the patient's efforts, the therapist applies just enough lateral force to the buttocks to cause motion. As the patient's skill improves, the therapist should reduce the assistance given.

A transfer often requires more than one twist. To make a series of twists possible, the patient moves her head and upper torso back in the other direction between twists. This return motion should not be done forcefully or the buttocks will slide in the wrong direction.

Occasionally, an inexperienced patient twists in both directions with equal force. As a result, the buttocks move back and forth over the same spot. The therapist should give verbal and tactile cues to help her correct this problem.

Independent work. A patient can practice moving her buttocks to the side while long-sitting on a mat or short-sitting between mats.

In Sitting, Lift Buttocks by Pushing Down on Armrests

To perform this activity, an individual must be able to tolerate upright sitting. Functioning triceps are also required. A patient who has adequate strength should not have difficulty lifting her buttocks by pushing down on her armrests.

Independent work. A patient can practice lifting her buttocks whenever she is in her wheelchair. To develop balance skills while practicing this skill, she can short-sit between two mats and do pushups on blocks.

In Sitting, Lift on Armrests and Move Buttocks

Before practicing this skill, the patient must be able to lift her buttocks by pushing down on the wheelchair's armrests.

To perform this maneuver, a person with a complete spinal cord injury throws her head and upper torso forward, back, to the side, or in a rotary direction while lifting her buttocks off of the wheelchair's seat. A patient who moves too timidly while practicing should be encouraged by the therapist to move more forcefully.

Independent work.   This skill can be practiced independently while sitting in a wheelchair.

Lift Buttocks by Pivoting on Extended Arms

To lift her buttocks, a person must first be able to prop forward on extended arms in sitting and hold this position against resistance.

The patient should be shown how to lean forward over her extended arms while tucking her head and protracting her scapulae. It is often helpful for the therapist to assist her into position. This can give the patient a feel for the motion and a sense of just how far she needs to pivot forward to lift her buttocks. The patient should accept full weight on her upper extremities while the therapist helps her lift her buttocks from the mat by leaning forward over her arms, rolling her head down, and protracting her scapulae. Once in position, the patient can attempt to maintain the lift. As the individual gets a feel for the maneuver, she should progress to practicing with spotting and verbal cueing, and then to practicing independently.

One of the challenges of learning to lift the buttocks is finding the balance point. A person with a complete spinal cord injury must move her body fairly far forward over her arms to lift high enough for a transfer. If she tips too far forward, however, she will fall. When an individual is at her balance point, she has moved as far forward as she can (and thus has lifted as high as she can) without falling. The patient should learn to lift to her balance point and hold there briefly.

Moving past the balance point is not the only cause of falls while performing this maneuver; people lacking triceps can also fall forward due to an inability to stabilize their elbows in extension.

To correct this problem, a patient may need further strengthening, practice in locking her elbows, or both.

Often, a patient will develop the ability to pivot and raise her buttocks, but the lift will still be inadequate for a transfer without equipment. This problem can occur when the patient does not protract her scapulae enough during the lift. The therapist should check for scapular protraction as she attempts the lift.

An individual who does not protract her scapulae adequately when she attempts to lift her buttocks may have serratus anterior weakness. The problem may also be caused by improper technique. If the latter is the case, the therapist can call the person's attention to the problem and provide further instruction. One useful strategy involves placing a hand between the patient's scapulae as she pivots forward on her arms. While pivoting, the patient is asked to push against the therapist's hand by lifting her trunk between her scapulae. If the individual is still unable to perform the motion, the therapist can assist with the scapular protraction during the lift. As the patient pivots forward on her arms, the therapist lifts her thorax between her scapulae (Figure 11–19). The patient should attempt to hold the position. Once she gets a feel for the scapular protraction, she can attempt the motion on her own.

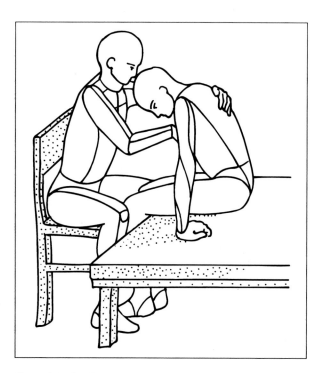

Figure 11–19.   *Therapist assisting with scapular protraction by lifting patient's thorax between his scapulae while he pivots forward on his arms.*

Independent work. This skill takes a good deal of practice to develop. Once a patient is able to initiate some lift, she can practice on her own while short-sitting between two mats. She should emphasize lifting her buttocks as high as she can, controlling the motion. She should also work on finding her balance point, getting a feel for the limit of her forward pivot.

Lift Buttocks and Move Laterally

Before working on this skill, a person must be able to lift her buttocks by pivoting forward on extended arms.

The therapist should explain and demonstrate how the buttocks can be moved laterally by throwing the head and upper torso to the side while lifting. The motion should be quick and forceful. While first learning the skill, the patient can lift her buttocks first, then twist to move laterally. She should progress to a single combined lift-and-twist motion.

A common problem that occurs while a patient learns this maneuver is that the buttocks drop as the patient attempts the lateral motion. This is due to a tendency to raise the head when throwing it to the side. The therapist should direct the patient's attention to this problem and encourage her to keep her head low.

Patients also tend to fall forward as they learn the skill. In some cases this is due to the difficulty of keeping the elbows locked in extension during the maneuver. A forward fall also happens

PROBLEM-SOLVING EXERCISE 11–2

Your patient has complete (ASIA A) tetraplegia. She is dependent in all functional activities, and is unable to tolerate an upright sitting position. One of her goals is to transfer independently to and from a bed without using equipment.

The patient's muscle test results are as follows.

Muscles	Left	Right
Deltoids (anterior, middle and posterior)	5/5	5/5
Shoulder external rotators	5/5	4+/5
Elbow flexors	5/5	5/5
Radial wrist extensors	5/5	3+/5
Serratus anterior	4/5	4–/5
Triceps brachii	2/5	1/5
Long finger flexors	0/5	0/5
Abductor digiti minimi	0/5	0/5
Trunk and lower extremity musculature	0/5	0/5

Pinprick and light touch on the left are intact in the C1 through C8 key sensory points, impaired in T1, and absent below T1. On the right, pinprick and light touch are intact in C1 through C7, impaired in C8, and absent below. Sensation and voluntary motor function are absent in the anal region.

The patient's joint range of motion and muscle flexibility are normal throughout.

- Identify this patient's motor level(s), sensory level(s), and neurological level of injury using the ASIA classification system.
- What are the physical prerequisites for even transfers without equipment?
- What strength and range should the therapeutic exercise program emphasize to facilitate the attainment of this goal?
- What are the skill prerequisites for even transfers without equipment?
- Describe a functional training program (for the goal of even transfers without equipment) that would be appropriate for this patient at this time.
- How would you progress the patient once she has developed tolerance to upright sitting?

when a patient pivots past her balance point. People who fall forward may require more practice in this activity, strengthening of the anterior deltoids, or practice in the prerequisite skill of raising the buttocks by pivoting on extended arms.

Independent work. The patient can practice this skill while short-sitting between two mats. She should start by hopping her buttocks over small distances and gradually increase the distance.

Lift Buttocks from Floor to Higher Surface (Side Approach)

Before working on a side-approach transfer from the floor, a patient should be proficient in even transfers without equipment. She should also be able to assume the starting position of the transfer. The skills required to get into this position are covered in Chapter 10.

At the start of the transfer, the person sits in front of the higher surface, at a 30- to 45-degree angle from the higher surface. Her knees should be flexed, pointing upward. One hand is on the higher surface and one is on the floor, slightly lateral and anterior to the hip. From this position, the person lifts her buttocks by pushing on her arms and throwing her head down and away from the higher surface.

To lift her buttocks high enough for a floor-to-wheelchair transfer, the person must execute her head and upper torso motions in a forceful and exaggerated manner. As can be seen in Figure 11–13, the head must angle toward the floor for the buttocks to lift high enough. During functional training, the therapist should emphasize the magnitude of the head motion required.

Initially, patients are often reluctant to throw their heads down far enough and with enough force. A therapist can help a patient to get a feel for the maneuver by moving her passively through the motion as she pivots on her arms.

When first working on this skill, it is best to start by transferring between the floor and a very low surface. The patient should transfer up and down, moving under control in both directions. As her ability improves, she can gradually increase the height of the surface.

Folding mats are useful for this process: the patient can transfer from a floor mat to progressively higher stacks of folded mats. Starting with minimal height, she can gradually build up to the full distance from the floor to a wheelchair seat. Mats should be added to increase the height of the transfer only when the individual has mastered

the technique at a given height, performing the transfer consistently and with good control.

An individual who runs into difficulty with higher transfers may need to throw her head further down to get a better lift. Another possibility is that she needs to protract her scapulae more forcefully as her buttocks approach the level of the higher surface.

The patient should remember that when she transfers from a higher to a lower surface, gravity provides the downward force. The head should not be thrown forcefully up to move the buttocks downward. Instead, the patient should resist the downward motion to control the descent.

During functional training, it can be useful to approach the transfer from both directions: in addition to practicing transfers between the floor and higher surfaces, a patient can practice moving between the wheelchair and progressively lower surfaces. During these transfers, her feet should rest on the floor rather than on the piled mats. This position more closely replicates the body's orientation at the end of a floor-to-chair transfer.

Once a patient is consistently able to move between the floor and mats stacked to the height of a wheelchair seat, she is ready for practice with a wheelchair. Because a seat cushion adds height to the transfer, the patient should first practice without it. A cushion can be added when the patient masters the transfer without it.

During practice of floor-to-wheelchair transfers, it is common for a patient to catch her buttocks under the wheelchair's seat. This occurs when the individual transfers from a position too close to the chair.

Independent work. Once she has developed some initial skill, a patient can work independently on transfers from a floor mat to higher surfaces or from a wheelchair to lower surfaces. Tumbles that occur while an individual transfers between the floor and higher surfaces are usually not a great problem. Early on, before she has become very skillful, a patient practices transfers to and from fairly low surfaces and does not have far to fall. By the time she works on higher transfers, she has developed some degree of control.

Transfer practice between a wheelchair and lower surfaces presents more of a problem. Early in the training, when potential falls would occur from the full height of the wheelchair seat, the patient will not yet have developed enough control to break her fall. Transfers should be practiced with guarding until the patient can perform them safely.

Straight Lift from Floor
(Front or Back Approach)

Before working on these maneuvers, a patient should be proficient in even transfers without equipment. She should also be able to push down with her arms to lift her body while in a sitting position, starting with her hands positioned close to her shoulders. This ability can be practiced while sitting in a wheelchair between parallel bars, or while sitting on a floor mat between two chairs.

Both front- and back-approach transfers from the floor to a wheelchair involve lifting the body by pushing down with the arms. Using the front approach, a person starts from a kneeling position facing the wheelchair, with her hands on the armrests or seat. In the back-approach transfer, the transfer's starting position is sitting on the floor facing outward, with the hands on the front of the wheelchair seat. Using either approach, the person lifts her body from the starting position by leaning toward the wheelchair and pushing straight downward. Once her buttocks have passed the seat and she has lifted as high as she can in this manner, she tucks her head and protracts her scapulae to lift her buttocks further.

The patient should practice this maneuver while being spotted. If she has adequate strength, it should not take many attempts to master. If the patient does not lift her buttocks high enough, the therapist may need to give her verbal and tactile cues to encourage her to tuck her head lower and protract her scapulae more forcefully.

Similar to side-approach floor-to-chair transfers, back-approach transfers can be practiced between the floor and progressively higher stacks of folding mats. Front-approach transfers cannot be developed in this manner because the postures and actions involved in this approach require a relatively tall surface on which to push.

Independent work. If an individual has some degree of control, this skill can be practiced independently over a floor mat. Someone who has difficulty with the lift facing away from the chair can start by practicing transferring from a raised surface to the chair and can work from progressively lower surfaces as her skill improves.

Turn Body to Drop onto Wheelchair Seat

Before practicing this maneuver, the patient should be able to lift her body above her wheelchair seat from a kneeling position. Once she has lifted high enough, she lets go of an armrest and throws her arm and head away from the armrest. This causes her body to turn and drop onto the wheelchair seat.

A patient who lands on a hip rather than on her buttocks may not have lifted her body high enough initially. Prior to releasing the armrest, she should lift her buttocks higher by tucking her head lower, and protracting her scapulae more. The problem may also occur when the height of the lift is adequate but the patient does not turn far enough before landing. In these instances, the

---

PROBLEM-SOLVING EXERCISE 11–3

Your patient is independent in even and slightly uneven transfers without equipment. He wants to learn to transfer from the floor to his wheelchair.

This individual has 5/5 strength in all of his upper extremity musculature. His hip flexors test 2/5 bilaterally, and all myotomes below this level test 0/5. When he attempts to perform a sit-up, his abdominal musculature has palpable contractions from the ribs to the pubis.

Pinprick and light touch are intact in the C1 through T12 key sensory points bilaterally, and impaired in L1 bilaterally. Both sensory modalities are absent below L1, with the exception that sensation is present at the anus.

The patient's joint range of motion and muscle flexibility are normal in all extremities, with the following exceptions: shoulder extension is 10 degrees bilaterally, and passive straight-leg raise is 70 degrees bilaterally.

- Classify this person's spinal cord injury using the ASIA classification system.
- Which method of floor-to-chair transfer is this patient likely to achieve most readily?
- What strength and range should the therapeutic exercise program emphasize to facilitate the attainment of this goal?
- Describe a functional training program for this patient.

patient should be instructed to throw her arm and head more forcefully.

Independent work.   Once a person has developed some degree of control over this maneuver, she can practice alone. The wheelchair should be placed on or in front of a floor mat.

TRANSFER TECHNIQUES AND THERAPEUTIC STRATEGIES FOLLOWING INCOMPLETE SPINAL CORD INJURY

The actions that an individual can use to perform transfers after sustaining an incomplete spinal cord injury will depend primarily on her voluntary motor function. A person who retains or regains only sensory function below her injury (ASIA B) will utilize the techniques that are used by people with complete spinal cord injuries, as just described. A person who has minimal motor sparing or return (ASIA C) is likely to utilize similar movement patterns, but may be able to add trunk or lower extremity actions to make the tasks easier. An individual who has significant motor function below her lesion (ASIA D) may be able to perform transfers using more normal movement patterns.

Another factor that can have an impact on the performance of transfers is spasticity. People with incomplete lesions tend to exhibit more spasticity than do people with complete lesions, and spasticity tends to be more severe among those with ASIA B and C lesions.[7, 10, 15] Involuntary muscle contractions can interfere with the functional use of voluntary motor function that is preserved below the lesion. When elevated muscle tone interferes with function, the rehabilitation team can work with the patient to reduce the abnormal tone.[j] In addition, the therapist and patient should note the conditions and bodily motions that tend to elicit involuntary muscle contractions. They can then work together in an effort to find ways in which the patient can transfer without causing these involuntary contractions. For example, the patient may find that she is less likely to experience involuntary contractions if she moves slowly during the transfer.

Perhaps the most challenging aspect of transfer training after an incomplete spinal cord injury is determining the methods that the individual can utilize to perform the skills. Each patient has

a unique pattern of muscle strength and weakness, spasticity, joint range of motion, muscle flexibility, and body build. It is often difficult to predict what methods of performing transfers will best suit the individual; some physical maneuvers will be within her potential and others will not. Functional training involves problem solving as the therapist works with the patient to help her discover and develop the movement strategies that will enable her to achieve her functional goals.

When deciding between transfer techniques, therapists should keep in mind the fact that incomplete spinal cord injuries are associated with a greater potential for motor return than are complete injuries.[3, 5] When motor function is preserved below the lesion, use of transfer techniques that utilize this function may help develop more normal movement patterns and enhance the individual's potential for future functional ambulation.[1]

When voluntary motor function is present below the lesion, the therapist and patient should work together to find ways to use this musculature functionally. With each task practiced, the patient should be encouraged to use her trunk and lower extremity musculature to the extent possible. When muscles below the lesion are strong enough that a patient has the potential to learn to perform a task without compensatory strategies, the patient and therapist should work together to develop this ability. When muscles are present but too weak to perform a task, their use can be combined with compensatory strategies during functional activities. For example, an individual who has 2+/5 or weaker strength in her hip flexors will be unable to lift her leg onto a mat or bed using just these muscles. She can, however, utilize this musculature to enhance her performance of the task, flexing her hip actively while lifting the leg with her arm.

Accessory Skills

Accessory skills include the various activities that are performed immediately before or after a person moves to or from a wheelchair: stabilizing and moving the body in a wheelchair, moving the feet on and off of the footrests, repositioning the footrests and an armrest, and moving the legs on and off of the mat or bed. A person who has either a complete injury or only sensory function below her lesion will use compensatory strategies, described earlier in the chapter, to perform these activities. A person who has voluntary motor function below her lesion will be able to use the

functioning trunk and lower extremity musculature to perform these skills more easily, with more
normal movement patterns, or both.

Therapeutic strategies. The therapeutic strategies used to develop accessory skills after incomplete injuries are similar to those used for patients
with complete injuries. The patient practices moving her body and manipulating the wheelchair's
components, using motions that make maximal
use of innervated musculature. The therapist can
provide assistance as needed, and engage the
patient in problem solving to discover movement
strategies that are most effective and efficient.

Even Transfers

People with complete injuries transfer by propping on their arms and using the head-hips relationship to move between surfaces. The transfer
techniques that people with incomplete injuries
can use depend largely on the motor function
present below their lesions. An individual who
has minimal sparing in her trunk and lower
extremity musculature can utilize techniques similar to those used by people with complete
injuries. She is likely to find transfers easier to
master, however, because she can use functioning
trunk and leg musculature to help lift her weight
and maintain her balance.

A person who retains or regains significant
innervation of her trunk and lower extremity musculature may be able to transfer using either a
stand-pivot or a squat-pivot technique. In these
transfer methods, most or all of the weight is supported on the legs.

A stand-pivot transfer involves coming to
stand, turning, and sitting on the mat or bed. The
arms may or may not be used to assist with these
maneuvers. In the sit-to-stand component of the
transfer, the individual moves her buttocks forward
in the chair, leans her trunk forward, and stands.
She can perform each of these actions as a discreet
step under control, or can combine the forward
lean and stand steps and move rapidly to utilize
momentum to make the task easier.[18] During the
stand-to-sit component of the transfer, the individual should control her descent through eccentric
contraction of her hip and knee extensors.

In a squat-pivot transfer, the person does not
come to a full standing position. Instead, she
remains in a "squat" position, leaning her trunk
forward and lifting her buttocks enough to clear
the wheel. During a squat-pivot transfer, the person can utilize both the head-hips relationship and

momentum to enhance her performance as she
moves between surfaces. With one hand on the
wheelchair and one on the mat or bed, she can use
her arms to help maintain her balance while she
lifts and turns her buttocks toward the mat or bed.

Therapeutic strategies. The patient should
practice even transfers, using techniques that
enable her to utilize her innervated musculature
and move between surfaces as safely and independently as possible. With the therapist's assistance and guidance, the patient can try various
strategies to discover ways in which she can move
her body most efficiently between surfaces.

Regardless of the transfer strategy used, the
patient may benefit from practicing the different
components of the task. If performing a stand-
pivot transfer, she can practice coming to stand
and returning to sit under control. If she has inadequate strength or control to perform these actions
from a wheelchair, she may benefit from practice
of sit-to-stand and stand-to-sit from an elevated
mat. Practice of these skills will be easiest if the
mat is elevated enough that the patient is close to
a standing position when her feet are on the floor
and her buttocks are on the mat. As her strength
and control improve, she can practice with the
mat in progressively lower positions until she can
stand up and return to sitting under control from
a surface the height of her wheelchair seat.

A patient learning a squat-pivot transfer may
benefit from practice lifting her buttocks and moving laterally while short-sitting on a mat. If she
has difficulty with this maneuver, she may benefit
from practice lifting her buttocks while sitting on
a mat that is elevated slightly. As her strength and
control improve, she can practice with the mat in
progressively lower positions until she can lift her
buttocks and move laterally on a surface the
height of her wheelchair seat.

In addition to functional training, the therapeutic program should include strengthening of the
muscles involved in transfers. The strengthening
program should emphasize scapular protraction
and depression, elbow extension, and hip and knee
extension. Exercise of these muscles in closed-
chain positions may be most beneficial because
these positions will simulate the conditions in
which the muscles function during transfers. Innervated muscles in the trunk should also be strengthened[k] to enhance the patient's ability to control her
trunk during transfers. Strengthening exercises for

---

[k] Chapter 10 presents strategies for strengthening trunk musculature.

limb and trunk musculature should address both concentric and eccentric contractions, since transfers involve both types of contraction.

Floor Transfers

Three methods of floor-to-wheelchair transfers are presented earlier in this chapter: side-, front-, and back-approach. Of these transfers, the back-approach is most easily adapted to utilize lower extremity musculature. In this transfer, the individual sits facing away from her chair, places her palms on the front of the seat, and pushes down to lift her buttocks. An individual who has some capacity to extend her hips and knees forcefully can do so while pushing with her arms to lift her buttocks onto the seat.

An alternate floor-to-wheelchair transfer technique utilizes the lower extremities to a greater extent. To perform this transfer, the individual assumes a half-kneeling position in front of the wheelchair, facing sideways to the chair (Figure 11–20). If lower extremity strength is asymmetrical, the stronger limb should be in the forward position (foot planted), as the forward limb will perform most of the work of the transfer. Once she is in a half-kneel position, the person can either place both hands on the wheelchair seat, or place one hand on the seat and one on her knee. Pushing down with her arms and legs, she lifts and turns her buttocks onto the seat. She may

find this maneuver to be easier if she rocks her head and trunk forward and laterally away from the wheelchair during this lift.

Therapeutic strategies. The back-approach transfer can be practiced using the strategies presented earlier in the chapter: the patient can practice transferring between the floor and progressively higher stacks of folding mats until she can transfer to and from a surface the height of a wheelchair seat. During this practice, the patient should be encouraged to use her leg musculature as much as possible. She and the therapist can experiment with different placements of her feet (at various distances from the buttocks) to determine the foot position that makes the transfer easiest. They can also try different strategies such as leaning the trunk toward or away from the chair during the lift, or starting the transfer with the elbows (instead of the hands) on the wheelchair seat. Because the legs can be used to support the body's weight, the arms can be repositioned during the transfer.

A patient who plans to learn the half-kneeling transfer approach may benefit from preparatory practice in quadruped, kneeling, and half-kneeling. She can practice assuming each of these positions, as well as stabilizing against resistance applied by the therapist, weight-shifting under control, and moving between positions.[13, 17] In this manner, she can develop her ability to control her body and move between the various postures involved in the transfer.

The patient can also practice lifting her buttocks from the half-kneel position. This task can be practiced with the patient half-kneeling in front of a stack of folding mats. Initial practice may begin with a stack of mats that is lower than the height of a wheelchair seat. As the patient's ability develops, she can practice lifting her buttocks onto progressively higher stacks of mats. Once she has developed the ability to transfer onto a stack of mats the height of her wheelchair seat, she can practice transferring onto the chair itself.

In addition to functional training, the therapeutic program should include strengthening of the muscles involved in transfers. The strengthening program should emphasize scapular depression, elbow extension, hip and knee extension, and trunk musculature. Exercise of the extremity muscles in closed-chain positions may be most beneficial, as these positions simulate the conditions in which the muscles function during transfers. Strengthening exercises for limb and trunk musculature should address both concentric and

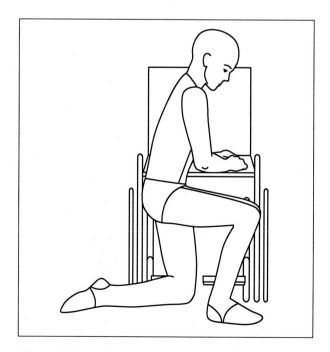

Figure 11–20.   *Half-kneeling position for floor-to-wheelchair transfer using lower extremities.*

eccentric contractions because transfers involve both types of contraction.

SUMMARY

- Transfers involve moving the body from one surface to another. The ability to transfer in and out of a wheelchair is a crucial functional skill for anyone who uses a wheelchair for mobility.

- A person with a complete spinal cord injury who wishes to function independently must learn compensatory strategies for performing transfers. This chapter presents a variety of techniques that can be used to perform even and uneven transfers to and from a wheelchair.

- The movement strategies possible for a person with an incomplete spinal cord injury will depend on the extent of motor sparing or return below her lesion. If she has little or no voluntary motor function below her lesion, she will use movement strategies similar to those used by people with complete injuries. If she has more significant motor function in her trunk and lower extremities, she may be able to use more normal movement strategies to perform transfers.

- During rehabilitation, the therapist and patient work together to discover the movement strategies that will enable the patient to perform transfers most effectively. The therapeutic program then consists of activities directed at developing the strength, range of motion, and skill needed to perform these functional tasks. This chapter presents a variety of strategies for developing the skills involved.

- The therapist and patient should take appropriate precautions during transfer training to prevent motion of unstable vertebrae, skin abrasions and pressure ulcers, overstretching of the long finger flexors and the low back, and injury from falls.

12

Wheelchairs and Wheelchair Skills

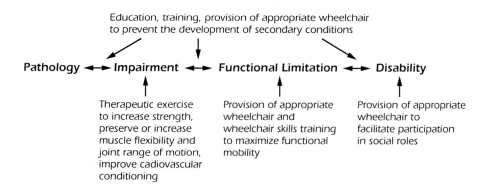

Education, training, provision of appropriate wheelchair to prevent the development of secondary conditions

Pathology ⟷ Impairment ⟷ Functional Limitation ⟷ Disability

Therapeutic exercise to increase strength, preserve or increase muscle flexibility and joint range of motion, improve cadiovascular conditioning

Provision of appropriate wheelchair and wheelchair skills training to maximize functional mobility

Provision of appropriate wheelchair to facilitate participation in social roles

Most people with spinal cord injuries use wheelchairs as their sole means of locomotion. This is true even for those who learn to walk with knee-ankle-foot orthoses (KAFOs) and assistive devices during their rehabilitation.[18] If ambulation is impaired, a wheelchair provides a faster and more energy-efficient means of mobility than does walking. Even people who have such low lesions that they retain active hip flexion and knee extension, and are able to walk with ankle-foot orthoses (AFOs) and assistive devices, find wheelchair mobility to be faster and to require less energy than walking.[59, 60]

When ambulation is impaired, an appropriate wheelchair and cushion are essential for preservation of the individual's physical health and maximization of his functional independence. During rehabilitation after spinal cord injury, the rehabilitation team works together with the patient to select a wheelchair and cushion[a] that will best meet his needs. They also work together to develop the patient's ability to function optimally with this equipment. These tasks, equipment

selection and training in its use, are inextricably linked; the individual's capabilities influence the selection and adjustment of his wheelchair, and the wheelchair's characteristics in turn influence the skills that its user will need to develop.

This chapter presents information on wheelchair selection and adjustment, wheelchair skills, and training strategies for these skills. The descriptions of equipment, techniques, and training presented here should be used as a guide, not as a set of hard-and-fast rules. The equipment required and motions used to perform any functional task vary among people. This variability is due to differences in body build, skill level, range of motion, muscle tone, and patterns of strength and weakness. During rehabilitation, the therapist and patient should work together to determine the equipment and functional techniques that best suit that particular individual.

PRECAUTIONS

Following spinal cord injury, activities performed in a wheelchair can cause a variety of problems if appropriate precautions are not taken. Table 12–1

---

[a] Wheelchair cushions and their selection are addressed in Chapter 6.

269

TABLE 12–1.   PRECAUTIONS DURING WHEELCHAIR USE AND WHEELCHAIR SKILL TRAINING

Potential Problems	Wheelchair Activities that Place Patients at Risk	Precautions
Excessive motion at site of vertebral instability, potentially causing additional neurologic and orthopedic damage	Any activity involving excessive motion or muscular action at or near site of unstable spine. Examples: Upright activities while the spine remains unstable, practice falling backward from wheelie position when spine is not fully healed.	• Strictly adhere to orthopedic precautions. • Check fit of vertebral orthosis with patient sitting in wheelchair. • When the spine is unstable, avoid activities that may cause motion or strong muscular contraction at site of instability.
Skin abrasions and pressure ulcers	Sitting in wheelchair more than 15 to 20 minutes.	• Provide patient with pressure-relieving wheelchair cushion and appropriately fit and adjusted wheelchair. • Pressure reliefs every 15 to 20 minutes when first sitting, with possible increase in time between reliefs if skin tolerance allows. • Proper sitting posture whenever in wheelchair. • Monitor skin status and adjust sitting time, pressure reliefs, and equipment as indicated.
	Stair negotiation on buttocks.	• Protective padding over buttocks and sacral region during this activity.
Overstretched low back, resulting in diminished capacity for functional independence	Prolonged sitting in wheelchair with lumbar spine in kyphotic posture.	• Proper sitting posture whenever in wheelchair. • Adequate postural support provided by wheelchair and cushion.
Postural deformity	Chronic positioning in wheelchair with improper posture.	• Proper sitting posture whenever in wheelchair. • Adequate postural support provided by wheelchair and cushion. • Access devices of power wheelchairs positioned so that rider can utilize them while maintaining good sitting posture.
Shoulder pain	Chronic use of manual wheelchair.	• Proper sitting posture whenever propelling wheelchair. • Properly fit and adjusted wheelchair. • Training in efficient propulsion pattern. • Exercise program to develop strength, endurance, and flexibility in shoulders.
Injury from tip or fall from wheelchair	Reaching outside of base of support; negotiation of environmental obstacles such as inclines, curbs, curbcuts, doorways, or uneven terrain; sports[13,24,26]	• Properly fit and adjusted wheelchair, with seat belt and antitipping devices when indicated. • Education and training in safe use of wheelchair and safe falling techniques. • Appropriate guarding during functional training.

presents a summary of precautions for wheelchair use and wheelchair skill training. These precautions should be taken whenever the individual sits in a wheelchair, starting as soon as out-of-bed activities are initiated after the injury. Sitting posture and shoulder pain are discussed in more detail as follows.

Sitting Posture

Because people with spinal cord injuries typically spend a good deal of time sitting in wheelchairs, their posture while using wheelchairs is important. Proper sitting posture (Figure 12–1A and B) will greatly enhance functional status and physical health.

Poor sitting posture is a prime source of overstretched low backs. A person who habitually sits with his buttocks forward on the wheelchair seat is likely to stretch his lumbar area (Figure 12–1C). The resulting excessive flexibility in his low back will interfere with his ability to perform functional activities such as independent transfers or rolling in bed.[b] To preserve beneficial tightness in his low back, an individual with a spinal cord injury should sit with his buttocks well back on the seat whenever he is in a wheelchair.

During the acute and early rehabilitation phase after spinal cord injury, it can be tempting to place a patient in a poor sitting posture, especially if the individual has a high lesion and has not yet developed the ability to maintain an upright sitting posture. Pulling the patient's buttocks out (forward) on the seat places him in a more stable position and enables him to stay upright more easily. Although this practice may seem to be sensible in the short run, it is likely to stretch the patient's back. In addition, it can encourage the habit of sitting in this posture. To preserve low back tightness, the therapist and patient should work together to develop the patient's ability to sit (and habit of sitting) upright with his buttocks well back on the seat.

In addition to over stretching the low back, poor sitting posture can lead to the development of pressure ulcers. Pelvic obliquity, lateral trunk lean, and posterior pelvic tilt alter the distribution of pressure on the skin,[28, 45] resulting in increased risk of skin breakdown over the areas of elevated pressure. Habitual improper positioning in a wheelchair can also result in scoliosis, thoracic kyphosis, and forward head. These postural abnormalities can, in turn, lead to reduced functional capacity, impaired respiratory function, and increased vulnerability to skin breakdown.

To avoid the development of posture-related problems, the patient should receive instruction on the risks of sitting with his spine and extremities improperly aligned, and should develop the skills

---

[b] Chapter 9 explains the link between low back tightness and the performance of functional skills.

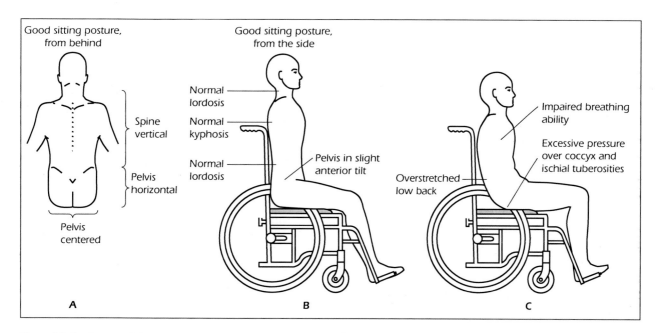

Figure 12–1. Impact of sitting posture on pressure distribution, low back flexibility, and breathing ability. **(A)** Good sitting posture, posterior view. **(B)** Good sitting posture: pressure distributed well, low back protected by proper positioning, and torso positioned to optimize breathing ability. **(C)** Poor sitting posture: low back overstretched, excessive pressure borne over coccyx and ischial tuberosities, and breathing ability impaired.

needed to maintain appropriate posture. He must also utilize a wheelchair and cushion that provide adequate postural support. The wheelchair and cushion should be configured so that they enable the patient to propel his wheelchair while maintaining proper postural alignment. For example, a power wheelchair with a hand-operated joystick control should be aligned so that the patient can access the joystick without leaning his trunk laterally.

Shoulder Pain

Shoulder pain is a common problem among people with chronic spinal cord injury.[c] Its incidence increases with time after injury. Repetitive stress from manual wheelchair propulsion is one of the causes of this problem.[2, 14, 27, 31, 44, 49, 52] Because the upper extremities are used to perform virtually all activities when the legs are paralyzed, many tasks involved in independent functioning at home and in the community are painful for individuals with shoulder pain.[9, 44] For this reason, shoulder pain is associated with a reduction in functional independence.[15]

Although the link between manual wheelchair use and shoulder pain has been well established, the solutions to this problem are not as clear. Exercise programs to develop endurance, balanced strength, and flexibility in the shoulder girdle musculature may help wheelchair users avoid the development of shoulder pain.[27, 44, 49] Sitting posture is another important consideration; abnormal alignment of the spine and shoulder girdle may interfere with the shoulder's functioning, resulting in abnormal stresses and increased risk of injury.[27] Thus, a properly fit and adjusted wheelchair may help prevent the development of chronic shoulder pain by providing good postural support. Moreover, training in efficient propulsion techniques, and a wheelchair with components and alignment that allow for propulsion with reduced stress at the shoulder joint, are likely to be beneficial.[2, 27] Finally, follow-up care for people with spinal cord injuries should include monitoring for the development of upper extremity overuse injuries, and appropriate treatment when these injuries occur.

WHEELCHAIRS

Wheelchair selection involves deciding between dozens of options in size, style, and components.

The wheelchair's size and features must be chosen carefully; an improperly prescribed wheelchair can result in pressure ulcers, deformity, chronic shoulder pain, and impaired functional status. A properly prescribed and adjusted wheelchair will maximize its owner's function and health.

The ideal wheelchair would provide its user with optimal postural support and safety while allowing independent mobility in all environments, with minimal stress to the upper extremities. It would also be affordable, durable, and stylish. Unfortunately, this ideal wheelchair does not exist, as many of the qualities listed are mutually exclusive. For example, a manual wheelchair with an anterior axle position is easier to propel but is less safe because it will tip over backwards more easily, a chair that provides superior postural support may restrict function, and a wheelchair made of durable materials is likely to be more expensive. Because each option for wheelchair alignment and components has both benefits and drawbacks, wheelchair selection and adjustment involve compromises. The rehabilitation team should work with the wheelchair user to obtain a chair that best matches that individual's abilities, physical characteristics, home and community environments, lifestyle, preferences, and priorities.[29, 51]

When the prospective user has a recent spinal cord injury, wheelchair prescription should *ideally* be delayed until functional training is well under way. During the weeks and months after injury, an individual's physical status and functional abilities are likely to change dramatically. As a result, his equipment needs will change significantly: a wheelchair that is appropriate for someone just beginning his rehabilitation may be completely unsuitable two months later. If a wheelchair is prescribed prematurely, it is not likely to be optimally matched to the individual's ultimate needs. This is particularly true when there is significant motor return. Unfortunately, the trend toward increasingly shortened inpatient rehabilitation stays necessitates the selection of equipment earlier post injury.

Options

Power wheelchairs. Power wheelchairs can provide a means of independent mobility for people who are unable to propel manual chairs at home or in the community. Models with power tilt, recline, or tilt and recline are available for people who cannot perform independent pressure

---

[c] The other upper extremity joints are also often painful, but the shoulders are most commonly affected.[2, 14]

reliefs without these features. Different control options are available for power chairs, allowing the user to control the chair using his breath or motions of his upper extremities, head, chin, or mouth. Because of the different control options, power chairs can make independent mobility possible for virtually anyone with a spinal cord injury, no matter how high the lesion.

Power wheelchairs are necessary equipment for people who cannot function independently using manual wheelchairs. They have drawbacks, however, that make their use unwise for individuals who are capable of functioning without them. Power chairs are bulky, requiring more space to maneuver than manual wheelchairs. They are also extremely heavy. Because of their size and weight, power chairs cannot be transported in cars[d] and are restricted to wheelchair-accessible environments. (A manual wheelchair can often be propelled through narrow doorways and taken up and down stairs or curbs independently or with assistance.) Perhaps the major disadvantage of a power chair is that its user does not receive the physical benefits that are gained from propulsion of a manual wheelchair.

Despite the drawbacks of power wheelchairs, a number of factors may make a power chair the most appropriate choice for independent mobility. These factors include inadequate motor function for manual wheelchair propulsion, vocational or educational activities that involve negotiation of long distances or hilly terrain, and medical or orthopedic conditions that preclude the use of a manual wheelchair for functional distances.

People with C4 and higher complete tetraplegia lack the motor function needed to propel a manual chair and clearly require power chairs. People with C5 tetraplegia are often able to propel manual wheelchairs for limited distances indoors, but require power chairs for mobility in the community. Some individuals with C6 tetraplegia function well with manual chairs and choose not to utilize power chairs. Others find that, although they can propel manual chairs over even surfaces, they are unable to function independently in all of the environments that they encounter during the course of a typical day or week. These "marginal pushers" may find manual wheelchair propulsion

to be too slow or too tiring, and decide that powered mobility is more suitable to their priorities and lifestyles.

Power chairs come in a variety of styles. The major choices when selecting a power wheelchair are its base, seating system, controller, and input device(s). These components are described in the following sections. The commonly prescribed options are summarized in Table 12–2.

Integrated frame and seat vs. power base. Conventional power wheelchairs are made with the seat and frame of the chair constructed as an integrated unit. In more recent designs of power wheelchairs, the seat and the main chassis of the chair are separate systems. The power base includes the chair's frame, drive wheels, casters, motors, controllers, and battery. A separate seating system is attached to this base.

Seating system. The seating system includes the seat, back, armrests, and legrests of the chair. It is mounted on the wheel base. Seating systems may be stationary or have the capacity to tilt, recline, or both tilt and recline. Pressure-relieving and contoured backrests, postural supports, and armrest troughs can be incorporated in the system to promote optimal function, posture, and skin integrity.

Access device. Access devices, also called input devices or drive controls, are the components that wheelchair riders use to drive their chairs. They are also used to direct other functions performed by the chair, such as legrest elevation or seating system tilt or recline, and can be used to interface with environmental control units and computers. A chair may have one or more access devices, depending on its user's needs and abilities.

Controller. The controller is the electronic "brain" of the wheelchair. It receives the signals sent by the patient through the input device, and directs the wheelchair's motors to carry out their various functions. Programmable controllers allow for the adjustment of a variety of parameters such as maximum speed and rate of acceleration and deceleration.

Manual wheelchairs. Manual wheelchairs are lighter and smaller than power chairs, so they can be transported in cars and can be taken into environments that are not accessible to wheelchairs. More importantly, manual wheelchair propulsion can result in improved physical fitness,[6, 54] which can lead to enhanced performance of functional

---

[d] For this reason, a manual wheelchair should be prescribed in addition to the power chair, for use when travel in a car is necessary. The exceptions are "transportable" power chairs and power packs that can be added to manual wheelchairs. Both of these can be disassembled and loaded into a car, but they are heavy and difficult to load.

TABLE 12-2.   OPTIONS AVAILABLE IN POWER WHEELCHAIR COMPONENTS

Components	Options	Characteristics
Power bases	Casters in front	Larger turning radius.
	Casters in rear	Smaller turning radius.
Seating systems	Stationary (standard)	Simpler mechanics and electronics, less expensive. Does not require long wheelbase for stability. Appropriate only for individuals who can independently perform pressure reliefs without tilt or recline feature.
	Tilt	Provides pressure relief while maintaining constant angle between seat and back. Less likely than recline to elicit spasticity, less likely to alter user's sitting posture upon return to upright. Requires long wheel base for posterior stability of chair during tilt.
	Recline	Provides pressure relief by reclining backrest. Knees and hips extend when back reclines, with possible benefits to joint range of motion. Intermittent catheterization easier in reclined position. Creates shear forces on back, although these forces may be minimized with "zero shear" models. Reclining motion may elicit spasticity, causing user's sitting posture to shift. Requires long wheel base for posterior stability of chair during recline.
	Tilt/recline combination	Allows either tilt or recline. Indicated for individuals who need tilt feature for pressure reliefs due to spasticity, but need recline feature for intermittent catheterization. Requires long wheel base for posterior stability of chair during tilt or recline.
Control options	Proportional	Works like the gas pedal of a car: commands can be graded, with the chair's response proportional to the magnitude of the signal. Example: the rider pushes a joystick over a short arc of motion to make the chair go slowly, pushes the joystick further to go faster.
	Microswitch	Works like a light switch: commands cannot be graded; the signal can provide an "on" or "off" command to a function. Example: the rider sips on a straw to make the chair go forward. The chair's speed is preset, and not proportional to the strength of the sip.
Control options	Momentary	The chair performs a function while the rider delivers the command, but stops performing the function when the rider stops. Example: the chair goes forward while the rider holds the joystick forward, but stops when the rider releases the joystick.
	Latched	Once signaled, the chair performs a function until it receives a signal to stop. Example: the rider sips on a straw to signal the chair to go forward, but does not have to keep sipping to continue going forward.
Access devices	Joystick	Typically proportional control, functioning in momentary mode. Joystick swivels on its base, wheelchair user pushes it forward, backward, right, left, or any angle between these directions to control the direction and speed of the chair's motion. Due to the joystick's simplicity, is the preferred input device for those who are capable of using it. Can be mounted for driving using motions of the hand, chin, mouth or head. Joystick/user interface can be adapted to maximize comfort and function.
	Peachtree head control	Proportional control, typically functions in momentary mode. Sensors embedded in headrest detect wheelchair driver's head position. Driver moves head to control the chair.
	Breath control (sip and puff)	Microswitch control, typically functions in both momentary and latched modes. Wheelchair driver signals chair through a straw, using hard and soft sips and puffs. Can be difficult for some drivers to master, due to the relative complexity of the commands.

TABLE 12–2. *(Continued)*

Components	Options	Characteristics
	Tongue-touch keypad	Microswitch control, functions in latched mode. Sensors embedded in custom-molded device resembling orthodentic retainer worn in roof of mouth. Driver signals chair by contacting sensors with tongue. Can be difficult for some drivers to master, due to the relative complexity of the commands.
	Additional input devices	Additional input devices may be used in combination with any of the devices listed above. These devices can be used to signal the chair to stop ("kill switch"), change modes (between driving and reclining, for example), or to perform functions such as legrest control and pressure relief. These switches can be mounted anywhere on the chair, depending on what motions the driver will use to operate the switch. Some of the more commonly used types of auxiliary switches are:
		Toggle switch: switch pivots in one plane, operated by pushing it.
		Proximity switch: sensor detects when body part comes close; operated by moving a body part close to switch.
		Button switch: switch is a button or pad that can be depressed; operated by pressing or hitting it.
		Leaf switch: thin ribbon-like switch, activated when bent; operated by pressing it.

Sources: references 1, 8, 22, 33, 56.

tasks. A significant disadvantage of manual wheelchair propulsion is that it can lead to the development of upper extremity pain due to chronic overuse.

Manual wheelchairs are available in standard weight, lightweight, and ultralight models. Standard weight chairs are heavy, and they have relatively limited options in size, components, and adjustability. Lightweight chairs are somewhat lighter but are still relatively heavy and have limited options. Ultralight wheelchairs are made of durable lightweight materials and are generally available with more options in size, components, and adjustability. Ultralight chairs allow more efficient propulsion, reducing the energy demands on the user[20] and making independent propulsion possible for some individuals who are unable to propel standard weight chairs.[30, 43] The ultralight models also tend to look better than other chairs. Their sporty colors and designs can make the user look less impaired, which can facilitate his reintegration into the community.

The components of a manual wheelchair are illustrated in Figure 12–2. Virtually all of these components have several options from which to choose when selecting a wheelchair. The commonly prescribed options for these components are summarized in Table 12–3.

Selecting Wheelchair Components and Manufacturers

In choosing between the available options for wheelchair components, the prospective owner and the rehabilitation team should weigh the benefits and drawbacks of each option. Trial runs in wheelchairs that have the features under consideration are critical to this choice. Different manufacturers have their own designs for each component, and seemingly minor differences between components may impact significantly on the wheelchair user's comfort, safety, and ability to function. What seems to be a good option when looking at the manufacturer's literature may turn out to be unsuitable when the chair arrives. Until an individual (particularly one with impaired upper extremity function) tries out a given design, it is often impossible to determine with certainty that he will be capable of using it. Someone who tries a "similar" wheel-

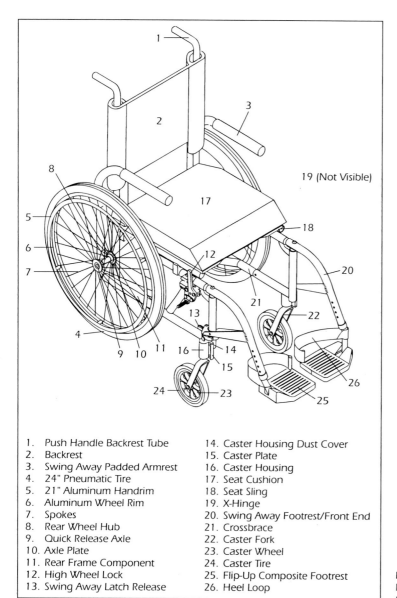

19 (Not Visible)

1. Push Handle Backrest Tube
2. Backrest
3. Swing Away Padded Armrest
4. 24" Pneumatic Tire
5. 21" Aluminum Handrim
6. Aluminum Wheel Rim
7. Spokes
8. Rear Wheel Hub
9. Quick Release Axle
10. Axle Plate
11. Rear Frame Component
12. High Wheel Lock
13. Swing Away Latch Release
14. Caster Housing Dust Cover
15. Caster Plate
16. Caster Housing
17. Seat Cushion
18. Seat Sling
19. X-Hinge
20. Swing Away Footrest/Front End
21. Crossbrace
22. Caster Fork
23. Caster Wheel
24. Caster Tire
25. Flip-Up Composite Footrest
26. Heel Loop

Figure 12–2. Manual wheelchair components labeled. (Reproduced with permission from Sunrise Medical, Fresno, CA.)

chair but does not actually sit in, propel, and transfer in and out of the exact model being considered for purchase may find that he cannot function optimally when his own chair arrives.

When selecting a wheelchair, the prospective user and the clinicians determine the size, style, and components most suitable to the individual's dimensions, abilities, activities, preferences, and the environments in which he will function. Another important choice is the manufacturer of the wheelchair. The manufacturer of choice will in part be determined by the wheelchair's specifications. Generally, a limited number of manufacturers will produce a chair with the desired characteristics. Other factors to consider when selecting

brands include cost, durability, chair weight, the overall dimensions of the chair, availability of replacement parts and service facilities, warranty specifications, and reputation of the manufacturer. When selecting a power wheelchair, the chair's maximum speed, stopping distance, obstacle climbing ability, range, maneuverability, static and dynamic stability, and performance in different climate conditions are also important considerations.[1,8] This information is available from manufacturers.

Although aesthetics were not formerly considered to be an important consideration in wheelchair design or selection, the significance of this area is now recognized.[55] Modern wheelchairs come in a variety of colors and styles. Wheelchair

TABLE 12–3. OPTIONS AVAILABLE IN MANUAL WHEELCHAIR COMPONENTS

Components	Options	Advantages	Disadvantages
Frame	Folding	Requires less space when folded, does not require good hand function to load into car, provides shock absorption, allows all wheels to contact the ground on uneven terrain.	Heavier, less durable. Propulsion less efficient.
	Rigid	Frame stiffness makes propulsion more efficient. More durable, lighter. Angle between seat and backrest often adjustable.	Wheels must be removed to load into car. Propulsion over uneven terrain more difficult.
Backrest	Fixed height	May be lighter and more durable.	Back height cannot be adjusted.
	Adjustable height	Allows custom adjustment to maximize function and comfort; can change back height as needs change.	May be heavier and less durable.
Backrest	Standard upholstery	Allows convenient folding.	Stretches over time, resulting in discomfort and reduced postural support.
	Solid back	Provides superior postural support.	Some designs cause wheelchair user to sit in more anterior position on seat, resulting in reduced propulsion efficiency and reduced area for distributing pressure on sitting surface. Must be removed to fold chair.
Seat	Standard upholstery (sling)	Allows folding.	Causes hip adduction and inward rotation, reducing postural stability and comfort, and altering pressure distribution.
	Solid	Provides superior postural support. Some models allow folding.	
Wheel attachments	Standard	Less expensive.	Require tools for removal and replacement.
	Quick release	Wheels easily removed and replaced for car transfers or adjusting axle position.	More expensive.
Axle position	Fixed	Lighter.	Axle position cannot be altered.
	Adjustable	Allows custom adjustment for optimal function, posture, and minimizing stress on shoulders.	Anterior and superior axle positions can increase risk of tips/falls.
Wheel camber	Vertical (standard)	Overall chair width narrower.	Less lateral stability than cambered, propulsion over side slope more difficult.
	Cambered	Gives chair superior lateral stability. Reduced rolling resistance and downward turning tendency on side slope make propulsion easier.	Increases overall width of chair.
Wheel locks	High-mount	Easier to reach, can be equipped with extensions to make operation easier.	Can injure thumb, especially during obstacle negotiation.
	Low-mount	Will not injure user's thumb.	More difficult to reach and operate.

(Cont.)

TABLE 12–3.   *(Continued)*

Components	Options	Advantages	Disadvantages
Wheel and caster design	Wire spokes	Lighter weight.	Require periodic adjustment.
	MAG	More durable, do not lose true, more easily cleaned.	Heavier. Entire wheel or caster must be replaced if damaged.
Anti-tipping devices	Present on wheelchair	Reduce (*but do not eliminate*) risk of tipping/falling over backwards in wheelchair.	Prevent wheelies, interfere with obstacle negotiation. Anti-tippers cannot be removed or repositioned by person sitting in wheelchair.
	Absent from wheelchair	Allows obstacle negotiation using wheelies.	Greater risk of injury from backwards tips/falls.
Handrims	Standard	Durable surface.	Most difficult handrim for propulsion with impaired hand grasp.
	Vinyl coated	Increase friction, making propulsion easier when hand function is impaired.	Surface not durable; gets nicks with sharp edges. Increased friction causes heat when descending incline.
	With handrim projections	Handrim projections make propulsion easier when arms are very weak.	Interfere with pushing rhythm, increase overall chair width.
Tires	Pneumatic	Less rolling resistance on soft surfaces such as sand or soft soil, making propulsion on these surfaces easier. Best shock absorption, providing smoother ride. Treaded pneumatic provide superior traction.	Require more maintenance (puncture, require periodic inflation), make chair's overall width greater.
	Solid	Less rolling resistance on hard surfaces, making propulsion easier indoors. Most durable tires, do not go flat or require inflation, add less width to chair.	Less cushioned ride, "bog down" in sand or soft soil, make obstacle negotiation more difficult.
Caster tires	Pneumatic	Best shock absorption, providing smoother ride. Do not "bog down" in sand or soft soil. May extend the life of the wheelchair due to shock adsorption.	Require more maintenance (puncture, require periodic inflation).
	Semipneumatic	Intermediate shock absorption, do not puncture or require inflation, do not "bog down" in sand or soft soil.	Heaviest caster tires.
	Solid	Most durable, do not puncture or require inflation, lightest.	Less cushioned ride, "bog down" in sand or soft soil, make obstacle negotiation more difficult.
Caster size	Large diameter	Easier to propel over uneven terrain, provide wheelchair with superior forward stability (chair less likely to tip over forward).	Heavier.
	Small diameter	Lighter, easier to maneuver on even surfaces. Provide greater clearance between casters and user's heels.	Reduce chair's forward stability, make propulsion over uneven terrain more difficult.

TABLE 12–3. *(Continued)*

Components	Options	Advantages	Disadvantages
Front rigging	Rigid nonremovable	Shorter frame length, stronger.	Can interfere with level and floor-to-wheelchair transfers.
	Swing-away detachable footrests	Can be repositioned easily for transfers.	Increase frame length, less durable than rigid nonremovable.
	Swing-away detachable legrests (elevating)	Allow propulsion with legs elevated.	Heavy and awkward to reposition, add more to length of chair than all other options, must be removed (not just repositioned) for lateral transfers.
	Heel loops (on footrests)	Keep feet from sliding off of footplates.	Make removal of feet from footplates more difficult.
Armrests	Present on wheelchair	May reduce risk of developing skin breakdown because of: (1) reduced seating pressure due to partial support of body weight, (2) promotion of upright sitting posture, and (3) enhanced stability promoting the performance of more pressure reliefs. Can be used functionally when reaching for high objects, and when narrowing chair to negotiate narrow doorways.	May restrict mobility. Can increase overall width of chair.
	Absent from wheelchair	Preferred by some experienced wheelchair users due to enhanced freedom of trunk and arm motions without armrests.	May increase risk of skin breakdown. Precludes use of armrests for functional tasks.
Armrests	Desk length	Allows closer approach to tables and desks.	
	Full length	Provides support to entire length of forearm.	
Armrests	Fixed		Only stand-pivot or mechanical lift transfers are possible. Add to chair's overall width.
	Removable, swing away, or pivoting	Can be removed or repositioned for transfers.	Some styles add to chair's overall width. Different styles have varying difficulty of management.
Armrests	Fixed height	Lighter, more durable.	Armrest height cannot be altered.
	Adjustable height	Can be adjusted to the individual to promote optimal posture, can be raised to make standing from wheelchair easier.	Heavier, may be less durable.

Sources: references 1, 8, 13, 16, 20, 21, 22, 24, 25, 30, 37, 58, 61, 62.

selection should include consideration of the chair's aesthetics, as it can affect both the user's acceptance of the chair and his integration in the community.

> Wheelchairs have become less institutional-looking. The new chairs are sporty-looking, lighter, faster, and take up less space, making me look less conspicuous. The first chair I had made me look like a tank.
>
> Dean Ragone[46]

Additional considerations specific to power wheelchairs. Wheelchair selection is particularly challenging for the individual with high tetraplegia. Profoundly impaired voluntary motor function will limit his ability to manipulate access devices. It will also limit his ability to correct his sitting posture if it shifts. A shift in sitting posture may result in an inability to reach the chair's access devices, and can cause skin breakdown due to alteration of sitting forces. To complicate the picture further, the individual may have spasticity that is elicited when the chair reclines.

An appropriate wheelchair will enable its user to independently, safely, and comfortably propel the chair, perform pressure reliefs, return to upright after a pressure relief, and maintain a good sitting posture. The rehabilitation team and wheelchair user work together to determine which combination of components will make this outcome possible. This selection process must involve trial periods and training with the components under consideration, to ensure that the individual will be able to function optimally with them.

Probably the most challenging aspect of the selection process is the choice of access device(s). The user must be able to direct his chair to perform all of its necessary tasks. For example, he must be able to signal the chair to tilt or recline enough to achieve adequate pressure relief, and *he must be able to return to an upright position.* When he is tilted or reclined he will be in a different position relative to gravity, and may find it difficult or impossible to operate an access device that he uses without difficulty when sitting upright. For this reason, he may need to drive the wheelchair and perform pressure reliefs with two or more separate access devices.

The various components included in a power wheelchair are often made by different manufacturers. Before prescribing a wheelchair, the rehabilitation team should make sure that the components being recommended are all compatible with each other. They should also take into consideration whether the individual will use the chair's input device to control an environmental control unit or computer. Finally, if the rider will utilize a portable ventilator, the wheelchair prescription must specify the incorporation of a vent tray on the back of the wheel base.

Size Selection

The fit of a wheelchair is important to both function and health. Use of a wheelchair that has the wrong dimensions can cause deformity, skin breakdown, impaired lower extremity circulation, and physical discomfort. It can also make independent propulsion more difficult, leading to reduced functional status and increased stress on the upper extremities. Table 12–4 presents information on optimal wheelchair dimensions, the benefits of appropriate fit, and the problems that can result from the use of a poorly fitting chair.

Tentative wheelchair dimensions can be determined using a tape measure with the patient sitting or lying on a mat. Figure 12–3 illustrates the measurements to be taken. These measurements are subject to error, due to the difficulty inherent in taking linear measures of a three-dimensional person. If the measurements are taken carefully, however, they should make it possible to fairly accurately determine the wheelchair dimensions that will be most appropriate for the individual.

The dimensions of a chair being ordered should be verified by having the wheelchair user sit in and operate a wheelchair with these dimensions. The trial wheelchair should also have the components that are to be included in the chair being ordered because differences in components may influence the fit of the chair. For example, rigid backrests or elevating legrests can alter the wheelchair user's position on the seat, and may necessitate ordering a chair with different dimensions.[1]

The height of cushion on which a person sits will affect his requirements for backrest, seat, and armrest height. For this reason, the cushion should be selected before the wheelchair is ordered.

Additional Considerations for People with Incomplete Injuries

Wheelchair selection and adjustment are very important components of the rehabilitation program of any patient with impaired ambulation.

TABLE 12-4.   WHEELCHAIR DIMENSIONS

Feature	Optimal Dimensions	Benefits of Proper Dimensions	Potential Problems from Improper Dimensions
Seat width	**Less than** 1¼ inches wider than wheelchair user's width at greater trochanters or widest portion of thighs. *Hips should not contact wheels, armrests or clothing guards.* If the wheelchair user plans to use lower extremity braces or bulky clothing, or if significant weight gain is likely, consider extra width.	Optimal postural support, propulsion efficiency.	**Too wide:** Increased difficulty of wheelchair propulsion, scoliosis, pressure ulcers from improper distribution of pressure over buttocks; overall chair width increased, limiting access through doorways. **Too narrow:** Pressure ulcers from pressure over greater trochanters.
Seat depth	1 to 2 inches less than distance between the posterior aspect of the buttocks and the popliteal fossa.	Optimal postural support, distribution of pressure on buttocks.	**Too deep** (seat too long from front to back): Lumbar kyphosis, impaired circulation below knees. **Too shallow** (seat too short from front to back): Pressure ulcers from excessive pressure on buttocks, due to limited area over which sitting pressure can be distributed.
Seat height	**Measure with cushion in place.** Power chair or manual chair propelled using arms: seat should be high enough to allow proper adjustment of footplates with at least 2 inches of clearance between floor and footplates. Manual chair propelled using legs: feet should rest flat on the floor while the wheelchair user remains in a good sitting posture.	Optimal postural support, safety, functional performance.	**Too low:** Proper leg positioning impossible, causing excessive pressure over ischial tuberosities with resulting pressure ulcers; if low seat height causes inadequate clearance between footrests and floor, footrests more likely to "bottom out" on uneven terrain or at base of inclines, resulting in tips and falls. **Too high:** Elevated center of gravity reduces chair's anteroposterior stability, increasing risk of tips and falls; can limit access to vans by increasing overall height of chair and rider; may make propulsion and transfers more difficult.
Backrest height	**Measure with cushion in place.** Appropriate height will depend on the wheelchair user's ability to stabilize his trunk in a wheelchair. Find optimal fit by experimenting with different back heights.	Optimal postural support, ease and comfort of manual wheelchair propulsion.	**Too high:** Impedes shoulder motion, making manual wheelchair propulsion uncomfortable and more difficult. **Too low:** Inadequate postural support, with resulting deformity and problems in breathing, skin integrity, and functional status.
Backrest width	Approximately ¾ inches wider than chest width at level of top of backrest.	Comfort, minimal interference with manual wheelchair propulsion.	**Too wide:** Backrest impedes shoulder motions, increasing difficulty of manual wheelchair propulsion. **Too narrow:** Discomfort.
Footrest-to-seat distance	**Measure with cushion in place and shoes on.** Middle range of adjustable footrest should allow proper adjustment of footrest height with at least 2-inch clearance between floor and footplates.	Optimal pressure distribution, safety.	**Too long:** Inadequate support of feet and legs results in reduced postural support and excessive pressure on postero-distal aspect of thighs. **Too short:** Reduced weight-bearing on thighs increases pressure on ischial tuberosities, threatening skin integrity.

(Cont.)

TABLE 12-4. *(Continued)*

Feature	Optimal Dimensions	Benefits of Proper Dimensions	Potential Problems from Improper Dimensions
Armrest height	**Measure with cushion in place.** In upright sitting posture with arms at sides and elbows flexed 90°, forearms should rest comfortably on armrests. (Measure from wheelchair seat to bottom of elbow.)	Comfort, postural support, pressure reliefs.	**Too high:** Cause scapular elevation, discomfort. **Too low:** Inadequate postural support, inadequate support for glenohumeral joint (relevant for individuals with severe upper extremity weakness), increased risk of skin breakdown due to inadequate postural support.

Sources: references 1, 8, 61, 62.

Two factors complicate this process when the individual involved has an incomplete spinal cord injury: the potential for motor return, and the potential for use of the lower extremities for wheelchair propulsion.

Potential for motor return. Significant motor return is more likely to occur when a spinal cord injury is incomplete. The likelihood of eventual functional ambulation[e] is greater among younger individuals, those who have injuries that are less complete at the time of the initial evaluation, and those with spared pin sensation.[17]

Unfortunately, it is not possible to predict with certainty the amount of motor return or the level of independence in ambulation that a given individual will experience. This uncertainty makes wheelchair selection difficult. For example, a person who has a high lesion with minimal motor sparing may require a power wheelchair with a tilt and recline seating system at the time of discharge from inpatient rehabilitation. A year down the road, he could require the same equipment, a

[e] Table 13-16 presents factors associated with future ambulatory potential.

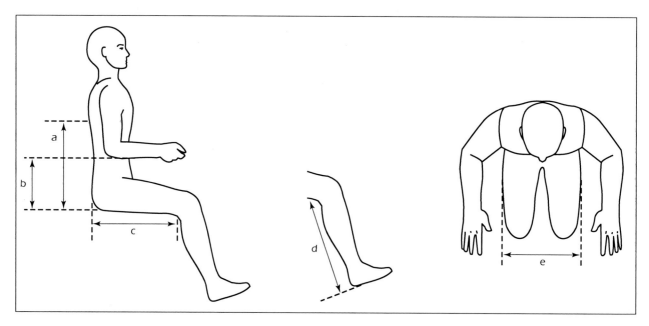

Figure 12-3. *Measurements for wheelchair prescription.* **(a)** Seat to inferior border of scapula. **(b)** Seat to elbow. **(c)** Posterior aspect of buttocks to popliteal fossa. **(d)** Posterior thigh to sole. **(e)** Width at greater trochanters or widest portion of thighs.

power chair without the tilt/recline feature, a manual chair, or even no wheelchair at all for independent mobility in the community.

Ideally, the patient will be provided with equipment that is appropriate for his current needs, with changes in equipment as his needs change. One option is the use of a rental wheelchair at first, with purchase of a chair once enough time has passed that the individual's ultimate functional potential is more clear. This solution may not be possible because of funding restrictions or a lack of availability of appropriate rental equipment. When it is not possible to delay the purchase of a wheelchair, the patient and rehabilitation team must do their best to select a chair that is most likely to meet both his current and future needs.

Lower extremity propulsion. A second consideration in wheelchair selection and adjustment for people with incomplete lesions is the use of the lower extremities for propulsion. An individual who uses his feet for propulsion is likely to require a chair with a lower than standard floor-to-seat height. This feature will enable him to propel without sliding his buttocks forward on the seat; he will be able to maintain a good sitting posture while propelling if his feet can rest flat on the floor while his buttocks remain positioned well back on the seat.

The drawback of a low seat height is that it can make bed transfers more difficult because the person will have to transfer from a low surface to a higher one. A low seat height will also make sit-to-stand transfers more difficult. This problem will be a concern for individuals who both walk and use wheelchairs for their functional mobility.

When selecting and adjusting a wheelchair, the patient and rehabilitation team should consider the impact of seat height on propulsion, transfers, and posture.

Examination and Evaluation

When a wheelchair is delivered, the physical therapist should examine and evaluate it, addressing the following questions. Are the chair's dimensions appropriate, and are its features suitable? Does the chair match the prescription? If not, are the substitutions acceptable to both the clinician and the person for whom the chair was ordered? If the wheelchair meets the criteria listed above, the therapist should adjust the wheelchair to ensure that it provides the user with proper postural support and enables him to function optimally.

Adjustment

Proper adjustment of a wheelchair is critical to its user's functional status and health. Improper adjustment can limit the individual's capacity to function independently with his manual or power chair, and can cause skin breakdown, postural deformity, injury from tips and falls, and increased stress on the upper extremities.

Footrest height. Virtually all wheelchairs have at least one adjustable feature: footrest height. This adjustment is critical to both posture and pressure distribution. The footrests should be adjusted with the person sitting in the wheelchair on his cushion and wearing shoes. If the cushion is ever changed, the footrest height should be checked and readjusted if needed. The footrests should be positioned at a height that places the knees at or slightly below the level of the hips when the feet are flat on the footplates. This position will help to optimize posture and pressure distribution. Footplates that are positioned too high lift the thighs off the seat, resulting in excessive pressure over the ischial tuberosities. Footplates positioned too low cause excessive pressure on the distal thighs and reduce postural support.

Backrest height. If the wheelchair has an adjustable backrest, the optimal backrest height should be determined. To find the best backrest height, the wheelchair user can sit in and propel the chair with the backrest adjusted to various heights. He should also perform functional activities that involve reaching, as backrest height influences a chair's anteroposterior stability. The patient should sit on his cushion during this assessment, as cushion height will influence optimal backrest height. The clinician and wheelchair user should determine which height results in the best posture, comfort, function, and safety.

Armrest height. The armrests should be positioned so that the rider can rest his arms comfortably on them while maintaining an erect sitting posture. With his back against the backrest and his scapulae in a neutral position (not elevated), he should be able to sit with his forearms on the armrest pads with his shoulders flexed approximately 30 degrees and his elbows flexed approximately 60 degrees.[37] This armrest height promotes proper sitting posture and reduces sitting pressure.

Axle position. If the manual wheelchair has an axle with adjustable position, the clinician and wheelchair user should work together to find the optimal axle position. Anteroposterior adjustments can have a profound effect on function, especially in cases where the wheelchair user is only marginal in his propulsion ability.[57] A relatively anterior wheel position makes propulsion easier by increasing the chair's propulsion efficiency, reducing the chair's rolling resistance and tendency to turn downhill,[f] making it easier to turn, and reducing caster flutter (vibration) during propulsion. Posterior placement of the axle has the opposite effect. Anteroposterior adjustments of the wheel's position also affect the chair's "tippiness." Anterior placement of the axle reduces the chair's posterior stability. This reduced stability makes it easier to lift the casters for obstacle negotiation, but also increases the risk of tipping the chair over backwards.[3, 8, 13, 30, 37] Optimal adjustment for an individual may involve finding a balance between propulsion efficiency and stability.[57]

Vertical axle adjustments can affect the tilt of the seat and backrest: a more superior axle position effectively tilts the seat and backrest backward.[8] A slight backward tilt can be helpful to the wheelchair user who has difficulty maintaining trunk stability. The drawback of this adjustment is that it increases the pressure over the ischial tuberosities and greater trochanters.[8]

Vertical axle adjustments can be combined with change in the height of the caster fork to alter the seat height relative to the wheel without changing the tilt of the seat. (In other words, the seat can be raised or lowered without altering its angle.) A lower seat will result in superior anteroposterior stability.[13]

Unfortunately, axle position adjustments that benefit propulsion and posture can interfere with transfers to and from the wheelchair. Moving the wheels to an anterior or superior position reduces the distance that the seat extends anterior to the wheels. This reduces the space available for lateral transfers to and from the wheelchair.[57] For the individual who is marginal in both transfer and propulsion skills, optimal wheelchair adjustment will involve finding a balance between transfer and propulsion abilities.

Alterations in axle position change the position of the wheel locks relative to the wheels,

interfering with the locks' function. Thus the locks must be adjusted after the axles have been positioned. Axle position also affects the orientation of the casters, which impacts on wheelchair propulsion. When adjustments are made in a wheelchair's axle position, the caster angle should be adjusted to achieve a vertical orientation of the caster stems.[30, 57]

Wheel alignment. A manual chair's rear wheels should be aligned so that the distance between their front and rear aspects is equal. If the two wheels are angled so that they are closer to each other in the front than in the back (toe-in), or are closer in the back than in the front (toe-out), propulsion will be more difficult. To check this alignment, the therapist should measure the distance between the right and left wheels' rims at the height of the axle. This measurement should be taken at the front and rear aspects of the wheels.[30]

Tire pressure. If the casters or rear wheels have pneumatic tires, they should be inflated to their recommended pressures. Underinflated tires can increase rolling resistance, making propulsion more difficult.[30]

Adjustments specific to power wheelchairs. In addition to the adjustments just described, the adjustment of a power wheelchair includes the chair's access devices. The access devices should be positioned where they enable the rider to utilize them most effectively. If either a joystick or toggle switch is used, it may require modification. For example, a modified handle may be added to the device to enhance the rider's ability to manipulate it. During the period of training in wheelchair skills, a fair number of adjustments may be required. The patient and rehabilitation team must work together to find the spatial orientation and physical configuration of the access devices that enable the patient to utilize them efficiently and comfortably to perform all of the chair's actions.[42]

The control parameters also require adjustment to suit the needs of the individual involved. A number of adjustments can be made, including the chair's maximum speed, turning speed, rate of acceleration and deceleration, and rate of tilt or recline. These parameters can be set to accommodate the individual's skill level, preferences, and physical response to motion. Optimal settings are likely to change as training progresses.

---

[f] Sidewalks usually have a cross slope, with the sidewalk surface tilting slightly toward the street. A wheelchair being propelled over this slope tends to turn in the downhill direction, making propulsion more difficult.

[g] Moving the axle superiorly is the same as moving it UP relative to the back of the seat. This adjustment can also be conceptualized as moving the back of the seat DOWN relative to the position of the axle.

PROBLEM-SOLVING EXERCISE 12–1

Your patient has C7 tetraplegia, ASIA B. She propels her wheelchair independently over even surfaces for long distances, and is interested in learning how to negotiate small (1- to 2-inch) curbs. She has difficulty "popping" her casters from the floor.

- Assuming that the wheelchair has adjustable rear wheel axles, what adjustment could you make to the axle position to make it easier to lift the chair's casters from the floor?
- What effect will this change in axle position have on the chair's stability?
- What could be added to the chair to make it safer (assuming that they are not already present)? What impact will this addition have on curb negotiation?
- What effect will the change in axle position have on the patient's ability to propel the chair?
- What effect could the change in axle position have on transfers?
- So should you move the wheels or not?

WHEELCHAIR SKILLS

Someone who uses a wheelchair for mobility must possess a variety of skills to function independently. These skills include propulsion of the wheelchair over even surfaces and negotiation of obstacles, as well as the more basic skills of pressure reliefs, positioning the trunk and buttocks within the wheelchair, and handling the chair's parts. Chapter 11 addresses the skills required for positioning and the management of wheelchair parts.

Wheelchair skills can provide freedom and mobility. In addition, manual wheelchair propulsion can be good exercise, resulting in cardiovascular conditioning and muscle strengthening. The increased strength gained through manual wheelchair propulsion may benefit other areas of function, such as transfers and mat skills.

Physical and Skill Prerequisites

Each method of performing a functional activity involves a particular set of skills. Each activity also has strength, joint range of motion, and muscle flexibility requirements. A deficiency in any of these skills or physical requirements will impair a person's performance of the activity.

The descriptions of functional techniques that follow are accompanied by tables that summarize the physical and skill prerequisites. Exact values for the physical prerequisites are not given because the requirements vary among individuals. For example, someone who is very skillful in curb negotiation will require less strength

for this activity than another person who is less skillful and must use sheer strength rather than momentum.

PROGRAM DESIGN

The therapeutic program is designed to enable the patient to achieve all of his functional goals. The steps of program planning follow.

1. Identify the functional goals.[h]
2. Determine the methods that the patient will utilize to perform the activities identified in the goals. This determination will involve choosing the methods that provide the best match between the patient's characteristics and the physical and skill requirements of the activities.
3. Consider the patient's impairments and functional limitations as they compare to the physical and skill requirements of the activities to be achieved.
4. Devise a therapeutic program to develop the needed strength, range of motion, and skills.

For the purposes of program planning, it may be best for the therapist and patient first to consider each goal separately and devise a plan for achieving each goal. The different goals and their plans can then be considered together. Fortunately, there is much overlap of physical and skill prerequisites for the different functional activities. Thus, a person working on maintaining a balanced

[h] Goal-setting is addressed in Chapter 8.

USING CHAPTER 12 AS A RESOURCE FOR PROGRAM PLANNING

When using this chapter as a resource to assist in designing a program to work toward a functional goal, the therapist should first read the description of that functional activity. These descriptions are located under the headings "Wheelchair Skills Following Complete Spinal Cord Injury" in the first half of the chapter, and "Wheelchair Skills and Therapeutic Strategies Following Incomplete Spinal Cord Injury" at the end of the chapter. Based on the description of the functional activity, the corresponding tables, or both, the therapist can determine what physical and skill prerequisites are required to perform the activity. Taking into consideration the patient's evaluation results, the therapist can determine where the patient has deficits relevant to the functional goal. The program should then be designed to address these deficits, developing the needed physical and skill prerequisites.

This chapter presents functional training strategies for each prerequisite skill listed in the tables that accompany the description of wheelchair skills. These functional training strategies are presented under the headings, "Therapeutic Strategies Following Complete Spinal Cord Injury," and "Wheelchair Skills and Therapeutic Strategies Following Incomplete Spinal Cord Injury." The therapist can use these suggestions, coupled with his or her own imagination, clinical expertise, and problem solving, to design a functional training program. The program should aim first at developing the most basic prerequisite skills and build to more advanced skills as the patient's abilities develop.

wheelie position is potentially progressing himself toward independence in negotiating ramps, curbs, stairs, and uneven terrain in a wheelie. Furthermore, work aimed at developing one ability can benefit other, seemingly unrelated, activities. For example, the strengthening and motor learning that result from practicing manual wheelchair propulsion may help a patient's transfer abilities.

Practice in Department and "Real World"

The physical therapy department in a rehabilitation center should be equipped with curbs of varying heights, stairs, and a ramp. This equipment is useful for initial practice of obstacle negotiation; however, practice should not end with mastery of these artificial obstacles. Many obstacles that a wheelchair user will encounter outside of the department will be more difficult to negotiate. For example, ascending a cement curb from a street is likely to be more difficult than ascending a wooden curb from a linoleum floor. The "real world" is full of uneven sidewalks, long and steep staircases, heavy doors, elevators that snap shut with a death grip, and uneven surfaces such as grass and sand. Functional training should include practicing wheelchair skills outside of the department so that the individual will be better prepared to function in the "real world" after rehabilitation.

WHEELCHAIR SKILLS FOLLOWING COMPLETE SPINAL CORD INJURY

The motor function that an individual has following spinal cord injury will influence to a large degree the manner in which he will be able to utilize a wheelchair. Table 12–5 presents a summary of the level of independence in wheelchair skills that can be achieved by people who have complete spinal cord injuries at different motor levels (motor component of neurological level of injury). When prognosticating about an individual's capacity to develop wheelchair skills, the clinician should take into consideration the many other factors that also impact on functional gains.[i]

The characteristics of the wheelchair itself will have a strong impact on the individual's ability to function. For this reason, wheelchair selection, adjustment, and skill training are intertwined processes.

Upright Sitting Tolerance

When upright activities are first initiated, people with spinal cord injuries may experience orthostatic hypotension. This is a transient problem

---

[i] Chapter 8 presents factors that can influence functional outcomes.

TABLE 12–5. FUNCTIONAL POTENTIALS

Motor Level	Significance of Innervated Musculature	Potential for Independence in Wheelchair Skills
C3 and higher	Inadequate voluntary motor function to utilize upper extremities to propel manual wheelchair or control power chair using hand-held joystick.	**Typical Functional Outcomes** **Propelling manual wheelchair:** unable to propel chair. **Driving power wheelchair:** independent driving power chair using motions of the head or chin, tongue, or breath to access the input device. **Pressure reliefs:** independent in pressure reliefs using power tilt and/or recline. **Positioning in wheelchair:** dependent.
C4	Inadequate voluntary motor function to utilize upper extremities to propel manual wheelchair. **Full innervation of trapezius and partial innervation of rhomboids and levator scapulae** enhances capacity for (limited) postural control. When some voluntary motor function is present in the C5 myotome, this musculature plus that listed above makes it possible to utilize a hand-held joystick to control power wheelchair in exceptional cases. (Using the ASIA classification system, people with a C4 motor level can have limited function in the C5 myotome.)	**Typical Functional Outcomes** **Propelling manual wheelchair:** unable to propel chair or perform pressure reliefs. **Driving power wheelchair:** independent driving power chair using motions of the head or chin, tongue, or breath to access the input device. **Pressure reliefs:** independent in pressure reliefs using power tilt and/or recline. **Positioning in wheelchair:** dependent. **Exceptional Functional Outcomes** **Power wheelchair:** independent in driving power chair and controlling specialty seating system using hand-held joystick. **Positioning in wheelchair:** able to shift trunk laterally from upright and return to upright from slight lateral lean.
C5	**Partial innervation of the deltoids** makes it possible to extend the elbows using muscle substitution. **Partial innervation of the biceps brachii, brachialis, and brachioradialis** plus partial innervation of the deltoids makes it possible to use elbow and shoulder flexion to pull. Minimal serratus anterior function is inadequate to stabilize the scapulae against the thorax.	**Typical Functional Outcomes** **Propelling manual wheelchair:** independent to some assist indoors on uncarpeted level floors; may use either high-friction or pegged handrims; manual wheelchair propulsion ability inadequate for mobility in the community. **Obstacle negotiation:** unable to propel over uneven surfaces or obstacles. **Driving power wheelchair:** independent using hand-held joystick. **Pressure reliefs:** independent in power wheelchair using power tilt and/or recline; some assist to independent in pressure relief in manual wheelchair using lateral lean method. **Positioning in wheelchair:** some assist to dependent in positioning buttocks and trunk in wheelchair. **Exceptional Functional Outcomes** **Pressure reliefs:** independent in pressure reliefs without specialty seating system. **Positioning in wheelchair:** independent in positioning buttocks and trunk in wheelchair.

(Cont.)

TABLE 12-5.   *(Continued)*

Motor Level	Significance of Innervated Musculature	Potential for Independence in Wheelchair Skills
C6	**Fully innervated deltoids, infraspinatus, teres minor, and clavicular portion of the pectoralis major** allow for stronger elbow extension using muscle substitution. **Fully innervated deltoids, biceps brachii, brachialis and brachioradialis** allow strong shoulder and elbow flexion for pulling. **Partial innervation of the serratus anterior** makes it possible to stabilize the scapulae against the thorax. Scapular protraction and stability enhance propulsion capability and capacity to position self in wheelchair. **Partial innervation of the latissimus dorsi** enhances shoulder girdle depression, allowing greater lift of the buttocks during pressure reliefs. Minimal innervation of the triceps brachii is inadequate to contribute significantly to wheelchair skills.	**Typical Functional Outcomes** **Propelling manual wheelchair:** independent indoors on uncarpeted level floors; may use high-friction handrims; manual wheelchair propulsion ability likely to be inadequate for mobility in the community. **Obstacle negotiation:** some to total assist negotiating mild obstacles such as carpeted floors, sidewalks, 1:12 grade ramps. **Driving power wheelchair:** independent using hand-held joystick. **Pressure reliefs:** independent in power wheelchair either without specialty seating system or using power tilt and/or recline. Some assist to independent in pressure relief in manual wheelchair using depression, forward lean, or lateral lean method. **Positioning in wheelchair:** some assist to independent in positioning buttocks and trunk in wheelchair. **Exceptional Functional Outcomes** **Propelling manual wheelchair:** independent on even and slightly uneven surfaces for long distances, allowing independent mobility in the community using a manual wheelchair. **Obstacle negotiation:** independent in negotiation of mild obstacles such as 1:12 grade ramps, slightly uneven (outdoor) terrain, 2- to 4-inch curbs. **Pressure reliefs:** independent in pressure relief in manual wheelchair using depression, forward lean, or lateral lean method. **Positioning in wheelchair:** independent in positioning buttocks and trunk in wheelchair.
C7	**Partial innervation of the triceps brachii** allows for stronger elbow extension. **Full innervation of the serratus anterior** provides more stable scapula, stronger protraction and upward rotation. **Partial innervation of the latissimus dorsi and sternocostal portion of pectoralis major** enhance shoulder girdle depression, enhancing propulsion, pressure reliefs, and positioning in wheelchair.	**Typical Functional Outcomes** **Propelling manual wheelchair:** independent indoors and outdoors on level terrain for long distances, allowing independent mobility in the community using manual wheelchair. **Obstacle negotiation:** independent to some assist negotiating 1:12 ramps. Some to total assist negotiating unlevel terrain and curbs. **Pressure reliefs:** independent using depression method. **Positioning in wheelchair:** independent in positioning buttocks and trunk in wheelchair.

TABLE 12–5. *(Continued)*

Motor Level	Significance of Innervated Musculature	Potential for Independence in Wheelchair Skills
		Exceptional Functional Outcomes **Obstacle negotiation:** independent in negotiation of mild obstacles such as ramps with slightly steeper than 1:12 grade, slightly uneven (outdoor) terrain, 4-inch curbs.
C8	**Full innervation of the triceps brachii** provides normal strength in elbow extension. **Full innervation of the latissimus dorsi and nearly full innervation of pectoralis major** allow strong shoulder girdle depression, enhancing propulsion, pressure reliefs, and positioning in wheelchair. **Partial innervation of the long finger flexors allows grasp of wheelchair handrims**, resulting in greater ease in wheelchair propulsion and obstacle negotiation.	**Typical Functional Outcomes** **Propelling manual wheelchair:** independent indoors and outdoors on level terrain for long distances, allowing independent mobility in the community using manual wheelchair. **Obstacle negotiation:** independent negotiating 1:12 ramps. Some assist negotiating unlevel terrain and curbs. **Pressure reliefs:** independent using depression method. **Positioning in wheelchair:** independent in positioning buttocks and trunk in wheelchair. **Exceptional Functional Outcomes** **Obstacle negotiation:** independent in negotiation of mild obstacles such as ramps with slightly steeper than 1:12 grade, slightly uneven (outdoor) terrain, 4-inch curbs, narrow doorways, fall safely.
T1 and lower	**Fully innervated upper extremities** make all wheelchair skills more easy to achieve.	**Typical Functional Outcomes** **Propelling manual wheelchair:** independent indoors and outdoors on level terrain for long distances, allowing independent mobility in the community using manual wheelchair. **Obstacle negotiation:** independent negotiating 4- to 6-inch curbs, uneven terrain, ramps with grade steeper than 1:12, narrow doorways; can descend stairs backwards holding handrail, ascend on buttocks and bring chair; can fall safely and return wheelchair to upright while remaining in chair. **Pressure reliefs:** independent using depression method. **Positioning in wheelchair:** independent in positioning buttocks and trunk in wheelchair. **Exceptional Functional Outcomes** **Obstacle negotiation:** independent in negotiating curbs higher than 6 inches, ascending stairs while remaining in wheelchair, descending stairs in wheelie.

Sources: references for innervation: 23, 36, 39, 40, 50. For more complete innervation information, see Appendix B *(www.prenhall.com/somers).*

that is most prevalent among people with lesions above T6.[4, 7, 32, 64] Especially after prolonged bed rest, moving directly to an upright sitting position can cause a drop in blood pressure, with resulting dizziness, vomiting, and loss of consciousness. Before an individual becomes independent in any wheelchair skills, he must first develop the capacity to sit upright in a wheelchair without experiencing these problems. Although upright sitting tolerance involves physiological accommodation rather than skill development, it is included in this chapter because all wheelchair skills depend upon it. Strategies for developing upright sitting tolerance are presented in the skill development strategy section of the chapter.

Positioning in the Chair

The ability to position one's self and to maintain that position within a wheelchair is one of the most basic requirements for the independent use of a wheelchair. To use a wheelchair independently, a person needs to be able to maintain an upright sitting posture.[j] He should also be able to reposition his trunk and buttocks in the chair so that he can adjust his posture in the event that his position shifts during the day.

With functioning biceps and deltoids. Chapter 11 presents techniques for stabilizing the trunk in a wheelchair and for moving the trunk and buttocks. These techniques require functional strength in the deltoids and biceps.

In the absence of functioning biceps and deltoids. Without functioning biceps and deltoids, the potential for stabilizing and moving the trunk is limited; however, a person with high tetraplegia can gain some skills in this area. Through motions of his head and scapulae, he can exercise some control over his position in the wheelchair.

To maintain an upright sitting posture, a person with a high lesion can hold his head upright and his scapulae adducted. This posture can be a useful adjunct to trunk stability for anyone with a spinal cord injury.

A person with functioning trapezius, sternocleidomastoid, and cervical paraspinal musculature (present with C4 tetraplegia) can also make limited adjustments in his trunk's position, tilting his trunk laterally by throwing the head and

shoulders. For example, he can tilt his trunk to the left by repeatedly throwing his head to the left while simultaneously elevating his right scapula. These neck and scapular motions are performed forcefully to maximize momentum. This technique can be used to tilt to the side from an upright position or to return to upright from a slight lateral lean.

The physical and skill prerequisites required for positioning in the chair in the absence of functioning biceps and deltoids are presented in Tables 12–6 and 12–7.

Pressure Reliefs

In terms of survival value, the ability to perform pressure reliefs is probably the most important functional skill that a person with a spinal cord injury can acquire. When someone with a complete injury sits for more than a few minutes, he requires periodic relief of pressure over his buttocks to prevent skin breakdown. This is true regardless of the quality of cushion on which he sits.[45] An individual who cannot perform pressure reliefs independently must depend upon assistance from others throughout the period of sitting.

The purpose of a pressure relief is to reduce the pressure on tissues that have been bearing weight, allowing circulation in areas that have been ischemic during weight bearing. When sitting with good posture, the bulk of weight bearing occurs on the ischial tuberosities. It is the skin over these boney prominences that must be relieved during a pressure relief.

People vary in their requirements for pressure relief. During rehabilitation, each must discover his skin's requirements for the duration of each pressure relief and the length of time that can pass between reliefs.[k]

Sitting pushup. Perhaps the quickest and most effective method of pressure relief is the sitting pushup. Someone with adequate strength in his triceps can eliminate pressure over his ischial tuberosities by lifting his buttocks completely off of the supporting surface. To do so, he places his hands lateral to his buttocks on the wheelchair's seat, armrests, or wheels. He then lifts his body by pushing down, extending his elbows and depressing his shoulders.

Weight shift. Pressure reliefs do not require complete elimination of pressure on the ischial

---

[j] An individual who is unable to do so without equipment may use a strap or lateral supports, but this equipment will interfere with independent pressure reliefs.

[k] Additional information on skin care is presented in Chapter 6.

TABLE 12–6. HIGH-LESION SKILLS: POSITIONING IN WHEELCHAIR AND CONTROL OF POWER WHEELCHAIR—PHYSICAL PREREQUISITES

		Positioning in wheelchair	Hand-held joystick	Chin-control and head-control joystick	Mouth-control joystick or tongue-touch keypad	Breath-control	Peachtree head control
Strength							
Cervical paraspinals		√	√	√			√
Sternocleidomastoid		√		√			√
Trapezius		√	√–	√			√
Anterior deltoids		•	•				
Middle deltoids		•	•				
Posterior deltoids		•	•				
Serratus anterior		•	•				
Oral musculature					√	√	
Biceps, brachialis, and/or brachioradialis			√–				
Range of Motion							
Cervical	Lateral flexion	√–					√–
	Rotation			√–			√–
	Flexion			√–			√–
	Extension	√–		√–			√–
Scapular	Elevation	√–					
	Abduction		√–				
	Adduction		√–				

√– = At least 2–/5 to 2+/5 strength is needed for this activity, or severe limitations in range will inhibit this activity.

• = Not required, but helpful.

√ = At least 3/5 strength is needed for this activity.

TABLE 12–7. HIGH-LESION SKILLS: POSITIONING IN WHEELCHAIR AND CONTROL OF POWER WHEELCHAIR—SKILL PREREQUISITES

	Positioning in wheelchair	Hand-held joystick	Chin-control and head-control joystick	Mouth-control joystick or tongue-touch keypad	Breath-control	Peachtree head control
Sitting in wheelchair, move trunk using head and scapular motions (p. 318)	√					
Place hand on joystick (p. 319)		√				
Move joystick in all directions using arm and scapular motions (p. 319)		√				
Signal wheel chair using chin, head, or tongue motions (p. 320 & 321)			√	√		
Signal wheelchair by sipping and puffing in appropriate pattern (p. 320)					√	
Signal wheelchair by moving head toward/away from sensors in headrest (p. 321)						√
Drive power wheelchair over even surfaces and mild obstacles (p. 321)		√	√	√	√	√

tuberosities. Adequate relief can be obtained by redistributing weight bearing and reducing pressure on the ischial tuberosities by moving the pressure to different areas.[53] A person with a spinal cord injury can perform an effective pressure relief by leaning forward enough to unweight his ischial tuberosities.[19, 28] He can also perform a pressure relief by leaning to one side and then the other, unweighting one side at a time.[28] Chapter 11 presents techniques for moving the trunk forward or laterally in a wheelchair.

Power tilt or recline. A person with a power tilt or recline feature on his wheelchair can independently perform pressure reliefs by using an access device to signal his chair to tilt or recline. He can use the same input device that he uses to drive the chair, or he may use one or more alternate inputs. Regardless of the number of switches used, he needs to be able to direct the chair to tilt or recline fully, *and return to upright after the pressure relief.* Strategies for developing this skill are presented below in the chapter's section on therapeutic strategies following complete spinal cord injury.

Wheelchair Mobility over Even Surfaces

Independence in propulsion over even surfaces brings the freedom to move about within a wheelchair-accessible environment. The functional use of a wheelchair requires the ability to propel forward and backward, and to turn.

The methods used for propulsion depend upon the type of wheelchair used; different techniques are used to propel manual wheelchairs with standard or pegged handrims and the various

types of power wheelchairs. One task of the rehabilitation team involves working with the patient to determine the propulsion mode that is most appropriate for that individual. This analysis involves weighing the advantages and disadvantages of the different options for the individual concerned. Table 12–8 presents a comparison of some of the advantages and disadvantages of power wheelchairs and manual chairs with pegged and standard handrims.

Driving power wheelchair. Manual wheelchair propulsion requires the presence of functioning deltoids and biceps. An individual who lacks innervation or adequate strength in this musculature will require a power wheelchair for independent mobility. A variety of options are available to enable people with limited physical capabilities to control powered wheelchairs. Ac-

TABLE 12–8. COMPARISON OF WHEELCHAIR PROPULSION OPTIONS

Options	Advantages	Disadvantages
Power wheelchairs	• Make independent mobility possible for people who cannot propel manual wheelchairs. • When daily activities necessitate propulsion over long distances, conserves time and energy for other tasks. • Do not cause chronic shoulder pain.	• No cardiovascular or muscular conditioning occurs with propulsion. • Restricted to accessible environments. • Cannot be transported in car.
Manual wheelchairs with handrim projections	• Not restricted to wheelchair-accessible environments. • Cardiovascular conditioning and muscle strengthening occur with propulsion. • Can be transported in car.	• Handrim projections make wheelchair wider. • Handrim projections interfere with efficient propulsion rhythm. • Strengthening limited to shoulder and elbow flexors. • Some people are unable to propel manual wheelchairs. • Prolonged use of manual wheelchair can cause chronic upper extremity pain.
Manual wheelchairs with standard handrims	• Not restricted to wheelchair-accessible environments. • Cardiovascular conditioning and muscle strengthening occur with propulsion. • Muscle strengthening optimal for enhancement of transfer skills. • Can be transported in car.	• Some people are unable to propel manual wheelchairs. • Prolonged use of manual wheelchair can cause chronic upper extremity pain.

cess devices commonly used to drive are joysticks, Peachtree head control, breath control, and tongue-touch keypads. These inputs, and the manner in which the wheelchair driver uses them, are described in Table 12–2. The physical and skill prerequisites required to drive a power wheelchair using these input devices are summarized in Tables 12–6 and 12–7.

Propulsion using manual wheelchair with standard handrims. A person with functioning finger flexors can propel his wheelchair by grasping the handrims and pulling forward or backward. The following descriptions of techniques for propelling forward, backward, and turning are appropriate for people who lack functional finger flexors. In these techniques, friction is used to move the handrims. Adequate strength is required in the deltoids and biceps.

The physical and skill prerequisites required to propel a manual wheelchair with standard handrims are summarized in Tables 12–9 and 12–10.

Forward. To propel forward without grasping the wheelchair's handrims, a person with a spinal cord injury starts by placing his palms against the lateral surface of the handrims. His elbows are flexed and his shoulders are internally rotated slightly. Using elbow extension and combined shoulder adduction, external rotation, and flexion, he stabilizes his palms against the handrims and pushes forward.[1] In the absence of functioning triceps, the anterior deltoids are used to extend the elbows.

The wheelchair user starts with his hands well back on the handrims and pushes until they are well forward (Figure 12–4). As he reaches back to start another stroke, the wheelchair continues to glide forward. By using long strokes for propulsion, the wheelchair user may subject his upper extremities to lower levels of stress.[47]

Backward. Backward propulsion without innervated finger flexors can be accomplished by reversing the technique for forward propulsion. The person places his palms on the outer surface of the handrims, squeezes in, and pulls back (Figure 12–5A).

Figure 12–5B illustrates an alternate method of backward propulsion. The person places his

---

[1] People who cannot grasp the handrims must use a medially directed force to stabilize their palms against the handrims. This requirement makes wheelchair propulsion less efficient than propulsion with intact upper extremities.[10, 11]

TABLE 12–9. PROPULSION OF MANUAL WHEELCHAIR WITH STANDARD HANDRIMS— PHYSICAL PREREQUISITES

		Forward	Backward pulling handrims	Backward pushing tires	Turning
Strength					
Trapezius		√	√	√	√
Anterior deltoids		☑	√	√	√
Middle deltoids		√	√	√	√
Posterior deltoids		√	√	√	√
Infraspinatus, teres minor		√		√	√
Pectoralis major, teres major		•	•		•
Biceps, brachialis, and/or brachioradialis		√	√	√	√
Serratus anterior		•			•
Triceps		•		•	•
Hand musculature (active grasp)		•	•	•	•
Range of Motion					
Scapular	Elevation			√	
	Depression			√	
	Abduction	√			
	Adduction	√	√	√	√
Shoulder	Flexion	√	√		√
	Extension	√	√	√	√
	Internal rotation	√	√		√
	External rotation	√		☑	√
	Abduction			√	
Elbow	Flexion	√	√		√
	Extension	√	√	√	√

√ = Some strength is needed for this activity, or severe limitations in range will inhibit this activity.

☑ = A large amount of strength or normal or greater range is needed for this activity.

• = Not required, but helpful.

TABLE 12–10. PROPULSION OF MANUAL WHEELCHAIR WITH STANDARD HANDRIMS— SKILL PREREQUISITES

	Forward	Backward pulling handrims	Backward pushing tires	Turning
Maintain upright sitting position[a]	√	√	√	√
Place palms against standard handrims (p. 322)	√	√		√
Push standard handrim(s) forward (p. 323)	√			√
Pull standard handrim(s) backward (p. 324)		√		
Place palms on tires, behind seat (p. 325)			√	
With palms on tires behind seat, propel wheelchair backwards using elbow extension and scapular depression *or* using only scapular depression (p. 325)			√	
Propel manual wheelchair over even surfaces (p. 326)	√			

[a] Refer to Chapter 11 for a description of this skill and therapeutic strategies.

palms on top of the tires, just posterior to his buttocks. With his hands facing backward and his shoulders externally rotated, he pushes backward on the tires by extending his elbows, using either triceps or anterior deltoids.

Someone who is unable to extend his elbows against the resistance supplied by his chair's wheels may be able to propel backward using a third method, illustrated in Figure 12–5C. When using this method, the person starts by placing his palms against the medial-superior surfaces of his tires, posterior to his buttocks. His shoulders should be externally rotated and elevated and his elbows locked[m] in extension. By depressing his scapulae, he then pushes the wheels backward.

[m] Elbow locking is addressed in Chapter 11.

Turning. The technique used to turn will depend upon the turning radius desired. Turning in a long arc simply involves pushing harder with one hand than the other, or pushing one wheel while applying resistance to the other wheel. To turn sharply, the wheelchair user can pull one wheel backward while he pushes the other one forward. The techniques for pushing the wheels forward and backward are the same as those described in the preceding paragraphs.

Propulsion using manual wheelchair with handrim projections. Inadequate strength or range of motion can make propulsion with standard handrims impossible or prohibitively difficult. Handrim projections, also called pegs, may make propulsion easier in these instances. Functional deltoids and biceps are required.

The physical and skill prerequisites required to propel a manual wheelchair with pegged handrims are summarized in Tables 12–11 and 12–12.

Forward. To propel forward using pegged handrims, each palm or forearm is placed behind a peg. Using shoulder and elbow flexion, the wheelchair user pulls forward on the pegs. Propulsion will be more efficient if he uses long strokes, starting with his hands on pegs that are posterior to his buttocks (Figure 12–6).

Backward. Backward propulsion can be accomplished by pulling back on the handrim projections. With his shoulders internally rotated, the person places his hands or forearms against the front aspects of anteriorly located pegs. He then pulls back using glenohumeral extension and scapular adduction.

An individual who is strong enough may be able to propel backward by pushing against the backs of his tires, as described earlier.

Turning. Turning is accomplished in the same manner as turning a wheelchair with standard handrims. Using the techniques described above, the person pushes one wheel harder than the other or pushes one wheel forward while pulling the other backward.

Negotiation of Obstacles

Independent wheelchair propulsion over even surfaces will enable a person to be mobile indoors within the confines of a single-level home or work environment, provided that there are no narrow doorways or elevated thresholds in the doors. For independent and safe mobility within a greater

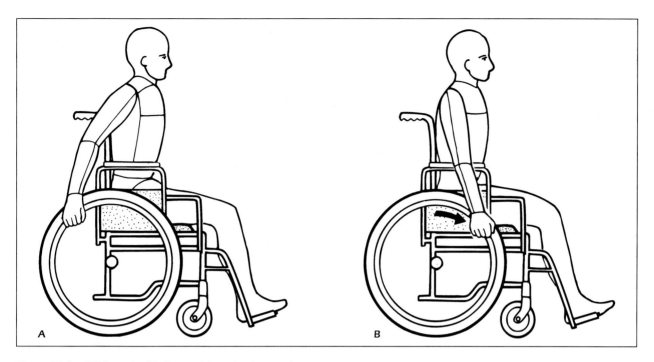

Figure 12–4. Efficient wheelchair propulsion using long strokes.

variety of environments, obstacle negotiation skills are necessary.

Techniques for negotiation of inclines, curbs, uneven terrain, stairs, and narrow doorways are presented in this section. The descriptions apply to manual wheelchairs with standard handrims but can be adapted to pegged handrims.

Tables 12–13 through 12–20 summarize the physical and skill prerequisites for independent negotiation of obstacles.

Inclines: Ramps, curb cuts, and hills. Ramps, curb cuts, and hills present similar challenges to wheelchair riders: propelling up a slope involves a risk of tipping/falling over backwards, and requires greater force than does propelling on a horizontal surface. Descending a slope in a wheelchair involves controlling the chair as gravity causes it to roll downhill.

Training in negotiation of inclines often focuses on ascending because this is the more difficult part of the task. Skill in descending inclined surfaces should also be developed. To be safe when descending a ramp or hill in a wheelchair, the wheelchair user should maintain control of the chair for the entire length of the slope. He should be able to steer to the right or left and stop at will. If he does not have this level of control, he may eventually collide with someone or something that gets in the way. There is no guarantee that a clear path will stay clear as a wheelchair descends a slope.

Practice in ramp negotiation should *not* be limited to the gentle 1:12 grade of a standard public incline. Many, if not most, ramps found in the community are far steeper than this. People undergoing rehabilitation should develop the skills needed to ascend and descend slopes as steep as possible within their potentials.

Ascending. Fully innervated upper extremities make ramp ascension easier but are not required for this activity. Someone with C6 tetraplegia may be able to negotiate mild slopes. More and stronger innervated musculature will make it possible to negotiate steeper and longer inclines.[5]

Propulsion up an incline is accomplished on four wheels, using variations of the techniques described previously for forward propulsion. The techniques are altered to enable the wheelchair user to propel up the ramp without tipping over backward or rolling backward between pushes. To ascend a ramp without tipping over backward, the wheelchair user pushes forward forcefully but avoids jerking the wheels abruptly. A forward lean of the head and (when possible) trunk will also help prevent backward tipping. To avoid rolling backward between pushes, he uses shorter strokes and repositions his hands rapidly between pushes.

Descending on four wheels. When a wheelchair descends a slope, gravity provides the force that moves the chair. The wheelchair user *controls* the

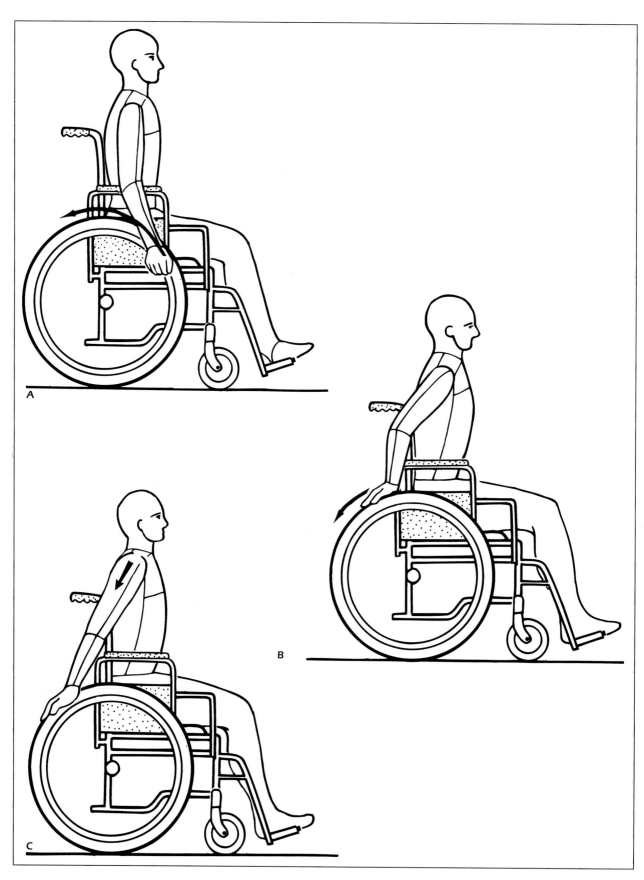

Figure 12–5. Backward propulsion without innervated finger flexors, using standard handrims. **(A)** Squeezing in and pulling back on handrims. **(B)** Pushing back on tires using elbow extension. **(C)** Pushing back on tires using scapular depression.

TABLE 12–11. PROPULSION OF MANUAL WHEELCHAIR WITH PEGGED HANDRIMS—PHYSICAL PREREQUISITES

	Forward	Backward	Turning
Strength			
Trapezius	√	√	√
Anterior deltoids	√	√	√
Middle deltoids	√	√	√
Posterior deltoids	√	√	√
Biceps, brachialis, and/or brachioradialis	√	√	√
Pectoralis major, teres major		√	
Range of Motion			
Scapular adduction		√	
Shoulder Flexion	√	√	√
Extension	√	√	√
Internal rotation		√	
Elbow Extension	√	√	√

√ = Some strength is needed for this activity, or severe limitations in range will inhibit this activity.

TABLE 12–12. PROPULSION OF MANUAL WHEELCHAIR WITH PEGGED HANDRIMS—SKILL PREREQUISITES

	Forward	Backward	Turning
Maintain upright sitting position[a]	√	√	√
Place palms or forearms against handrim projections (p. 326)	√	√	√
Pull handrim projections forward (p. 326)	√		√
Pull backward on handrim projections (p. 326)		√	√
Propel manual wheelchair over even surfaces (p. 326)	√		

[a] Refer to chapter 11 for a description of this skill and therapeutic strategies.

chair rather than propels it. During the descent, he keeps the chair under control by resisting its motion. He can slow or turn the chair while descending by applying resistance to the wheel rims.

A person who has functioning hand musculature can control the chair by gripping the handrims loosely and allowing them to slide through his hands. His grip should provide enough resistance to the handrims to slow and control the chair's descent.

An individual who lacks functioning finger flexors can control the chair's descent by pressing his palms against the handrims. The palms should be slightly in front of the hips, with the elbows slightly flexed and the shoulders internally rotated.

Descending in a wheelie position. Many ramps and curb cuts are steep, with an abrupt angle at the bottom where they meet the street or sidewalk. When a person descends such a ramp or curb cut on four wheels, the footplates may "bottom out," striking the street or sidewalk. The chair comes to an abrupt stop, and the rider may be thrown out of the chair. This problem can be avoided by descending the slope in a wheelie (balanced on the rear wheels).

Descending an incline in a wheelie is an easy skill to master for anyone who can glide on two wheels. The wheelchair user approaches the slope in a wheelie, then grips the chair's handrims loosely and allows them to slide through his hands as he descends the slope. His grip should provide just enough resistance to slow and control the chair's descent. Good hand function is required for this skill.

Curbs. Although ramps and curb cuts have become fairly common, many public places remain inaccessible to wheelchairs. Certainly most private residences are inaccessible. Thus, it is likely that many places where an individual wants to go will not have ramps or will have ramps that are obstructed or placed in inconvenient locations.

Curb negotiation skills can be used to get over a variety of obstacles that block a wheelchair's path with a vertical obstruction. Examples

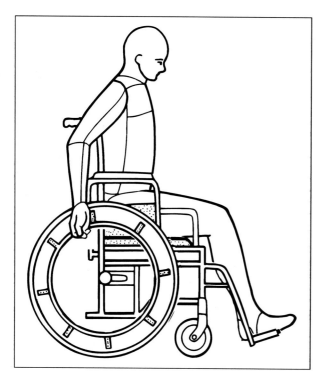

Figure 12–6. *Forward propulsion using pegged handrims.*

of such obstacles include curbs at the junctures between streets and sidewalks, irregularities in sidewalks, elevated thresholds or weather stripping in doorways, and entranceways in which the floor on one side of the doorway is higher than on the other side.

Ideally, someone who uses a wheelchair for mobility in the community will be able to negotiate tall curbs—the taller the better. *Any* skill in curb negotiation will be helpful, however, no matter how limited. Even the ability to negotiate a 1-inch curb will be useful, making it possible to get over weather stripping or an irregularity in the sidewalk.

The height of curb that an individual will be able to master will be influenced by his lesion level as well as his strength and skill. It is possible for people with tetraplegia as high as C6 to ascend 2-inch, even 4-inch, curbs using either of the following methods. Curb negotiation is challenging, however, with such a high lesion. It is more readily accomplished by people with fully innervated upper extremities. For many people with paraplegia, independent negotiation of 6-inch or higher curbs is a reasonable goal.

Ascending from stationary position. This curb ascension technique utilizes strength more than momentum. It requires less space than ascending using momentum because it does not involve a running start. It also requires less skill than ascending using momentum; the timing of motions is not as critical. However, this technique is more limited: higher curbs can be negotiated using momentum.

To ascend a curb from a stationary position, the wheelchair user approaches the curb front-on and stops a few inches shy of the curb (Figure 12–7A). From this position, he pops his casters onto the curb: starting with his hands well back on the handrims, he pulls forward forcefully and abruptly (Figure 12–7B). To lift his casters, he may need to throw his head back simultaneously with the pull.

Once the casters are on the curb, the person backs his chair until the casters are at the edge (Figure 12–7C). Positioning the chair in this manner makes it possible to gain some momentum in the next step.

When the casters are positioned appropriately, the wheelchair user places his hands well back on the handrims (Figure 12–7D). He then pulls forward forcefully and throws his head and trunk forward. If the wheels hit the curb with enough force, the chair will ascend (Figure 12–7E). During this step, the trunk may fall forward. This should not pose a problem; the person can return to an upright sitting position once the chair is past the curb.

Ascending using momentum. Ascending a curb using momentum involves finesse rather than sheer muscle power. It is faster than ascending from a stationary position because the wheelchair user does not stop in front of the curb before ascending. Taking advantage of momentum also makes it possible to get up higher curbs than can be ascended from a stationary position.

Using this method, people with C6 tetraplegia can ascend low curbs. An *exceptionally* skillful person with fully innervated upper extremities can ascend 10-inch or higher curbs.

To ascend a curb using momentum, the wheelchair user approaches the curb head-on, with speed. At the last moment, he pops his casters up onto the curb: without slowing the chair, he reaches back and pulls forward on the wheel rims abruptly and forcefully. He may need to throw his head back at the same time to lift the casters. The caster pop should be timed so that the casters lift over the curb and land just before the rear wheels hit the curb. Momentum will carry the chair up the curb if the maneuver is timed correctly and the curb is approached with adequate speed.

TABLE 12–13. NEGOTIATION OF INCLINES AND UNEVEN TERRAIN—PHYSICAL PREREQUISITES

		Ascend incline	Descend incline on four wheels	Descend incline in wheelie position	Negotiate uneven terrain on four wheels	Negotiate uneven terrain in wheelie
Strength						
Trapezius		√	√	√	√	√
Anterior deltoids		☑	√	√	☑	☑
Middle deltoids		√	√	√	√	√
Posterior deltoids		√	√	√	√	√
Infraspinatus, teres minor		√			√	
Pectoralis major, teres major		•	•	√	•	√
Biceps, brachialis, and/or brachioradialis		√	√	√	√	√
Serratus anterior		•			•	√
Triceps		•		√	•	√
Hand musculature (active grasp)		•	•	√	•	√
Range of Motion						
Scapular	Abduction	√		√	√	√
	Adduction	√		√	√	√
Shoulder	Flexion	√		√	√	√
	Extension	√	√	√	√	√
	Internal rotation	√	√	√	√	√
	External rotation	√			√	
Elbow	Flexion	√	√	√	√	√
	Extension	√			√	√
Finger	Flexion			√		√

√ = Some strength is needed for this activity, or severe limitations in range will inhibit this activity.

☑ = A large amount of strength or normal or greater range is needed for this activity.

• = Not required, but helpful.

Descending backwards. This method of descending curbs does not involve a wheelie. Thus, it is the method of choice for people who cannot glide in a wheelie.

Like ascending from a stationary position, descending backwards is most appropriate for lower curbs. On higher curbs, the chair may tip over backwards. To descend a curb backwards, the wheelchair user first backs his chair to the edge of the curb (Figure 12–8A). After the wheels pass the curb's edge, he controls the chair's descent by resisting the handrims' motion. Leaning the trunk and head forward will reduce the likelihood of the chair tipping over backward when the wheels hit the ground (Figure 12–8B).

After lowering the chair's rear wheels, the wheelchair user removes the casters from the curb. He can roll the casters straight back off of the curb *only* if the curb is a very low one. If he rolls his chair straight back from too high a curb, the footplates will catch on the curb. Once the footplates are caught, it will be difficult to free the chair from the curb.

TABLE 12–14.   NEGOTIATION OF INCLINES AND UNEVEN TERRAIN—SKILL PREREQUISITES

	Ascend incline	Descend incline on four wheels	Descend incline in wheelie position	Negotiate uneven terrain on four wheels	Negotiate uneven terrain in wheelie
Propel wheelchair over even surfaces (p. 326)	✓			✓	
Propel wheelchair up a slope (p. 327)	✓				
Descending slope on four wheels, control wheelchair by applying friction to handrims (p. 327)		✓			
Assume wheelie position (p. 328)			✓		✓
Maintain balance point in wheelie position (p. 328)			✓		✓
Descending slope in wheelie, control wheelchair by applying friction to handrims (p. 331)			✓		
Negotiate uneven terrain on four wheels (p. 337)				✓	
Propel wheelchair forward (glide) in wheelie position (p. 331)			✓		✓
Turn in wheelie position (p. 331)					✓
Propel backward in wheelie position (p. 331)					✓
Negotiate uneven terrain in wheelie position (p. 337)					✓

Most curbs are high enough that backing the casters off is not possible. To avoid catching his footplates on the curb, the wheelchair user lowers the casters by turning the chair rather than backing up (Figure 12–8C). He should turn his chair in a tight arc, pushing one wheel forward while pulling the other back. Once the casters move past the curb, they will drop safely to the lower surface.

Descending in a wheelie position. Descending curbs in a wheelie is faster than descending backwards. To descend backwards, the individual must interrupt his chair's forward motion to turn around and approach the curb backwards, and must turn again after descending the curb. Descending in a wheelie does not involve this interruption of forward motion. Good hand function is required for this method.

To descend a curb using this method, the wheelchair user pops his chair into a wheelie position as he approaches the curb. He glides toward the curb in a wheelie and maintains that position as the chair descends the curb (Figure 12–9). The curb descent itself simply involves letting the handrims slide through the hands as the chair descends. The wheelie may be maintained after the curb has been descended, but that is not necessary for safe curb negotiation.

Uneven terrain.   Slightly uneven terrain, such as bumpy asphalt or a well-groomed lawn, may be negotiated using the same techniques as are used for propulsion over even surfaces. Propulsion on these surfaces will be more difficult, requiring more strength. Someone who is only marginally functional pushing on even surfaces will not be able to propel on uneven terrain.

Very uneven terrain is more challenging. A wheelchair's casters tend to get caught in ruts or bog down in deep gravel or sand. Because the

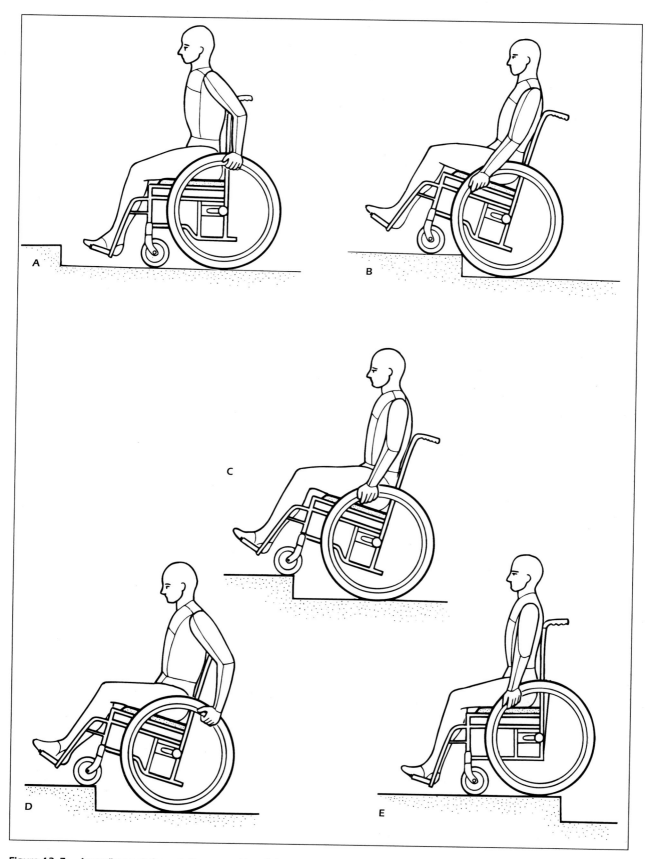

Figure 12–7. *Ascending curb from stationary position.* **(A)** *Starting position: facing the curb, a few inches from curb.* **(B)** *Casters popped onto curb.* **(C)** *Casters backed to edge of curb.* **(D)** *Hands placed well back on handrims.* **(E)** *Curb ascended.*

TABLE 12–15. NEGOTIATION OF CURBS—PHYSICAL PREREQUISITES

	Ascend from stationary position	Ascend using momentum	Descend backwards	Descend in wheelie
Strength				
Trapezius	√	√	√	√
Anterior deltoids	☑	☑	√	√
Middle deltoids	√	√	√	√
Posterior deltoids	√	√	√	√
Infraspinatus, teres minor	√	√		
Pectoralis major, teres major	•	•	•	√
Biceps, brachialis, and/or brachioradialis	√	√	√	√
Serratus anterior	•	•	•	•
Triceps	•	•	•	√
Hand musculature (active grasp)	•	•	•	√
Range of Motion				
Scapular Abduction	√	√	√	√
Adduction	√	√	√	√
Downward rotation	√	√		
Shoulder Flexion	√	√		
Extension	√	√	√	√
Internal rotation	√	√	√	√
External rotation	√	√		
Elbow Flexion	√	√	√	√
Extension	√	√	√	√
Finger Flexion				√

√ = Some strength is needed for this activity, or severe limitations in range will inhibit this activity.

☑ = A large amount of strength or normal or greater range is needed for this activity.

• = Not required, but helpful.

TABLE 12–16. NEGOTIATION OF CURBS—SKILL PREREQUISITES

	Ascend by muscling up	Ascend using momentum	Descend backwards	Descend in wheelie
Position trunk in wheelchair[a]	√	√	√	
Propel manual wheelchair over even surfaces (p. 326)	√	√	√	
From stationary position, lift casters from floor (p. 333)	√			
Pop casters onto curb from stationary position (p. 333)	√			
Position casters at edge of curb (p. 333)	√			
Ascend curb from stationary position (p. 333)	√			
Lift casters off floor while chair moves forward (p. 334)		√		
Pop casters onto curb while chair moves forward (p. 335)		√		
Ascend curb using momentum (p. 335)		√		
Backing down curb, control rear wheels' descent (p. 336)			√	
Lower casters from curb by turning wheelchair (p. 336)			√	
Assume wheelie position (p. 328)				√
Glide forward in wheelie (p. 331)				√
Descend curb in wheelie position (p. 336)			√	

[a] Refer to Chapter 11 for a description of this skill and therapeutic strategies.

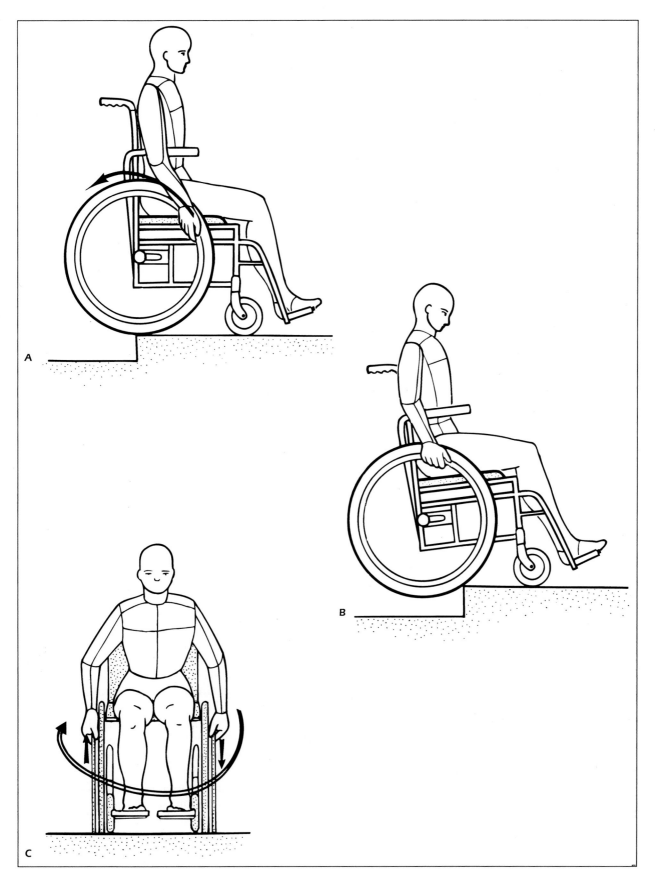

Figure 12–8.   Descending curb backwards. **(A)** Starting position: chair backed to edge of curb. **(B)** Controlling chair's descent. **(C)** Turning the wheelchair in a tight arc to lower casters from curb.

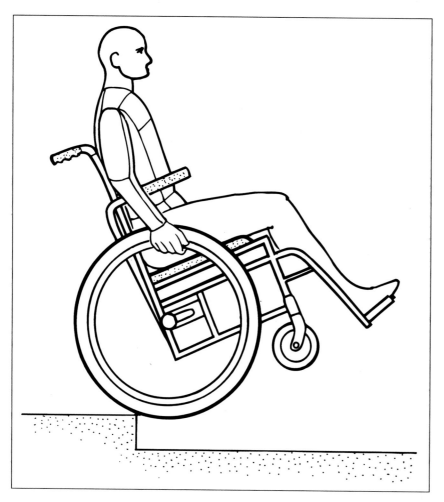

Figure 12–9. Descending curb in a wheelie.

greatest difficulty in propelling over uneven terrain involves catching or sinking of the casters, uneven surfaces are often easier to negotiate with the casters off the ground. The wheelchair user assumes a wheelie position and maintains it as he propels over the rough surface.

Stairs. Why should a person who uses a wheelchair learn to negotiate stairs in this day and age? Most public buildings have elevators. Most private buildings, however, do not. Someone who wants to visit friends and relatives, or the second floor of his own home, is likely to have to negotiate stairs. And even public buildings with elevators *do not* have functioning elevators when there is a power outage or a fire.

Independent stair negotiation is more convenient than assisted stair negotiation; someone capable of helping may not always be available. Independent stair negotiation is also safer. An attendant, family member, or helpful stranger can slip or lose his grasp. A wheelchair user who can

ascend and descend stairs without help will be in control, rather than dependent on the skill, strength, and sobriety of another.

Ascending on buttocks. This method of ascending stairs is slow but requires less strength than ascending in a wheelchair. In *rare* cases it is possible for an individual with C8 tetraplegia to perform this skill, but it is more feasible for people with fully innervated upper extremities. Ascending stairs on the buttocks requires the ability to transfer independently between a wheelchair and the floor.[n]

The first task in ascending stairs on the buttocks is a transfer from the wheelchair to a low step (Figure 12–10A). The transfer can be to the lowest step or to the one above it, depending on the individual's ability. Once on the step, the per-

---

[n] Transfers between the wheelchair and floor are presented in Chapter 11.

TABLE 12-17. NEGOTIATION OF STAIRS—PHYSICAL PREREQUISITES

	Ascend on buttocks	Ascend in wheelchair	Descend on buttocks	Descend in wheelchair holding rail	Descend in wheelie
Strength					
Fully innervated upper extremities	•	☑	•	•	√
Anterior deltoids	☑	☑	☑	☑	√
Middle deltoids	√	√	√	√	√
Posterior deltoids	√	√	√	√	☑
Biceps, brachialis, and/or brachioradialis	☑	√	☑	☑	☑
Serratus anterior	☑	☑	☑		√
Latissimus dorsi	☑	☑	☑		
Triceps	☑	☑	☑	•	√
Hand musculature (active grasp)	√	•	√	•	√
Range of Motion					
Scapular — Abduction	√	√	√	√	√
Adduction	√	√	√		√
Downward rotation	√	√	√		
Upward rotation	√	√	√	√	
Shoulder — Flexion	√	√	√	√	
Extension	☑	☑	☑	√	√
Internal rotation	√	√	√	√	√
External rotation				√	
Elbow — Flexion	√	√	√	√	√
Extension	√	√	√	√	√
Finger — Flexion	√		√		√

√ = Some strength is needed for this activity, or severe limitations in range will inhibit this activity.

☑ = A large amount of strength or normal or greater range is needed for this activity.

• = Not required, but helpful.

son positions his buttocks and legs. His buttocks should be securely on the step, with the legs facing down the steps and the knees bent. The step-to-step transfers that follow will be easiest to perform if the legs are aligned with the body's midline, instead of leaning to the side. To maintain this alignment, the person can position his feet laterally and lean his knees against each other.

After aligning his buttocks and legs on the step, the person positions his chair. Maintaining his balance by propping on one arm, he grasps the chair with the other hand. He then turns the chair so that it faces away from the stairs, with the rear wheels against the lowest step. Tilting the chair back, he places the push handles on the highest step that they will reach (Figure 12–10B).

From this point, the individual ascends the stairs by transferring up one step at a time and pulling the chair along. To transfer up a step, he places both hands on the next higher step and leans back while pushing down (Figure 12–10C).

TABLE 12-18.   NEGOTIATION OF STAIRS—SKILL PREREQUISITES

	Ascend on buttocks	Ascend in wheelchair	Descend on buttocks	Descend in wheelchair holding rail	Descend in wheelie
Transfers between wheelchair and floor[a]	✓		✓		
Position buttocks and legs on step[a]	✓		✓		
Sitting on step or floor, tilt wheelchair back to position to ascend or descend stairs (p. 337)	✓		✓		
Sitting on step, stabilize wheelchair by pushing down through push handles (p. 337)	✓		✓		
Transfer up a step while stabilizing wheelchair (p. 337)	✓				
Sitting on step, position buttocks and legs while stabilizing wheelchair (p. 338)	✓		✓		
Sitting on step or landing, pull wheelchair up (p. 338)	✓				
Sitting on floor, pull wheelchair to upright position (p. 338)	✓		✓		
Lower chair into position to ascend stairs in wheelchair (p. 338)		✓			
Sitting in wheelchair tilted back onto steps, reposition hands (p. 339)		✓			
Sitting in wheelchair, push on step to lift wheelchair up a step (p. 339)		✓			
Return wheelchair to upright (p. 345)		✓			
Sitting on a step, lower wheelchair down a step (p. 339)			✓		
Sitting on a step, transfer down a step while stabilizing wheelchair (p. 339)			✓		
Sitting in wheelchair holding stair handrail(s), lower chair down stairs (p. 340)				✓	
Assume wheelie position (p. 328)					✓
Glide forward, back, and turn in wheelie (p. 331)					✓
In wheelie, position wheels at top of step (p. 340)					✓
In wheelie, stabilize wheels against step (p. 340)					✓
Descend step, remaining in wheelie position (p. 340)					✓

[a] Refer to Chapter 11 for a description of this skill and therapeutic strategies.

As his buttocks clear the edge of the higher step, he lifts them onto the step by depressing his shoulders and tipping his head forward.

Once the person has transferred up a step, he moves his legs. He should place them with the knees flexed and the feet flat on a lower step (Figure 12–10D). Positioning the legs in this manner will make it easier to transfer to the next step.

It may be possible to transfer up a step before moving the chair. As the individual moves further up the stairs, he must bring the chair along. The chair will remain beside him as he ascends. To pull the wheelchair up a step, he first places his buttocks well back on the step and positions his legs as just described. He then places his free hand (the one farthest from the chair) on the step above the one on which he sits. The hand should be slightly lateral to his trunk. Propping on this arm, he leans back and pulls the chair up a step, placing the push handles on the step above the one on which he sits (Figure 12–10E and F).

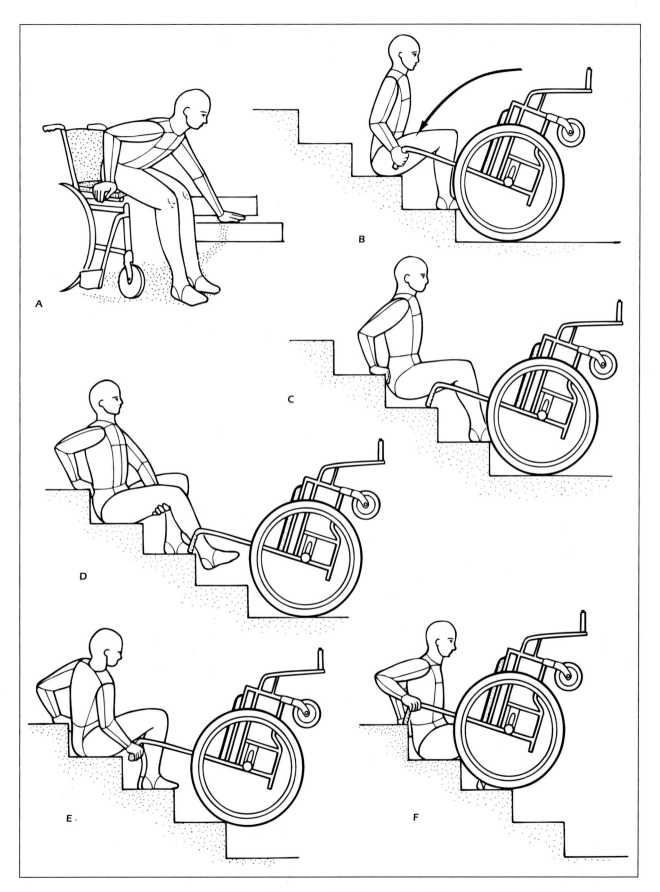

Figure 12–10.   Ascending stairs on buttocks. **(A)** Transferring to step. **(B)** Tilting wheelchair back onto step. **(C)** Transferring up a step. **(D)** Repositioning legs. **(E)** Pulling wheelchair up a step. **(F)** Transferring up a step while stabilizing wheelchair.

Once a person has brought his wheelchair up onto the steps so that the wheels rest on a step, he must hold the chair to keep it from falling down the stairs. If he lets go even briefly, it will fall. Maintaining a hold on the chair while transferring from step to step is most easily accomplished by bearing weight through the push handle when transferring. The force on the push handle must be directed straight downward.

Ascending stairs involves repeating the process of pulling the wheelchair up a step, transferring up, and repositioning the legs. Once the person has reached the landing at the top of the stairs, he pulls the wheelchair onto the landing. He then rights the chair (away from the edge, please!) and transfers into it.

Ascending in a wheelchair.

Ascending stairs in a chair is faster than ascending on the buttocks. In addition, when ascending in his chair, a person does not risk traumatizing the skin over his ischial tuberosities or sacrum on the stairs and will not get his clothes wet or dirty. Unfortunately, not everyone can ascend stairs in this manner. *Strong, fully innervated upper extremities are required.*

Ascending stairs in this manner requires the use of either a seat belt (preferably) or a belt that encircles the proximal thighs and the wheelchair seat (Figure 12–11A). The wheelchair user backs up to the stairs, grasps the rail(s), and pulls on the rail(s) to tip the chair back. He lowers himself until the chair's push handles rest on a step (Figure 12–11B). From this position, he pulls himself up the stairs, one step at a time.

To ascend a step, the person first places his hands on the step above the one on which the push handles rest (Figure 12–11C). He then lifts his buttocks and the wheelchair by pushing down forcefully (Figure 12–11D). He will feel the chair's resistance reduce substantially as the wheels get up over the edge of the step.

Once an individual has lifted his wheelchair up a step, he moves his hands to the next step. To keep the chair from falling back down the stairs, he must move his hands one at a time. This involves balancing first on one arm and then the other and moving the free hand up a step.

The stairs are ascended one step at a time by the repeated process of pulling the wheelchair up a step and repositioning the hands to the next step. Once an individual has reached the landing at the top of the stairs, he pulls the wheelchair well onto the landing. After pulling his chair a safe distance from the top of the stairs, he can right the chair while remaining in it. Alternatively, he can get out of the wheelchair, return it to an upright position, and perform a floor-to-chair transfer.

Descending on buttocks.

To descend stairs on his buttocks, the wheelchair user performs in reverse the sequence of maneuvers used to ascend stairs on his buttocks.

Descending in a wheelchair, holding rail.

Using this technique to descend stairs, a wheelchair user holds the rail and lowers the chair backwards. Because he stays in his wheelchair, he does not risk traumatizing his skin on the stairs or getting his clothes dirty. This skill would be very helpful in the event of an emergency because it enables a person to descend stairs safely and quickly without assistance.

Virtually anyone with fully innervated upper extremities should be able to master this technique. Full use of the upper extremities, however, is not required for the exceptional individual.

To descend stairs using this method, the wheelchair user positions his chair close to one rail at the top of the stairs, facing away from the stairs (Figure 12–12A). He grasps the rail firmly with both hands.° The hand of the arm closest to the rail should be positioned lower on the rail than the other hand. Figure 12–12C illustrates the hand positions.

Pulling on the rail, the person moves his chair to the edge of the top step. As the wheels move past the edge, he leans his trunk forward. Once the tires move past the step's edge, gravity provides the force to move the chair. The wheelchair user's task is to control the chair's descent. He does so by maintaining his grasp on the rail and lowering the chair (Figure 12–12B). As the chair progresses down the stairs, he moves his hands down the rail, sliding one hand at a time.

Descending in a wheelie.

This stair negotiation technique involves maintaining the chair in a wheelie position during the descent. The wheelchair user faces down the stairs and holds the wheelchair's handrims rather than the stair rails. This technique is safest when the steps have large horizontal surfaces and small vertical rises. It is also safer on a small series of stairs rather than a long flight.

Like descending holding a rail, descending stairs in a wheelie is fast and does not require the person to leave the chair. Descending in a wheelie is

---

° On a narrow stairway, it may be possible to reach both rails. A person may then choose to position his chair in the center of the stairs and hold both rails as he lowers himself.

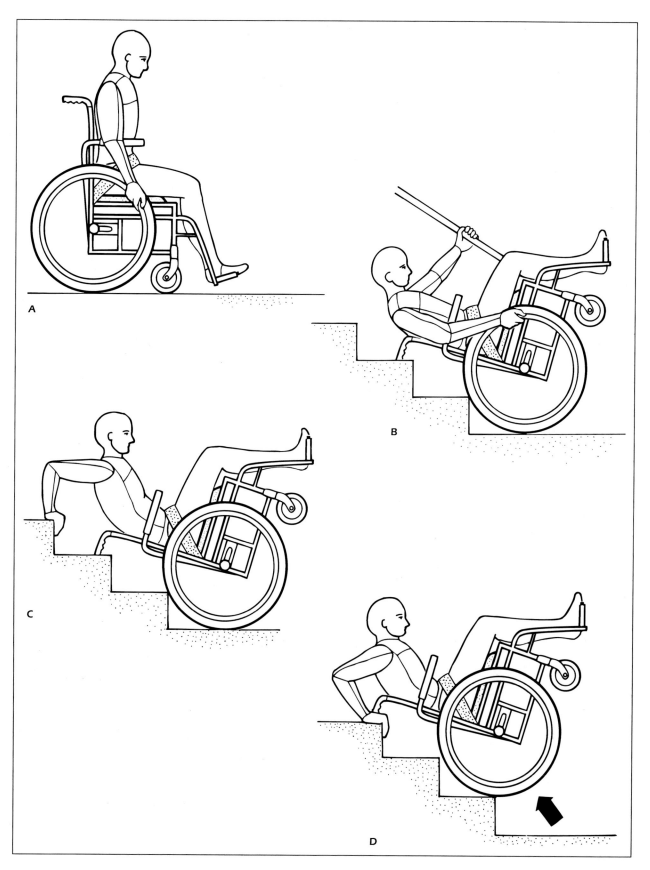

Figure 12–11. *Ascending stairs in wheelchair.* **(A)** *Belted into wheelchair.* **(B)** *Chair lowered onto step.* **(C)** *Hands positioned for ascending step.* **(D)** *Ascending step.*

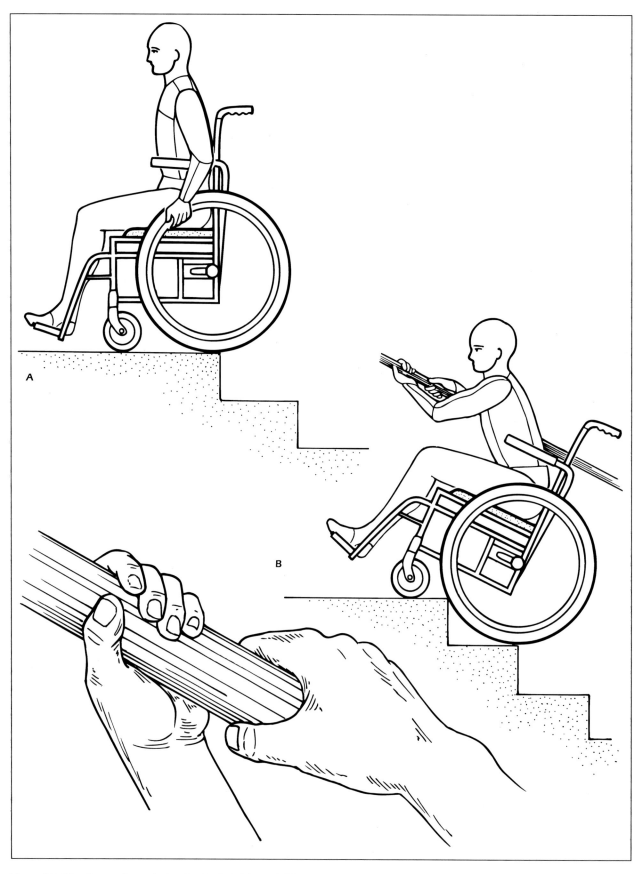

Figure 12–12. Descending stairs in wheelchair, holding rail. **(A)** Starting position: chair backed to top step. **(B)** Lowering wheelchair down stairs. **(C)** Hand positions.

more difficult, however, and involves a greater risk of falling. This maneuver can be performed only by people with fully innervated upper extremities who are exceptionally proficient in wheelchair skills. Its greatest advantage is that it makes it possible to descend stairs quickly when rails are absent.

When descending stairs in a wheelie, the person maintains a wheelie as he lowers the chair down one step at a time. He first approaches the stairs in a wheelie and positions the wheels at the edge of the top step (Figure 12–13A). From this position, he pushes forward on the handrims until the tires move over the edge and he feels the chair begin to descend. At this point, he stops pushing forward and works to control the chair's descent as gravity pulls it down the step (Figure 12–13B). He maintains control by gripping the handrims loosely and allowing them to slide through his grasp. When the wheels reach the next step, he can stabilize the chair by pulling back on the handrims until the wheels press against the vertical surface of the higher step (Figure 12–13C). He is then ready to repeat the process on the next step. In this manner, the wheelchair user descends the stairs one step at a time.

Narrow doorways. Many doorways in private homes are too narrow for wheelchairs to pass through. This is especially true of bathroom doors and of doors in mobile homes. Even if an individual has the financial resources to adapt his own home, he is likely to encounter narrow doorways when he leaves his home.

Fully innervated upper extremities and a wheelchair with a folding frame are needed to negotiate narrow doorways using the techniques described in this section.

Sitting on an armrest. In preparation for getting his wheelchair through a narrow doorway, the person positions his chair. If possible, his footplates should extend into the doorway and the doorjamb should be within reach (Figure 12–14A). After positioning the chair, he removes his foot from one footplate and folds the footplate up (Figure 12–14B). (Otherwise the footplates will collide as the chair narrows, limiting the amount that the chair can be narrowed.)

Once the chair is positioned, the person places his hands on the armrests so that he can transfer onto an armrest. The hand toward which he plans to transfer should be well forward, to leave room for his buttocks.[p] The transfer is

---

[p] When sitting on an armrest, the person actually balances on his proximal thighs.

TABLE 12–19. NEGOTIATION OF NARROW DOORWAYS— PHYSICAL PREREQUISITES

		Sitting on armrest	Remaining on the seat
Strength			
Fully innervated upper extremities		√	√
Range of Motion			
Scapular	Abduction	√	
	Adduction	√	
	Downward rotation	√	
	Upward rotation	√	
Shoulder	Flexion	√	
	Extension	√	
	Internal rotation	√	√
Elbow	Flexion	√	√
	Extension	√	
Finger	Flexion	√	√

√ = Some strength is needed for this activity, or severe limitations in range will inhibit this activity.

achieved by pushing down forcefully and throwing the head down and away from the armrest (Figure 12–14C).

After the transfer to the armrest, balance is maintained by propping with one arm on the opposite armrest. With his free hand, the wheelchair user grasps the seat and pulls upward forcefully and abruptly (Figure 12–14D). As he does so, he shifts his weight off of his supporting hand. When he pulls on the chair in this manner, it narrows slightly. Repeated pulls will narrow the wheelchair to the desired width.

Once he has narrowed his chair sufficiently, the wheelchair user is ready to move through the doorway. Still balancing on one arm, he pulls on the doorjamb (Figure 12–14E) or propels through the door by pushing the handrims with his free hand.

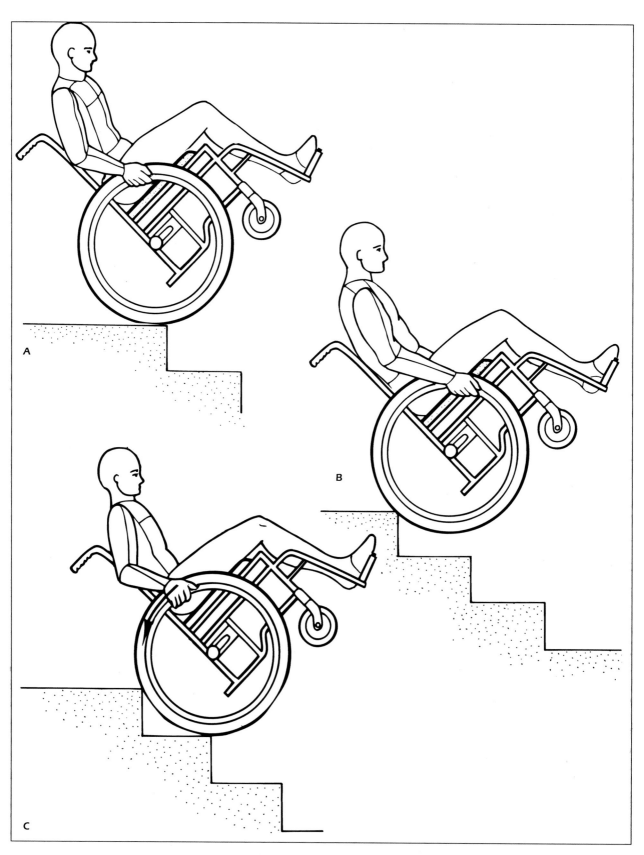

Figure 12–13.   *Descending stairs in a wheelie.* **(A)** *Starting position: in wheelie, wheels positioned at edge of top step.* **(B)** *Controlling chair's descent.* **(C)** *Stabilizing wheelchair by pulling wheel against stair.*

TABLE 12-20. NEGOTIATION OF NARROW DOORWAYS— SKILL PREREQUISITES

	Sitting on armrest	Remaining on the seat
Transfer to armrest (p. 341)	✓	
Maintain balance while sitting on armrest (p. 341)	✓	
Narrow wheelchair while sitting on armrest (p. 343)	✓	
Sitting on armrest, pull doorjamb to move narrowed wheelchair through door (p. 343) *or* Sitting on armrest, propel narrowed wheelchair (p. 343)	✓	
Transfer from armrest to wheelchair seat (p. 343)	✓	
Narrow wheelchair by rocking side-to-side (p. 343)		✓
Propel wheelchair over even surfaces (p. 326)		✓

After passing through the door, the person transfers back into the wheelchair's seat. With one hand on each armrest, he pushes down and tucks his head to lift his buttocks and swings his head laterally toward the armrest on which he has been sitting.

Remaining on the seat. This method of negotiating tight spaces enables people to remain seated while narrowing their wheelchairs. A chair's width cannot be reduced a great deal using this technique, so it is not useful with very narrow doorways. This technique provides a means of narrowing a chair for the many users who choose not to use armrests on their folding-frame chairs.

Reducing a wheelchair's width while remaining seated involves rocking the chair side to side while pulling up on the sides of the seat. The wheelchair user initiates the process by throwing his head to one side, simultaneously pulling up on the opposite side of the seat. (If rocking to the left, he throws his head to the left and pulls up on the right side of the seat.) The head motions and pulls on the seat must be performed forcefully and abruptly. As this maneuver is repeated, the chair rocks to one side and then the other. With each rock and pull, the chair narrows slightly. Once the chair's width has been reduced sufficiently, it can be propelled through the doorway.

Falling safely. Many advanced wheelchair skills involve propelling the chair with the casters lifted off the ground. These activities involve a risk of falling. A person who negotiates curbs independently or propels his chair in a wheelie is likely to fall eventually. While performing the maneuver, he will inadvertently move past his balance point, and the wheelchair will tip over backward. To minimize the risk of injury, anyone who learns to lift his casters off the ground should learn to respond appropriately when falling. Tables 12–21 and 12–22 present the physical and skill prerequisites for falling safely in a wheelchair.

Falling backward involves some risk, but appropriate action during the fall may reduce the risk of injury. When falling backward, a wheelchair rider should tuck his head and hold the wheels. When a person falls in this manner, he is not likely to injure himself or even experience discomfort. The chair's push handles, not the person's back or head, take the brunt of the force when the chair lands.[q]

When the wheelchair lands, the legs' momentum may cause the person's knees to hit his face. An alternate method of falling can prevent this. Using this method, the wheelchair user tucks his head and maintains his hold on one wheel. He quickly reaches his free arm across his legs and grasps the opposite armrest or seat. This arm blocks his thighs as they fall, keeping his knees from hitting his face (Figure 12–15).

Returning to upright after fall. After someone has fallen safely in his wheelchair, he faces the task of getting back up and into his chair. One option is to get out of the chair, place it in an upright position, and transfer back into it. A faster alternative involves staying in the chair while pushing it back to upright. Fully innervated upper extremities are required to perform this maneuver. Tables 12–21 and 12–22 present the physical and skill prerequisites for returning the wheelchair to upright after a fall.

---

[q] A wheelchair that lacks push handles, has a low backrest, or has a backrest with badly stretched upholstery will not provide this protection during a fall.

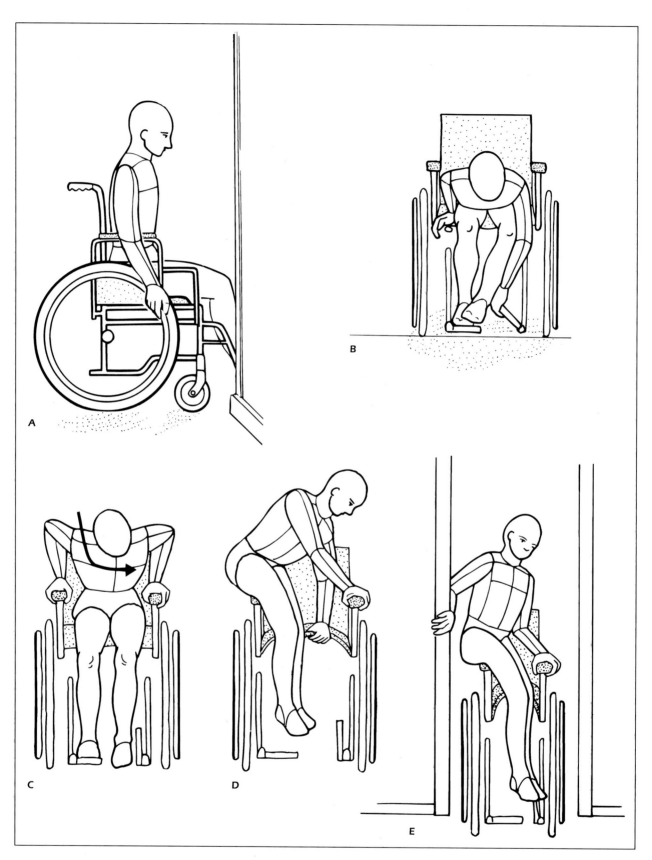

Figure 12–14.   Negotiating narrow doorway, sitting on an armrest. **(A)** Initial position of wheelchair. **(B)** Folding footplate after removing foot. **(C)** Transferring onto armrest. **(D)** Narrowing wheelchair by pulling upward on the seat. **(E)** Pulling on doorjamb to pull wheelchair through doorway.

TABLE 12–21. FALLING SAFELY AND RETURNING TO UPRIGHT— PHYSICAL PREREQUISITES

		Falling safely	Block lower extremities while falling safely	Return to upright while remaining in wheelchair
Strength				
Fully innervated upper extremities		•	✓	✓
Sternocleidomastoid		✓		
Biceps, brachialis, and/or brachioradialis		✓		
Hand musculature (active grasp)		•		
Range of Motion				
Scapular	Abduction		✓	✓
	Adduction			✓
	Upward rotation			✓
Shoulder	Flexion			✓
	Extension			✓
	Internal rotation		✓	✓
	External rotation			✓
	Abduction			✓
Elbow	Flexion	✓	✓	✓
	Extension	✓	✓	✓

√ = Some strength is needed for this activity, or severe limitations in range will inhibit this activity.

• = Not required, but helpful.

TABLE 12–22. FALLING SAFELY AND RETURNING TO UPRIGHT— SKILL PREREQUISITES

	Falling safely	Return to upright while remaining in wheelchair
While falling backward in wheelchair, tuck head and hold wheels (p. 343)	✓	
or		
Tuck head and block legs (p. 345)		
After falling backward in wheelchair, position self in chair (p. 345)		✓
Sitting in overturned wheelchair, lock brakes (p. 345)		✓
Sitting in overturned wheelchair, lift upper trunk from floor (p. 345)		✓
Sitting in overturned wheelchair, balance on one hand (p. 345)		✓
Sitting in overturned wheelchair, rock chair to upright (p. 345)		✓

Righting a wheelchair while remaining in it requires proper positioning: buttocks on the seat and legs looped over the front edge of the seat (Figure 12–16A). If the wheelchair user is wearing a seat belt or has held on during his fall, he should be fairly well positioned already. If he has slid out slightly or if his legs have fallen off of the seat, he will need to position himself in the chair before righting it. To move his buttocks back onto the seat, he pulls on the wheels. He can then grasp his legs and position them, looping them over the seat.

Once positioned appropriately, the person locks the chair's brakes. He then lifts his upper trunk from the floor by pulling on the front of the chair (Figure 12–16B). Once he has lifted his trunk, he releases one hand, turns, and places this hand on the floor (Figure 12–16C). For simplicity, this hand will be called "the supporting hand" for the rest of this description. The other hand will be called "the free hand."

The supporting hand should be positioned directly beneath the trunk, so that weight can be shifted onto it. Balancing on the supporting hand, the person releases the chair. He then reaches his free hand across his body and grasps the opposite wheel (Figure 12–16D).

Righting the chair from this position involves rocking it forward repeatedly and walking the supporting hand around to the side toward the front of the wheelchair. Rocking the chair is accomplished by bending the elbow of the supporting arm and then extending it (Figure 12–16E and F). The push against the floor should be forceful and abrupt enough to thrust the chair

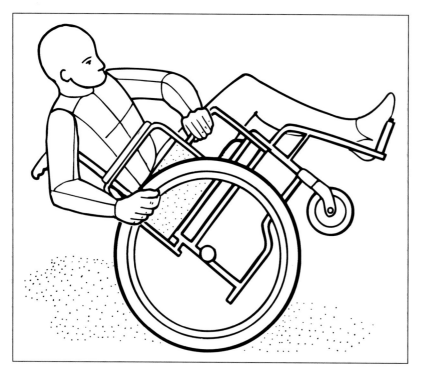

Figure 12–15. *Falling backward safely.*

toward an upright position. Each time the chair rocks forward, the supporting hand is inched forward around the side of the chair.[r] When the chair falls back from its forward rock, the person balances on his supporting arm and repeats the process.

As the wheelchair user rocks the chair and inches his supporting hand forward, his chair gradually assumes a more upright position (Figure 12–16G). Eventually, he will reach a position from which he can thrust hard enough to rock the chair forward past its balance point, returning it to an upright position (Figure 12–16H).

THERAPEUTIC STRATEGIES FOLLOWING COMPLETE SPINAL CORD INJURY

To accomplish a functional goal, a patient must acquire both the physical and skill prerequisites for that activity. For example, when working on driving a power wheelchair with a hand-held joystick, a person with a spinal cord injury must develop adequate strength in his shoulder girdle, as well as developing the ability to push the chair's joystick in various directions.

When developing skill prerequisites for a functional goal, the patient should start with the most basic prerequisite skills and progress toward more challenging activities. (A person had best develop skill in maintaining a wheelie before attempting to negotiate stairs in this position!)

Before asking a patient to attempt a new skill, the therapist should explain and demonstrate the technique.[s] The demonstration should provide a clear idea of the motions involved and the timing of these motions. The therapist should also demonstrate how the new skill will be used functionally.

During functional training, the therapist should remember that every person with a spinal cord injury will perform a particular activity differently. Each has a unique combination of body build, coordination, strength, and flexibility, and these characteristics influence the manner in which he performs functional tasks. As a result of these individual variations, each person is unique in the exact motions that he uses and the timing of these motions as he ascends a curb or rights his wheelchair after a fall. What works for one patient may be a total disaster for the next. The challenge

---

[r] This maneuver will be easier if the armrest has been removed, particularly if the wheelchair user is short.

[s] This demonstration can also be provided by another person with a spinal cord injury, if someone is available who has similar impairments but a higher level of functional ability. Alternatively, the patient may watch a videotaped demonstration of the skill.

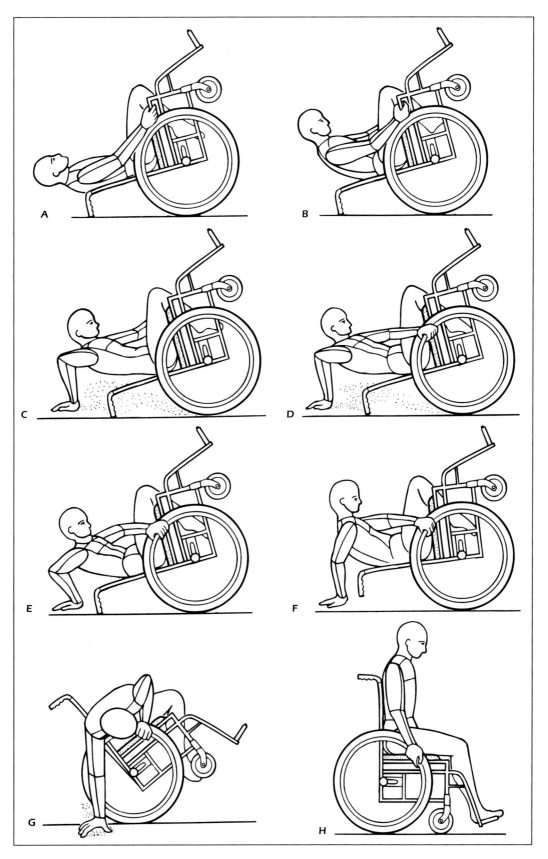

Figure 12–16.   Returning to upright after fall. **(A)** Starting position: buttocks on seat, legs looped over front edge of seat. **(B)** Trunk lifted by pulling on front of wheelchair. **(C)** Hand placed on floor. **(D)** Opposite wheel grasped. **(E** and **F)** Rocking wheelchair toward upright by pushing with supporting arm. **(G)** Hand inched forward. **(H)** Upright.

of functional training is finding the timing and maneuvers that best suit the individual involved.

As a therapist and patient work together on a skill, they can learn from failed attempts by analyzing the problem. Is the patient strong enough to perform the maneuver? Did he drop his casters too early or too late as he attempted to ascend the curb? Did he approach the curb with adequate speed?

Strategies for addressing the various prerequisite skills are presented in the following sections.

Upright Sitting Tolerance

The development of upright sitting tolerance involves a gradual accommodation to elevation of the head and torso above horizontal. A reclining wheelchair is useful for this process. When a recently injured person is first placed in this type of wheelchair, the chair's back can be almost fully reclined and the legrests elevated. As the patient adapts to sitting, the wheelchair's back can be raised in small increments to a progressively more vertical position, and the legrests can be lowered.

If a reclining wheelchair is not available, sitting tolerance can be developed in bed. The patient should be able to accommodate to increasingly upright positions by sitting with the head of his bed elevated and his feet dangling over the side of the bed. When his sitting tolerance has increased sufficiently, the patient can use a nonreclining wheelchair.

Thigh-high antiembolic stockings and an abdominal binder[t] can be worn initially to reduce orthostatic hypotension by facilitating venous return. Unless it is required to enhance the individual's breathing ability,[u] the binder can be discontinued once the patient has accommodated to sitting. The patient can be weaned gradually from its use through loosening over a period of days.

During the period of adjustment to upright sitting, mild dizziness is common and will need to be tolerated as the individual adjusts to sitting. If the patient becomes very nauseated, loses consciousness, or loses vision or hearing, these symptoms can be eliminated by elevating the legs, tipping the wheelchair back into a more reclined position, or both. It is important to remember that the above-described symptoms are not dangerous

and to treat them accordingly.[v] A calm attitude on the therapist's part can result in an easier and more rapid adjustment to sitting.

The time allotted to developing sitting tolerance need not be spent with the patient passively watching the clock and waiting for nausea or dizziness (or sudden death from boredom) to strike. While the patient adjusts to sitting, he can perform strengthening exercises and begin working on wheelchair propulsion. He can also practice stabilizing his trunk and leaning from side to side in the wheelchair, controlling the motion by pulling on the armrests.

Sitting in a Wheelchair, Move Trunk Using Head and Scapular Motions

Training in this skill will be easiest if the patient is able to tolerate upright sitting. In a reclined sitting position, weight bearing through the back makes it more difficult to move the trunk laterally.

During initial practice of this skill, the patient can work on moving laterally from a midline sitting position. The therapist can demonstrate the technique and then manually guide him through the motions. The patient then practices throwing his head and shoulder vigorously and repeatedly in one direction at a time. In this manner, he can practice moving laterally past his balance point in one direction and then the other.

Early training should also include practice in returning upright from a lateral lean. This practice should start with the patient sitting with a *slight* lean, in a position barely lateral to midline sitting. The therapist should encourage him to move his trunk back to upright using vigorous head and scapular motions.

Once the patient is able to move both toward and away from an upright position, he can combine practice of the two skills, shifting a short distance to the side and returning to upright. As his ability improves, he can gradually increase the arc of motion. He should practice moving laterally toward and away from upright over increasing arcs until he achieves his maximal capability.

Independent work.   Once able to move laterally in and out of upright sitting over small arcs, the patient can practice alone. He should be encour-

---

[t] An abdominal binder is an elasticized band that encompasses the entire abdomen.

[u] See Chapter 7 for respiratory issues.

---

[v] Orthostatic hypotension should not be confused with autonomic dysreflexia, which is a dangerous condition. Autonomic dysreflexia is characterized by a *rise* in blood pressure rather than a fall and is brought on by noxious stimulation below the lesion. Its management is addressed in Chapter 3.

aged to shift as far as he can while maintaining control over the motion; he should move far enough to make the activity challenging but not so far that he cannot return to upright independently.

Place Hand on Joystick

A person who has enough strength in his deltoids and biceps to move well against gravity should be able to learn to place his hand on his wheelchair's joystick without difficulty. He may require only a demonstration and brief practice.

Someone with limited ability to move against gravity in elbow flexion and shoulder flexion and abduction may be able to learn this skill but will require more practice. An individual with such pronounced upper extremity weakness places his arm on the joystick using a combination of scapular, shoulder, and elbow motions. The maneuvers used are determined by the arm's starting position. If the arm is initially positioned hanging down outside of the armrest, the person elevates his scapula to lift his arm. By partially abducting and internally rotating his shoulder, he places his elbow in a gravity-reduced position for elbow flexion. He can then place his hand on the joystick by flexing his elbow.

If the person's arm is positioned in his lap, he uses a combination of scapular elevation and retraction, shoulder abduction and external rotation, and elbow flexion to place his hand on the joystick. Alternatively, he can use these motions to position his hand outside of the armrest, then lift it onto the joystick using the maneuver described above.

When an individual has limited ability to move his shoulder and elbow against gravity, practice of the required motions may begin with the arm suspended in a sling or supported by a skateboard placed on a board (Figure 12–17). Using this equipment, the patient can practice moving repeatedly through gravity-eliminated arcs. As his strength and skill improve, he can progress to moving up a slight slope and increase the slope as appropriate. With different positions of the sling or board, he can work on moving his shoulder and elbow through the various motions required to place his hand on a joystick. In this manner, he can build the strength required for this skill.

Skill training can begin with the patient working on moving his hand onto the joystick from a position just lateral to the stick. As his ability improves, he can move his hand from positions progressively lateral and inferior to the joystick. In this manner, he can gradually develop the ability to lift his hand onto the joystick, starting with his arm hanging at his side lateral to the armrest. The ability to perform this skill with the arm initially positioned in the lap can be developed using the same strategy: the patient begins by repeatedly placing his hand from a position just medial to the joystick. As his skill builds, he works from progressively medial and inferior starting positions.

Independent work. The strengthening and skill practice just described are ideal independent exercises.

Move Joystick in All Directions Using Arm and Scapular Motions

When a joystick is mounted for hand control, it is mounted in a vertical or nearly vertical position. To control his wheelchair, the person must be able to move his hand in all directions in a horizontal or nearly horizontal plane. Independent place-

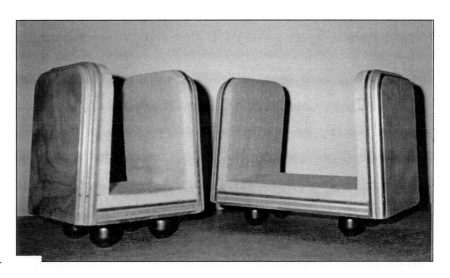

Figure 12–17. Skateboards.

ment of the hand on the joystick is not necessary for practicing this skill.

Practice in moving a joystick should be done with the wheelchair's motor off or disconnected from the wheels (clutch disengaged). The patient can then work on pushing the stick in various directions without having the chair whirl about uncontrollably.

People with good scapular and shoulder control are not likely to need much training to master this skill. They may require only a demonstration and brief period of practice.

Individuals with weaker proximal musculature require more extensive training. Before learning to push a joystick, they must develop the ability to perform the necessary motions. Practice may begin with the arm suspended in an overhead sling or supported by a skateboard placed on a board (Figure 12–17). Using this equipment, the patient can practice moving his hand in all directions in the horizontal plane. Backward and forward motion can be accomplished using scapular adduction and abduction.[w] Glenohumeral rotation and horizontal adduction and abduction are used for lateral motions. Diagonal motions are performed by combining these glenohumeral and scapular motions.

The patient can practice using a joystick once he is able to move his hand well with his arm supported by a sling or skateboard. If he remains unable to move the joystick, the therapist can facilitate practice by making the task easier. This can be done by suspending the arm in an overhead sling or mobile arm support, splinting the elbow and wrist, and strapping the hand to the joystick. These "crutches" can be removed[x] as the patient's skill improves with practice.[34, 42]

Particularly if the patient has very limited upper extremity strength, the training period with the wheelchair is likely to involve a fair amount of equipment adjustment. The joystick can be moved in any plane: it can be placed in a more medial, lateral, anterior, or posterior position; rotated in the horizontal plane; or tilted from vertical in any direction. By altering the joystick's position, the therapist can place it so that the motions required to control the chair are most suited to the individual's patterns of strength and weakness. In addition to placing the joystick optimally in space, the therapist can alter the joystick/user interface. The

stick can be made taller, or a grip shaped like either a "T" or a goal post can be added to enhance the individual's capacity to manipulate it. The therapist and patient should work together to determine the joystick position and configuration of the joystick/user interface that will be most comfortable and functional.

Independent work. The strengthening and skill practice just described are ideal independent exercises.

Move Joystick in All Directions Using Head, Chin, or Tongue Motions

When a joystick is mounted for head control, the headrest is the interface between the patient and the joystick. The patient controls the wheelchair by pushing the headrest backward or to the side. When a joystick is mounted for chin or mouth control, it is placed in a position close to horizontal; the end of the joystick moves in a nearly vertical plane. To control his wheelchair, the person moves the end of the joystick in all directions within this plane. With chin control, neck and jaw motions are used to move the stick up, down, laterally, and diagonally. With mouth control, the patient uses his tongue to push the joystick.

The therapist should explain and demonstrate the motions and allow the patient to practice pushing the stick in all directions. Practice moving the joystick should be done with the wheelchair's motor off or disconnected.

Mastery of this ability is likely to be more a matter of equipment adjustment than skill development. The therapist and patient should work together to determine the joystick position and configuration of the joystick/user interface that will be most comfortable and functional.

Signal Wheelchair by Sipping and Puffing in Appropriate Pattern

The therapist should explain and demonstrate the sipping and puffing pattern and allow the patient to practice. The patient will need to develop both the technique of delivering hard and soft sips to the straw with the appropriate force, and will need to learn the "code" of sips and puffs that are used to signal the chair.

Initial practice should be done with the wheelchair's motor off or disconnected. The wheelchair typically has a visual display that can be used to provide feedback to the patient about the signal that he has provided.

---

[w] In the absence of active scapular abduction, the patient can adduct actively using the middle trapezius and allow passive abduction upon relaxation of the trapezius.

[x] These "crutches" should be removed one at a time as skill increases. With each removal, the patient's performance can be expected to deteriorate temporarily until his skill improves.

Signal Wheelchair by Pressing Tongue Against Sensors in Tongue-Touch Keypad

The therapist should show the patient the sensors embedded in the tongue-touch keypad, and explain how it works. The patient will need to develop his skill in contacting the desired sensors with his tongue, and will need to learn how the sensors are used to signal the chair.

Initial practice should be done with the wheelchair's motor off or disconnected. The wheelchair typically has a visual display that can be used to provide feedback to the patient about the signal that he has provided.

Signal Wheelchair by Moving Head Toward and Away from Sensors in Headrest

The therapist should explain and demonstrate how head motions can be used to signal the chair by activating sensors in the headrest. The patient can practice initially with the wheelchair's motor off or disconnected.

Tilt or Recline Power Wheelchair and Return to Upright

Training in the performance of pressure reliefs should begin as soon as possible after out-of-bed activities are initiated. Early emphasis on this skill may promote the development of good pressure relief habits.

If the patient utilizes a power wheelchair with a tilt or recline feature, the manner in which he signals the chair to perform this function will depend on the type of access device used. The type of access device will in turn be influenced by the patient's ability to utilize the various devices available. Functional training goes hand in hand with equipment selection and adjustment as the therapist and patient analyze the available options, select the input device that appears to best match the patient's abilities, and try the device.

An access device that does not require the patient to move against gravity will be as easy to utilize whether the patient is sitting upright or is tilted or reclined. Tongue-touch keypads and sip-and-puff devices are examples. With these devices, functional training involves instruction in the manner in which the individual will give commands to the chair, and practice of the skills involved.

An input device that is accessed through upper extremity motions may be more difficult to utilize when the patient sits in a tilted or reclined position. As the seating system tilts or reclines from upright, the user's body moves relative to the line of gravity and the input device may also move relative to gravity. For example, a hand-held joystick is likely to be manipulated using arm motions performed in a horizontal plane when the seat is upright. The plane of motion of the joystick moves as the seat tilts back, and the patient must move his hand and arm against gravity to push the joystick forward. As a result, a person with severely limited upper extremity strength may be unable to signal the chair to perform a tilt through its full excursion or return to upright from a tilted position. When this is the case, the patient can practice tilting and returning to upright over a small arc of motion, increasing the excursion as his ability increases. He may also improve his performance by strengthening his shoulder and elbow musculature. An alternative solution is the use of a different input device to control the chair's tilt function.

Drive Power Wheelchair

Before practicing driving a power wheelchair, a person should have developed some initial skill in signaling the wheelchair using the access device. Driving practice should begin in a large area that is free of obstacles and potential victims. A therapist should be present to override the controls when necessary. Ideally, the therapist will have access to a "kill switch" that can be used to stop the chair if it appears that a collision is imminent.

When training first begins, the controller should be adjusted so that the chair's maximum velocity, turning speed, and rates of acceleration and deceleration are all slow. These parameters can be adjusted as the patient's skill improves.

During early work on driving, emphasis should be placed on gaining *control* of the chair. The patient should practice starting, stopping, and maneuvering in all directions. Once he has mastered these tasks, he can progress to driving over greater distances, maneuvering around obstacles, and driving over inclines, uneven terrain, and doorsills.

People with C4 tetraplegia who retain minimal sparing in the C5 myotome can learn to use a hand-held joystick, but this can be a challenging task. The therapist and patient will need to work together to find the position and configuration of the joystick that enable the individual to function most optimally. During early practice, the patient may require added equipment to make the task easier. An overhead sling or mobile arm support

PROBLEM-SOLVING EXERCISE 12-2

Your patient has normal joint range of motion and muscle flexibility throughout his upper and lower extremities bilaterally. His upper extremity muscle test results are as follows.

Muscles	Left	Right
Trapezius (upper, middle, and lower)	4/5	4/5
Deltoids (anterior, middle, and posterior)	2/5	2+/5
Elbow flexors	2/5	2+/5
Radial wrist extensors	0/5	0/5
Serratus anterior	1/5	1/5
Pectoralis major (clavicular)	1/5	1/5
Triceps	0/5	0/5
Flexor digitorum profundus	0/5	0/5

The patient is learning to perform pressure reliefs by tilting the seating system of a power wheelchair, controlling the chair using a hand-held joystick. He can independently place his hand on the joystick, and can move the joystick through its full excursion in all directions when the seating system is in its upright position. When he attempts to perform a pressure relief, however, his hand falls off of the joystick after he has tilted approximately 45 degrees from upright. He is then unable to lift his hand to place it back on the joystick to tilt further or to return to upright.

- Why is the patient unable to maintain his hand on the joystick while he tilts the chair through its full excursion?
- What equipment changes could enhance this patient's ability to perform a pressure relief and return to upright independently?
- What muscle strength could the therapeutic exercise program emphasize to facilitate the attainment of this goal?
- Describe a functional training activity for this patient.

to suspend the arm, splints to stabilize the elbow and wrist, and a strap to hold the hand on the joystick may facilitate practice. These "crutches" can be removed, one at a time, as skill and strength improve with practice.[34, 42]

Independent work. Once an individual has gained some ability to control his chair, he can practice without constant supervision. He may first practice within the department, where assistance is available when needed. As his skill and confidence improve, he can practice in other areas, further removed from assistance. When driving a chair independently, the wheelchair user should have a means of effecting an "emergency stop." If he is driving with a hand-held joystick, and if he is consistently able to remove his hand from the joystick while driving, he can stop the chair by lifting his hand from the joystick. Otherwise, he will need a separate "kill switch,"

typically a leaf switch or button switch that can be activated using head or scapular motions.

Place Palms Against Standard Wheelchair Handrims

This prerequisite skill rarely requires much, if any, training. Most people who have the physical potential to propel a manual wheelchair are able to place their palms against their chairs' handrims without practice. A few, however, have difficulty recognizing when their palms are in contact with the handrims. These patients require training in this prerequisite skill.

When training is required, the patient should be encouraged to focus on alternative sensory cues to recognize when his hands are placed appropriately. He can concentrate on proprioceptive and tactile sensations from his hands and arms while the therapist places his hands passively on the chair's handrims. He can progress to placing his hands with assistance and finally, practice placing his hands without help.

Push Standard Handrim(s) Forward

To practice this skill, a patient should be able to place his palms against the wheelchair's handrims. Most people with intact upper extremity musculature are able to push their wheelchair handrims forward without extensive training. At most, they may require brief instruction and practice.

People who lack functioning finger flexors require more training to acquire this skill. They must learn to compensate for their lack of active grasp, moving the handrims by pressing their palms inward against the rims and pushing forward. Handrims with a high-friction surface will make this task easier. During early practice, therapists may move their patients' hands passively to give them a feel for the motions involved. The patient can then assist with the motions and progress to pushing without assistance.

Because moving a wheelchair's handrims involves moving the wheelchair, this skill is difficult for many who have impaired upper extremity function. Initially, an individual with impaired upper extremity function may not be strong enough to move his handrims. When this is the case, the therapist can make the task easier by placing the chair's casters in a trailing position (Figure 12–18). If an individual remains unable to move his handrims despite this positioning, the therapist can assist with the chair's motion. While the patient attempts to push the handrims forward, the therapist pushes the chair, providing just enough force to enable him to move the

wheelchair. As his ability and strength improve, the assistance should be decreased.

The functional training strategy just described is appropriate if the individual is on the verge of being able to propel without assistance. This approach has the advantage of enabling the patient to develop propulsion skills using the type of handrims that he will ultimately use. Unfortunately, this training strategy does not allow for independent practice.

A different approach may be needed for weaker individuals. When a patient lacks the strength to propel his wheelchair without assistance, the therapist can make the task easier by wrapping the chair's handrims with rubber tubing (Figure 12–19). The tubing provides small handholds for the patient, making it easier to push the handrims. Because the handholds are small, he must use the same motions to propel the chair as he would without the tubing: he squeezes in and pushes forward. Thus, while he practices pushing his chair with the handrims wrapped, he develops the musculature and skills required for propulsion without tubing.[y]

Some people initially lack the strength to push a chair, even with the handrims wrapped in tubing. When this is the case, the therapist may resort to placing pegged handrims on the patient's chair. Handrim projections can enable a weak individual to propel his chair, making practice possible. The patient should grow stronger with

---

[y] One nice thing about rubber tubing is that it deteriorates. Thus as the patient's strength and skill are improving, the tubing is gradually disintegrating. Often, the individual's readiness to progress to propulsion without tubing coincides with the tubing's deterioration. This can make the transition to propulsion without tubing easier.

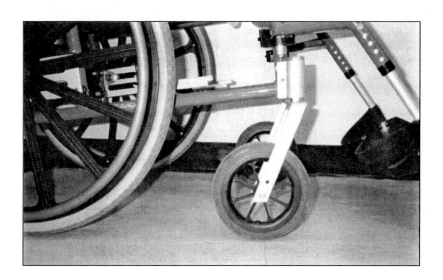

Figure 12–18. Caster in trailing position.

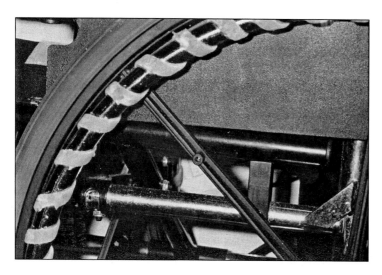

Figure 12–19. *Wheelchair handrim wrapped in rubber tubing.*

practice and may eventually build his strength enough to enable him to propel with standard handrims. The disadvantage of practicing with pegged handrims is that the motions used are different from those used to propel with standard handrims. Instead of squeezing in and pushing forward, the wheelchair user simply pulls forward on the handrim projections. Because the musculature and skills involved are different, the transition from pegged to standard handrims will be more difficult than a transition from wrapped to unwrapped standard handrims.

If upper extremity strength is impaired, propulsion will be slow and laborious at first. Therapists should resist the temptation to alter the handrims to make the task easy. A patient will gain maximal benefit from practice in pushing his wheelchair handrims if he practices at the point where the activity is challenging but possible with effort. If a patient can propel his chair, albeit slowly, with unwrapped standard handrims, then he should practice with the handrims unwrapped. If he is unable to do so, wrapping the handrims with rubber tubing is appropriate. If the individual remains unable to push his handrims, a period of practice and strengthening with pegged handrims is indicated.

Regardless of the type of handrim used, wheelchair propulsion practice should begin on hard and smooth floor surfaces such as linoleum tile. Propelling over this type of surface is easier than propelling over carpet.[41, 63]

Independent work. Once an individual is able to push his handrims forward without assistance, he can develop his skill by practicing alone.

Pull Standard Handrim(s) Backward

Before working on this skill, a patient should be able to place his palms against the wheelchair's handrims.

Most people with intact upper extremity musculature are able to pull their wheelchair handrims backward without extensive training. At most, they may require brief instruction and practice.

People who lack functioning finger flexors require more training to acquire this skill. They must learn to compensate for their lack of active grasp, moving the handrims by pressing their palms inward against the rims and pulling backward. During early practice, therapists may move their patients' hands passively to give them a feel for the motions involved. The patients can then assist with the motions and progress to pulling their handrims backward without assistance.

Because moving a wheelchair's handrims involves moving the wheelchair, this skill is difficult for many people who have impaired upper extremity function. Initially, an individual with impaired upper extremity function may not be strong enough to move his handrims. When this is the case, the therapist can make the task easier by positioning the chair's casters anteriorly (Figure 12–20). If an individual remains unable to move his handrims despite this positioning, the therapist can assist. While the patient attempts to pull the handrim(s) backward, the therapist helps move the chair, providing just enough force to enable him to move the wheelchair. As the patient's ability and strength improve, the assistance should be decreased.

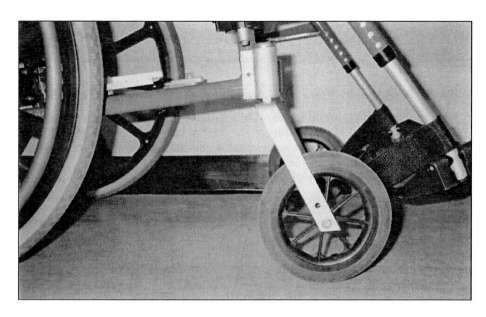

Figure 12–20. Caster positioned anteriorly.

Independent work. Once an individual is able to pull his handrims backward without assistance, he can develop his skill by practicing alone.

Place Palms on Tires, Behind Seat

A patient must be able to place his arms behind his chair's push handles before he begins work on this skill.[z] Once he has acquired that prerequisite skill, learning to place his palms on the tires should require only demonstration and a brief period of practice.

With Palms on Tires Behind Seat, Propel Backwards Using Elbow Extension and Scapular Depression

To practice this skill, a patient should be able to place his palms on his wheelchair's tires, behind the seat. An individual who lacks functional strength in his triceps must be able to extend his elbows using muscle substitution.[aa]

The therapist should first demonstrate the skill, pushing the tires backward using elbow extension and scapular depression. During initial practice, therapists may move their patients' arms passively to give them a feel for the motions

involved. The patients can then assist with the motions and progress to pushing their wheels backward without assistance.

Initially, a person with impaired upper extremity function may not be strong enough to push his chair backwards. When this is the case, the therapist can make the task easier by positioning the casters anteriorly (Figure 12–20). If an individual remains unable to propel his chair backwards despite this positioning, the therapist can assist. While the patient attempts to push the chair, the therapist provides just enough force to enable him to move the wheelchair. As his ability and strength improve, this assistance should be decreased.

Independent work. Once a patient is able to push his handrims backwards without assistance, he can develop his skill by practicing alone.

With Palms on Tires Behind Seat, Propel Backwards Using Scapular Depression

People who are unable to propel their wheelchairs backward using combined elbow extension and scapular depression may learn to do so using scapular depression alone. To practice this skill, a patient should be able to place his palms on the wheelchair's tires, behind the seat. Training can be done using the strategy described above for backward propulsion using elbow extension and scapular depression.

---

[z] Strategies for developing the ability to place the arms behind the push handles are described in Chapter 11.

[aa] Strategies for developing the skill of elbow extension using muscle substitution are described in Chapter 11.

Place Palms or Forearms Against Handrim Projections

This prerequisite skill rarely requires much, if any, training. Most people who have the physical potential to propel a manual wheelchair are able to place their palms or forearms against their chairs' handrim projections without practice. A few, however, have difficulty recognizing when their palms or forearms are in contact with the pegs. These individuals require training in this prerequisite skill.

When training is required, the patient should be encouraged to focus on alternative sensory cues to recognize when his arms are placed appropriately. The wheelchair user can concentrate on proprioceptive and tactile sensations from his hands and arms while the therapist places his palms or forearms passively on the chair's handrims. He can progress to placing his hands with assistance and finally practice placing his hands without help.

Pull Handrim Projections Forward

Once a patient has developed the ability to place his palms or forearms against the posterior aspects of his chair's handrim projections, he can work on pulling these projections forward.

Training in this skill should begin with a demonstration of how a wheelchair can be propelled by placing the hands or forearms behind posteriorly located handrim projections and pulling forward. During early practice, therapists may move their patients' arms passively to give them a feel for the motions involved. Patients can then assist with the motions and progress to pushing without assistance.

Because moving a wheelchair's handrims involves moving the wheelchair, this skill is difficult for many people who have impaired upper extremity function. As is true with standard handrims, initial practice with pegged handrims should begin on a hard floor surface such as linoleum.

Initially, an individual with impaired upper extremity function may not be strong enough to move his chair's handrims. When this is the case, the therapist can make the task easier by placing the casters in a trailing position (Figure 12–18). Propulsion will also be easier if the handrim projections are positioned symmetrically on the two sides of the chair. If an individual remains unable to move his handrims despite this positioning of the casters and pegs, the therapist can assist with the chair's motion. While the patient attempts to push the handrims forward, the therapist pushes

the chair, providing just enough force to enable him to move the wheelchair. As the patient's ability and strength improve, this assistance should be decreased.

If a patient is able to propel his wheelchair forward easily, he is probably ready to work with standard handrims.

Independent work. Once a patient is able to pull his handrim projections forward without assistance, he can develop his skill by practicing alone.

Pull Backward on Handrim Projections

Before practicing this skill, a person should be able to place his palms or forearms against the anterior aspects of his chair's handrim projections.

Training in this skill should begin with a demonstration of how a wheelchair can be propelled backward by placing the hands or forearms in front of anteriorly located handrim projections and pulling backward. During early practice, therapists may move their patients' arms passively to give them a feel for the motions involved. Patients can then assist with the motions and progress to pushing without assistance.

Initially, an individual with impaired upper extremity function may not be strong enough to move his chair's handrims. When this is the case, the therapist can make the task easier by positioning the casters anteriorly (Figure 12–20). Propulsion will also be easier if the handrim projections are positioned symmetrically on the two sides of the chair. If a patient remains unable to move his handrims despite this positioning of the casters and pegs, the therapist can assist with the chair's motion. While the patient attempts to pull the handrims backward, the therapist pushes the chair, providing just enough force to enable him to move the wheelchair. As his ability and strength improve, this assistance should be decreased.

Propel Manual Wheelchair over Even Surfaces

Once an individual is able to push his handrims forward, with or without assistance, he is ready to begin work on forward wheelchair propulsion. The training strategy is the same whether the patient uses pegged or standard handrims.

People who can push their handrims forward easily can readily achieve efficient propulsion. The therapist should demonstrate, showing how long strokes make propulsion less energy consuming. The patient should be encouraged to start each push with his hands well back, then push through and allow the chair to glide between strokes. During early practice, the therapist should give the patient feedback on his propulsion technique. The patient can then practice on his own.

Wheelchair propulsion training is more time consuming for people who have difficulty pushing their handrims forward. Before learning the finer points of efficient propulsion, these patients must learn to propel. This takes practice, practice, and more practice. Propulsion is likely to be painfully slow at first, but the patient should grow stronger and faster with practice. He should be encouraged to push wherever he goes in the course of each day. As his ability improves, he can work on developing a more efficient pattern of propulsion.

The therapist and patient should remember that wheelchair propulsion is difficult initially if upper extremity musculature is impaired. Pushing is likely to be too slow to be functional at first, but the patient should keep at it. The only way to become more proficient is to practice.

Independent work. Once an individual is able to propel his chair forward and turn without assistance, he can practice independently. He should be encouraged to push to therapies and meals during the day, and can propel during his free time in the evenings. In addition to practicing propulsion, the patient can exercise on an arm cycle ergometer to improve his wheelchair propulsion endurance.[12]

Propel Manual Wheelchair up a Slope

To practice this skill, a person must be able to propel a manual wheelchair independently over even surfaces. Because ascending a slope takes greater strength and skill than does propelling on a horizontal surface, the patient should be fairly proficient in wheelchair propulsion prior to beginning ramp negotiation practice.

Before attempting to ascend a ramp, the patient should be shown proper technique: each push is forceful but not abrupt, and the hands are repositioned rapidly between pushes. When pushing and repositioning, he should move his hands simultaneously and symmetrically. The strokes are shorter than those used for propulsion over even surfaces. Forward flexion of the head, and, if possible, trunk can help prevent backward tipping of the wheelchair.

Practice in ramp negotiation should begin on an incline with a very gentle slope. Initially, the patient may not be able to push the chair forcefully enough to ascend. When this is the case, the

therapist can assist, applying just enough force to the chair's push handles to enable the patient to push up the ramp with maximal effort. The assistance should be reduced as the patient's ability improves with practice.

People learning to push their wheelchairs up ramps often reposition their hands too slowly between pushes, allowing their chairs to roll backward excessively. Guarding is required to ensure safety at this point. While guarding, the therapist should allow a slight backward roll between pushes. The chair's motion, combined with verbal cueing, can provide feedback to the patient regarding his technique.

As a patient's skill in ascending slopes increases, the assistance given should be reduced. Once the individual masters a slope of a particular grade, he should progress to steeper slopes. Training in ramp negotiation can continue in this manner until the patient has reached his maximal potential.

Descending Slope on Four Wheels, Control Wheelchair by Applying Friction to the Handrims

When descending a slope on four wheels, the wheelchair user controls his chair's descent by applying friction to the handrims as they slide past his hands. He does this by gripping the handrims loosely or by pressing his palms inward against the rims, depending on whether or not his finger flexors are innervated.

During functional training, emphasis should be placed on *controlling* the chair's descent. To negotiate a ramp safely, a person must be able to stop the chair or turn while descending. This is possible only if he maintains control throughout the descent rather than releasing the handrims and trying to regain control when the need arises.

Practice in descending ramps should begin on gentle slopes at low speeds. Once an individual has developed the ability to slow, stop, and turn a manual wheelchair while slowly descending a gentle slope, he can progress to practicing at higher speeds and on steeper inclines.

Even on a mild incline and at a slow speed, a patient may be unable to control his chair's descent at first. When this is the case, the therapist can help to slow the chair. The therapist should apply just enough force to the push handles (resisting the chair's downhill motion) to enable the person to control the chair with maximal effort. This assistance can be reduced as the patient's ability improves.

Maintain Balance Point in Wheelie Position

The balance point in a wheelie is the position in which a wheelchair is on its rear wheels and is in equilibrium, falling neither forward nor backward. A patient need not be able to assume his balance point independently before beginning practice in maintaining this position.

The first step in teaching a person how to maintain his balance point in a wheelie is showing him where that point is located. If the individual has an inaccurate understanding of where his balance point is located, he will be unable to maintain the correct position. (If his notion of the balance point is tilted forward from the correct position, he will resist tipping back his chair far enough. As a result, he will constantly fall forward.) To teach a person where his balance point is located, the therapist can demonstrate in his own chair and then tip the patient back[bb] and allow him to feel the position (Figure 12–21A).

After showing the patient his balance point, the therapist should teach him how to control his chair in a wheelie. With the therapist guarding closely, the patient can pull his handrims forward and back while in a wheelie position, paying attention to the effects that these maneuvers have on the chair's position (Figure 12–21B and C). Gross motions are acceptable at this point; the purpose of this exercise is to familiarize the patient with the control motions.

Once the patient has learned how to tip his chair forward and back in a wheelie, he is ready to begin working on maintaining his balance point. The therapist can assist the patient to the balance point and encourage him to keep the chair balanced. The therapist should spot closely while the patient makes adjustments in his position. The patient is likely to overcorrect at first. He should be encouraged to maintain his balance with smaller corrections.

From this point on in the functional training, hands-off guarding is best (Figure 12–21D). If the therapist's hands remain on the push handles while the patient works to maintain his balance, the therapist is likely to make corrections for him. This will deprive the patient of practice and can make it difficult for him to discern when he has moved off of his balance point. The therapist should allow the chair to fall a short distance when it moves out of the balance point, so the patient can feel that he has lost his balance and needs to make corrections.

Fear is often the largest barrier to learning this skill. Someone who is afraid of falling over backwards is unlikely to allow himself to remain tipped far enough back to balance. He will attempt to maintain the chair's wheelie in a position tilted too far forward and, as a result, will not be able to balance. This tendency is compounded by the fact that wheelchairs balance at a point that is tilted further back than most would expect. A patient may feel as though he is about to fall backward when he is at his balance point. Therapists can aid the process of learning to maintain a balanced wheelie by attending to their patients' feelings during functional training. The therapist should remain reassuring and calm and should encourage the patient to relax. When assisting a fearful patient to his balance point, the therapist should avoid quick, jerky motions that may increase the patient's fear. In addition, the therapist can assure the patient that he will catch him if he starts to fall.

Independent work. If a patient is able to get into a balanced wheelie position without assistance, he can practice maintaining that position independently. Figure 12–22 illustrates a setup in which the wheelchair's push handles are secured to suspended straps. The straps are attached with enough slack to allow the patient to move slightly past his balance point but without enough slack to allow him to fall to the floor.

Assume Wheelie Position

In a wheelie, the wheelchair rests on its rear wheels with the casters off the ground. To assume a wheelie position, the wheelchair user essentially tips his chair over backwards. This skill may be easier to acquire if the patient has initiated (not necessarily completed) training in maintaining his balance in a wheelie. This prior exposure to wheelies can give him an understanding of how far back he must tip his chair, and it can make him less fearful about falling over backwards.

A wheelchair's construction and alignment influence the difficulty of this task. An ultralight wheelchair with its axles positioned relatively anteriorly is easy to tip backwards. With a heavier wheelchair or more posteriorly located axles, the task is more difficult.

[bb] The therapist should take care to show the patient his true balance point. The balance point is easily found if the therapist pays attention to the force that he must exert on the chair to keep it tipped back on the rear wheels. At the balance point, the chair will remain in position (briefly) without any assistance from the therapist. If the chair is tipped too far back or forward, the therapist will have to apply force to keep the chair from tipping further back or forward, respectively.

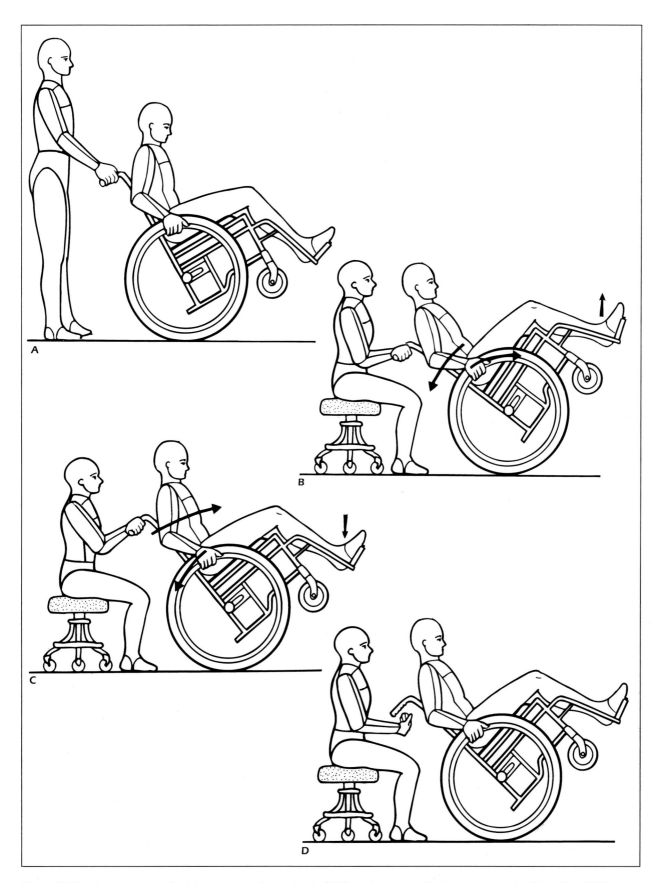

Figure 12–21. Instruction in maintaining balance point in wheelie. **(A)** Therapist assists patient into balanced wheelie position. **(B)** Chair tips further back when wheels are pushed forward. **(C)** Chair tips toward upright when wheels are pulled back. **(D)** Non-contact guarding for wheelie practice.

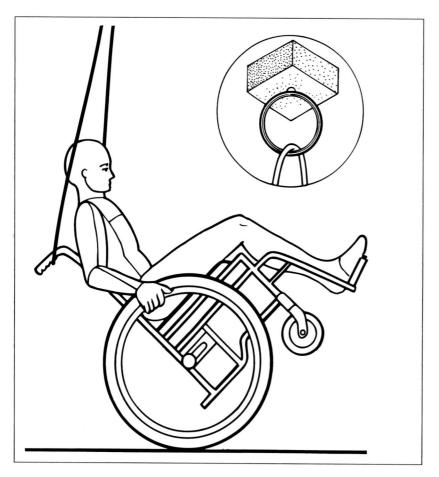

Figure 12–22.   *Safety rigging for independent practice of achieving and maintaining wheelie position.*

With intact upper extremities and an ultra-light wheelchair, the wheelie position can be attained easily from a stationary position. The wheelchair user grasps[cc] the handrims posteriorly and pulls them forward abruptly and forcefully. If an individual is unable to lift his casters in this manner, he may be able to do so by throwing his head back when he pulls his handrims.

Impaired upper extremity function, a heavy wheelchair, or posteriorly located axles make it more difficult to tilt a chair back. People who are unable to "pop a wheelie" from a stationary position may be able to accomplish the task using the following technique: grasp the handrims anteriorly, pull backward, then abruptly and forcefully reverse the direction of pull. The person may find the task easier if he throws his head back when he pulls the handrims forward.

During early practice, the therapist should encourage the patient to use abrupt, forceful motions. The aim is to disturb the wheelchair's balance, tipping it over backwards. The patient will not accomplish this if he "eases into" his motions. To gain enough momentum to tilt his chair, he may need to exaggerate his motions at first. He can refine his motions as he develops a feel for the maneuver.

An individual who is unable to lift his casters may be pulling his handrims in the wrong direction, throwing his head in the wrong direction, or timing his maneuvers incorrectly. The therapist should observe him closely as he makes his attempts and give him feedback on his technique.

Independent work.   For some, this skill takes a good deal of practice to achieve. Independent work will make this extensive practice feasible. Safety rigging, described earlier and illustrated in Figure 12–22, is required to keep the patient from falling backwards. With this safety rigging, an individual who has been instructed and has received some initial practice and feedback can independently practice attaining his balance point.

[cc] An individual who lacks functioning finger flexors moves his handrims using friction, pressing in on the rims instead of grasping them.

Glide Forward in Wheelie Position

Before beginning training in this skill, a person should be able to assume and maintain his balance point in a wheelie.

To initiate a forward glide in a wheelie, the wheelchair user positions his chair at its balance point (Figure 12–23A) and tips the chair forward slightly. The forward tilt will make the chair start to fall forward (dip; Figure 12–23B). The person counteracts this fall and propels the chair by pushing forward on the handrims (Figure 12–23C). He should allow the rims to slide through his hands as his chair glides forward in its balance point (Figure 12–23D). From the balance point, he can repeat the dip and push. By repeating this sequence of actions, the wheelchair user glides forward in a wheelie.

After demonstrating and explaining how to glide in a wheelie, the therapist should allow the patient to practice with guarding.[dd] The chair's motions are likely to be jerky at first, with exaggerated up and down motions. As the patient gains skill and confidence, the therapist should encourage him to smooth out the motion. The patient should also work to gain *control* of his glide; to use a glide functionally, he will need to be able to glide at various speeds, turn, and stop his chair at will. With practice, he should gain the capacity to glide faster, with greater control, and with less vertical motion of the casters.

Independent work. A patient should practice this skill independently *only after he has learned to fall safely.* Once he can fall safely and has developed some initial skill in a wheelie glide, he can practice on his own.

Turn in Wheelie Position

Before initiating practice of this skill, the patient should be able to assume and maintain his balance point in a wheelie.

Turning while balanced on two wheels can be accomplished by pushing one handrim forward while pulling the other back. To turn while propelling forward or backward in a wheelie, the wheelchair user can push or pull one handrim more forcefully than the other. As he turns, he must make adjustments as necessary to keep his chair in a balanced position.

After demonstrating and explaining how to turn in a wheelie, the therapist should allow the patient to practice with guarding.[ee] At first, the chair's motions are likely to be jerky, with excessive vertical motions of the casters. As the patient gains skill and confidence, the therapist should encourage him to smooth out the motion.

Independent work. A patient should practice this skill independently *only after he has learned to fall safely.* Once he can fall safely and has developed some initial skill in turning in a wheelie, he can practice on his own.

Propel Backward in Wheelie Position

To practice this skill, a patient should be able to assume and to maintain his balance point in a wheelie.

Propelling backward in a wheelie is like gliding forward, with the actions performed in reverse. From a balanced wheelie position, the wheelchair user tips his chair back slightly. The backward tilt will make the chair start to fall backward. The person counteracts this fall and propels the chair backward by pulling back on the handrims.

After demonstrating and explaining how to propel backward in a wheelie, the therapist should allow the patient to practice with guarding.[ff] At first, the chair's motions are likely to be jerky. As the patient gains skill and confidence, the therapist can encourage him to smooth out the motion.

Independent work. A patient should practice this skill independently *only after he has learned to fall safely.* Once he can fall safely and has developed some initial skill in backward propulsion in a wheelie, he can practice on his own.

Descending Slope on Two Wheels, Control Wheelchair by Applying Friction to Handrims

When descending a slope in a wheelie, the wheelchair user controls the chair's descent by applying friction to the handrims as he allows them to slide through his hands. The force applied to the handrims should be light, giving slight resistance to the rims' forward motion.

This skill can be taught using the functional training strategies used to teach descending a

---

[dd] As was explained previously, the therapist should avoid touching the wheelchair while guarding. His hands should be poised under the push handles, ready to catch if needed.

[ee] As was explained earlier, the therapist should avoid touching the wheelchair while guarding. His hands should be poised under the push handles, ready to catch if needed.

[ff] As was explained earlier, the therapist should avoid touching the wheelchair while guarding. His hands should be poised under the push handles, ready to catch if needed.

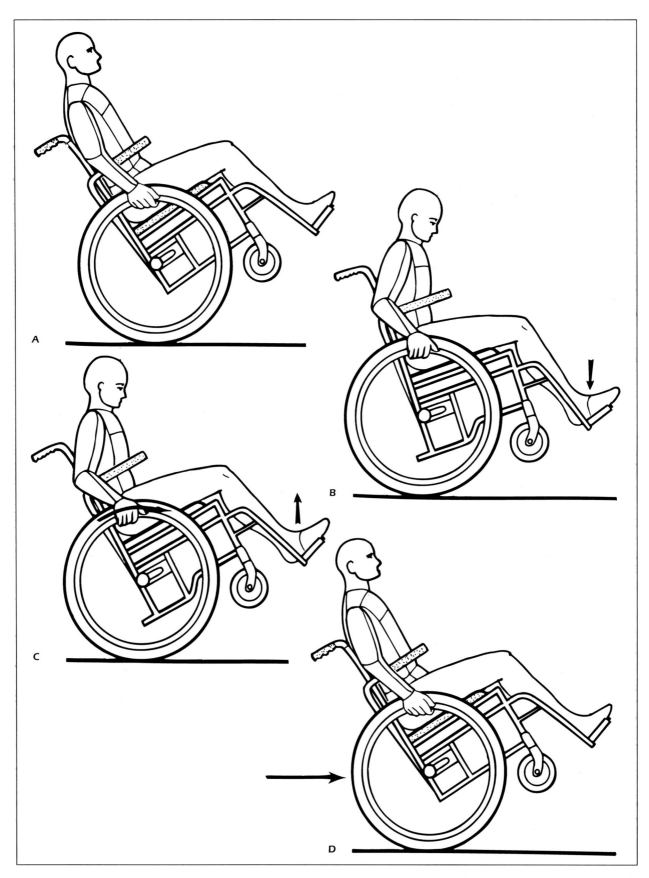

Figure 12–23.   Forward glide in a wheelie. **(A)** Starting position: balanced wheelie position. **(B)** Wheelchair falls forward slightly. **(C)** Forward push on handrims propels chair forward and lifts casters. **(D)** Glide in balance point.

Your outpatient has complete T8 paraplegia. His range of motion is normal in all extremities, and his strength is normal in all musculature innervated above the lesion. He reports that he has fallen twice while descending steep curb cuts. On both occasions, his footplates hit the pavement at the bottom of the curb cut and his chair tipped over forward.

- What technique can this person learn for safe descent of curb cuts?
- What are the physical prerequisites for this skill?
- What strength and range of motion should the therapeutic exercise program emphasize to facilitate the attainment of this goal?
- Describe a functional training program for this patient.

ramp on four wheels. Before beginning training, the patient should be skillful in gliding forward and turning in a wheelie.

From Stationary Position, Lift Casters from Floor

Before learning to lift his casters from the floor, the patient should be proficient in forward propulsion over even surfaces. He need not be able to assume or to maintain a balanced wheelie position.

Lifting a wheelchair's casters from the floor is a lesser version of assuming the wheelie position; the same maneuvers are used, but they are performed less forcefully. To teach a patient to lift his casters, the therapist can use the training strategies presented above for teaching a patient to assume a balanced wheelie position.

Pop Casters onto Curb from Stationary Position

Training in this skill should begin after the patient has acquired the ability to lift his wheelchair's casters from the floor from a stationary position. Once an individual can lift his casters consis-

tently, he can practice popping his casters onto small (1-inch) curbs. As his skill develops, he can progress to taller curbs.

Independent work. A patient who is independent in lowering his chair's casters from a curb and has developed some initial skill in popping his casters onto a curb can practice alone. If his skill level is such that he may tip his chair over backward and if he has not learned to fall safely, he can practice while using safety rigging as shown in Figure 12–22.

Position Casters at Edge of Curb

Ascending a curb from a stationary position involves popping the chair's casters onto the curb and then backing them to the edge of the curb. This repositioning requires proficiency in backward propulsion and turning. Training in repositioning the casters on the curb will be easier if the patient is able to place his casters on the curb.

A person with the physical potential to ascend curbs should be able to master this prerequisite skill with minimal practice. During training, the therapist should emphasize placing the casters right at the edge of the curb (Figure 12–24A). This position maximizes the distance between the curb and the chair's rear wheels (Figure 12–24B), making it possible to gain more momentum for ascending the curb.

Independent work. This skill can be practiced concurrently with placing the casters on and lowering them from a curb if the patient has developed some ability in each of these maneuvers. If his skill level is such that he may tip his chair over backward and if he has not learned to fall safely, the patient can practice using safety rigging, as shown in Figure 12–22.

Ascend Curb from Stationary Position

To practice ascending a curb from a stationary position, a patient must be proficient in forward propulsion. Training will be easier if he can place his casters on the curb and position them at the curb's edge.

Once a wheelchair user has lifted his casters onto a curb and positioned them at the edge of the curb, he grasps[gg] the chair's handrims posteriorly

---

[gg] A person who lacks functioning finger flexors moves his handrims using friction, pressing in on the rims instead of grasping them.

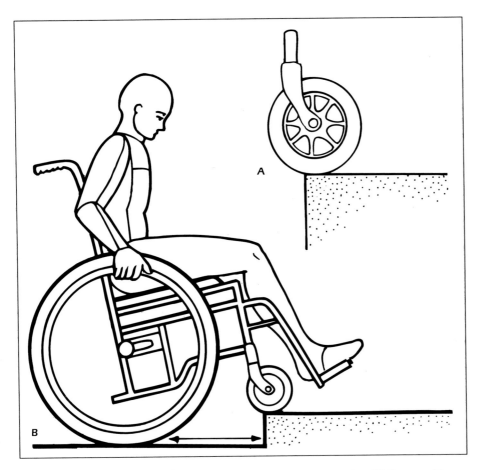

Figure 12–24. Positioning casters at edge of curb. **(A)** Correct caster position. **(B)** Caster position maximizes distance between curb and rear wheels.

and pulls forward forcefully. To add to the chair's forward momentum, he throws his head and (if possible) trunk forward as his chair approaches the curb. This added momentum is especially important with higher curbs or when the individual's upper extremity musculature is impaired.

Training should start on a small (1-inch) curb. As the person's skill improves, he can progress to taller curbs. The curb height should be increased in small increments, with the patient progressing only when he is able to ascend a curb of a given height consistently.

Independent work. A patient should practice this skill independently *only after he has learned to fall safely.* Once he can fall safely and has developed some initial skill in curb negotiation, he can practice on his own.

Lift Casters off of Floor while Chair Moves Forward

Lifting a wheelchair's casters while propelling forward is more difficult than doing so from a sta-

tionary position. Impaired upper extremity function, a heavy wheelchair, or posteriorly located axles will make it difficult to accomplish this task. These factors, however, will not necessarily prevent acquisition of this skill.

This maneuver requires appropriate timing rather than the application of brute force. To lift his casters while propelling forward, a wheelchair user grasps[hh] his handrims posteriorly and pulls them forward abruptly and forcefully. If he is unable to lift his casters in this manner, he may be able to do so by throwing his head back when he pulls his handrims.

With intact upper extremities and an ultra-light wheelchair, many patients are able to master this skill without excessive difficulty. During early practice, the therapist can encourage the patient to make abrupt, forceful motions. The aim is to disturb the wheelchair's balance, tipping it backwards. The patient will not accomplish this if

[hh] A person who lacks functioning finger flexors moves his handrims using friction, pressing in on the rims instead of grasping them.

he "eases into" his motions. To gain enough momentum to lift his casters, he may need to exaggerate his motions at first. He can refine his technique as he develops a feel for the maneuver.

An individual who is unable to lift his casters may be pulling his handrims in the wrong direction, throwing his head in the wrong direction, or timing his maneuvers inappropriately. The therapist should observe him closely as he makes his attempts, and give him feedback on his technique.

Fear is a potential roadblock to acquiring this skill; someone who is afraid that he will fall over backward may not pull on the handrims forcefully enough. For this reason, this skill may be easier to acquire if the patient has initiated (not necessarily completed) training in maintaining his balance in a wheelie. This prior exposure to wheelies can give him an understanding of how far back he must tip his chair to fall, and it can make him less fearful about falling over backward when lifting his casters from the floor.

During early practice lifting his casters while propelling his chair forward, the patient can work at low speeds. As his skill develops, he can increase his speed.

Independent work. A person should practice this skill independently *only after he has learned to fall safely.* Once he can fall safely and has developed some initial skill in lifting his casters while propelling forward, he can practice on his own.

Pop Casters onto Curb while Chair Moves Forward

Popping a wheelchair's casters onto a curb while propelling forward requires more than the ability to lift the casters high enough. The wheelchair user must time the maneuver appropriately: the casters must lift before the footplates hit the curb and must lower just after crossing the curb.

After a patient has developed the ability to lift his casters while propelling forward, he should work on his timing. During early work on timing, he can practice popping his casters over a mark on the floor, propelling toward the mark, and popping his casters just before his footplates reach it. When he is consistently able to time his caster lift in relation to a floor mark, he will be ready to work on curbs.

Curb training should begin on a small (1-inch) curb, with the patient progressing to higher curbs as his skill develops. Once he has

developed some skill in popping his casters onto a curb of a given height, he can practice this maneuver concurrently with ascending the curb using momentum.

Independent work. When a patient performs this maneuver with improper timing, he may fall forward out of his chair or tip the chair over backward. For this reason, this skill should be practiced independently only after the patient has had a good deal of practice and is not likely to fall. In addition, he should practice this skill independently *only after he has learned to fall safely.*

Ascend Curb Using Momentum

Before initiating practice in ascending curbs using momentum, a patient must be able to lift his casters off of the floor while propelling forward. He must also have developed some skill in popping his casters onto a curb while his chair moves forward, but he need not have perfected this maneuver.

To ascend a curb using momentum, a wheelchair user approaches the curb front-on and pops his casters onto the curb at the last moment. Timing is crucial; the casters should lift over the curb and land just before the rear wheels hit the curb. If the maneuver is timed correctly and the wheelchair has approached the curb with enough speed, momentum will carry the chair up the curb. During functional training, the therapist should carefully observe the patient's timing so that he can provide feedback. He should also encourage the patient to be aware of the timing.

For most people, a good deal of practice is required to learn this skill. Training should start on a small (1-inch) curb. As the patient's skill improves, he can progress to taller curbs. The curb height should be increased in small increments, with the patient progressing only when he is able to ascend a curb of a given height consistently.

Close guarding is required as the patient works on ascending curbs using momentum. If the chair is not tipped back enough or if it drops too early as it approaches the curb, the casters will hit the curb's vertical surface (Figure 12–25A). The chair will stop abruptly, and the rider may be thrown forward out of the chair. If the casters drop too late, the rear wheels will hit first while the chair is still tipped back (Figure 12–25B). Again, the chair is likely to stop abruptly. On a tall curb, an abrupt stop can cause the chair to tip over backward.

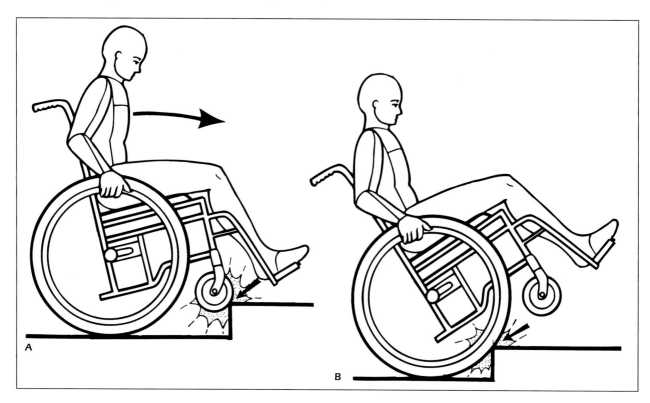

Figure 12-25. *Problems resulting from improper technique when ascending curb using momentum.* **(A)** *Caster strikes curb's vertical surface.* **(B)** *Rear wheel strikes curb while chair is still tipped back.*

Because a patient can fall forward or backward during curb negotiation practice, the therapist must be prepared to catch in either direction. The therapist can guard from behind, following closely as the patient propels toward the curb. Alternatively, the therapist can guard from the front. This involves standing beside the curb prepared to catch when the patient reaches it.

Practice in curb ascent and descent can be combined: after an individual succeeds in popping his casters onto the curb or ascending the curb, he can practice getting back down.

Independent work.   This skill should be practiced independently only after the patient has had a good deal of practice and is not likely to fall. In addition, he should practice this skill independently *only after he has learned to fall safely.* He should also be able to descend curbs without assistance.

Backing Down Curb, Control Rear Wheels' Descent

Backing a wheelchair down a curb under control requires the ability to apply a strong forward force on the wheels. A patient should be skillful in

manual wheelchair propulsion before beginning practice backing down a curb.

Functional training in this skill should emphasize developing control. The patient should practice backing just past the curb's edge and resisting the chair's motion as gravity pulls it downward. Training should begin on small (1-inch) curbs, progressing to higher curbs as skill develops. Curb descent can be practiced concurrently with curb ascent.

Lower Casters from Curb by Turning Wheelchair

To perform this maneuver, a person need only be able to turn his wheelchair in a tight arc. Anyone who is able to propel a manual wheelchair independently should be able to learn, with minimal practice, to lower his casters from a curb by turning his chair.

Descend Curb in a Wheelie Position

Before practicing this skill, a patient must be able to glide forward in a wheelie with good control. Training should begin with small (1-inch) curbs, progressing to higher curbs as the patient's skill develops.

Negotiate Uneven Terrain on Four Wheels

To practice negotiating uneven terrain on four wheels, the patient should be proficient in propulsion over even surfaces. Propelling over slightly uneven terrain is primarily a matter of pushing hard. If the wheelchair's progress is impeded by a tough spot, such as a clump of grass, the person may be able to get past it by backing up and ramming the obstacle.[ii]

Practice should start with slightly uneven terrain, such as a level sidewalk that is in good condition. As the patient's strength and skill improve, he can progress to more challenging surfaces such as grass, sand, gravel, and sidewalks in disrepair. The patient should practice propelling over the various surfaces that he is likely to encounter after his rehabilitation.

Independent work.   A patient can work on this skill independently once he has gained some ability. He should practice where he can obtain assistance when needed, in case he gets stuck.

Negotiate Uneven Terrain in a Wheelie

The challenge of negotiating uneven terrain in a wheelie is maintaining one's balance. While pushing hard to propel his chair over irregularities in the supporting surface, the wheelchair user must compensate for the effects that these irregularities have on the chair's equilibrium.

Before beginning work on this skill, a patient should be proficient in propulsion forward, backward, and turning in a wheelie on even surfaces. Once skillful on even surfaces, he can begin work on a slightly uneven surface such as a sidewalk that is in good condition. As his strength and skill improve, he can progress to more challenging surfaces, such as grass, sand, gravel, and sidewalks in disrepair. The patient should practice propelling over the various surfaces that he is likely to encounter after his rehabilitation.

Independent work.   A patient should practice this skill independently *only after he has learned to fall safely*. Ideally, he should also be able to right his chair after a fall. Once he can fall safely and has developed some skill in negotiating uneven terrain in a wheelie, he can practice on his own. He should practice in a location where he can obtain assistance when needed.

Sitting on Step or Floor, Tilt Wheelchair Back to Position to Ascend or Descend Stairs

This skill requires good dynamic balance in sitting propped on one arm.[jj] A person with intact upper extremity musculature who has good balance in this posture should find it easy to position his wheelchair in preparation to ascend or to descend stairs on his buttocks. He simply grasps a push handle and pulls on it to turn and tip the chair. A brief period of practice should be sufficient to master this maneuver.

Sitting on Step, Stabilize Wheelchair by Pushing Down through Push Handles

Before beginning work on this skill, a patient must have good balance when positioned in short-sitting propped forward on two arms.[kk] People with the physical potential to ascend stairs on their buttocks should learn without difficulty to stabilize their wheelchairs.

During functional training, the patient should be encouraged to push straight downward through the chair's push handle. An obliquely directed push may cause the chair to slide on the step. Practice should start with the patient sitting on a step that is close to the base of the stairway. A wheelchair is easier to stabilize in this location because it is supported by the floor (Figure 12–26A). After brief practice at the base of the stairs, the patient can progress to practicing on higher steps, where the chair is not supported by the floor (Figure 12–26B).

Transfer Up a Step while Stabilizing Wheelchair

Training in this skill should begin after the patient can stabilize his wheelchair while sitting on stairs. He must also be proficient in using the head-hips relationship and performing step-high back-approach uneven transfers from the floor.[ll]

Before an individual becomes skillful in this maneuver, he may have difficulty stabilizing his chair while transferring. While concentrating on the transfer between stairs, the inexperienced patient may apply an obliquely directed force to the chair's push handle, causing it to slide. The therapist should encourage him to push straight downward through the push handle as he transfers.

[ii] Alternatively, he may pop his casters from the ground to lift them over the obstacle. Strategies for developing this skill are described above.

[jj] This skill is addressed in Chapter 11.
[kk] This skill is addressed in Chapter 11.
[ll] Training strategies for the head-hips relationship and transfer skills are presented in Chapter 11.

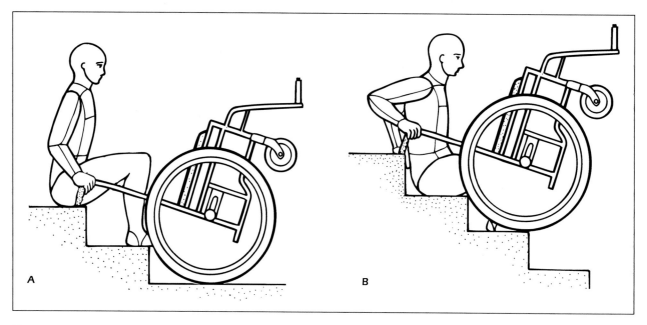

Figure 12–26.   *Stabilizing wheelchair while ascending stairs.* **(A)** *Early practice on lower step, with rear wheel on floor.* **(B)** *Practice on higher step, wheelchair's rear wheel resting on stairs.*

Practice should begin on a low step, where the chair is supported by the floor. As the patient's skill develops, he should progress to transferring from higher steps, where the chair is not supported by the floor (Figure 12–26). After he has developed some skill in transferring up a step while stabilizing his chair, he can practice this skill concurrently with the skill of pulling the chair up a step.

Sitting on Step, Position Buttocks and Legs while Stabilizing Wheelchair

Training in this skill should begin after the patient can stabilize his wheelchair while sitting on stairs. He should also be independent in gross mat mobility and leg management.[mm]

A person who has the required prerequisite skills should learn without difficulty to position his buttocks and legs while stabilizing his wheelchair on stairs. Practice should begin on a low step, where the chair is supported by the floor. As the patient's skill develops, he should progress to transferring from higher steps, where the chair is not supported by the floor (Figure 12–26).

Sitting on Step or Landing, Pull Wheelchair Up

A patient must have good dynamic balance in one-hand-supported short-sitting before begin-

ning training in this skill.[nn] If he has good balance, he should learn to pull his wheelchair up a step or onto a landing with minimal practice. The patient is likely to find the task easier if he leans away from the chair as he pulls it up.

Sitting on Floor, Pull Wheelchair to Upright Position

To right a wheelchair while sitting on the floor, a person with a complete spinal cord injury first gets into a long-sitting position. Propping on one arm, he pulls upward on one of the wheelchair's push handles to right the chair.

A patient must have good dynamic balance in one-hand-supported long-sitting to practice this skill.[oo] If he has good balance, he should learn to right his wheelchair with minimal practice.

Lower Chair into Position to Ascend Stairs in Wheelchair

Someone who has the physical potential to ascend stairs in a wheelchair should learn with minimal practice to lower his chair into position. If a patient has difficulty at first, he can practice lowering and raising himself through a small arc of motion, gradually increasing the arc as his skill and confidence develop (Figure 12–27).

[mm] Training strategies for gross mat mobility and leg management are presented in Chapter 10.

[nn] This skill is addressed in Chapter 11.

[oo] Functional training strategies for these skills are presented in Chapter 10.

Sitting in Wheelchair Tilted Back onto Steps, Reposition Hands

In this maneuver, a person who is sitting in a wheelchair that is tilted back onto a step moves his hands from one step to another. This maneuver is made challenging by the fact that he must support himself and the chair while he does so. To do this, he supports himself on one hand at a time, repositioning his free hand to the step above.

Practice should start at the base of the stairway. A wheelchair is easier to stabilize in this location because it is supported by the floor. After brief practice at the base of the stairs, the patient can progress to practicing on higher steps, where the chair is not supported by the floor (Figure 12–26). This skill can be practiced concurrently with pulling the chair up a step.

Sitting in Wheelchair, Push on Step to Lift Wheelchair Up a Step

Lifting a wheelchair up a step while sitting in the chair is more a matter of strength than skill. This maneuver will be easier to learn if the patient is skillful in back-approach uneven transfers[pp] and can reposition his hands between steps.

Training should start at the base of a stairway, with the patient belted into a wheelchair that is tilted back onto the stairs. If the patient is both strong and able to reposition his hands between steps, he may practice pulling himself up the stairs without prior preparation. He is likely to find the maneuver easier if he lifts one wheel at a time up the step. A patient who has difficulty pulling his chair up the steps may first practice raising and lowering his chair over a single step at the base of the stairs.

Sitting on a Step, Lower Wheelchair Down a Step

A patient must have good dynamic balance in one-hand-supported short-sitting before beginning training in this skill.[qq] If he has good balance in this position, he should learn to lower his wheelchair down a step with minimal practice. To avoid losing his balance forward, the patient should be encouraged to lean away from the chair as he lowers it.

Sitting on a Step, Transfer Down a Step while Stabilizing Wheelchair

Training in this skill should begin after the patient can stabilize his wheelchair and reposition his hands while sitting on stairs. He must also be proficient in using the head-hips relationship and performing step-high back-approach uneven transfers to the floor.[rr]

---

pp These transfers are presented in Chapter 11.

qq This skill is addressed in Chapter 11.
rr Training strategies for the head-hips relationship and transfer skills are presented in Chapter 11.

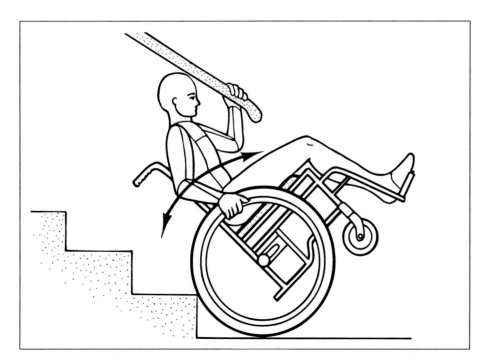

Figure 12–27.   Practice lowering wheelchair into position to ascend stairs in wheelchair.

Before a patient becomes skillful in this maneuver, he may have difficulty stabilizing his wheelchair while transferring. While concentrating on the transfer between stairs, the inexperienced person often applies an obliquely directed force to the chair's push handle, causing it to slide. The therapist should encourage the patient to push straight downward through the push handle as he transfers.

Practice should begin on a low step, where the chair is supported by the floor. As the patient's skill develops, he should progress to transferring from higher steps, where the chair is unsupported by the floor. After he has developed some skill in transferring down a step while stabilizing his chair, the patient can practice this skill concurrently with lowering the chair.

Sitting in Wheelchair and Holding Stair Handrail(s), Lower Wheelchair Down Stairs

This maneuver is very easy to learn, requiring neither great amounts of strength nor skill. The greatest obstacle to overcome during functional training is fear: understandably, many people are afraid at first that they will lose control of the chair and fall down the stairs.

To reduce a patient's fear during functional training, the therapist should stress the maneuver's safety and make a point of modeling comfort while demonstrating the technique. The therapist should also make it clear to the patient that he is guarding carefully during practice. The patient may feel more secure during initial practice if it takes place on a short (2- or 3-step) stairway. He can progress to working on longer stairways as his comfort level increases.

In Wheelie, Position Wheels at Top of Step

Before working on this skill, a patient must be proficient in gliding forward, backward, and turning in a wheelie. Functional training then simply involves demonstration and practice. A patient who has difficulty positioning his chair at the top edge of a step may start with practice positioning the chair relative to a mark on the floor. He can progress to positioning his chair at the top edge of a low (1-inch) curb, then practice on higher curbs, and finally, work on positioning his chair at the top of a series of steps.

In Wheelie, Stabilize Wheelchair against Step

To practice this skill, a patient should be proficient in maintaining a balanced wheelie position.

During initial practice, the patient should work on stabilizing his chair against a curb rather than against a step, as this will make guarding easier. After demonstrating the technique, the therapist can position the patient in a wheelie with the back of the chair's wheels resting against a curb. Once positioned, the patient can practice stabilizing the chair by pulling back on the wheels' handrims. He can work on maintaining the chair's position and lowering and raising (tilting) the chair through small arcs of motion (Figure 12–28).

Once an individual is able to stabilize his chair well, he should learn to get his chair into position. Starting positioned in a wheelie with the chair a small distance (a few inches) from the curb, he should practice backing until the wheels make contact with the curb, then practice stabilizing the wheels. Once he can perform these maneuvers well at a curb, he can practice on the bottom step of a stairway.

When a patient has developed skill in stabilizing his chair against a curb and descending a curb while remaining in a wheelie, he can practice the two skills concurrently.

Independent work. A patient who has good control in a wheelie, can fall safely, and is independent in propelling backward in a wheelie can practice stabilizing his chair against a curb.

Descend Step, Remaining in Wheelie Position

A patient should be able to stabilize his wheelchair against a step in a wheelie position before beginning practice in this skill. He should also be skillful in balancing, gliding, and descending curbs in a wheelie.

When descending a curb in a wheelie, one does not have to remain in the wheelie position; once the chair's rear wheels have reached the base of the curb, the casters can drop without threat to the rider's safety. In contrast, one *must* remain in a wheelie when descending steps forward. If the chair tips forward before it has reached the bottom of the steps, it and the rider will fall down the stairs. It is this risk of falling that makes descending stairs in a wheelie hazardous to all but the most skillful riders.

During functional training, the patient should develop the ability to descend a step under control, remaining in a wheelie during and after the descent. He should develop his skill on curbs first because practice there will be safer than on stairs. The patient may start on low curbs, pro-

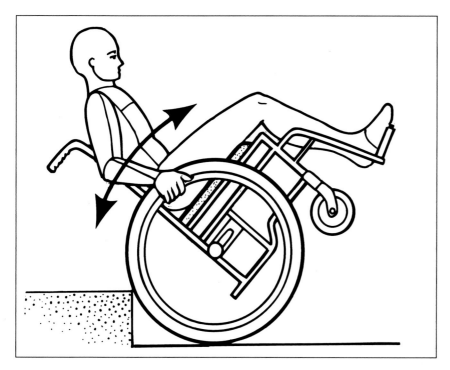

Figure 12–28. *Practice stabilizing wheelchair against a curb.*

gressing to higher curbs as his skill develops. Once he is consistently able to remain in a wheelie while and after descending a step-high curb, and can stabilize his wheelchair against the step, he can practice on stairs. The patient should practice on a small series of steps. He can start on stairs with a small vertical rise per step, progressing to higher steps and longer stairways as his skill improves.

Independent work. A patient who can independently descend a curb in a wheelie can practice remaining in a wheelie after descending.

Transfer to Armrest

To practice transferring to an armrest, a patient should be adept in even and slightly uneven transfers without a sliding board and in using the head-hips relationship to move his buttocks.[ss]

The therapist should demonstrate and then have the patient practice transferring from his wheelchair seat to the armrest. The patient should be encouraged to push down hard and throw his head and upper trunk down and to the side to lift his buttocks. Emphasis should be placed on exaggerated motions of the head and upper trunk. Dur-

ing initial practice, many patients will be able to get onto their armrests with only guarding. These individuals can develop their skill by practicing with spotting until they become independent. Other patients have more difficulty learning the transfer. When this is the case, the therapist can make the task easier by placing cushions on the wheelchair's seat, reducing the distance that must be traversed in the transfer. As the patient's skill increases with practice, he can reduce the number of cushions on the seat, transferring from progressively lower levels until he can transfer directly from the seat to the armrest.

Maintain Balance while Sitting on Armrest

Before working on this skill, the patient should have good dynamic balance while propped forward on one extended arm in short-sitting.[tt]

Practice should start with the patient sitting on an armrest, with one hand on each armrest (Figure 12–29). From that position, he shifts his weight and lifts the hand that is propped next to his buttocks. Once he can maintain this position, the patient can begin working on dynamic balance, shifting his weight while propping on one arm. Finally, he can practice maintaining his balance while reaching in all directions.

[ss] These skills are addressed in Chapter 11.

[tt] This skill is addressed in Chapter 11.

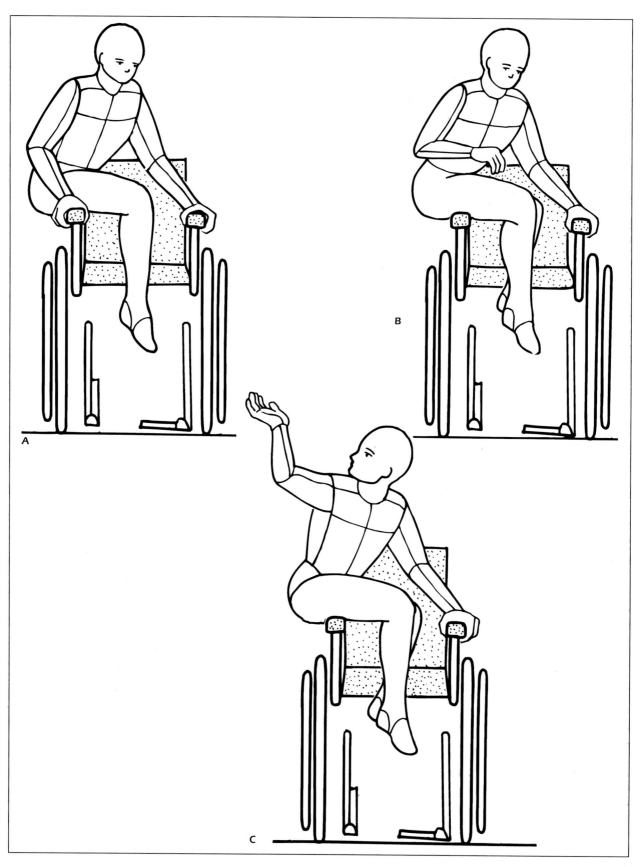

Figure 12–29.   Practice maintaining balance while sitting on armrest.

Initial functional training in this skill will be most practical if the patient works on it concurrently with transfers to the armrest: he can alternate transferring onto the armrest and balancing there. Once he has become skillful in maintaining his balance while sitting on an armrest, he should practice this skill with the chair narrowed. This can be done concurrently with practice narrowing the chair.

Narrow Wheelchair while Sitting on Armrest

To practice narrowing his wheelchair while sitting on an armrest, a patient must first be able to maintain his balance while sitting on an armrest, propped on one arm. Once he has dynamic balance in that position, narrowing the chair is not particularly difficult.

The therapist should demonstrate narrowing the wheelchair, then have the patient practice with guarding. The patient should be encouraged to pull forcefully and abruptly upward on the wheelchair seat while maintaining his balance. The chair will be easier to narrow if he shifts his weight off of his supporting arm each time he pulls on the seat. He should be encouraged to regain his balance between pulls.

In preparation for negotiating narrow doorways, the patient can combine practice narrowing the chair with practice balancing on the narrowed wheelchair. To reopen the chair, he can transfer from the armrest onto the seat.

Sitting on Armrest, Pull on Doorjamb to Move Narrowed Wheelchair through Door

This skill requires the ability to maintain dynamic balance while sitting on the armrest of a narrowed wheelchair, propped on one arm. A patient who can maintain his balance in this position should learn without difficulty to pull the chair through a doorway. After demonstrating the maneuver, the therapist should guard the patient while he practices grasping the doorjamb and pulling himself through the doorway.

Sitting on Armrest, Propel Narrowed Wheelchair

This skill requires the ability to maintain dynamic balance while sitting on an armrest of a narrowed wheelchair, propped on one arm. A patient who can maintain his balance in this position should learn without difficulty to propel his chair through a doorway. After demonstrating the maneuver, the

therapist should guard the patient while he practices propelling the chair by pushing on one handrim at a time with his free hand.

Transfer from Armrest to Wheelchair Seat

This maneuver is initiated with the wheelchair user sitting on an armrest, with one hand on each armrest. From this position, he pushes down on the armrests and tucks his head to lift his buttocks. As his buttocks lift, he twists his head and shoulders laterally away from the seat.

Before practicing this skill, a patient should be adept in even and slightly uneven transfers without a sliding board and in using the head-hips relationship to move his buttocks.[uu] A patient who has these prerequisite skills should be able to transfer from an armrest to the wheelchair seat without difficulty, after a brief period of practice with guarding. During initial practice, the wheelchair should remain open. As his skill develops, the patient can progress to transferring into the seat of a narrowed wheelchair.

Narrow Wheelchair by Rocking Side to Side

The therapist should demonstrate this technique and have the patient practice with guarding. The patient should be encouraged to use forceful and abrupt motions, synchronizing his head throws with upward pulls on the seat.

While Falling Backward in Wheelchair, Tuck Head and Hold Wheels

For most people, the automatic reaction when tipping over backward in a wheelchair is to turn and reach out a hand, with the elbow extended. A person who reaches in this manner when falling lands on his palm, taking the force of the fall through his upper extremity. In the process, he may injure himself. During functional training, this automatic reaction must be replaced by a safer falling technique.

Falling safely is a simple ability, without any true skill prerequisites. Functional training in this instance is more a matter of developing a new habit than of acquiring a new skill.

Fear can be a barrier to developing the habit of falling safely. To reduce a patient's fear, the therapist should model comfort with falling and demonstrate that it does not hurt. The therapist can also help the patient overcome his fear by intro-

---

[uu] These skills are addressed in Chapter 11.

ducing the fall gradually. The patient can first practice the appropriate actions to take when falling, tucking his head and holding the chair's wheels. He can then perform these maneuvers while the therapist simulates a fall, lowering the chair backward from a balanced wheelie position (Figure 12–30A). At first, these simulated falls can be slow, with warning, and over a small arc. As the patient's tolerance to this activity increases, the therapist can increase the speed and distance of the chair's "fall" and finally, omit the warning.

In the activity just described, the therapist should remain in control of the wheelchair, preventing a true fall. Once the patient develops some tolerance to falling and demonstrates the ability to respond appropriately, he can practice true falls. A fearful patient can develop his tolerance to falling by building up the distance over which he falls. Starting with a short fall onto a pile of floor mats, he can fall over progressively larger distances as his tolerance and habit develop (Figure 12–30B).

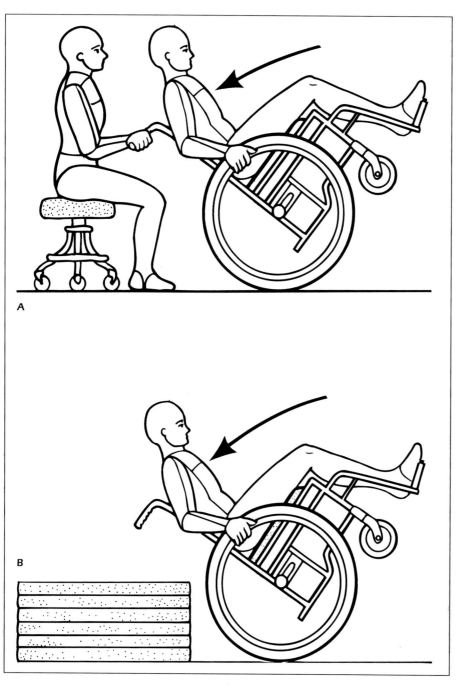

Figure 12–30. *Practice safe falling technique.* **(A)** *With therapist assisting.* **(B)** *Onto floor mats.*

While Falling Backward in Wheelchair, Tuck Head and Block Legs

This skill can be taught using the strategies just described for developing the habit of tucking the head and holding the wheels during a fall.

After Falling Backward in Wheelchair, Position Self in Chair

This skill involves pulling on the chair's wheels to slide the buttocks back onto the seat, grasping the legs, and placing them so that they hang over the front edge of the seat. A person who has the physical potential to right his chair after a fall should be able to master this prerequisite skill with minimal practice.

Independent work. Once a patient has been shown this technique and has had some initial practice, he can practice independently. The maneuver can be practiced concurrently with the other skill prerequisites for returning a chair to upright after a fall.

Sitting in Overturned Wheelchair, Lock Wheel Locks

To lock his brakes while sitting in an overturned wheelchair, the person simply grasps his brakes and locks them. He will probably need to lift his trunk to reach the wheel locks. He can do this by pulling on an armrest or the frame of his wheelchair. These maneuvers may be awkward when sitting in an overturned chair, but they should be readily accomplished with practice.

Independent work. Once a patient has been shown this technique and has had some initial practice, he can practice independently. This maneuver can be practiced concurrently with the other skill prerequisites for returning a chair to upright after a fall.

Sitting in Overturned Wheelchair, Lift Upper Trunk from Floor

A person who has the physical potential to right his chair after a fall should be able to master this prerequisite skill with minimal practice.

Independent work. Once a patient has been shown this technique and has had some initial practice, he can practice independently. The ma-

neuver can be practiced concurrently with the other skill prerequisites for returning a chair to upright after a fall.

Sitting in Overturned Wheelchair, Balance on One Hand

Before beginning training in this skill, a patient must have good dynamic balance when sitting propped back on one arm.[vv]

Appropriate hand placement is the key to balancing on one hand while sitting in an overturned wheelchair. The hand should be positioned directly behind the trunk, so that the person can support his weight on it. The patient should practice placing his hand, shifting his weight onto it, and releasing the other hand's grasp on the chair. When he has developed the ability to release the chair and balance on one hand, he should practice reaching his free hand toward the opposite wheel.

Independent work. Once a patient has been shown this technique and has had some initial practice, he can practice independently. This skill can be practiced concurrently with the other skill prerequisites for returning a chair to upright after a fall.

Sitting in Overturned Wheelchair, Rock Chair to Upright

Before beginning training in this skill, a patient must have good dynamic balance when sitting in an overturned wheelchair propped back on one arm.

Starting in the position shown in Figure 12–16D, the patient should practice rocking the chair toward upright. The therapist should encourage him to use forceful and abrupt motions to thrust the chair upward from the floor. When the patient has rocked the chair forward enough to unweight his supporting hand, he should inch this hand forward around the side of the chair. He should reposition the hand rapidly and over short distances, so that he can support himself and maintain his balance when the chair rocks back. The therapist can facilitate practice at first by assisting with the chair's forward rock, pulling up on the chair's push handles while the patient pushes. The therapist can also help support the chair if the patient does not regain his one-hand support quickly enough when the chair rocks back. As the patient's skill develops, this assistance should be withdrawn.

vv This skill is addressed in Chapter 10.

Independent work. Once a patient has been shown this technique and has had some initial practice, he can practice independently. He can practice rocking his wheelchair to upright concurrently with the other skill prerequisites for returning a chair to upright after a fall.

WHEELCHAIR SKILLS AND THERAPEUTIC STRATEGIES FOLLOWING INCOMPLETE SPINAL CORD INJURY

The actions that an individual can use to perform functional tasks after sustaining an incomplete spinal cord injury will depend primarily on his voluntary motor function. A person who retains or regains only sensory function below his injury (ASIA B) will utilize the techniques that are used by people with complete spinal cord injuries, described in this chapter. A person who has minimal motor sparing or return (ASIA C) is likely to utilize similar movement patterns, but may be able to add trunk or lower extremity motions to make the tasks easier. An individual who has significant motor function below his lesion (ASIA D) may be able to function independently without a wheelchair. If he does use a wheelchair, he is likely to be able to use his lower extremities to perform many wheelchair skills.

Another factor that can have an impact on the performance of wheelchair skills is spasticity. People with incomplete lesions tend to exhibit more spasticity than do people with complete lesions, and spasticity tends to be more severe among those with ASIA B and C lesions.[35, 38, 48] Involuntary muscle contractions can interfere with the functional use of voluntary motor function that is preserved below the lesion. When elevated muscle tone interferes with function, the rehabilitation team can work with the patient to reduce the abnormal tone.[ww] In addition, the therapist and patient should note the conditions and bodily motions that tend to elicit involuntary muscle contractions. They can then work together in an effort to find ways in which the patient can utilize a wheelchair without causing these involuntary contractions. In some cases, they may also find ways in which abnormal muscle tone can be used to enhance the performance of some activities. For example, this author had a patient (with C4 tetraplegia, ASIA C) who exhibited spasms in his trunk muscles that were brought on by tactile stimulation of his thighs: when the anterior aspect of either thigh was touched, the patient's trunk flexed laterally toward the side that had been touched. The patient learned to elicit these spasms to shift his trunk laterally from midline and to return to midline from a lateral lean.

Use of Power Wheelchair

A person who has motor return below his lesion may have the capacity for more actions that he can use to access input devices. The therapist and patient should work together to determine what body motions can be utilized, and which input devices will enable him to function most independently and comfortably.

Manual Wheelchair Propulsion over Even Surfaces

When motor sparing or return occurs in one or both of an individual's legs, he may be able to use his leg(s) to propel a manual wheelchair. Depending on the relative strength of his arms and legs, he may use his legs as the primary source of power for propulsion or use them in combination with his arms. He may propel his wheelchair using only his legs, or any combination of one or both arms and one or both legs.

The patient should be encouraged to maintain good sitting posture while propelling his wheelchair, with his buttocks well back on the seat. To use a single leg to propel forward, he should reach his foot forward and plant his heel on the floor. He can then pull the chair forward using knee flexion. Backward propulsion involves performing the reverse of these actions, and turning can be accomplished by exerting a laterally or diagonally directed force while propelling. If using two legs to propel, the patient should move his legs reciprocally: one leg pulls while the other reaches out.

Strategies for functional training are similar to those presented above for people with complete lesions. The therapist can demonstrate and provide assistance as needed. If propulsion is very difficult for the individual, the therapist can make the task easier at first by prepositioning the casters, altering the handrims if necessary, and having the patient practice on a hard floor surface such as linoleum. The patient should be encouraged to propel himself to his various activities in the course of the day. With practice, he should become faster and more proficient.

Obstacle Negotiation in Manual Wheelchairs

An individual who has significant motor sparing or return in one or both legs is likely to find nego-

---

[ww] Strategies for treating spasticity are presented in Chapter 3.

tiation of curbs, ramps, and uneven terrain easier if he approaches these obstacles backwards.

Inclines: Ramps, curb cuts, and hills.

Inclines can be negotiated using one or both legs, with or without one or both arms. Descending and ascending steep inclines is likely to be easiest and safest if performed with the chair facing down the slope. This position eliminates the risk of falling over backwards down the ramp. It also enables the wheelchair rider to push with his foot or feet to provide power for ascending the incline or controlling the descent.

Strategies for functional training are similar to those presented earlier for people with complete lesions. The therapist can demonstrate and provide assistance as needed. Practice should start on mild and short inclines, and progress to progressively steeper and longer ramps as the patient's skill develops.

Curbs.

Curbs can be ascended backwards using one or both legs and one or both arms. The wheel-chair rider should use as many extremities as are strong enough to contribute to the effort. To ascend a curb backwards, the individual backs his chair to the curb so that the rear wheels contact the curb. He should then plant his foot or feet on the floor in a position posterior to his knees, lean his trunk forward, and grasp the chair's hand-rim(s) (Figure 12–31A). The forward lean unweights the chair's rear wheels, making it easier to lift them onto the curb. The forward lean also makes it possible to reach further forward/inferiorly on the handrims.

While maintaining a forward lean, the individual should push with his foot or feet and pull on the handrim(s) to roll the rear wheels up onto the curb (Figure 12–31B). After positioning the rear wheels on top of the curb, he should continue rolling the chair to position the casters at the edge of the curb (Figure 12–31C).

Once the casters are positioned at the edge of the curb, the patient should plant his foot or feet at the base of the curb. He can then lean back to

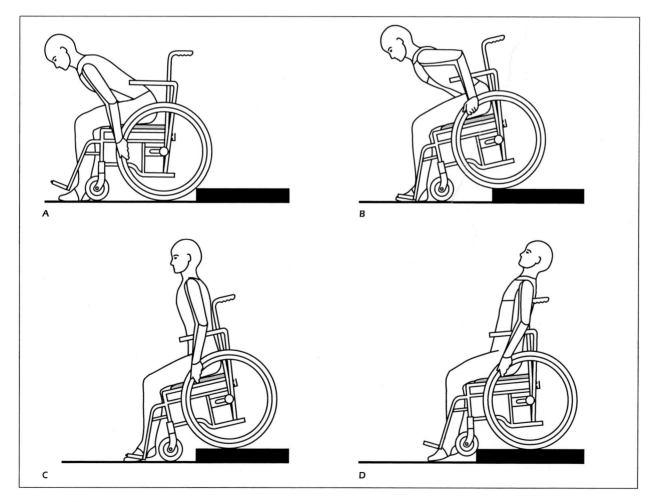

Figure 12–31. Ascending curb using upper and lower extremities. **(A)** Starting foot, trunk, and hand position. **(B)** Push/pull rear wheels onto curb. **(C)** Casters positioned at edge of curb. Foot, trunk, and hand position in preparation for lifting casters onto curb. **(D)** Push/pull casters onto curb.

unweight the casters, and position his hand(s) anteriorly on the push rims. To lift the casters onto the curb, he can simultaneously pull on the hand-rim(s) and push with his foot or feet (Figure 12–31D). The curb can be descended by performing the same motions in reverse.

Strategies for functional training are similar to those presented earlier for people with complete lesions. The therapist can demonstrate and provide assistance as needed. Curb negotiation training should start on short (1-inch) curbs, and progress to progressively higher curbs as the patient's skill develops.

Uneven terrain. To negotiate slightly uneven terrain, an individual may simply propel his chair using the technique that he utilizes over even surfaces, pushing/pulling harder to move the wheels over irregularities in the surface. Alternatively, he may find it easier to propel his chair backwards over uneven terrain. If the casters sink into soft soil or get caught on an irregularity in the surface, he can try leaning backward to shift his weight off of the casters.

Stairs. Stair negotiation strategies are essentially the same as those used by people with complete lesions, although functioning trunk or lower extremity musculature may make some maneuvers easier. Functional training involves the same approaches as were presented earlier for patients with complete lesions.

Falling Safely and Returning to Upright After a Fall

When the legs are used for propulsion and obstacle negotiation, backward tips and falls may be less likely to occur. The techniques used to negotiate obstacles using the combined action of the legs and arms do not involve wheelies or popping the casters from the ground and, as a result, may involve less risk of tipping over backwards than do the techniques performed using the arms only. Moreover, the wheelchair's seat is likely to be lower to allow propulsion with the legs, and the resulting lower center of gravity will make the chair more stable.

If a patient is likely to perform any activities involving a risk of tipping over backwards in his wheelchair, he should learn to fall safely. The techniques used are the same as those described above for people with complete spinal cord injuries.

The method used to return a chair to upright after a fall will depend on the individual's motor function. If his upper extremities are stronger than his lower extremities, he is likely to be more functional using the technique described above for people with complete lesions. If his lower extremities are stronger than his upper extremities, he may find it easier to get out of the chair, right it, and perform a floor-to-chair transfer.[xx]

SUMMARY

- When ambulation is impaired, the selection and adjustment of a wheelchair is necessary for the individual's physical health and independent functioning. The patient should play a central role in the wheelchair selection and adjustment process, working with the rehabilitation team to determine which of the many options will be most appropriate for him.

- Wheelchair skills are critical for the physical health and independent functioning of individuals who use wheelchairs for mobility. This chapter presents techniques for positioning the trunk in a chair, pressure reliefs, propulsion over even surfaces, negotiation of obstacles, falling safely, and returning the chair to upright after a fall.

- The manner in which a person with a spinal cord injury utilizes a wheelchair will depend on the extent of motor sparing or return below his lesion. If he has little or no voluntary motor function below his lesion, he must use muscles innervated above the lesion to perform wheelchair skills. If he has significant motor function in his trunk and lower extremities, he may be able to use his legs or trunk to assist in these activities.

- During rehabilitation, the therapist and patient work together to discover the movement strategies and equipment components and adjustment that will enable the patient to function independently, safely, and comfortably in a wheelchair. The therapeutic program then consists of activities directed at developing the strength, range of motion, and skill needed to perform these functional tasks. This chapter presents a variety of strategies for developing the skills involved.

- The therapist and patient should take appropriate precautions to prevent motion of unstable vertebrae, pressure ulcers, overstretching of the low back, postural deformity, shoulder pain, and injury due to tips or falls.

---

xx Floor-to-wheelchair transfers are presented in Chapter 11.

13

Ambulation

Pathology ◄─► Impairment ◄─► Functional Limitation ◄─► Disability

Therapeutic exercise
to increase strength,
preserve or increase
muscle flexibility and
joint range of motion,
develop balance and
motor control

Maximization of ambulatory
ability through gait training
and provision of
appropriate equipment

Ambulation is a priority concern for many people following spinal cord injury. This is common knowledge among health professionals who work with patients with spinal cord injuries. Especially during the early weeks and months after injury, much of a patient's questioning often centers on her future capacity to walk.

The high priority of walking is understandable when one considers the value that our society places on standing and walking. Our attitudes about different postures are reflected in our language. Sitting down epitomizes passivity. ("I'm not going to take that sitting down.") In contrast, standing is seen as a measure of power, competence, and potency. ("Stand up and take it like a man.")

AMBULATION AFTER COMPLETE INJURY: TO WALK OR NOT TO WALK?

Walking is clearly a priority for patients. However, it is an area of controversy for many health professionals. Ambulation with assistive devices and knee-ankle-foot orthoses or hip-knee-ankle-foot orthoses is a good deal slower than normal ambulation, and is profoundly more energy-consuming.[16, 57, 66, 67, 94, 99, 100] In contrast, the speed and energy costs of wheelchair propulsion[a] are similar to those of normal walking.[16] As a result, people with complete spinal cord injuries are likely to abandon their ambulation skills after rehabilitation.[28, 34, 42, 89, 94] This is true even for people who can walk with two ankle-foot orthoses and assistive devices.[96]

A reasonable question arises: If research and experience have shown that a person with a spinal cord injury is likely to abandon ambulation, why should the rehabilitation team spend time, money, and energy gait training? The answer is twofold.

First, though most patients with complete injuries give up ambulation following rehabilitation, some *do not*.[16, 35, 108] Is it ethical to deny people the opportunity to walk because they *probably* will give it up? If we do, some would-be walkers will never get the chance. Second, a patient may receive psychological benefit from gait training even if she ultimately uses a wheelchair. Until she has had the opportunity to experience ambulation after her injury, she may not be able to accept wheelchair mobility. ("They wouldn't let me try. I know if I could just try. . . .") Once she has tried walking with orthoses and assistive devices and has seen

---

[a] For people with paraplegia, the speed and energy requirements of wheelchair propulsion are comparable to normal ambulation. People with tetraplegia are likely to propel more slowly and with greater difficulty.

how difficult it is, she may be more ready to accept the alternative. Wheelchair mobility then becomes a matter of choice, representing independent and convenient mobility rather than symbolizing disability.

Ideally, any person with a spinal cord injury who wishes to attempt ambulation should be given the opportunity to do so, as long as there is no medical or orthopedic contraindication. Even a patient who has a high lesion may benefit from the attempt. Even if one agrees in theory that everyone should be given a chance to walk, however, the high cost of orthoses remains a barrier. It is hard to justify spending over a thousand dollars on a pair of orthoses for a person with a cervical lesion, knowing that she is likely to give up ambulation after a few gait training sessions.

Offering the opportunity for gait training to patients with spinal cord injuries will be more practical if the cost can be minimized. This can be done by postponing the purchase of orthoses until patients have demonstrated the capacity to walk functionally. If the physical therapy department has adjustable orthoses or a bank of donated orthoses, patients can begin gait training without purchasing orthoses. The individual's equipment can then be purchased toward the end of gait training, after she has shown the ability and drive required to walk independently.

Although patients should be provided with the opportunity to try walking, they should not be pressured into attempting ambulation if they are not interested. Unlike transfers, mat activities, and wheelchair skills, walking with orthoses is not a "survival" skill required for independent living. (A patient who is not motivated to pursue survival skills should not be forced to, but certainly a therapist should make every attempt to convince her of the need to learn these skills). Similarly, gait training should not supersede functional training in survival skills. If a patient has limited funding for functional training, more practical skills should take precedence.

When a patient with a complete spinal cord injury expresses interest in attempting ambulation, she should be given a clear understanding of the potential usefulness of this skill. The therapist should provide the patient with a realistic assessment of her potential for functional ambulation, and explain to her both the difficulty of ambulation with orthoses and assistive devices, and the extremely low rate of continued ambulation after completion of rehabilitation. If the patient chooses to attempt ambulation despite this information, the therapist should make it clear that if she discontinues walking in the future, that deci-

sion will be a reasonable and practical choice, not a failure.

THERAPEUTIC APPROACHES TO RESTORATION OF AMBULATION

People with complete lesions in the thoracic and lumbar regions of the spinal cord have inadequate voluntary motor function for ambulation using only their innervated musculature. To walk, they require orthoses (sometimes referred to as mechanical orthoses), functional electrical stimulation, or a combination of the two. Gait training with orthoses remains the most prevalent approach to ambulation following spinal cord injury. For this reason, the bulk of this chapter will focus on ambulation using orthoses.

People who have incomplete lesions may retain or regain adequate motor function to walk using more normal movement patterns than is possible following complete injury. Therapeutic interventions work toward restoration of locomotor ability rather than the provision of equipment and training in compensatory movement strategies.

The descriptions of equipment, ambulation techniques and gait training presented in this chapter should be used as a guide, not as a set of hard and fast rules. The equipment required and motions used to walk and perform other ambulation-related skills vary between people. This variability is due to differences in body build, skill level, range of motion, muscle tone, and patterns of strength and weakness. During functional training, the therapist and patient should work together to find the exact equipment and movement strategies that best suit that particular individual.

PRECAUTIONS

Following spinal cord injuries, ambulation can cause problems if appropriate precautions are not taken. Gait activities can result in excessive motion in unstable segments of the spine, skin damage, and injuries from falls. Table 13–1 presents a summary of precautions for gait training with orthoses.

LOWER EXTREMITY ORTHOSES

When motor function is inadequate for ambulation, mechanical orthoses can be used to provide stability and, in some cases, motion to the joints of the lower extremities. An orthosis can control the motion of the joints that it crosses in a variety of

TABLE 13–1.   PRECAUTIONS DURING AMBULATION AND AMBULATION TRAINING

Potential Problems	Ambulation Activities That Place Patients at Risk	Precautions
Excessive motion at site of vertebral instability, potentially causing additional neurologic and orthopedic damage	Any activity involving excessive motion or muscular action at or near site of unstable spine. Example: Upright activities while the spine remains unstable.	• Strictly adhere to orthopedic precautions. • Check fit of vertebral orthosis with patient in upright postures.
Pressure ulcers	Use of orthoses.	• Assess fit of orthoses and shoes to ensure that skin is not subjected to excessive pressure. • Ensure that any orthotic joints allowing motion are aligned with anatomic joints, to prevent shear forces and friction on skin from orthoses moving relative to limb. • Assess fabrication of orthoses and shoes to ensure that skin does not come in contact with sharp or rough surfaces. • When orthoses are first worn, gradually increase wearing time. • Monitor skin status for signs of damage from orthoses, and teach patient to monitor skin status.
Injury from fall	Ambulation with orthoses and assistive devices involves some risk of falling.	• Education and training in safe ambulation and falling techniques. • Appropriate guarding during gait training. • Provide patient with properly functioning orthoses and assistive devices.

ways. It can prevent, limit, cause, or resist movement.[49] Table 13–2 presents the terminology used to describe the different types of control that an orthosis can provide.

Lower extremity orthoses can be made of metal, plastic, or a combination of the two. Table 13–3 summarizes the characteristics of orthoses made of the different materials. Orthoses in each of these classes (metal, plastic, and metal-plastic) can provide each type of control: they can limit (stop), prevent (hold), or cause (assist) motion in the joints that they span.

Orthotic Prescription

A large variety of lower extremity orthoses are available for restoring ambulation after spinal cord injury. When prescribing an orthosis, the rehabilitation team selects the anatomic joints that the orthosis will span, the control that it will provide at each joint, and the orthotic components and materials that will be most appropriate for the individual.

Considerations for orthotic prescription. When an orthosis is used to aid in ambulation, its purpose is to provide stability during stance, enhance swing, or both. When choosing between various orthotic designs, the control that a given orthosis can provide is of primary importance; an orthosis should be selected that best meets the individual's biomechanical needs. These needs can be determined through assessment of the individual's capacity for lower extremity and trunk control during ambulation. If the individual is able to walk

TABLE 13-2.   ORTHOTIC CONTROL TERMINOLOGY

Control	Impact on Movement	Examples
Stop	Prevents motion beyond a certain degree in a given direction.	• An ankle dorsiflexion stop set at 5 degrees of dorsiflexion will allow dorsiflexion to 5 degrees, and prevent further dorsiflexion beyond this point. • An ankle plantar flexion stop set at 5 degrees of plantar flexion will allow plantar flexion to 5 degrees, and prevent further plantar flexion beyond this point. • An orthosis that has an ankle plantar flexion stop set at 5 degrees and a dorsiflexion stop set at 5 degrees will allow motion between these two positions, but will prevent motion past 5 degrees in either direction.
Hold	Prevents motion in either direction in a given plane.	• An ankle with a hold at 5 degrees of dorsiflexion will position the ankle at that angle and will not allow either dorsiflexion or plantar flexion.
Assist	Causes the joint to move in a given direction.	• A dorsiflexion assist moves the ankle into dorsiflexion. Plantar flexion occurs when muscular action or external forces are strong enough to overpower the dorsiflexion assist. A dorsiflexion assist *resists* this motion, but does not prevent it.
Lock	Prevents motion of a joint when locked, allows motion when unlocked.	• A knee lock holds the knee in extension when engaged (locked), allows free flexion when disengaged (unlocked).
Adjustable, or variable	Allows the control provided at the joint to be adjusted.	• An adjustable dorsiflexion stop set at 5 degrees of dorsiflexion prevents dorsiflexion beyond 5 degrees, but that position can be altered so that either more or less motion is allowed.

without orthoses, the therapist should perform a careful gait analysis[b] to identify the gait deviations that may require orthotic intervention.

A second consideration when choosing between orthotic designs is adjustability. Especially when a patient receives her first orthosis, adjustability can be useful because it allows the rehabilitation team to "fine tune" the appliance to the individual. The orthotic component that is most frequently adjustable is the ankle joint. An ankle joint that allows significant changes in the control that it provides will make it possible to make adjustments that enhance the patient's gait pattern and capacity to perform other functions such as balancing in standing or moving from a sitting

position to standing. Adjustability also makes it possible to alter the control that the orthosis provides as the patient's needs change. A disadvantage of an adjustable joint is that it is likely to add weight and bulk to the orthosis.

A third consideration when selecting orthoses is weight. The weight of an orthosis influences the energy cost of walking; heavier orthoses increase the oxygen consumed per meter of ambulation.[8] If all other things are equal, then, a lighter orthosis may result in the ability to walk greater distances before tiring.

A fourth consideration in orthotic prescription is the potential for damage to the patient's skin. A plastic or combined metal-plastic orthosis, because of its intimate fit, can exert excessive pressure on the skin if the patient's limb swells. These types of orthoses can also cause skin maceration if the patient perspires excessively. Thus metal orthoses are indicated for patients who have fluc-

---

[b] A thorough presentation of gait analysis is beyond the scope of this text. The following references provide comprehensive information on gait analysis: 1, 73, 74, 77.

TABLE 13–3.   CHARACTERISTICS OF METAL, PLASTIC, AND METAL-PLASTIC ORTHOSES

Materials	Weight	Adjustability of Control	Shoes	Additional Considerations
Metal	Heaviest	Depending on the type of ankle joint, it may allow a large degree of adjustability of joint position and type of control provided.	Shoes are built into the orthoses, so the wearer cannot readily change shoes. Shoes must be sturdy, so there is little choice in shoe design.	When there is fluctuating edema or excessive perspiration, metal orthoses may be preferable to other designs because they are least likely to cause skin breakdown.
Plastic	Lightest	As a rule, plastic orthoses are the least adjustable. Some ankle joints are adjustable, but do not allow as much adjustment as metal ankle joints allow.	Shoes are *not* built into the orthoses, so a variety of shoes may be worn. (Heel height must remain the same, to provide appropriate alignment.)	The control that a plastic orthosis provides is determined by the rigidity of the plastic used, the configuration of the orthosis, and the joints included. Fluctuating edema may cause skin breakdown, due to the intimate fit of orthoses. Excessive perspiration may cause skin breakdown, due to the nonabsorbent nature of plastic.
Metal-plastic	Intermediate weight	If the ankle joint is metal, it may allow a large degree of adjustability of joint position and type of control provided.	Similar to plastic, as plastic-metal orthoses are typically constructed with plastic shoe inserts.	Fluctuating edema and excessive perspiration can cause skin breakdown, as can occur with plastic orthoses.

Sources: references 61, 64, 65, 75, 83, 109.

tuating edema or excessive perspiration in their lower extremities.

Additional considerations in orthotic prescription include durability, ease of donning and doffing, cosmesis, cost, and impact on other functional activities such as transfers. Unfortunately, the funding source should also be considered in orthotic selection; third-party payers frequently provide limited funding for orthoses.

Choosing between orthotic options.   For any biomechanical deficit, there are a variety of possible orthotic solutions. For example, a patient who is unable to dorsiflex her ankles during swing due to muscle weakness could utilize metal, plastic, or metal-plastic ankle-foot orthoses (AFOs) to assist

dorsiflexion or stop plantar flexion. Moreover, each of these types of orthosis has a number of different designs that could provide the needed control.

When selecting an orthosis, it is best to keep in mind that every orthosis has both advantages and disadvantages. The various orthotic options differ in their adjustability, weight, risk of causing skin breakdown, durability, ease of donning and doffing, cosmesis, cost, and impact on overall functional independence. For example, a given orthosis may be light but not adjustable, or light and adjustable but expensive or potentially harmful to the wearer's skin. Clinicians involved in prescribing orthoses should investigate the benefits and drawbacks of the various orthotic options. Orthotic prescription should then be based on an analysis of the advantages and disadvantages of the various orthotic options, taking into consideration the needs and priorities of the patient.

When possible, it can be helpful to try orthoses before ordering them. Since most lower extremity orthoses that are appropriate for people with spinal cord injuries are custom-made, it is generally not possible to obtain trial orthoses that are *identical* to the ones being ordered. It may be possible, however, to utilize a *similar* orthosis for a trial period. Many physical therapy departments have a collection of orthoses for this purpose. During the trial period, the clinicians and wearer should note the influence of the orthosis on the individual's gait pattern, endurance in ambulation, standing balance, and performance of other tasks such as sit-to-stand or car transfers. Although a trial orthosis cannot perfectly replicate a custom-made orthosis, its use can provide some information on the impact that an orthosis will have on the individual's capacity to function.

Orthotic selection is a team process. Physical therapists, orthotists, and prospective wearers play key roles, each bringing a different perspective and knowledge base. Physical therapists contribute an understanding of the pathomechanics of gait, as well as knowledge about the patient's physical status, functional capacity, and vulnerabilities relevant to orthotic use. Orthotists bring information on the characteristics of the currently available orthotic components, materials, and designs. Prospective orthotic wearers bring their preferences, values, and priorities. The physical therapist, orthotist, and prospective wearer should work together to determine the orthotic design that will be most appropriate for the wearer.

Ankle-Foot Orthoses

Ankle-foot orthoses (AFOs) are primarily used for people who have the ability to stabilize their knees in stance using their quadriceps but need stabilization at their ankles. The orthotic control needed at the ankle will depend on the motor function present.

When the dorsiflexors are weak, a dorsiflexion assist at the ankle will prevent excessive plantar flexion during swing. By moving the ankle into neutral dorsiflexion during swing, an AFO can prevent toe drag and position the ankle for heel-first contact at the beginning of stance. A dorsiflexion assist will also allow plantar flexion after heel strike, resulting in a more normal gait pattern.

In the presence of gastrocnemius and soleus spasticity, a plantar flexion stop should be used instead of a dorsiflexion assist because the plantar

flexors are likely to overpower a dorsiflexion assist and place the ankle in a plantar flexed position. A plantar flexion stop will prevent this motion, enhancing foot clearance during swing and reducing the occurrence of knee hyperextension during stance. The disadvantage of a plantar flexion stop is that it increases the flexion moment at the knee during early stance,[107] increasing the demand on the quadriceps. Modification of the shoe's heel may be required to avoid excessive knee flexion during loading response.[96]

Weakness in the plantar flexors may necessitate a dorsiflexion stop to stabilize the tibia on the foot during stance, preventing excessive dorsiflexion as the person's center of gravity passes anterior to her ankle. A stop limiting dorsiflexion to 10 degrees will provide adequate stability and allow a relatively normal gait pattern.[75]

In addition to controlling ankle motions, an AFO can be used to provide control at the knee. When the quadriceps are weak, an AFO that stops dorsiflexion can help to prevent knee flexion during stance. This type of orthosis is often called a floor-reaction AFO[c] because it utilizes floor reaction forces to control the knee.[58] An AFO that stops plantar flexion can have the opposite effect on the knee: an ankle held in a neutral or slightly dorsiflexed position can prevent genu recurvatum.[69]

Metal orthosis with double action ankle joint. One type of orthotic ankle joint that is frequently used because of its adjustability is a double action ankle joint. This design is also called a dual-channel ankle joint, double-adjustable ankle joint, or bichannel adjustable ankle. This metal ankle has channels that are located anterior and posterior to the joint's axis (Figure 13–1).

A double action ankle joint can be used to limit, prevent, or assist motion in the sagittal plane.[83, 109] The control that it provides will depend on the contents of the channels; pins (small metal rods) in the channels stop motion and springs in the channels assist motion. The pins and springs are held in place by set screws. The control provided by the orthotic joint can be adjusted by tightening or loosening the set screws, turning them clockwise or counter-clockwise, respectively.[d] The type of control that the orthosis provides can be altered by changing the contents of the channels. For example, a plantar flexion stop can be converted to a dorsi-

---

c Also called a ground-reaction AFO.
d The medial and lateral set screws should be adjusted the same amount. Otherwise, the orthotic ankle will be subjected to excessive stress.

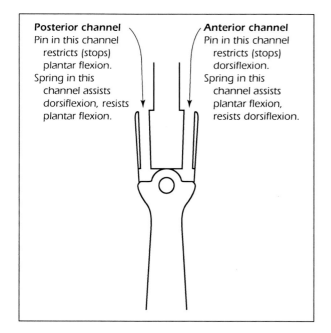

Posterior channel
Pin in this channel restricts (stops) plantar flexion.
Spring in this channel assists dorsiflexion, resists plantar flexion.

Anterior channel
Pin in this channel restricts (stops) dorsiflexion.
Spring in this channel assists plantar flexion, resists dorsiflexion.

Figure 13–1. Double action ankle joint, interior view.

flexion assist by removing the pins in the posterior channels and replacing them with springs. Table 13–4 summarizes the control options and adjustment for a double action ankle joint.

Plastic. Custom-molded plastic AFOs are commonly prescribed because they are lighter than metal AFOs. They can also be worn with a variety of shoes, making them more cosmetically acceptable to many wearers.[109] A plastic AFO can provide the same types of control that metal orthoses can provide.

A plastic AFO can be made with or without an articulating ankle. When an articulating ankle is incorporated in the orthosis, the ankle's design and materials determine the control that it provides and the degree to which it can be adjusted. When an AFO does not contain an articulating ankle, the control that the orthosis provides is determined by its trim lines[e] and materials: An orthosis that is designed to hold the ankle firmly in place typically extends anteriorly to encase the medial and lateral malleoli, and is constructed of rigid and thick materials. An orthosis that is designed to provide a dorsiflexion assist will have

more posteriorly located trim lines and will be made of more flexible and thinner plastic.

Knee-Ankle-Foot Orthoses

Knee-ankle-foot orthoses (KAFOs) are used when orthotic stabilization is required at the knees and the ankles. This stabilization may be required due muscle weakness or deficits in proprioception.[109] KAFOs are often used by people who lack muscular stabilization not only of the knees and ankles but of the hips and trunk as well. These individuals use compensatory motions of their upper bodies to control their hips and the portions of their trunks that are not innervated.

Conventional metal KAFOs. A conventional metal KAFO has double uprights that are connected posteriorly by two thigh bands and a calf band. Anterior thigh and leg cuffs and a knee cap stabilize the leg in the orthosis. Typically, drop-ring locks are used at the knees. The ankles generally stop plantar flexion, and dorsiflexion may be stopped or left unrestricted.

Scott-Craig KAFOs. A Scott-Craig KAFO (also called a Craig-Scott KAFO) is designed to provide maximal stability at the ankle and foot (Figure 13–2). A T-shaped foot plate is embedded in the sole of the shoe, extending from the heel to the level of the metatarsal heads. This plate provides excellent anteroposterior and mediolateral stability, making the shoe a stable base for the rest of the orthosis. An adjustable double-stop ankle[f] holds the ankle immobile in approximately 10 degrees of dorsiflexion. This fixed dorsiflexion at the ankles places the hips in a stable position during stance.[g] The optimal angle for a given individual's ankle is determined during initial gait training.

The knee locking mechanism of a Scott-Craig orthosis is a pawl lock with a bail control. The bail control is a U-shaped lever that circles posteriorly around the back of the leg, attached medially and laterally at the mechanical knee joints. Upward pressure on the bail control unlocks the orthotic knee, allowing flexion. The wearer who is in a sitting position can unlock the orthotic knee by pulling upward on the bail. Alternatively, she can unlock the knees while she sits down from a

---

[e] "Trim lines" refers to the edges of the orthosis. An AFO with more anterior trim lines extends more anteriorly around the ankle, so that the orthosis encases more of the circumference of the lower leg and ankle. An AFO with more posterior trim lines does not extend as far anteriorly around the lower leg and ankle.

[f] A double-stop ankle is a double-action ankle joint with anterior and posterior stops.

[g] When the feet are flat on the floor and the ankles are held in dorsiflexion, the hips are placed in an anterior position. The effect of hip position on stability is discussed later in this chap-

TABLE 13–4. DOUBLE ACTION ANKLE JOINTS: CONTROL OPTIONS AND ADJUSTMENT

Control	Pin or Spring Location	Adjustment
Dorsiflexion stop	Pins in anterior channels	**To allow more dorsiflexion:** turn set screws in anterior channels counter-clockwise.
		To allow less dorsiflexion: turn set screws in anterior channels clockwise.
Plantar flexion stop	Pins in posterior channels	**To allow more plantar flexion:** turn set screws in posterior channels counter-clockwise.
		To allow less plantar flexion: turn set screws in posterior channels clockwise.
Hold	Pins in posterior and anterior channels, adjusted to prevent any motion in sagittal plane	**To hold the ankle in a more dorsiflexed position:** turn set screws in anterior channels counter-clockwise, reposition ankle to the more dorsiflexed position, then turn set screws in posterior channels in clockwise direction.
		To hold the ankle in a more plantar flexed position: turn set screws in posterior channels counter-clockwise, reposition ankle to the more plantar flexed position, then turn set screws in anterior channels in clockwise direction.
Dorsiflexion assist	Springs in posterior channels	**To increase force of dorsiflexion assist:** turn set screws in posterior channels in clockwise direction.
		To reduce force of dorsiflexion assist: turn set screws in posterior channels in counter-clockwise direction.
Free motion in sagittal plane	Anterior and posterior channels left empty	

standing position. To do so, she stands with the bails positioned on top of the sitting surface and then sits down. When the sitting surface pushes upward on the bails, the knees will unlock.

In addition to the knee locking mechanism and the specialized shoe and ankle, a Scott-Craig KAFO has two metal uprights, a single posterior thigh band, a hinged pretibial band, and a cushioned heel. The sole of the shoe is shaped to allow both stability and a smooth roll-over in stance. After the orthotic user has developed her ambulatory skills and the optimal ankle position has been determined, a sturdy plastic AFO can be substituted for the components below the knee.[47, 64, 69]

Whether a Scott-Craig orthosis or a conventional KAFO is used, an orthosis with a long sole plate and an ankle that is positioned rigidly in dorsiflexion makes walking easier for people with complete paraplegia who require KAFOs. The stability provided by these features makes it possible to maintain a balanced standing posture without

upper extremity effort. (Once in a balanced standing posture, the individual may be able to balance with both hands lifted.) Additionally, the magnitude of the vertical oscillations of the individual's center of gravity during gait are less than occur with KAFOs which allow free dorsiflexion. The end result is that less energy is consumed during ambulation.[47, 69]

Hip-Knee-Ankle-Foot Orthoses

Hip-knee-ankle-foot orthoses (HKAFOs) provide orthotic control to the hips and joints caudal to this point. The various types of HKAFO differ most in the type of hip control that they provide. During gait, the hip mechanisms of HKAFOs can lock the hips in extension, allow a limited range of flexion and extension, or cause reciprocal motion at the hips. HKAFOs are less functional than KAFOs in terms of capacity for stair and curb negotiation, transfers in and out of cars, and toileting.[63]

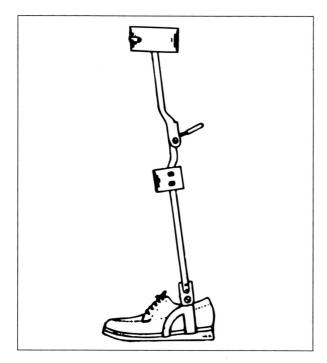

Figure 13–2. Scott-Craig orthosis. *(Reproduced with permission from Lower-Limb Orthotics [1986], Sidney Fishman, PhD, and Norman Berger, eds., Prosthetic-Orthotic Publications, New York.)*

Conventional HKAFOs. A conventional HKAFO is made of the components used in KAFOs plus locking hip joints and a pelvic band to provide hip and pelvic stability. A spinal orthosis can be added to provide trunk stability. Because of the orthotic stabilization at the hips, ambulation with conventional HKAFOs is limited to a swing-to or swing-through gait.[83] Because of their weight and the high energy requirements of ambulation with these orthoses, conventional HKAFOs are rarely prescribed for adults with spinal cord injuries.[42]

Hip Guidance Orthoses. A Hip Guidance Orthosis (HGO), also called a ParaWalker, allows free flexion and extension of the hips within a limited range. This metal orthosis includes metal foot plates, locking knees, hip joints with flexion and extension stops, a pelvic band, and a chest strap. The wearer walks with a reciprocal gait by unweighting one leg at a time and allowing gravity to pull the unweighted leg forward like a pendulum suspended at the hip.[14, 63] The wearer relies heavily on her arms during ambulation.[36] This type of orthosis has limited usefulness in terms of functional ambulation.[63]

Reciprocating Gait Orthoses. A Reciprocating Gait Orthosis (RGO) is a type of HKAFO that immobilizes the knees, ankles and feet and causes reciprocal motions of the hips during ambulation. The

orthosis consists of plastic KAFOs with locking knees and reinforced ankles, attached proximally to a molded pelvic band with thoracic extensions (Figure 13–3). Hip motions are controlled by cables that connect the hip joints. These cables are designed to transfer forces between the hips. Motion at one hip causes motion in the opposite direction to occur in the contralateral hip: to take a step forward, the wearer shifts her weight off of the leg and extends the contralateral hip. [12, 47, 64]

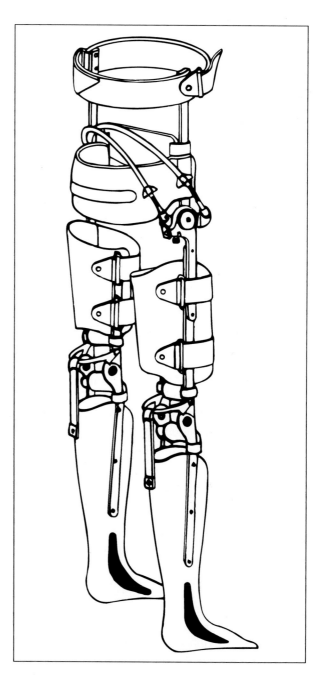

Figure 13–3. Reciprocating gait orthosis. *(Reproduced with permission from Nick Rightor, CO, and the LSU Medical Center. [1983]. In LSU Reciprocating Gait Orthosis: A Pictorial Description and Application Manual. Chattanooga, TN: Fillauer, Inc.)*

PROBLEM-SOLVING EXERCISE 13-1

Your patient has L5 paraplegia, ASIA A. He uses Lofstrand crutches to walk without orthoses, bearing excessive weight on his upper extremities. When he attempts to walk without the crutches, he is unstable due to excessive knee flexion during late stance.

The patient's joint range of motion and muscle flexibility are normal throughout. His light touch and pin prick sensation are normal in the C1 through L5 dermatomes, impaired in S1, and absent below. Proprioception is normal in his upper extremities, hips, knees, and ankles. The muscle test results are as follows.

Muscles	Left	Right
Abdominals and upper extremities	5/5	5/5
Hip flexors	5/5	5/5
Hip abductors	4/5	4/5
Quadriceps	5/5	5/5
Hamstrings	4/5	4/5
Ankle dorsiflexors	5/5	5/5
Long toe extensors	4/5	4/5
Ankle plantar flexors	2/5	2/5

- What is the most likely cause of this patient's knee instability during late stance? Explain your answer.
- Would AFOs or KAFOs be most beneficial for this patient? Why?
- What control should these orthoses provide? Explain.

Alternative HKAFO designs that provide a reciprocating gait include the Advanced Reciprocating Gait Orthosis (ARGO) and the Isocentric RGO. An ARGO couples the hips through one cable, in contrast to the two cables in an RGO. An Isocentric RGO utilizes a bar and tie rod mechanism to couple the hips.[3, 59, 105] Both types of orthosis cause hip flexion in the swing limb when the stance limb extends.

The various designs of reciprocating gait orthoses (RGO, ARGO, and Isocentric RGO) have several disadvantages when compared to KAFOs. They are bulkier and more cumbersome, making donning, doffing and transfers more difficult. These orthoses are also more expensive than KAFOs.[42, 92] These disadvantages are not counterbalanced by functional advantages; as is true with KAFOs and other types of HKAFO, ambulation with reciprocating gait orthoses is slow and requires a high energy expenditure.[12, 42, 105] Reciprocating gait orthoses are more likely to be used for exercise than for functional mobility, especially outside of the home.[28]

FUNCTIONAL POTENTIALS

After a spinal cord injury, an individual's potential for achieving independence in ambulation, and the orthotic support that she will require, is determined largely by her voluntary motor function. People with more intact voluntary motor function in their lower extremities are able to bear less weight on their arms while walking. This decreased dependence on the arms for support reduces the energy costs of ambulation.[95, 99, 100, 106]

With complete injuries, the voluntary motor function present in the lower extremities is determined by the level of the lesion and, thus, lesion level has a strong impact on ambulatory potential. Table 13–5 presents a summary of the level of independence in ambulation that can be achieved by people who have complete spinal cord injuries at different motor levels (motor component of the neurological level of injury).

With incomplete lesions, ambulatory potential is related more to the degree of completeness than the neurological level of injury. Greater preservation or return of voluntary motor function below the lesion leads to a better potential for functional ambulation.

When prognosticating about an individual's capacity to walk, the clinician should take into consideration the many other factors that also impact on functional gains. These factors include muscle tone, range of motion, pain, motivation, age, physical condition, medical complications, obesity, access to services and equipment, and physical coordination.[63, 72, 80, 91, 92, 95, 100]

PHYSICAL AND SKILL PREREQUISITES

Every functional activity involves a particular set of skills. Each activity also has strength, joint range of motion, and muscle flexibility requirements. A deficiency in any of these skill or physical requirements will impair a person's performance of the activity.

The descriptions of ambulation skills that follow are accompanied by tables that summarize the physical and skill prerequisites. Exact values

Motor Level	Significance of Innervated Musculature	Potential for Independence in Ambulation
C8 and higher	Inadequate voluntary motor function for functional ambulation.	Functional ambulation not feasible.
T1-9	**Fully innervated upper extremities** make it possible to lift the body's weight using elbow extension and scapular depression. Trunk musculature inadequate to provide trunk control.	**Ambulation potential:** unlikely to walk functionally; may walk for exercise, independently or with assistance. **Assistive devices:** Lofstrand crutches or walker. **Orthoses and movement strategies:** KAFOs with locked knees and ankles held in slight dorsiflexion are required for ambulation; swing limb advancement and hip and trunk stability during stance are achieved using compensatory movements of the head and upper extremities. Alternative orthoses: HKAFOs, various designs.
T10-12	**Partial innervation of trunk musculature** (T6-L1 innervation) enhances ambulation ability. Lack of lower extremity motor function limits ambulation potential.	**Ambulation potential:** independent functional ambulation within the home and for limited distances in the community is possible, although *most choose wheelchairs for mobility* due to the high energy requirements of ambulation. **Assistive devices:** Lofstrand crutches or walker. **Orthoses and movement strategies:** KAFOs with locked knees and ankles held in slight dorsiflexion are required for ambulation; swing limb advancement and hip stability during stance are achieved using compensatory movements of the head and upper extremities; trunk stability during stance is achieved using trunk musculature and/or compensatory movements, depending on the motor function present in the trunk. Alternative orthoses: HKAFOs, various designs.
L1	**Full innervation of trunk musculature** enhances ambulation ability. **Minimal innervation of psoas major** may provide active hip flexion (<3/5 strength[a]) during swing.	**Ambulation potential:** independent functional ambulation is possible within the home and for limited distances in the community; *most choose wheelchairs for mobility* due to the high energy requirements of ambulation. **Assistive devices:** Lofstrand crutches or walker. **Orthoses and movement strategies:** KAFOs with locked knees and ankles held in slight dorsiflexion are typically required for ambulation; swing limb advancement is accomplished using either compensatory movements (for swing-through or swing-to gait) or active hip flexion (for four-point gait); hip stability during stance is achieved using compensatory movements

(Cont.)

359

TABLE 13–5. *(Continued)*

Motor Level	Significance of Innervated Musculature	Potential for Independence In Ambulation
L1		of the head and upper extremities; trunk stability during stance is achieved using trunk musculature. Alternative orthoses: HKAFOs, various designs.
L2	**Partial innervation of psoas major, iliacus, sartorius, and pectineus** provide active hip flexion (≥3/5 strength[a]) for swing limb advancement. **Partial innervation of sartorius and gracilis** provide limited capacity for knee flexion for swing limb advancement (relevant only if AFOs are used instead of KAFOs.) Minimal innervation of the quadriceps (<3/5 strength[a]) is inadequate to contribute significantly to ambulation.	**Ambulation potential:** independent functional ambulation is possible within the home and for limited distances in the community; *most choose wheelchairs for mobility* due to the high energy requirements of ambulation. **Assistive devices:** Lofstrand crutches or walker. **Orthoses and movement strategies:** KAFOs with locked knees and ankles held in slight dorsiflexion are typically recommended for ambulation; swing limb advancement is accomplished using either compensatory movements (for swing-through or swing-to gait) or active hip flexion (for four-point gait); hip stability during stance is achieved using compensatory movements of the head and upper extremities; trunk stability during stance is achieved using trunk musculature. Potential for ambulation with ground-reaction AFOs.
L3	**Fully innervated iliacus and pectineus, and nearly full innervation of psoas major and sartorius** provide strong hip flexion for swing limb advancement. **Partial innervation of sartorius and gracilis** provide limited capacity for knee flexion for swing limb advancement (relevant only if AFOs are used instead of KAFOs.) **Partial innervation of the quadriceps** (≥3/5 strength[a]) provides potential for active knee control during stance.	**Ambulation potential:** potential for independent community ambulation; many choose wheelchairs for long distances due to the high energy requirements of ambulation. **Assistive devices:** Lofstrand crutches or walker. **Orthoses and movement strategies:** if quadriceps strength is adequate for knee control (typically ≥4/5), the knee may be left unbraced; AFOs with plantar flexion stops or dorsiflexion assists are required to allow toe clearance during swing; dorsiflexion stops are needed to prevent excessive ankle dorsiflexion during late stance. If quadriceps strength is not adequate for knee control (typically <4/5), KAFOs with locked knees and ankles held in slight dorsiflexion are usually recommended for ambulation; swing limb advancement is accomplished using either compensatory movements (for swing-through or swing-to gait) or active hip flexion (for four-point gait); hip stability during stance is achieved using compensatory movements of the head and upper extremities; trunk stability during stance is achieved using trunk musculature. Alternative orthoses if quadriceps strength is inadequate for knee stability: ground-reaction AFOs.

L4	Fully innervated **sartorius and gracilis** provide limited capacity for knee flexion for swing limb advancement. Fully innervated **quadriceps** provides knee control during stance. Partial innervation of the **tibialis anterior and peroneus tertius** allows active dorsiflexion (≥3/5 strength[a]) during swing limb advancement and potential for eccentric control of ankle plantar flexion during early stance. Partial innervation of **tensor fascia latae, gluteus medius, and gluteus minimus** provide limited capacity for hip abduction, likely to be inadequate to stabilize the pelvis in the frontal plane during stance.	**Ambulation potential:** may ambulate independently within the community; if significant weight is borne on the upper extremities (because of hip extensor and abductor weakness), likely to choose wheelchairs for long distances due to the high energy requirements of ambulation. **Assistive devices:** Lofstrand crutches or canes. **Orthoses:** AFOs with dorsiflexion stops are required to prevent excessive ankle dorsiflexion during late stance; if dorsiflexor strength is inadequate to provide eccentric control of plantar flexion after initial contact, or if dorsiflexors fatigue during ambulation and toe drag results, a dorsiflexion assist may be required.
L5	Nearly full innervation of the **tibialis anterior** provides ankle dorsiflexion during swing and eccentric control of plantar flexion during early stance. Nearly full innervation of the **tensor fascia latae and partial innervation of the gluteus medius and gluteus minimus** provide stronger hip abduction for stabilization of the pelvis in the frontal plane during stance. Partial innervation of the **hamstrings** enhances the capacity for active knee flexion for swing limb advancement. Nearly full innervation of **peroneus tertius and extensor digitorum longus, and partial innervation of the tibialis posterior, peroneus longus and brevis, extensor hallucis longus, flexor digitorum longus, and flexor hallucis longus** provide limited capacity for stabilization of the subtalar joint and foot during stance.	**Ambulation potential:** independent community ambulation. **Assistive devices:** standard canes. **Orthoses:** AFOs with dorsiflexion stops are indicated to prevent excessive ankle dorsiflexion during late stance.
S1	Full innervation of the **tensor fascia latae, gluteus medius, and gluteus minimus** provide strong hip abduction for stabilization of the pelvis in the frontal plane during stance. Nearly full innervation of the **hamstrings** provides strong knee flexion for swing limb advancement. Nearly full innervation of the **hamstrings and partial innervation of the gluteus maximus** provide sagittal plane stability for the hip in early stance. Partial innervation of the **gastrocnemius and soleus** provide active plantar flexion (≥3/5 strength[a]), with potential for eccentric control of dorsiflexion during midstance and terminal stance.	**Ambulation potential:** community ambulation. **Assistive devices:** no assistive devices, or standard cane(s). **Orthoses:** if plantar flexor strength is inadequate to control the forward progression of the tibias during late stance, AFOs with dorsiflexion stops are indicated.

(Cont.)

TABLE 13-5. *(Continued)*

Motor Level	Significance of Innervated Musculature	Potential for Independence in Ambulation
S1	**Full innervation of peroneus tertius and extensor digitorum longus, tibialis posterior, peroneus longus and brevis, and extensor hallucis longus; partial innervation of the flexor hallucis longus; and nearly full innervation of the flexor digitorum longus** provide strong inversion and eversion for stabilization of the subtalar joint and foot during stance.	
S2	**Full innervation of the hamstrings and gluteus maximus** provide strong hip extension for stabilization of the hip in the sagittal plane during early stance. **Full innervation of the gastrocnemius and soleus** provide strong plantar flexion for eccentric control of dorsiflexion during midstance and terminal stance.	**Ambulation potential:** community ambulation. **Assistive devices:** none. **Orthoses:** none.

KAFOs, knee-ankle-foot orthoses; HKAFOs, hip-knee-ankle-foot orthoses; AFOs, ankle-foot orthoses

[a] Strength grades indicate strength in key muscles according to American Spinal Injury Association classification system.

Sources: references 18, 39, 53, 56, 60, 63, 79, 92, 95, 97, 98, 99, 100. For more complete information on innervation, see Appendix B (www.prenhall.com/somers).

for the physical prerequisites are not given because the requirements vary among individuals. For example, a person who is very skillful in coming to stand from the floor may require less hamstring flexibility for this activity than does someone who is less skillful.

PROGRAM DESIGN

The therapeutic program is designed to enable the patient to achieve all of her functional goals. The steps of program planning follow.

1. Identify the functional goals.[h]
2. Determine the methods that the patient will utilize to perform the activities identified in the goals. This determination will involve choosing the methods that provide the best match between the patient's characteristics and the physical and skill requirements of the activities.
3. Consider the patient's impairments and functional limitations as they compare to the physical and skill requirements of the activities to be achieved.
4. Devise a therapeutic program to develop the needed strength, range of motion, and skills.

For the purposes of program planning, it may be best for the therapist and patient first to consider each goal separately and devise a plan for achieving each goal. The different goals and their plans can then be considered together. Fortunately, there is much overlap of physical and skill prerequisites for the different functional activities. Thus, a person working on maintaining a balanced standing position is potentially progressing herself toward independence in ambulation over even surfaces and obstacles. Furthermore, work aimed at developing one ability can benefit other, seemingly unrelated, activities. For example, the strengthening and motor learning that result from practicing ambulation may help a patient's transfer abilities.

Practice in Department and "Real World"

The physical therapy department in a rehabilitation center should be equipped with curbs of varying heights, stairs, and a ramp. This equipment is useful for the initial practice of obstacle negotiation; however, practice should not end with mastery of these artificial obstacles. Many obstacles that a patient will encounter outside of the department

USING CHAPTER 13 AS A RESOURCE FOR PROGRAM PLANNING

When using this text as a resource to assist in designing an ambulation program, the therapist should first determine whether the patient will utilize knee-ankle-foot orthoses (KAFOs) to walk. If so, the therapist can find descriptions of walking and ambulation-related skills under the heading "Ambulation with Knee-Ankle-Foot Orthoses" in the first half of the chapter. Based on the description of the functional activity, the corresponding tables, or both, the therapist can determine what physical and skill prerequisites are required to perform the activity. Taking into consideration the patient's examination results, the therapist can determine where the patient has deficits relevant to the functional goal. The program should then be designed to address these deficits, developing the needed physical and skill prerequisites.

This chapter presents functional training strategies for each prerequisite skill listed in the tables that accompany the skill descriptions in the first half of the chapter. These functional training strategies are presented under the heading "Therapeutic Strategies for Gait Training with Knee-Ankle-Foot Orthoses." The therapist can use these suggestions, coupled with his or her own imagination, clinical expertise, and problem solving, to design a functional training program. The program should aim first at developing the most basic prerequisite skills and build to more advanced skills as the patient's abilities develop.

Patients who have the capacity to walk with ankle-foot orthoses (AFOs) or without orthoses will walk using more normal movement patterns. Descriptions of therapeutic strategies that may be useful for these patients are presented in the second half of the chapter under the headings "Ambulation and Therapeutic Strategies with Ankle-Foot Orthoses Following Complete Spinal Cord Injury" and "Ambulation and Therapeutic Strategies Following Incomplete Spinal Cord Injury."

---

[h] Goal-setting is addressed in Chapter 8.

will be more difficult to negotiate. For example, ascending a cement curb from a street is likely to be more difficult than ascending a wooden curb from a linoleum floor. The "real world" is full of carpeted floors, uneven sidewalks, long and steep staircases, and uneven surfaces such as grass and sand. Functional training should include practicing ambulation skills outside of the department so that the patient will be better prepared to function in the "real world" following rehabilitation.

AMBULATION WITH KNEE-ANKLE-FOOT ORTHOSES FOLLOWING COMPLETE SPINAL CORD INJURY

Complete spinal cord injury at and above the L3 or L4 neurological level of injury results in a loss of adequate voluntary motor function to control the knees and ankles during ambulation. When walking is a goal, KAFOs can provide a stable base during stance by immobilizing the ankles and knees. Standing and walking are accomplished using musculature innervated above the lesion. During gait training with KAFOs, the patient learns to use compensatory movement strategies to walk and perform other gait-related tasks. These compensatory strategies include muscle substitution, momentum, and the head-hips relationship.[i]

Functional ambulation involves more than walking over even surfaces. To use KAFOs functionally at home, an individual must be able to balance in standing, walk over even surfaces, rise from a wheelchair and sit back down, fall safely and get up from the floor, and don and doff the orthoses. To walk in the community, she must also be able to walk over obstacles. This chapter presents descriptions of these ambulation skills,[j] as well as suggestions on how to teach them.

Balanced Standing

Balanced standing is the most basic ambulation skill; before a person can walk, she must be able to remain upright in a standing position. With total paralysis of the lower extremities, knee-ankle-foot orthoses (KAFOs) provide stability at the feet, ankles, and knees. A person with this

level of paralysis uses her arms, head, and upper trunk to stabilize her hips.

In the absence of innervated lower extremities, posture is the key to balanced standing. The position of stability is illustrated in Figure 13–4A. In the balanced standing posture, the person stands with her pelvis forward so that her weight line falls posterior to her hip joints. This position results in an extension moment at the hips. Since hip extension is restricted by the Y ligaments, the hips are stable in this posture.

In contrast to extension, hip flexion is not limited by ligaments. In the absence of muscular control, the hips will flex without restriction if a flexion moment exists at the hips. Thus if a person who lacks hip extensors changes her posture so that her weight line falls anterior to her hips, she will lose her stability at the hips; she will "jack-knife" as a result of this unrestricted hip flexion (Figure 13–4B).

Attaining and maintaining a balanced standing posture is accomplished using the head-hips relationship. With her hands stabilized on parallel bars or Lofstrand crutches, the person can push her pelvis forward by retracting her scapulae and throwing her head back. Tucking the head forward and protracting the scapulae will move the pelvis posteriorly.

Functional ambulation requires the ability to stand balanced without weight on both hands, at least briefly. The functional ambulator must be able to free at least one hand to move her crutches, to open doors, and to reach for objects.

Ambulation over Even Surfaces

This chapter will focus on ambulation with Lofstrand crutches and two KAFOs. Tables 13–6 and 13–7 summarize the physical and skill prerequisites for independent ambulation over even surfaces.

Four-point gait. When walking with a four-point gait, a person moves one crutch or one foot at a time. This gait pattern is slow but safe because at least three points (crutches and feet) remain in contact with the floor at all times. A four-point gait pattern also requires less energy expenditure than does a swing-through gait.[100]

The person with a complete spinal cord injury preparing to walk with KAFOs should start in a balanced standing posture with her hips extended, pelvis forward, lumbar spine in lordosis, scapulae retracted, and head erect (Figure 13–5A). From this starting position, she shifts her weight off of one crutch. While balanced on her

---

[i] These movement strategies are explained in Chapter 9.
[j] This chapter does not attempt to present all possible ambulation skills. An individual who is unable to master a skill described in this chapter may fare better with a variation of that technique or with an altogether different method.

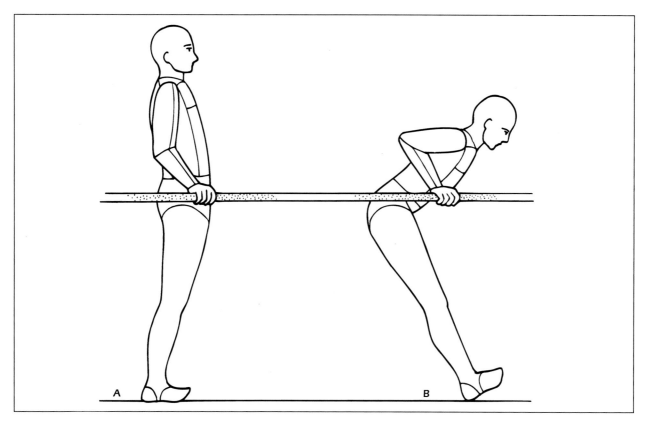

Figure 13–4. Balanced standing. **(A)** Position of stability: pelvis forward with weight line posterior to hip joints. **(B)** "Jacknifing": stability lost if weight line passes anterior to hips.

feet and one crutch, she lifts the unweighted crutch and moves it forward (Figure 13–5B).

After moving a crutch, the person steps with her contralateral foot. (For simplicity, the leg that is moving or about to be moved will be called the swing leg.) To step, she shifts her weight off of the swing leg, presses down on the crutches, and elevates the swing side of her pelvis (Figure 13–5C).

Elevation of the swing side of the pelvis can be accomplished using the latissimus dorsi, quadratus lumborum, or abdominal musculature if these muscles are innervated. The person can supplement this muscular action with the head-hips relationship: while shifting her weight and pushing on her crutches, she tucks her head down and laterally away from the swing leg. As the torso pivots on the shoulders, the swing side of the pelvis lifts.

With one side of the pelvis lifted, the leg swings forward as a pendulum (Figure 13–5D). If the individual's hip flexors are innervated, she can use them to step actively.

After stepping, the person regains a balanced standing posture, pushing her pelvis forward by lifting her head and retracting her scapulae (Figure 13–5E). From the balanced standing posture,

she repeats the process just described and steps with her other leg.

Swing-through gait. A swing-through gait is faster than a four-point gait but requires more energy and entails a greater risk of falling. A person with a complete spinal cord injury about to walk with KAFOs should start in a balanced standing posture with her hips extended, pelvis forward, lumbar spine in lordosis, scapulae retracted, and head erect (Figure 13–6A). While in this posture she lifts her crutches and moves them forward (Figure 13–6B).

To take a step, the person leans on her crutches and lifts her pelvis (and legs) by extending her elbows, depressing and protracting her scapulae, and tucking her head (Figure 13–6C). Once the pelvis lifts enough for the feet to leave the ground, the torso and legs will swing forward as a pendulum suspended at the shoulders (Figure 13–6D).

When the person's heels strike (Figure 13–6E), she should move quickly to stabilize herself. By retracting her scapulae, moving her head and upper trunk posteriorly, and pushing on the crutches, she moves her pelvis forward to return to a stable stand-

TABLE 13-6. AMBULATION OVER EVEN SURFACES—PHYSICAL PREREQUISITES

	Four-point Gait	Swing-through Gait	Swing-to Gait	Drag-to Gait	Stepping Back or to the Side
Strength					
Trapezius	√	√	√	√	√
Deltoids	√	☑	√	√	√
Biceps, brachialis, and/or brachioradialis	√	√	√	√	√
Serratus anterior	☑	☑	☑	☑	☑
Pectoralis major	☑	☑	☑	•	☑
Latissimus dorsi	☑	☑	☑	√	☑
Triceps	☑	☑	☑	•	☑
Wrist and hand musculature	•	√	√	•	•
Abdominals	•	•	•	•	•
Quadratus lumborum	•				•
Iliopsoas	•				
Range of Motion					
Scapular Elevation	√	√	√		
Depression	√	√	√	√	√
Abduction	√	√	√	√	√
Adduction	√	√	√	√	
Downward rotation	√	√			
Shoulder Flexion	√	√	√	√	√
Extension	√	√			
Elbow Extension	☑	☑	☑	√	√
Hip Extension	☑	☑	☑	☑	
Knee Extension	☑	☑	☑	☑	☑
Ankle Dorsiflexion	√	√	√	√	√

√ = Some strength is needed for this activity, or severe limitations in range will inhibit this activity.

☑ = A large amount of strength or normal or greater range is needed for this activity.

• = Not required, but helpful.

TABLE 13-7. AMBULATION OVER EVEN SURFACES— SKILL PREREQUISITES

	Four-point Gait	Swing-through Gait	Swing-to Gait	Drag-to Gait	Stepping Back or to the Side
Control pelvis using head-hips relationship[a]	√	√	√	√	√
Balanced standing (p. 390)	√	√	√	√	√
Weight shift in standing (p. 390)	√	√	√	√	√
Lift and move one crutch (p. 391)	√			√	√
Step forward with one leg (p. 391)	√				
Step to side or back with one leg (p. 392)					√
Lift and move two crutches (p. 392)		√	√	(√)	
Swing-through step (p. 392)		√			
Swing-to step (p. 392)			√		
Drag-to step (p. 392)				√	
Distance/efficient ambulation (p. 393)	√	√	√	√	

[a] Refer to Chapter 11 for a description of this skill and therapeutic strategies.

ing posture (Figure 13–6F). Once in this posture, she balances on her feet while she repositions her crutches forward. She is then in position to take another step.

Swing-to gait. A swing-to gait is similar to a swing-through gait. The difference is that the person steps to, not past, her crutches. This gait pattern is slower than swing through, but it involves a smaller risk of falling.

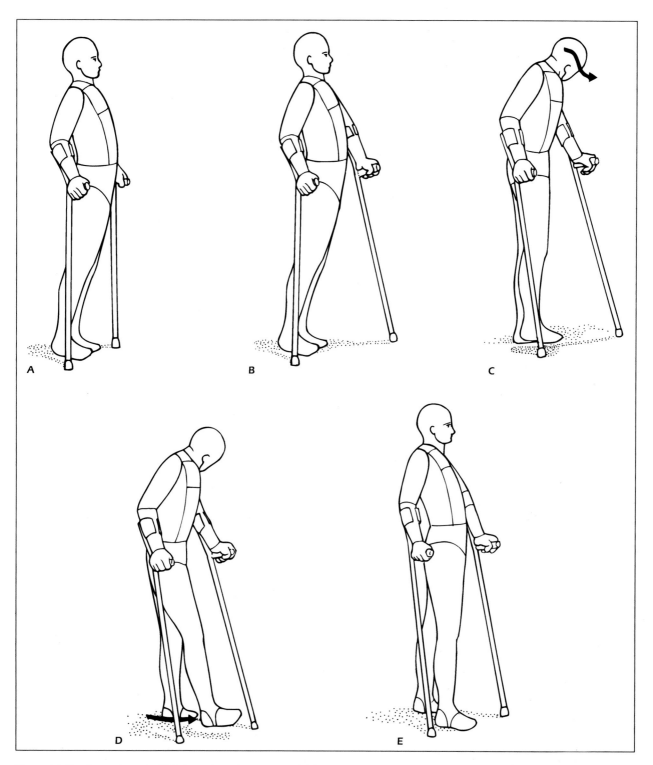

Figure 13–5.   Four-point gait. **(A)** Balanced standing posture. **(B)** One crutch advanced. **(C)** Lifting one leg by elevating pelvis on that side. Head tucked down and laterally away from swing leg. **(D)** Once lifted, leg swings forward as a pendulum. **(E)** Balanced standing posture with one leg advanced.

The maneuvers used to perform a swing-to gait are the same as those used for a swing-through gait, except that the person drops her feet before they swing past her crutches (Figure 13–7). At the end of the step, the feet and crutches are approxi-mately collinear. This is an unstable position, as the base of support is shallow in the anteroposterior dimension. To maximize her stability while walk-ing with a swing-to gait, the person should quickly reposition her crutches anteriorly once she has

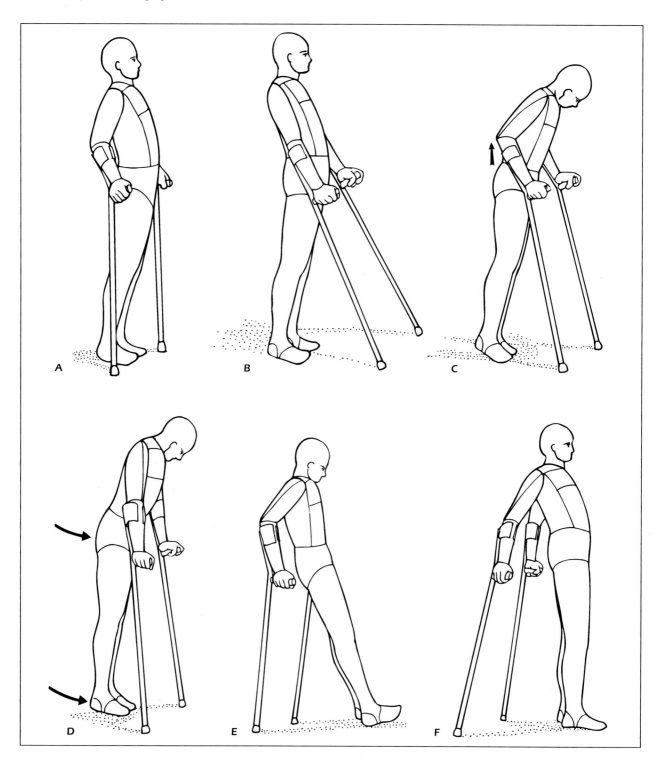

Figure 13–6. *Swing-through gait.* **(A)** *Balanced standing posture.* **(B)** *Crutches advanced.* **(C)** *Lifting pelvis and legs by extending elbows, depressing and protracting scapulae, and tucking head.* **(D)** *Once lifted, torso and legs swing forward as a pendulum.* **(E)** *Heels strike.* **(F)** *Balanced standing posture regained by lifting head, retracting scapulae, and pushing on crutches to push pelvis forward.*

completed a step and resumed a balanced standing posture.

Drag-to gait. Using a drag-to gait pattern, a person does not lift her trunk; her feet remain on the floor. The feet are dragged to, but not past, the crutches. This is a slow, energy-consuming gait. It requires less strength than the other gait patterns, however, and thus may be the only option for someone with a relatively high lesion.

As is true with the other gait patterns, the person walking with a drag-to gait starts in the balanced

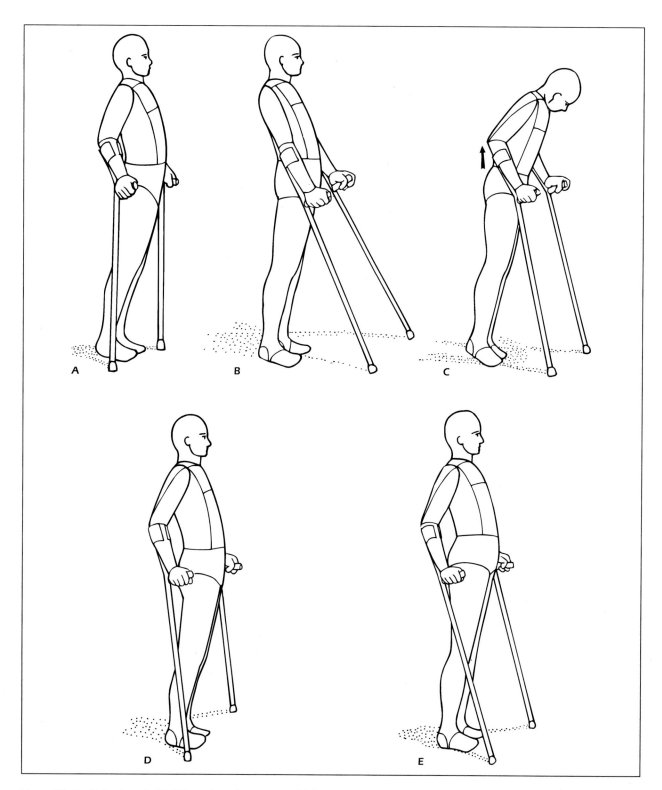

Figure 13–7. *Swing-to gait. (A) Balanced standing posture. (B) Crutches advanced. (C) Lifting pelvis and legs by extending elbows, depressing and protracting scapulae, and tucking head. (D) Feet are advanced to, not past, crutches. Balanced standing posture resumed. (E) Crutches quickly repositioned anteriorly for greater stability.*

standing posture and repositions her crutches anteriorly before taking a step. Depending on her stability in standing, she can reposition her crutches simultaneously or one at a time. After repositioning her crutches she leans forward, extends her elbows,

and depresses her scapulae enough to unweight her legs and drag her feet toward the crutches.

After moving her feet, the person uses head and scapular motions to regain a balanced standing posture. As with a swing-to gait, she should quickly reposition her crutches at this point to increase her anteroposterior stability.

Stepping backward or to the side. This skill is used when walking sideways or backwards. It is also used to reposition a single foot when, for example, a person places her feet in preparation to sit down in a wheelchair.

To step backward or to the side, the person lifts her leg using the same technique as is used in a four-point gait. She shifts her weight off one leg and lifts it using the latissimus dorsi, quadratus lumborum, abdominals, or motions of the head and upper trunk, or a combination thereof to lift that half of the pelvis.

With her leg lifted, the person positions her foot by moving her pelvis. Using head and upper trunk motions to move her pelvis, she swings the leg as a pendulum. To step to the side, she moves her head and upper trunk back and forth laterally. This motion causes the unweighted leg to swing medially and laterally. To step backward, she moves her head and upper trunk up and down. This motion causes the unweighted leg to swing forward and back. Whether stepping forward, backward, or to the side, the person drops her pelvis (by lifting her head) to place her foot when it has swung to the desired position.

Negotiation of Obstacles

Independence in ambulation over even surfaces will enable a person to walk indoors within the confines of a single-level home or work environment. To walk in the community, obstacle negotiation skills are necessary. Techniques for negotiation of ramps, curbs, and stairs are presented in this section.

Tables 13–8 and 13–9 summarize the physical and skill prerequisites for independent ambulation over obstacles.

Ramps. The greatest challenge when walking up or down a ramp is avoiding being thrown down the slope. When a person wearing orthoses with immobile ankle joints stands on a slope, her orthoses, and therefore her hips, are thrown in the downhill direction.

Practice in ramp negotiation should not be limited to the gentle 1:12 grade of a standard public incline. Many, if not most, ramps in the community are far steeper than this. The patient who intends to walk in the community should develop the skills needed to ascend and descend ramps as steep as possible within her potential.

TABLE 13–8. AMBULATION OVER OBSTACLES—PHYSICAL PREREQUISITES

	Ramps	Curbs	Stairs
Strength			
Trapezius	√	√	√
Deltoids	√	√	√
Biceps, brachialis, and/or brachioradialis	√	√	√
Serratus anterior	☑	☑	☑
Pectoralis major	☑	☑	☑
Latissimus dorsi	☑	☑	☑
Triceps	☑	☑	☑
Wrist and hand musculature	√	√	√
Abdominals	•	•	•
Quadratus lumborum	•	•	•
Iliopsoas	•	•	•
Range of Motion			
Scapular Elevation	√	√	√
Depression	√	√	√
Abduction	√	√	√
Adduction	√	√	√
Downward rotation	√	√	√
Shoulder Flexion	√	√	√
Extension	√	√	√
Elbow Extension	☑	☑	☑
Hip Extension	☑	☑	☑
Knee Extension	☑	☑	☑
Ankle Dorsiflexion	√	√	√

√ = Some strength is needed for this activity, or severe limitations in range will inhibit this activity.

☑ = A large amount of strength or normal or greater range is needed for this activity.

• = Not required, but helpful.

Ascend. When ascending a ramp, a person walking with KAFOs should keep her crutches well in front of her feet. To maximize hip stability, she should keep her body angled up the hill, with her pelvis well forward. She should use a

TABLE 13–9. AMBULATION OVER OBSTACLES—SKILL PREREQUISITES

	Ascend Ramps	Descend Ramps	Ascend Curbs	Descend Curbs	Ascend Stairs	Descend Stairs
Swing-to ambulation over even surfaces (p. 392)	✓					
Swing-to ambulation up a slope (p. 393)	✓					
Swing-through ambulation over even surfaces (p. 392)		✓	✓	✓	✓	✓
Swing-through ambulation down a slope (p. 393)		✓				
Balanced standing (p. 390)	✓	✓	✓	✓	✓	✓
Reposition crutches while standing (pp. 391 & 392)	✓	✓	✓	✓	✓	✓
Step up curb or step (p. 393)			✓		✓	
Step down from curb or step (p. 393)				✓		✓

step-to (or step-toward) gait, not a swing-through pattern.

Descend. When a person wearing KAFOs walks forward down a ramp, the slope tends to throw the hips toward a stable position. A swing-through gait pattern can be used.

Curbs. Curb negotiation skills are required for independent ambulation in the community. Although ramps have become common, they still are not universally present.

Ascend. To ascend a curb, the person approaches it face-on. She positions her feet with the toes at the edge of the curb (Figure 13–8A), assumes a balanced standing posture, then places her crutch tips on the higher surface of the curb, a few inches from the edge (Figure 13–8B).

From the starting position, the person lifts her feet onto the curb. She does this by leaning forward on the crutches, tucking her head, extending her elbows, and depressing her scapulae (Figure 13–8C). As her feet lift, the toes will drag up the vertical surface of the curb. When the toes lift past the curb, her torso and legs will swing forward as a pendulum.

A person ascending a curb can step to or past her crutches. When her feet land, she throws her head back and retracts her scapulae to push her pelvis forward and regain a balanced standing posture (Figure 13–8D).

Descend. When descending a curb, the person approaches it face-on. She assumes a balanced standing posture with her feet a few inches from the edge of the curb and places her crutch tips close to the edge of the curb (Figure 13–9A).

From the starting position, the person steps off the curb. She does this by leaning on the crutches, tucking her head, extending her elbows, and depressing her scapulae. When the feet lift, her torso and legs will swing forward as a pendulum (Figure 13–9B).

When the person's feet have swung past the edge of the curb, she drops them. (When "dropping" her legs, she quickly lowers her torso/legs/feet with eccentrically controlled elbow and shoulder motions.) When her feet land, the person regains a balanced standing posture, pushing her pelvis forward by throwing her head back and retracting her scapulae (Figure 13–9C).

Stairs. Anyone who walks in the community inevitably comes across stairs. Many public and private buildings have stairs at their entrances. Within buildings, elevators are not always present and working. Patients who learn to climb stairs during gait training are less likely to discontinue ambulation after discharge. [28]

In the following stair negotiation techniques, the person does not use a rail. The techniques are described in this way because rails are not always available in the community. The methods described can be adapted easily: when negotiating stairs using one crutch and one rail, the person holds the crutch not in use in the hand that holds the other crutch (Figure 13–10).

Ascend. Ascending stairs is similar to ascending a series of curbs. The curb-negotiation techniques described above can be used to ascend stairs front-on (facing up the stairs).

In an alternative approach, the crutch walker can ascend stairs backwards. In the starting position

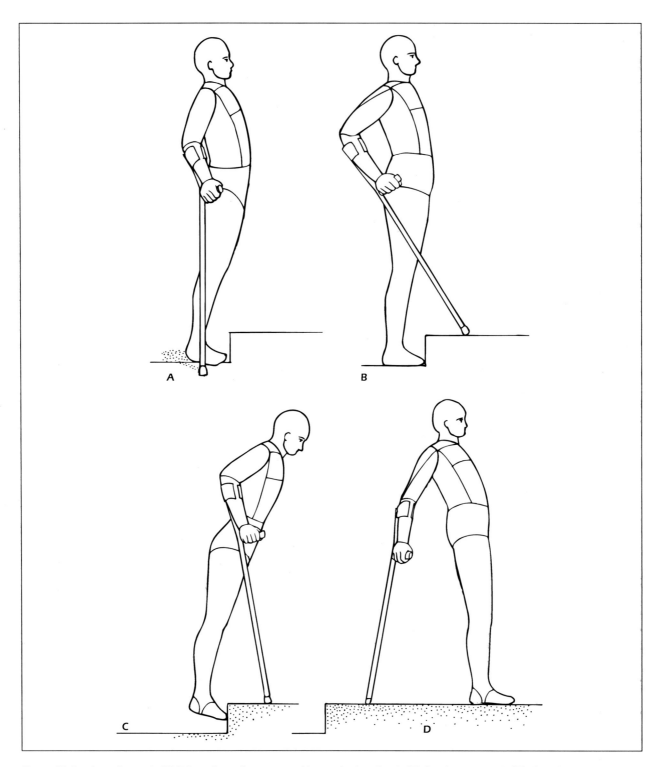

Figure 13–8. Ascending curb. **(A)** Balanced standing posture with toes at edge of curb. **(B)** Crutches onto curb. **(C)** Lifting feet onto curb by leaning on crutches, extending elbows, and depressing scapulae. **(D)** Pelvis pushed forward by throwing head back and retracting scapulae.

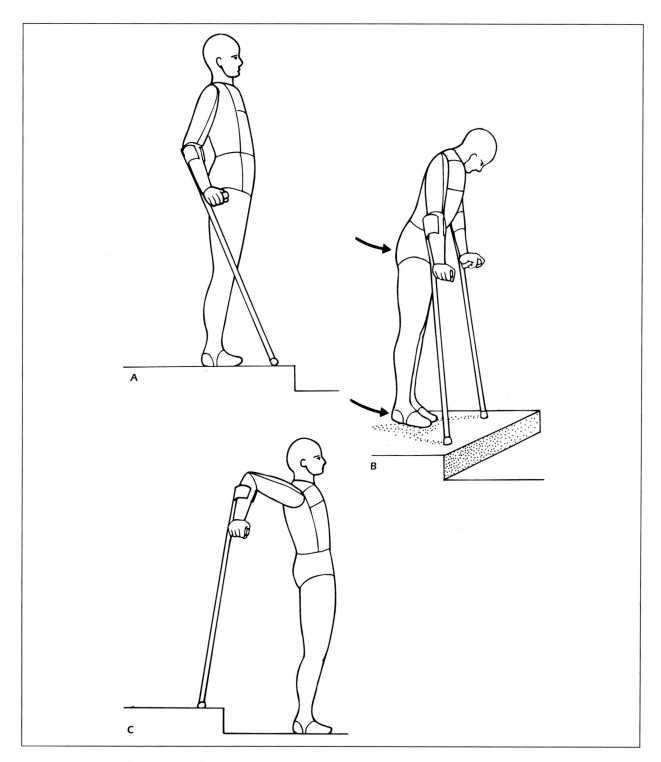

Figure 13–9. Descending curb. **(A)** Balanced standing posture with crutches close to edge of curb. **(B)** Swing-through step. **(C)** Pelvis pushed forward by throwing head back and retracting scapulae.

for this technique, the person stands facing away from the stairs. She should stand in a balanced posture with her feet in front of the first stair and her crutches anterior to her feet (Figure 13–11A).

From the starting position the person places her crutches on the lowest step (Figure 13–11B).

She then leans on the crutches, extends her elbows, and depresses her scapulae to lift her feet onto the step (Figure 13–11C). When her feet lift past the step, her torso and legs will swing backward as a pendulum. When her feet land, she throws her head back and retracts her scapulae to

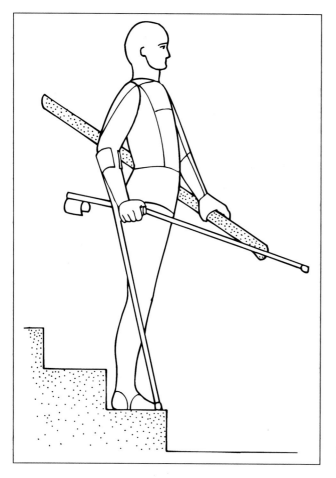

Figure 13–10. *Descending stairs using a rail and one crutch, carrying second crutch.*

push her pelvis forward and to regain a balanced standing posture (Figure 13–11D).

Descend. Descending stairs is much like descending a series of curbs. A technique similar to the curb-negotiation method described earlier can be used to descend stairs. The person places her crutches close to the edge of the step on which she stands, lifts her feet, and her torso and legs swing forward as a pendulum.

The difference between descending a step and a curb is that when descending a step in a stairway, the crutch walker has a limited area on which her feet can land safely. Thus when negotiating stairs, she must control the length of her step. If her feet land too far from their starting position, she will miss the next step. To avoid this problem, she should allow her feet to swing back over the step before she drops them.

Coming to Stand from a Wheelchair

Functional ambulation requires the ability to get into a standing position. The techniques described below center on rising from a wheelchair. They can be adapted to surfaces other than wheelchairs.[k]

Tables 13–10 and 13–11 summarize the physical and skill prerequisites for coming to stand from a wheelchair.

Both hands on armrests. This is the most readily achievable method of coming to stand from a wheelchair. Because the person gets onto her feet while both hands remain on the wheelchair, it is easier, steadier, and requires less skill than the other techniques presented. Rising from a wheelchair using this method takes longer, however, because more steps are involved.

To rise from her wheelchair using this method, the person first locks the chair's brakes and places her crutches where she will be able to reach them once she is on her feet. She then positions her buttocks so that she is sitting at the front edge of her seat, resting on the side of her pelvis.

---

[k] An individual who plans to ambulate in the community should practice getting up and down from other sitting surfaces such as car seats and standard chairs.

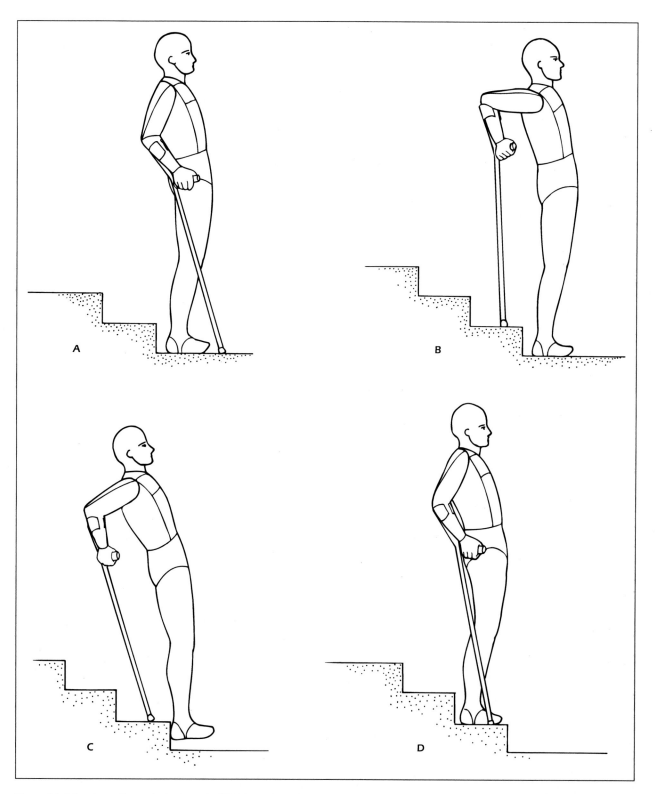

Figure 13–11.   Ascending stairs backwards. **(A)** Balanced standing posture with feet a few inches from lowest step. **(B)** Crutches onto step. **(C)** Lifting feet onto step by leaning on crutches, extending elbows, and depressing scapulae. **(D)** Balanced standing posture regained.

TABLE 13–10. COMING TO STAND FROM WHEELCHAIR—PHYSICAL PREREQUISITES

	Both Hands on Armrests	One Hand on Armrest and One on Crutch	Both Hands on Crutches
Strength			
Trapezius	√	√	√
Deltoids	☑	√	√
Biceps, brachialis, and/or brachioradialis	√	√	√
Serratus anterior	☑	☑	☑
Pectoralis major	☑	☑	☑
Latissimus dorsi	√	☑	☑
Triceps	☑	☑	☑
Wrist and hand musculature	√	√	√
Abdominals	•	•	•
Range of Motion			
Scapular Elevation	√	√	√
Scapular Depression	√	√	√
Scapular Abduction	√	√	√
Scapular Adduction	√	√	√
Scapular Upward rotation	√	√	√
Scapular Downward rotation		√	√
Shoulder Flexion	√	√	√
Shoulder Extension	√	√	√
Shoulder Internal rotation	√	☑	☑
Elbow Flexion	√	√	√
Elbow Extension	☑	☑	☑
Hip Flexion	√	√	√
Hip Extension	☑	☑	☑
Knee Extension	☑	☑	☑
Ankle Dorsiflexion	√	√	√
Combined hip flexion and knee extension	☑	☑	☑

√ = Some strength is needed for this activity, or severe limitations in range will inhibit this activity.

☑ = A large amount of strength or normal or greater range is needed for this activity.

• = Not required, but helpful.

TABLE 13–11. COMING TO STAND FROM WHEELCHAIR—SKILL PREREQUISITES

	Both Hands on Armrests	One Hand on Armrest and One on Crutch	Both Hands on Crutches
Move buttocks using head-hips relationship[a]	√	√	√
Position legs in preparation to stand (p. 393)	√	√	√
Hands on armrests, assume standing position from wheelchair (p. 393)	√		
Standing in front of wheelchair with hands on armrests, grasp crutch (p. 394)	√		
Standing with one hand on armrest and one on crutch, grasp second crutch (p. 394)	√	√	
Standing with crutches positioned forward, walk crutches back (p. 394)	√		
One hand on armrest and one on crutch, assume standing position from wheelchair (p. 395)		√	
Balanced standing (p. 390)	√	√	√
Both hands on crutches, assume standing position from wheelchair (p. 395)			√
While standing, lift and move both crutches (p. 392)			√

[a] Refer to Chapter 11 for a description of this skill and therapeutic strategies.

Once she is positioned appropriately in her seat, the person locks the orthotic knees and positions her legs in preparation to stand. The superior leg should rest on top of or slightly anterior to the other leg (Figure 13–12A).

In the next step the person turns and places her hands on the armrests (Figure 13–12B). She then gets onto her feet using the head-hips relationship: she presses down on the armrests, protracts her scapulae, and twists her head and upper trunk down and laterally. Her lateral twist should

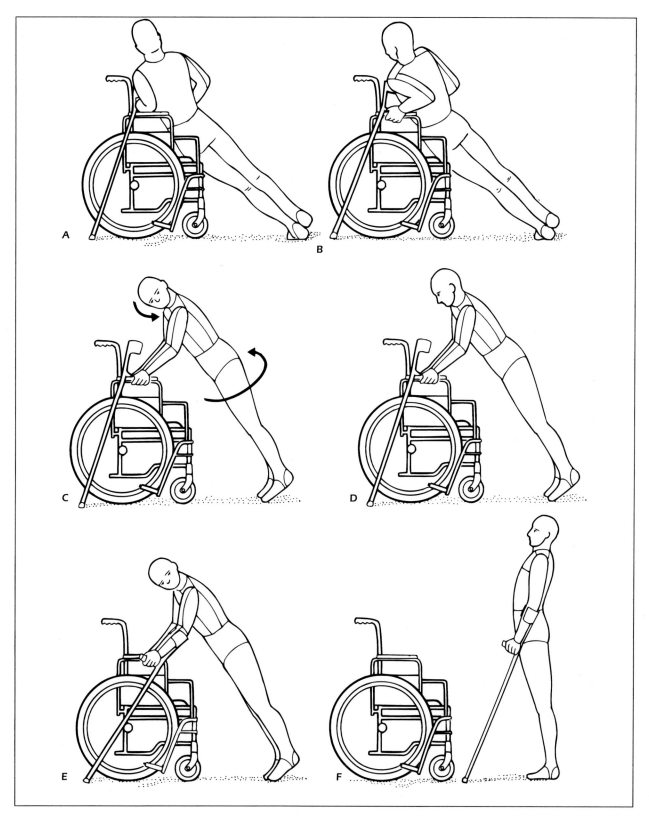

Figure 13–12. Coming to stand from a wheelchair, both hands on armrests. **(A)** Sitting at front edge of seat, resting on side of pelvis. **(B)** Hands on armrests. **(C)** Onto feet using head-hips relationship. **(D)** Standing with hands on armrests. **(E)** Crutch positioned on arm. **(F)** Upright standing.

be toward the side of the chair on which she sits (Figure 13–12C). As she twists her head and upper trunk, her pelvis will lift up and over her feet. Once on her feet, the person uses the head-hips relationship to attain her balance point.

The person now stands with her hands on the wheelchair's armrests (Figure 13–12D). Her next task is to substitute her crutches for the armrests. To grasp the first crutch, she shifts laterally to unweight one hand. While balancing on her feet and one hand, she grasps a crutch and positions it on her free arm (Figure 13–12E). She then places the crutch tip on the floor, lateral to the wheelchair. Shifting her weight onto the crutch, she unweights her other hand and grasps the remaining crutch. After positioning the second crutch on her arm, she places the crutch tip on the floor, lateral to the wheelchair. From this position, she achieves an upright standing posture by walking her crutches back (Figure 13–12F).

One hand on armrest, one on crutch. When standing up from a wheelchair using this method, the person gets onto her feet with only one hand on the wheelchair. The other hand rests on a crutch, which provides a much less stable base of support. For this reason, this method requires more skill than does coming to stand with both hands on a wheelchair. The advantage of the method presented here is that it is quicker than coming to stand with both hands remaining on the chair.

The person starts by locking the wheelchair's brakes and placing her crutches within easy reach. She then moves her buttocks to the front edge of the seat, locks the orthotic knees, and positions her legs and buttocks so that her legs extend diagonally from the seat.

After positioning her legs, the person grasps a crutch and positions it on her arm. The crutch should be held in the hand that is furthest from the chair. After grasping the crutch, the individual should place her free hand on the armrest that she faces (Figure 13–13A).

The person now sits diagonally at the front of her seat, with one hand on an armrest and one on a crutch. From this position she pushes down with both hands, keeping her head tucked. If she performs the maneuver correctly, her pelvis will lift and her feet will drag toward the chair (Figure 13–13B). When the legs reach a vertical or nearly vertical position, she pushes her pelvis forward to attain a balanced standing posture (Figure 13–13C).

Once on her feet in a balanced posture, the person shifts her weight laterally onto the crutch.

She then lifts her free hand, grasps the second crutch (Figure 13–13D) and positions her arm in it, and places the crutch tip on the floor (Figure 13–13E). After repositioning her crutches as necessary, she is ready to walk.

Both hands on crutches. This is the fastest method of rising to standing from a wheelchair using KAFOs. It also requires the most skill; rising from a chair while balancing on two crutches is a very challenging maneuver.

The person starts by locking her wheelchair's brakes, moving her buttocks to the front edge of the seat, locking her orthotic knees, and positioning her legs so that they extend straight forward from the seat. She then grasps both crutches, positions them on her arms, and places the crutch tips lateral to the wheelchair (Figure 13–14A).

To stand from her chair, the crutch walker pushes down forcefully on the crutches. As she first lifts from the chair, she should keep her trunk flexed forward at the hips (Figure 13–14B). As her legs move toward vertical, she extends her trunk toward and then past vertical by pushing on the crutches, lifting her head, and retracting her scapulae to push her pelvis forward (Figure 13–14C). As she reaches a vertical standing position, she quickly repositions her crutches anteriorly. In this manner she assumes a balanced standing posture (Figure 13–14D).

Sitting Down from a Standing Position

Functional ambulation requires the ability to sit down safely after walking. The following techniques center on sitting on a wheelchair. They can be adapted to surfaces other than wheelchairs.

The challenge of rising from a chair is obvious: the person must lift herself onto her feet, maintaining her balance throughout the maneuver. Returning to the chair has a less obvious challenge: the individual must lower herself into the chair without traumatizing her skin or tipping the chair. She does this by controlling her descent so that she lands squarely on the seat rather than on an armrest or on the backrest, and she lands without undue force.

Tables 13–12 and 13–13 summarize the physical and skill prerequisites for sitting down from a standing position.

Both hands on armrests. This maneuver is similar to coming to stand with both hands on the armrests, performed in reverse. While lowering herself to sitting, the person supports herself with both hands on the wheelchair. Because the wheelchair

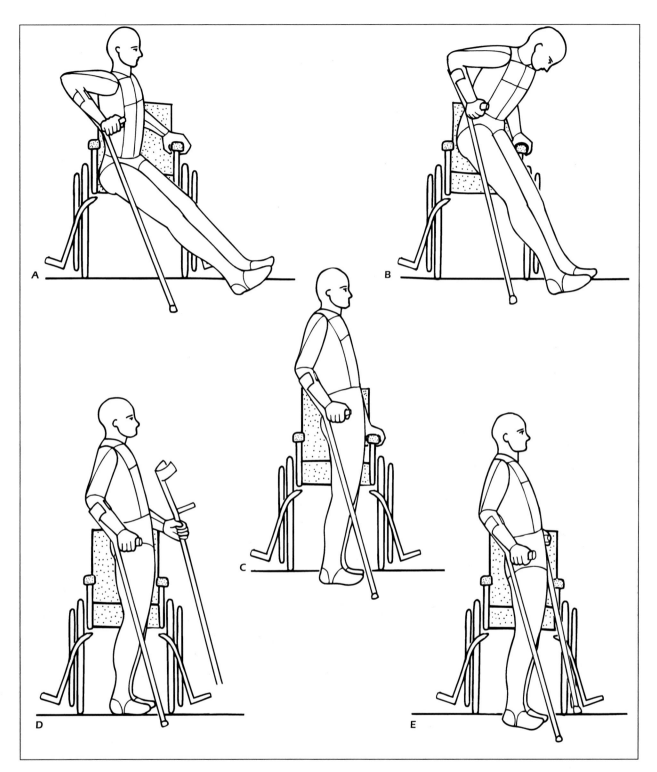

Figure 13–13.   Coming to stand from a wheelchair, one hand on armrest and one on crutch. **(A)** Sitting at front edge of seat with one hand on armrest and one on crutch. **(B)** Lifting pelvis by tucking head while pushing on crutch and armrest. **(C)** Balanced standing posture. **(D)** Grasping second crutch. **(E)** Second crutch placed on floor.

provides a relatively steady base of support, this method of sitting from a standing position requires the least skill to perform safely.

In the starting position the individual stands facing the wheelchair with her feet in front of and slightly lateral to the casters (Figure 13–15A). The appropriate foot position depends on the person's height. The feet should be placed so that when the crutch walker pivots on them, she will land squarely on the seat.

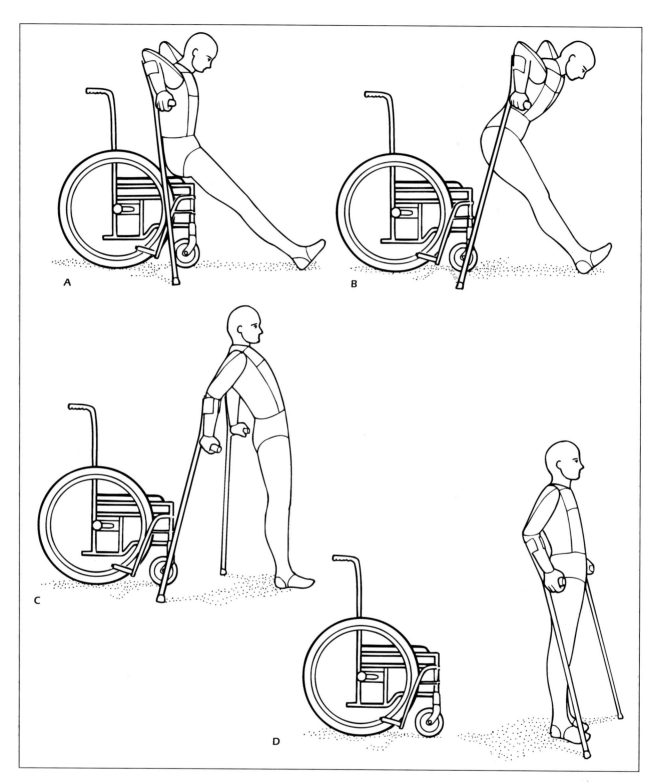

Figure 13–14.   Coming to stand from a wheelchair, both hands on crutches. **(A)** Sitting at front edge of seat with both hands on crutches. **(B)** Rising from wheelchair. **(C)** Scapular retraction and head-hips relationship used to push pelvis forward. **(D)** Balanced standing posture with crutches repositioned anteriorly.

Standing in front of the wheelchair, the person shifts her weight onto one crutch and removes her unweighted hand and forearm from the other crutch. She then leans the unused crutch against the wheelchair and places her free hand on an armrest. Shifting her weight onto the armrest, she removes her other hand and forearm from its crutch, leans the crutch against the wheelchair, and places her hand on the other armrest (Figure 13–15B).

TABLE 13–12. SITTING DOWN FROM A STANDING POSITION— PHYSICAL PREREQUISITES

	Both Hands on Armrests	Both Hands on Crutches
Strength		
Trapezius	√	√
Deltoids	√	√
Biceps, brachialis, and/or brachioradialis	√	√
Serratus anterior	☑	☑
Pectoralis major	☑	☑
Latissimus dorsi	√	☑
Triceps	☑	☑
Wrist and hand musculature	√	√
Abdominals	•	•
Range of Motion		
Scapular Elevation	√	√
Depression	√	√
Abduction	√	√
Adduction	√	√
Upward rotation	√	√
Downward rotation		√
Shoulder Flexion	√	√
Extension	√	√
Internal rotation	√	☑
Elbow Flexion	√	√
Extension	☑	☑
Hip Flexion	√	√
Extension	☑	☑
Knee Extension	☑	☑
Ankle Dorsiflexion	√	√
Combined hip flexion and knee extension	☑	☑

√ = Some strength is needed for this activity, or severe limitations in range will inhibit this activity.

☑ = A large amount of strength or normal or greater range is needed for this activity.

• = Not required, but helpful.

TABLE 13–13. SITTING DOWN FROM A STANDING POSITION— SKILL PREREQUISITES

	Both Hands on Armrests	Both Hands on Crutches
Position self in preparation to sit in wheelchair (p. 395)	√	√
Standing facing wheelchair, place hands on armrests (p. 395)	√	
Move pelvis using head-hips relationship[a]	√	√
Balanced standing (p. 390)	√	√
Facing wheelchair with hands on armrests, turn and lower self into chair (p. 396)	√	
Standing facing away from wheelchair, lower self into chair (p. 396)		√
While standing, lift and move both crutches (p. 392)	√	√
Step forward, back, and to the side (pp. 391 & 392)	√	√
Weight shift in standing (p. 390)	√	

[a] Refer to Chapter 11 for a description of this skill and therapeutic strategies.

The person is now standing in front of the wheelchair supporting herself with a hand on each armrest. In the next step, she turns and lowers herself into the chair. The direction of the turn is determined by the position of her feet in relation to the wheelchair. The turn should be toward the feet: if the feet are to the left of the chair, the head and upper trunk should turn toward the left. As she turns, she releases one armrest. (If turning to the left, she releases the right armrest.) She can either throw her free arm in the direction of the turn (Figure 13–15C) to add momentum to the turn or place her hand on the far rear corner of the seat. After landing, she unlocks the orthotic knees and repositions her buttocks on the seat as needed.

Both hands on crutches. Using this method to sit down from a standing position, a person sup-

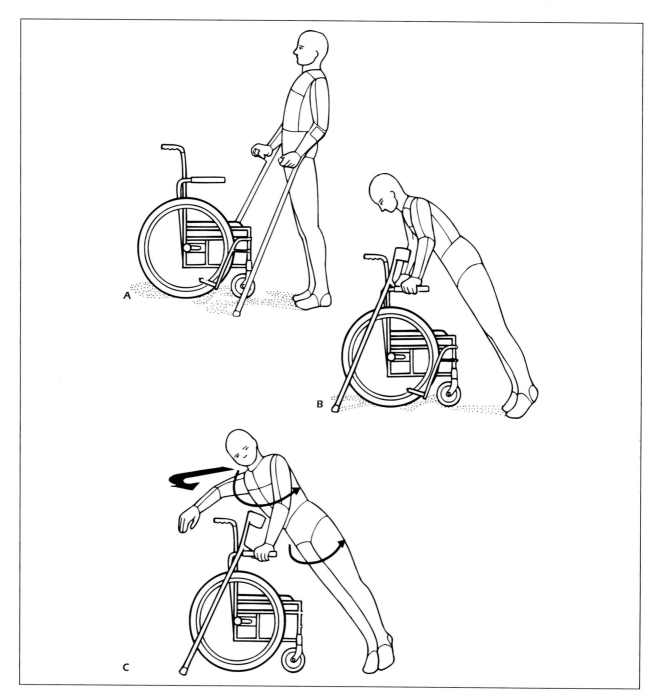

Figure 13–15. *Sitting down from standing position, both hands on armrests.* **(A)** *Standing facing wheelchair.* **(B)** *Both hands placed on armrests.* **(C)** *Turning toward hand on armrest.*

ports herself on two crutches while lowering herself into a wheelchair. This maneuver requires more skill than is required if she supports herself on the armrests.

In the starting position for this maneuver, the crutch walker stands well in front of the wheelchair, facing away from it (Figure 13–16A). The appropriate foot position depends on the individual's height. The person should place her feet so

that when she pivots on them, she will land squarely on the seat. It is critical that she places her feet an appropriate distance from the chair. If she stands too far from the chair, she will miss the seat when she sits. If she stands too close to the chair, she will hit the backrest instead of the seat and may tip the chair over backwards.

Standing facing away from the wheelchair, the crutch walker balances on her feet and repositions

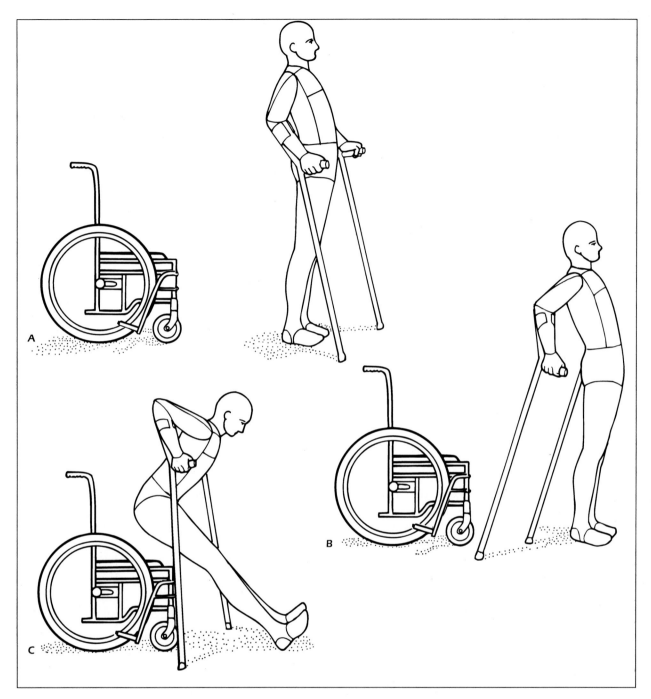

Figure 13–16. *Sitting down from standing position, both hands on crutches.* **(A)** *Standing facing away from wheelchair.* **(B)** *Crutches repositioned posteriorly.* **(C)** *Lowering self onto wheelchair seat.*

her crutches posteriorly (Figure 13–16B). The exact placement of the crutches will vary among individuals. The person should position the crutches so that she will be able to pivot on them and lower her buttocks onto the seat.

After positioning her crutches, the person lowers herself into the wheelchair. Supporting her weight on the crutches, she tucks her head for-

ward. This causes her pelvis to move backward out of the position of stable standing, and she jackknifes at the hips (Figure 13–16C). She then lowers herself onto the seat. After landing, she unlocks the orthotic knees and repositions her buttocks on the seat as needed.

A person who has orthoses that have knee mechanisms with bail controls (described earlier in this chapter) can use a slightly different technique to sit down. She first stands facing away from the chair with her legs against or close to the chair so that the bail controls are above the sitting surface. She then positions her crutches lateral to the chair, and leans back on them. This motion will cause the bail controls to press against the sitting surface and unlock the knees. When this occurs, the knees will flex. The person should control her descent by supporting her weight and balancing on her arms as she lowers her buttocks to the wheelchair seat. Because of the inherent instability of unlocking the knees while weight is being borne through the legs, this method of sitting down typically requires more practice than does sitting down with the knees locked.

Falling Safely

Ambulation involves a risk of falling. Anyone who walks, especially if she has impaired motor and sensory function, is likely to fall eventually. Anyone who learns to walk with orthoses and assistive devices should learn to fall in a way that will minimize the risk of injury.

When falling, there are two things that a crutch walker can do to minimize her risk of injury. First, she can move her crutches out of the way so that she does not injure herself by landing on a crutch or by having a crutch exert excessive force on her arm. While falling, the person throws her crutches laterally (or laterally and posteriorly) away from the path of fall. She should aim to get the crutch tips up off of the floor, so that the crutches do not act as fulcrums on her arms when she lands.

The second thing that a person can do when she falls is to break her fall with her arms. She should land on her palms and cushion the fall by allowing her elbows and shoulders to "give" when she lands. She must *not* hold her arms rigid as she falls onto them.

Tables 13–14 and 13–15 summarize the physical and skill prerequisites for falling safely and assuming a standing position from the floor.

Assume Standing Position from the Floor

After getting onto the floor, either by falling or by design, a person needs to be able to get back up. This task is challenging but feasible for people with intact upper extremity function.

To prepare to rise from the floor, the person gets into a prone position with her hips adducted and externally rotated, and her knees locked in extension. She then places a crutch on either side of herself. The crutch tips should point away from

TABLE 13–14. FALLING SAFELY AND STANDING FROM THE FLOOR— PHYSICAL PREREQUISITES

	Fall Safely	Stand from the Floor
Strength		
Trapezius		√
Deltoids	√	√
Biceps, brachialis, and/or brachioradialis	√	√
Serratus anterior	☑	☑
Pectoralis major	☑	☑
Triceps	☑	☑
Wrist and hand musculature	√	√
Abdominals		•
Range of Motion		
Scapular Elevation		√
Scapular Abduction	√	√
Scapular Adduction	√	√
Scapular Upward rotation	√	☑
Scapular Downward rotation		√
Shoulder Flexion	√	☑
Shoulder Extension		√
Shoulder Internal rotation		√
Shoulder Horizontal adduction		√
Shoulder Horizontal abduction	√	☑
Elbow Flexion	√	√
Elbow Extension	√	☑
Hip Flexion		√
Hip Extension		☑
Knee Extension		☑
Ankle Dorsiflexion		√
Combined hip flexion and knee extension		☑

√ = Some strength is needed for this activity, or severe limitations in range will inhibit this activity.

☑ = A large amount of strength or normal or greater range is needed for this activity.

• = Not required, but helpful.

TABLE 13–15. FALLING SAFELY AND STANDING FROM THE FLOOR— SKILL PREREQUISITES

	Fall Safely	Stand from the Floor
Throw crutches (p. 396)	✓	
Catch self on hands (p. 396)	✓	
Position self in prone[a]		✓
Position crutches in preparation to stand (p. 396)		✓
Assume plantigrade posture from prone (p. 396)		✓
Dynamic balance in plantigrade and modified plantigrade (p. 397)		✓
In plantigrade, walk hands toward feet (p. 397)		✓
In plantigrade, grasp and position crutch (p. 399)		✓
In modified plantigrade with one hand on crutch, grasp and position second crutch (p. 399)		✓
From modified plantigrade supported on two crutches, push torso to upright (p. 399)		✓
Standing with crutches positioned forward, walk crutches back (p. 394)		✓

[a] Refer to Chapter 10 for a description of this skill and therapeutic strategies.

her feet, and the grips should be at or caudal to the level of her greater trochanters. In this position, the crutches will be within reach when she is ready to use them.

After positioning her crutches and legs, the person places her palms on the floor next to her shoulders (Figure 13–17A). She then moves from prone to plantigrade by lifting her pelvis from the floor using the head-hips relationship, pushing down and forward (away from her feet) while tucking her head (Figure 13–17B). When she has lifted her pelvis as high as she can, she walks her hands toward her feet while keeping her head tucked. This maneuver will elevate the pelvis further (Figure 13–17C).

As the person walks her hands toward her feet, her legs become more vertical. By walking

her hands back, she moves her legs as far as she can toward (not past) vertical. The remaining steps involved in coming to stand will be easier with more vertically oriented legs.

Once the individual has elevated her pelvis maximally by walking her hands back, she shifts her weight and balances on one hand. She then grasps a crutch with her unweighted hand (Figure 13–17D).

In the next step the person balances on one crutch while grasping the remaining crutch with her free hand (Figure 13–17E). For many people, this is the most challenging part of coming to stand from the floor. Balancing on one crutch will be easiest if the crutch tip is aligned with the midline of the torso. Placement of the proximal aspect of the crutch varies between individuals. Three positions are illustrated in Figure 13–18.

While propping on one crutch, the person grasps the other crutch with her free hand and positions it on her forearm (Figure 13–17F). She then shifts her weight onto this crutch. If the forearm cuff of the first crutch is not on her forearm, she can now balance on the other crutch while repositioning this cuff. Supporting herself on both crutches, she then pushes to a standing position: using the head-hips relationship, she lifts her head and pushes her pelvis forward (Figure 13–17G). Once standing, she walks her crutches back until she is upright (Figure 13–17H).

Don and Doff Orthoses

Independent functioning with orthoses requires the ability to put them on and take them off. For people with intact upper extremity functioning, this is the easiest of the ambulatory skills to master.

A person can put on her orthoses while sitting in bed or in her wheelchair. The technique is essentially the same in either location. When donning an orthosis while sitting in a wheelchair, the person props the orthosis on furniture to support it with the knee in extension (Figure 13–19). Whether in bed or in a wheelchair, she first positions her orthosis and opens the shoe and all straps. She then lifts her leg and positions it over the orthosis, with her knee flexed. She slides her foot into the shoe, checks to make sure that her toes are positioned appropriately, then fastens the shoe and all straps.

Removing an orthosis is generally easiest if the individual remains seated in her wheelchair. This task simply involves opening all straps and the shoe and lifting the leg out of the orthosis.

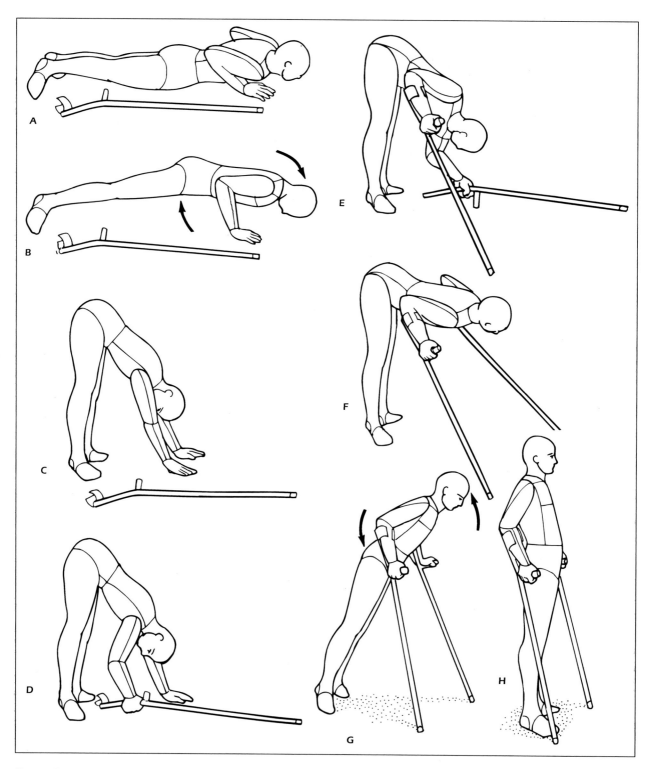

Figure 13–17. Assuming standing position from the floor. **(A)** Starting position: prone with legs and crutches positioned appropriately, palms on floor. **(B)** Lifting to plantigrade using head-hips relationship. **(C)** Pelvis elevated fully. **(D)** Grasping first crutch. **(E)** Balancing on one crutch while grasping second crutch. **(F)** Forearm cuffs positioned. **(G)** Pushing trunk upright. **(H)** Upright standing.

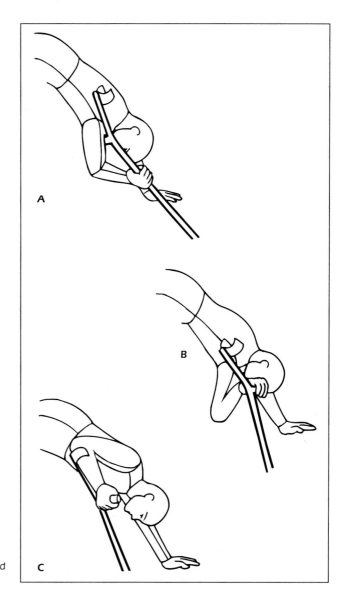

Figure 13-18. Three crutch-position options for coming to stand from the floor.

THERAPEUTIC STRATEGIES FOR GAIT TRAINING WITH KNEE-ANKLE-FOOT ORTHOSES FOLLOWING COMPLETE SPINAL CORD INJURY

General Strategies

To accomplish a functional goal, the patient must acquire both the physical and skill prerequisites for that activity. For example, when working on ambulation with a swing-through gait, she must develop adequate strength and range in the extremities, as well as develop the ability to balance in standing, lift the trunk by pushing down on Lofstrand crutches, and resume and maintain a balanced standing posture.

When developing skill prerequisites for a functional goal, the patient should start with the most basic prerequisite skills and progress toward more challenging activities. (A person had best develop the ability to maintain an upright standing posture before attempting to take a step.)

Before asking a patient to attempt a new skill, the therapist should explain and demonstrate the technique.[1] The demonstration should provide a clear idea of the motions involved and the timing of these motions. The therapist should also explain how the new skill will be used functionally.

During functional training, the therapist should remember that every person with a spinal

---

[1] This demonstration can also be provided by another person with a spinal cord injury, if someone is available who has similar impairments but a higher level of functional ability. Alternatively, the patient may watch a videotaped demonstration of the skill.

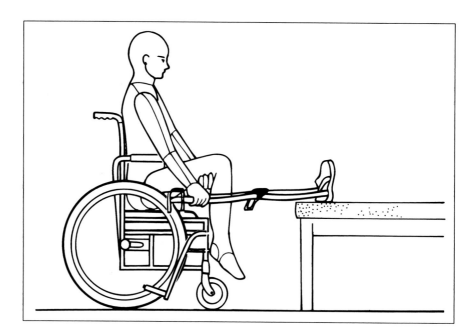

Figure 13–19. *Donning orthosis while sitting in wheelchair.*

cord injury will perform a particular activity differently. Each has a unique combination of body build, coordination, strength, and flexibility, and these characteristics influence the manner in which she performs functional tasks. For example, each person is unique in the exact motions that she uses and the timing of these motions as she stands up from the floor. What has worked for the last patient may be a total disaster for the next. The challenge of functional training is finding the timing and maneuvers that best suit the individual involved.

As a therapist and patient work together on a skill, they can learn from failed attempts by analyzing the problem. Is the patient strong enough to perform the maneuver? Is she flexible enough? Is she shifting her weight too far or not far enough? Are her crutches placed appropriately?

Strategies for addressing the various prerequisite skills are presented in the following sections.

Equipment. Before attempting any of these skills, the therapist should check the patient's equipment. The parallel bars or crutches should be adjusted to the appropriate height. The standard height for assistive devices is used: as the patient stands in a balanced posture with her shoulders relaxed and her hands on the parallel bars or on the crutches, her elbows should be in 20 to 30 degrees of flexion.

The therapist must evaluate the orthoses carefully to make sure that they fit and function well and are aligned appropriately. The ankles should be held in slight dorsiflexion, and the knees should lock securely in full extension. The

orthoses must not exert excessive pressure on any area of the skin. The therapist should check for potential sources of trauma to the skin, such as rough seams in leather components or nail points protruding from the soles of the shoes.

During gait training, the therapist and patient should check the patient's skin frequently for problems caused by abrasion or excessive pressure. The skin is at risk anywhere it comes in contact with the orthosis.

Parallel bars. Anyone with a complete spinal cord injury who lacks functioning hip extensors will be very unstable when she first gets onto her feet using KAFOs. For this reason, the most sensible place to initiate gait training is in the parallel bars. This equipment provides stable support for early practice; however, parallel bars are a double-edged sword. The very stability that makes them a secure place to begin standing and walking can cause problems. Parallel bars will support a person's weight regardless of whether she pulls, pushes, or leans on them. No other assistive device can provide this degree of support. A patient who develops the habit of leaning laterally or pulling on parallel bars is likely to have difficulty making the transition to ambulation with Lofstrand crutches.

To prepare a patient for the eventual transition to ambulation outside of the parallel bars, the therapist should encourage her to avoid leaning laterally or pulling on the bars. This should be stressed from the beginning of gait training, to avoid the development of bad habits. When pressing on the bars, the patient should direct the force vertically downward. By maintaining her hands in an open position while standing and walking, she can avoid inadvertently pulling on the bars.

No matter how careful a patient and therapist have been to avoid developing bad habits in the parallel bars, the transition from bars to crutches is a challenging one because crutches provide a much less stable base of support than do parallel bars. Even someone who walks independently and skillfully in the parallel bars is likely to require close guarding, even significant assistance, when she first ventures out of the bars. The therapist should keep the difficulty of this transition in mind. Deterioration in the patient's performance when she first practices with crutches is not necessarily an indication that she should utilize a walker or return to the parallel bars for further preparatory practice.

Guarding.   Guarding is required during much of gait training to ensure the patient's safety. The challenge of guarding well is to keep the crutch walker safe without interfering with her gait or motor learning.

Contact guarding while walking with a person with a complete injury is best done from behind. A therapist who stands behind the patient is less likely to get in the way of her head and trunk motions and feet as she steps. When practicing stairs or curbs, the therapist is likely to find it easier to guard the patient when standing below her.

When a patient loses her balance while walking, the natural reaction for many therapists is to pull her pelvis (via a gait belt) up and toward the therapist. This guarding technique is not effective for people with complete spinal cord injuries because a backward tug on a patient's pelvis will throw her hips into an unstable position. Uncontrolled forward flexion of the trunk on the hips (jacknifing) is likely to result.

A therapist should guard in such a way that the patient's balance is restored, not hindered, when assistance is given. When a person lacking innervated hip extensors loses her balance while walking with KAFOs, the therapist should push her pelvis forward and pull her upper trunk back. These forces will return her to a balanced standing posture (Figure 13–20).

When a therapist makes a postural correction for a patient or catches her when she starts to lose her balance, the patient should be made aware of this assistance. Especially if the therapist has a hand on an area with impaired sensation, the patient may not realize that the therapist has assisted her. As a result, she will not realize that she has made an error that needs to be corrected.

There are two ways in which a therapist can

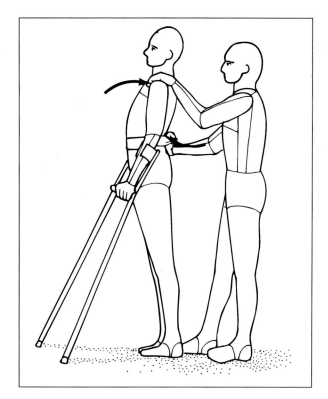

Figure 13–20.   Forces applied when helping a patient maintain or return to a balanced standing posture.

make a patient aware of her mistakes and of the assistance being given. First, the therapist can provide verbal feedback. ("I had to catch you just now. You were falling to the left.") Verbal feedback is especially important when a patient first attempts a skill. In the second strategy, the therapist guards in a way that enables the patient to feel her mistakes. Specifically, when the patient starts to jackknife or lose her balance to the side, the therapist does not catch her or correct her posture until she has fallen far enough that she can sense what has happened.[m] This strategy is not appropriate when the patient first attempts a skill. Standing for the first time, or walking outside of the parallel bars for the first time, can be frightening enough as it is. The therapist should begin allowing partial falls only after the patient has overcome her initial fear of the activity.

Close guarding is required during most of gait training. At some point, however, a person who plans to walk independently must practice walking without spotting. The transition from walking with

---

[m] This is not to say that the patient should be allowed to plummet halfway to the floor each time she starts to lose her balance. A few inches of free fall is generally enough to catch a person's attention.

guarding to walking alone can be a test of nerves for both the patient and the therapist. To ease this transition, and to maximize the patient's safety throughout the process, the shift should be gradual. As (and *only* as) an individual demonstrates that she can safely perform a skill unassisted, the therapist's guarding should be withdrawn. The patient and therapist first progress from walking with contact guarding to walking with the therapist's hands hovering inches away, ready to grab if needed. They then progress to walking with the therapist standing nearby, ready to dive and grab. When both parties are ready, the patient walks while the therapist watches from a distance[n] and prays, and finally just prays. In this manner, the patient and (perhaps more so) the therapist can be weaned from guarding.

Balanced Standing

Training in balanced standing should include practice maintaining a balanced standing posture as well as practice moving in and out of that posture while standing upright. Before a patient begins practice in balanced standing, she should have had prior practice using the head-hips relationship to control her pelvis.[o]

The therapist should demonstrate and explain the balanced standing posture, showing how head and shoulder motions can be used to move the pelvis and stabilize the hips. The patient should stand with her head erect, chest forward (scapulae retracted), and pelvis forward. Her feet should be a few inches apart.

During early training, the patient gains an awareness of her pelvis' motions in standing and develops skill in controlling these motions. She should practice moving her pelvis using head and scapular motions. As she moves in and out of a balanced posture, she should attend to sensory cues that tell her of her pelvis' position. Practice should include experiencing how her hips jackknife when her weight line falls anterior to her hips.

During initial training, the therapist can assist the patient to a balanced standing posture in the parallel bars. The therapist can help her to maintain the posture and give her feedback and suggestions. As the patient's skill develops, the therapist should reduce the assistance provided. Once the patient can balance well with both hands on the parallel bars, she can practice balancing with one hand, then both hands, lifted. If she has difficulty balancing, the alignment of the orthotic ankles may need to be adjusted. Aligning the ankles in a more dorsiflexed position will cause the pelvis to be positioned more anteriorly when the feet are flat on the floor. Conversely, aligning the ankles in a more plantar flexed position will cause the pelvis to be positioned in a more posterior position when the feet are flat on the floor. The ankles should be aligned in equal amounts of dorsiflexion; asymmetrically aligned ankle joints will cause lateral instability in standing.

When a person with a spinal cord injury walks, her feet do not always land where she wants them to. A patient will be better prepared for ambulation if she learns to balance, at least briefly, with her feet in less than optimal positions. Training in standing balance, then, should be done with the feet in various positions. The patient should start with her feet in the easiest position (close to parallel and a few inches apart) and progress to balancing with her feet in more challenging positions.

Initial practice of standing balance should take place in the parallel bars. Once the patient has progressed to walking in the bars and is ready to start working with Lofstrand crutches, she should practice standing with crutches. Because crutches provide less stable support than do parallel bars, balancing with them is more challenging.

Independent work. Once a patient has had initial practice in the parallel bars and has demonstrated that she can catch herself if she loses her balance, she can practice independently in the bars.

Weight Shift in Standing

Before practicing weight shifts in standing, the patient must be able to maintain a balanced standing posture. To practice shifting her weight while standing with a given assistive device (parallel bars or Lofstrand crutches), the person should be adept in balanced standing using that assistive device.

The patient can begin weight shifting with lateral shifts, with her feet side by side a few inches apart. As her skill improves, she can progress to shifting her weight with her feet in other positions. If she is to walk with a four-point gait, the patient must develop the capacity to stand with one foot diagonally in front of the other and shift her weight onto the forward foot.

During early weight-shifting practice, the therapist can assist the patient into position in the parallel bars and guard her as she shifts her

---

[n] Before walking alone, the patient must be proficient in falling safely.

[o] Strategies for developing skill in controlling the pelvis using head and shoulder motions are presented in Chapter 11.

weight. The therapist can help her get a feel for the motion by placing a hand against her trunk or shoulder and having her push against the hand. As the patient's skill improves, the therapist can withdraw the resistance and the guarding. When gait training has progressed to the point where the patient is ready to start ambulation outside of the parallel bars, she should practice weight shifting with Lofstrand crutches.

Independent work. Once an individual has had initial practice in the parallel bars and has demonstrated that she can catch herself if she loses her balance, she can practice weight shifting independently in the bars.

Lift and Move One Crutch

To lift a crutch while standing, a person must be able to maintain a balanced standing posture and weight shift while using crutches. She will be better prepared to practice moving a crutch if she has practiced lifting a hand while standing in the parallel bars.

The patient should practice lifting a crutch while the therapist guards and provides assistance as necessary. As her skill improves, the assistance can be withdrawn.

Step Forward with One Leg

Balanced standing and weight shifting are prerequisites for stepping forward with one leg. To practice stepping using a given assistive device (parallel bars or Lofstrand crutches), the patient should be adept in standing and weight shifting using that assistive device. She should also be skillful in the use of the head-hips relationship before attempting to step with one leg.

Practice should start with the patient standing in the parallel bars with one hand in front of the other. (The hand opposite the stepping leg should be more anterior.) From this position, she practices shifting her weight off of the leg and lifting her pelvis on the unweighted side. When her pelvis tilts enough to lift the foot off the ground, the leg swings forward as a pendulum or by muscle action, depending on whether or not the iliopsoas is innervated.

The patient elevates her pelvis using the quadratus lumborum, latissimus dorsi, abdominal musculature, or the head-hips relationship, or a combination thereof. Whichever method she uses, the therapist can help her to learn the motion by demonstrating, assisting with the motion, and providing verbal and tactile feedback during practice.

A patient with innervated quadratus lumborum, latissimus dorsi, or abdominals may build the groundwork for stepping by practicing elevating her pelvis in sidelying. Utilizing quick stretch and resistance, the therapist can facilitate motor learning and strengthening.

If using the head-hips relationship to elevate her pelvis, the patient may use exaggerated motions when first practicing, tucking her head far down and to the side. As she develops a feel for the maneuver, she can reduce her head and upper trunk motions.

Practice stepping should begin in the parallel bars, with the therapist guarding and assisting as needed. As the patient's skill improves, the assistance should be withdrawn. Once proficient in the parallel bars, the patient should progress to working outside of the bars with crutches. Before attempting to step with crutches, she should develop her dynamic balance skills in standing with these assistive devices.

Independent work. Once a patient has had initial practice in the parallel bars and has demonstrated that she can catch herself if she loses her balance, she can practice stepping independently in the bars.

Step to the Side or Back with One Leg

The patient must be proficient in using the head-hips relationship, balanced standing, and weight shifting before attempting to step to the side or back. To practice stepping using a given assistive device (parallel bars or Lofstrand crutches), the patient should be adept in standing and weight shifting using that assistive device. Prior practice in stepping forward should make learning to step back or to the side easier.

Practice should start with the patient standing in the parallel bars. From this position, she practices shifting her weight off of one leg and lifting her pelvis on the unweighted side. The techniques that she can use for elevating her pelvis and the therapeutic strategies for developing this skill are the same as described previously for stepping forward with one leg.

With her leg lifted, the patient practices swinging it laterally or forward and back using head and upper trunk motions to move her pelvis. She may use exaggerated motions when first practicing. As she develops a feel for the maneuver, she can reduce her head and upper body motions.

Once she has learned to swing her leg, the patient can practice placing her foot by lowering her pelvis when her foot has swung to the desired position.

Practice should begin in the parallel bars, with the therapist guarding and assisting as needed. As the patient's skill improves, the assistance should be withdrawn. Once proficient in the parallel bars, the patient should progress to working outside of the bars with crutches. Before attempting to step with crutches, she should develop her dynamic balance skills in standing with these assistive devices.

Independent work. Once a patient has had initial practice in the parallel bars and has demonstrated that she can catch herself if she loses her balance, she can practice stepping to the side and back independently in the bars.

Lift and Move Two Crutches

Before attempting to lift and move two crutches at once, a patient must be proficient in balanced standing with crutches. She should also be able to lift both hands simultaneously while maintaining a balanced standing posture in the parallel bars. An individual who has acquired these skills should not have difficulty learning to lift and move both crutches with a brief period of practice.

Swing-Through Step

Before practicing this maneuver, a patient must be skillful in balanced standing, including moving in and out of the balanced posture. She should also be skillful in the use of the head-hips relationship. To practice stepping using a given assistive device (parallel bars or Lofstrand crutches), the individual should be adept in standing using that assistive device.

Practice should start with the patient standing in a balanced posture in the parallel bars with her hands anterior to her hips. From this position, she should practice lifting her feet off of the ground by leaning forward onto her arms while extending her elbows, depressing and protracting her scapulae, and tucking her head. When her feet leave the ground, her trunk and legs will swing forward as a pendulum hanging from her shoulders. During gait training, the therapist should stress the passive nature of the feet's motion: the crutch walker's task is to lift her feet; gravity will provide the force to move them forward.

When the patient's heels strike, she should quickly regain the balanced standing posture. She does this by retracting her scapulae and throwing her head back, pushing her pelvis forward.

The therapist can help the patient learn the required motions by demonstrating, assisting with the motions, and providing verbal and tactile feedback during practice. The patient may use exaggerated motions when first practicing lifting her feet and regaining a balanced posture. As she develops a feel for the maneuver, she can reduce her head and upper body motions.

Practice should begin in the parallel bars, with the therapist guarding and assisting as needed. As the patient's skill improves, the assistance should be withdrawn. Once proficient in the parallel bars, the patient should progress to working outside of the bars with crutches. Before attempting to step with crutches, she should have developed her dynamic balance skills in standing with these assistive devices.

Independent work. Once a patient has had initial practice in the parallel bars and has demonstrated that she can catch herself if she loses her balance, she can practice stepping independently in the bars.

Swing-To or Drag-To Step

To practice a swing-to or drag-to step, a patient must be skillful in balanced standing and able to move in and out of a balanced standing posture. She should also be skillful in the use of the head-hips relationship. To practice stepping using a given assistive device (parallel bars or Lofstrand crutches), the patient should be adept in standing using that assistive device.

A swing-to step is like a swing-through step, except that the feet land even with, not past, the crutches. In a drag-to step, the patient lifts her trunk only enough to drag her feet to or toward the level of her crutches. Her feet do not leave the ground. Both gait patterns can be taught using the training strategies described for teaching a swing-through step.

Distance and Efficient Ambulation

Once a patient is able to walk with a given gait pattern using assistive devices, she will require practice to develop her endurance and perfect her skills. She should walk over increasing distances as her ability develops. She can also practice walking on carpet and uneven surfaces such as sidewalks and grass.

Independent work. When a patient is able to walk safely and to fall without guarding, she can practice independently. When her distance capabilities have increased enough, she should be encouraged to walk to her various activities during the day and to walk during her free time in the evenings.

Ambulation Up and Down Slopes

A patient must be proficient in ambulation over even surfaces before beginning practice on ramps. Even if she walks well on even surfaces, she is likely to be very unstable when first walking on ramps. This is especially true when ascending because the inclined surface tends to throw the pelvis into an unstable position. The patient should be encouraged to keep her crutches well in front of her feet when ascending and to keep her body angled up the hill with her pelvis well forward. She should use a step-to (or step-toward) gait, not a swing-through pattern. When descending, she may step past her crutches.

Practice in ramp negotiation should start on gentle slopes. Once the patient masters a slope of a particular grade, she should progress to steeper inclines. Training in ramp negotiation can continue in this manner until the individual has reached her maximal potential.

Step Up and Down Curb or Step

Before attempting ambulation over curbs or stairs, the patient must be proficient in ambulation over even surfaces.

During training, the therapist should emphasize maintaining control during ascent and descent, and rapid resumption of a balanced standing posture once the feet have landed. Practice should start on small curbs. As the patient's skill increases, the curb height can be increased. Once the patient is skillful in negotiating step-high curbs, she can progress to practicing on stairs.

Sitting in Wheelchair, Position Legs in Preparation to Stand

To practice positioning her legs in preparation to stand, a patient must be skillful in stabilizing her trunk in a wheelchair.[p] Prior practice in leg management on a mat[q] will make practice in a wheelchair easier.

If an individual has the physical potential to come to standing from a wheelchair, she should be able to learn to position her legs without much difficulty. The therapist should demonstrate the maneuver and encourage the patient to practice.

Independent work. After a brief period of supervised practice with feedback, the patient should be able to practice this skill independently.

With Hands on Armrests, Assume Standing Position from Wheelchair

Before a patient begins working on this skill, she must be proficient in using the head-hips relationship to move her pelvis.

During initial practice, the therapist can demonstrate and assist the patient as she pushes herself into a standing position. The therapist should encourage her to use forceful and abrupt head and upper trunk motions to lift her pelvis. As the patient's skill develops, the therapist's assistance should be reduced.

This maneuver is most difficult at its beginning, when the person lifts herself from the seat. If an individual has difficulty lifting herself to a standing position from a wheelchair, she can work on the skill in reverse in the following manner.

---

p This skill is addressed in Chapter 11.
q This skill is addressed in Chapter 10.

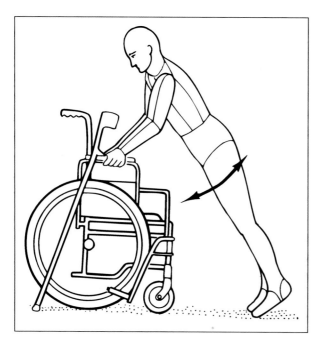

Figure 13–21. *Practice lowering buttocks toward seat and returning to standing.*

The therapist assists her to the starting position: standing facing the chair with one hand on each armrest. The patient's feet should be positioned in front of and slightly lateral to the casters. From this position she turns and lowers her buttocks slightly toward the seat and then pushes herself back to the starting position (Figure 13–21). She should move over a small arc at first, lowering herself only as far as she can retain control of the motion and push back up. As her skill improves, she should increase the arc of motion. She should challenge her limits as she practices, working in a range in which she experiences difficulty but can maintain control. By pushing her limits in this manner, the patient gradually builds to the point where she can lower herself to the seat and push back up to standing.

Standing in Front of Wheelchair with Hands on Armrests, Grasp Crutch

Anyone who has the physical potential to assume a standing position from a wheelchair should achieve this prerequisite skill without much difficulty. The patient can start by practicing weight shifting while standing in front of a wheelchair with her hands on the armrests. She can progress to lifting a hand, then grasping a crutch. The therapist can assist the patient into position and guard her as she practices.

Standing with One Hand on Wheelchair Armrest and One on Crutch, Grasp Second Crutch

To practice this skill, a patient must be able to weight shift while standing with crutches, and balance in standing with one hand lifted.

The patient stands in front of a wheelchair with one hand on an armrest and one on a crutch. She should face toward or sideways to the chair, depending on the method of coming to standing being practiced. From the starting position, the patient practices shifting her weight off of the hand on the armrest. She can progress to lifting the unweighted hand, then grasping the second crutch. The therapist can assist the patient into position and guard her as she practices.

Standing with Crutches Positioned Forward, Walk Crutches Back

To perform this maneuver. the person shifts her weight from one side to the other and repositions each crutch as it is unweighted. Before practicing this skill, a patient should be proficient in balanced upright standing and able to lift and reposition one crutch at a time while standing upright.

Walking the crutches back from a forward position is most difficult when the crutch tips are furthest from the feet. In this position, the person is furthest from upright, and the greatest amount of weight is being borne through the crutches. As she walks her crutches toward her feet, she assumes a more upright posture. Her weight is increasingly borne through her legs, and the task becomes easier.

Practice of this skill will be easiest if the patient starts in the least challenging position and works toward the most difficult. She should start with her legs close to vertical, with the crutch tips a few inches in front of her feet. From this position, she walks her crutches away from her feet and back again. As her skill improves, she walks her crutches over greater distances, walking the crutch tips as far anteriorly as she can while maintaining control and retaining the ability to return to upright.

This skill can be practiced concurrently with the other prerequisite skills for coming to stand from a wheelchair or from the floor.

Independent work. This skill is most readily practiced independently if the patient can get into position on her own. If she knows how to fall safely and has developed some skill in walking her crutches forward and back, she can practice independently over a floor mat. For added safety, she can practice in front of a wall. When practicing in front of a wall, she should face away from the wall and position her feet far enough from the wall that she does not touch it while she practices, but close enough that the wall will support her if she starts to fall backward.

With One Hand on Armrest and One on Crutch, Assume Standing Position from Wheelchair

Practice of this skill requires proficiency in using the head-hips relationship to move the pelvis. The patient must also be skillful in balanced standing with crutches, including moving in and out of a balanced standing posture.

During initial practice, the therapist can demonstrate and assist the patient as she lifts herself into a standing position. The therapist should encourage her to use forceful and abrupt head and upper trunk motions to lift her pelvis. As the patient's skill develops, the assistance should be reduced.

With Both Hands on Crutches, Assume Standing Position from Wheelchair

Before attempting this maneuver, the patient must be proficient in using the head-hips relationship to move her pelvis. She must also be skillful in balanced standing with crutches, including moving in and out of a balanced standing posture.

When teaching this skill, the therapist can demonstrate and then assist the patient as she lifts herself to standing. As the patient's skill develops, the therapist can reduce the assistance given.

The therapist should encourage the patient to push forcefully and abruptly on her crutches and to keep her head tucked as her pelvis lifts. As the patient's legs move toward vertical, she must push her pelvis forward to attain a balanced standing posture. As her legs move past vertical, she must reposition her crutches anteriorly. During practice, the patient can work on perfecting her motions and timing. She can also experiment with different crutch positions to determine which position enables her to come to standing most easily.

Position Self in Preparation to Sit in Wheelchair

When sitting down from a standing position, a person wearing KAFOs with the knees locked piv-

ots on her feet as she descends. Thus, if she does not position her feet appropriately prior to sitting, she will not land correctly in the wheelchair. Instead of landing on the seat, her buttocks may hit the chair's backrest or armrest, or even miss the wheelchair altogether.

A patient should be able to step in all directions before practicing this skill. Training in foot placement for sitting is then a matter of finding the position that is best for that individual.

To find the optimal foot position, the therapist and patient can first make an educated guess, judging from the individual's leg length and predicting the path of her buttocks as she pivots on her feet. The patient can then position her feet and, with the therapist guarding closely, sit down in the chair. If she does not land appropriately on the seat, the patient and therapist should determine what was wrong with her initial foot position. (Were her feet too close to the chair? Too far away? Too far lateral to the chair's midline? Not lateral enough?) She can then try again with her feet in a different position. By this informed trial and error and by learning from their mistakes, the patient and therapist can find an appropriate foot position for sitting down in the chair.

This skill can be practiced concurrently with other skill prerequisites for getting in and out of a standing position from a wheelchair.

Standing Facing Wheelchair, Place Hands on Armrests

To practice this skill, a patient must be proficient in the following balanced standing skills with Lofstrand crutches: moving in and out of a balanced standing posture, weight shifting, lifting a hand, and repositioning the crutches.

When working on this skill, the patient practices shifting her weight off of one crutch, leaning the crutch on the wheelchair, and placing her unweighted hand on an armrest. She then repeats these actions with her other hand.

During initial practice, the therapist provides guarding and assistance as needed. As the patient's skill improves, the assistance can be reduced.

When practicing this skill, the patient should get into the habit of leaning her crutches against the wheelchair where she can reach them. When crutches are placed in this manner instead of being tossed aside, they are less likely to be damaged. In addition, the crutch that is placed within reach remains retrievable. Once a crutch is tossed, the patient loses the option to change her mind about sitting down.

Facing Wheelchair with Hands on Armrests, Turn and Lower Self into Chair

Before practicing this maneuver, a patient should be proficient in using the head-hips relationship to move her pelvis.

When sitting down using this technique, the person standing in front of her wheelchair turns approximately 180 degrees and drops into the chair. Because she releases an armrest while descending, the descent is not truly controlled: the person drops into the seat instead of lowering herself.

The therapist should encourage the patient to use head and upper trunk motions that are forceful enough to generate the momentum required to turn her torso and land on her buttocks. The therapist should guard closely at first. As the patient's skill develops, the guarding can be withdrawn.

Standing Facing Away from Wheelchair, Lower Self into Chair

Practice of this skill requires proficiency in using the head-hips relationship to move the pelvis, and balanced standing skills with Lofstrand crutches.

In this maneuver, a crutch walker standing in front of a wheelchair flexes at the hips and lowers her buttocks into the chair. She should be able to control the descent to some degree, because both of her hands remain on her crutches while she descends. Because the crutches do not provide a stable base of support, she is not likely to be in total control of the descent, able to stop or reverse her motion at will. She should, however, have enough control to land without excessive force and with her buttocks squarely in the seat.

As the patient practices with guarding, the therapist should encourage her to control her motion as she lowers herself into the wheelchair. As her skill develops, the guarding can be withdrawn.

This skill can be practiced concurrently with other skill prerequisites for getting in and out of a standing position from a wheelchair.

When Falling, Throw Crutches and Catch Self on Hands

The two components of this maneuver, throwing the crutches and landing on the hands, can initially be practiced separately or in combination. Before training is complete, however, the patient must practice both together.

When throwing the crutches while falling, the aim is to position them so that they will not cause injury. The patient should be encouraged to

throw her crutches laterally, or laterally and posteriorly, out of her path of fall. The crutch tips should swing upward so that they do not catch on the ground. The throw should not be forceful. The goal is to position the crutches out of the way, but not to fling them out of reach. The forearm cuffs may remain on the arms.

To get a feel for the throw, the patient can practice throwing one crutch at a time while the therapist guards her. For added security while practicing throwing one crutch, the patient can stand outside of a set of parallel bars and hold the nearest bar.

When a patient practices falling and landing on her hands, the therapist should stress to the patient that she *must* allow her arms to "give" to absorb the shock. During initial practice, the force of the fall should be minimized. The therapist can accomplish this by having the person fall over a short distance and by lowering her instead of allowing her to fall unrestrained. As the patient's skill develops, she can progress to falling unrestrained over a short distance and gradually build the distance over which she falls.

Lying on the Floor, Position Crutches in Preparation to Stand

For a patient with the physical potential to get herself into a standing position from the floor, this prerequisite skill is not physically challenging. Training is simply a matter of determining the correct placement for the crutches.

When preparing to assume a standing position from the floor, the person should position her crutches so that she will be able to reach them easily when the time comes. The appropriate position will depend on how far back she walks her hands in plantigrade as she comes to stand. The crutches' hand grips are likely to be reached easily if they are positioned at or caudal to the level of the greater trochanters. The therapist and patient can determine the optimal crutch position through problem solving and trial and error, with the patient grasping the crutches in various positions while in plantigrade.

From Prone, Assume Plantigrade Posture

To move from prone to plantigrade, a person with a complete spinal cord injury must be proficient in moving her pelvis using the head-hips relationship. Prior practice in using head and upper trunk motions to assume a quadruped position from prone will facilitate acquisition of this skill.

During early practice, the therapist can assist the patient as she attempts to assume a plantigrade posture. The patient should be encouraged to push forcefully down and cephalad while tucking her head and upper torso to lift her pelvis. A strong and skillful individual may be able to move from prone to plantigrade with minimal practice. Others may require more training.

This maneuver is most difficult at its beginning, when the person lifts her pelvis from the floor. A patient who has difficulty assuming a plantigrade posture can work on the skill in reverse in the following manner. The therapist assists her into a plantigrade posture with her pelvis well off of the floor. From this position, the patient lowers herself slightly toward prone and pushes back to the starting position. She should move over a small arc of motion at first, lowering herself only as far as she can retain control of the motion and push back up. As her skill improves, she should increase the arc of motion. She should challenge her limits as she practices, working in a range in which she experiences difficulty but can maintain control. By pushing her limits in this manner, the patient gradually builds to the point where she can lower herself to prone and push back up to plantigrade.

Assuming a plantigrade posture can be practiced concurrently with other skill prerequisites used in coming to stand from the floor.

Independent work. After a patient has developed some ability in this maneuver, she can work independently on a floor mat to increase her skill and the consistency of her performance. If she has difficulty lifting her pelvis, she can work with her feet stabilized by a wall. She must progress to pushing into plantigrade without her feet stabilized if she is to become independent in coming to stand from the floor without her feet stabilized on an object.

Dynamic Balance in Plantigrade and Modified Plantigrade

In the plantigrade posture, a person is positioned with her feet and hands on the floor, her hips flexed, and her buttocks in the air (Figure 13–22A). Modified plantigrade includes a variety of postures in which a person's feet are on the floor, her hips are flexed, and her hands are supported by a surface that is higher than the floor. The hand placement in the modified plantigrade postures involved in coming to stand from the floor include one hand on the floor and one on a crutch, and both hands on crutches (Figure 13–22B and C).

A patient need not be independent in attaining plantigrade or modified plantigrade postures to practice dynamic balance in these positions. To practice dynamic balance in a given posture, she should have well-developed dynamic balance skills in less challenging postures. Thus to practice in plantigrade, an individual should have good dynamic balance in quadruped.[r] Before beginning balance practice in modified plantigrade with one or two crutches, she should have good dynamic balance in plantigrade.

To develop dynamic balance in plantigrade or modified plantigrade, the patient can start with practice maintaining the posture. The therapist can assist her into position and have her attempt to maintain the posture using head, scapular, and upper trunk motions to control her pelvis. The therapist helps at first, reducing the assistance as the patient's skill improves. The patient can progress to maintaining the position while the therapist applies resistance in various directions.

One task when practicing modified plantigrade with one hand on a crutch involves determining the crutch position that best suits the individual. Three crutch positions used in coming to stand from the floor are illustrated in Figure 13–18. While working on balance in modified plantigrade, the patient can try the different crutch positions to see which one affords her the best control.

Once an individual is able to stabilize herself in plantigrade or modified plantigrade, she can progress to shifting her weight in that posture, then weight shifting and lifting the unweighted hand, and finally maintaining her balance as she lifts a hand and reaches in different directions. All of these actions can be performed with and without resistance supplied by the therapist.

Independent work. If a patient can assume plantigrade or modified plantigrade without assistance, she can practice her dynamic balance on a floor mat independently.

In Plantigrade, Walk Hands Toward Feet

To practice walking her hands back while in a plantigrade posture, a patient should have well-developed dynamic balance skills in plantigrade. She does not have to be independent in assuming this posture.

---

[r] Strategies for developing dynamic balance in quadruped are presented in Chapter 11, under the heading, "Control Pelvis Using Head and Shoulders."

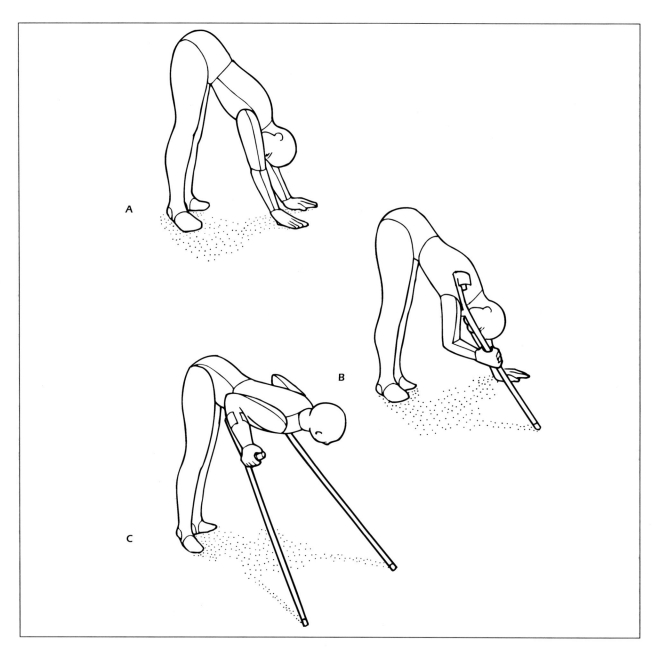

Figure 13–22. Plantigrade and modified plantigrade postures. **(A)** Plantigrade. **(B** and **C)** Modified plantigrade postures involved in coming to stand from the floor with KAFOs and Lofstrand crutches.

An individual with good dynamic balance in plantigrade should be able to learn to walk her hands back with minimal practice. During early training, the therapist may help her control her pelvis as she attempts the maneuver. This assistance can be decreased as the patient's skill develops.

This skill can be practiced concurrently with other skill prerequisites used in coming to stand from the floor.

Independent work. If a patient can assume a plantigrade posture without assistance, she can practice this skill independently on a floor mat. For added safety, she can practice near a wall. When practicing near a wall, she should face away from the wall and position her feet far enough from the wall that she does not touch it while she practices, but close enough that the wall will support her if she starts to fall backward.

In Plantigrade, Grasp and Position Crutch

In this maneuver the person moves from plantigrade to modified plantigrade. In the end posture she supports her weight with one hand on the floor and one on a crutch (Figure 13–22B). A patient need not be independent in assuming a plantigrade posture to practice this skill, but she should have well-developed dynamic balance skills in plantigrade. The therapist can help the patient maintain her balance during early practice. As her skill builds, this assistance can be decreased.

This skill can be practiced concurrently with other skill prerequisites used in coming to stand from the floor.

Independent work. If a patient can get into plantigrade and walk her hands toward her feet without assistance, she can practice grasping and positioning a crutch independently on a floor mat. For added safety she can practice near a wall. When practicing near a wall, she should position herself so that the wall is close enough to prevent a backward fall but does not support her as she practices.

In Modified Plantigrade with One Hand on Crutch, Grasp and Position Second Crutch with Free Hand

In this maneuver, the patient moves from one modified plantigrade posture to another. In the end posture she supports her trunk with two crutches (Figure 13–22C). Before attempting this skill, she should have well-developed dynamic balance skills in modified plantigrade.

This skill is likely to require a moderate amount of practice, even for a skillful patient. The therapist and patient can use the strategies just described for learning to move from plantigrade to one-crutch-supported modified plantigrade.

From Modified Plantigrade Supported on Two Crutches, Push Torso to Upright

The starting position for this maneuver is illustrated in Figure 13–22C. From this posture, the person lifts her trunk by pushing downward on the crutches. While raising her trunk, she pushes her buttocks forward by lifting her head.

During early practice, the therapist can help the patient stabilize her pelvis as she lifts her torso. This assistance can be removed as the patient's skill improves.

This skill can be practiced concurrently with other skill prerequisites used in coming to stand from the floor.

Independent work. If a patient can get into two-crutch-supported modified plantigrade without assistance and if she is able to fall safely, she can practice pushing her torso to upright independently on a floor mat. For added safety, she can practice near a wall. When practicing near a wall, she should position herself so that the wall is close enough to prevent a backward fall but does not support her as she practices.

Donning and Doffing Orthoses

This skill should be readily achievable by anyone with the potential for independent ambulation. During early practice, the therapist can provide suggestions and assist the patient as needed.

Independent work. After a brief period of supervised practice with feedback, the patient should be able to practice this skill independently.

PROBLEM-SOLVING EXERCISE 13–3

Your patient has L2 paraplegia, ASIA B. He is able to walk independently with KAFOs and Lofstrand crutches over even surfaces for 200 feet, using either a swing-through or four-point gait pattern. His goal is to come to standing from the floor. He is able to assume a modified plantigrade position, but is unable to lift a hand and reach for a crutch without losing his balance.

- What range-of-motion or muscle flexibility limitations could cause this problem?
- What strength limitations could cause this problem?
- If strength and range are adequate for this task, what skill prerequisites may be lacking?
- Describe a functional training program to address this problem.
- How would you progress the program?

AMBULATION AND THERAPEUTIC STRATEGIES WITH ANKLE-FOOT ORTHOSES FOLLOWING COMPLETE SPINAL CORD INJURY

Standard AFOs (as opposed to floor-reaction AFOs) are typically recommended for individuals who have adequate quadriceps strength and proprioception to enable them to stabilize their knees during stance without KAFOs. This group includes people with complete paraplegia with neurologic level of injury ranging from L3 through S1, and thus includes individuals with a wide range of lower extremity function. Table 13–5 includes information on the motor function present and the orthotic control typically required at different levels of complete paraplegia.

The ambulatory capabilities of people with complete paraplegia using AFOs are influenced by the motor function in their lower extremities. Those with higher lesions have less functioning musculature with which to stabilize their hips in the frontal and sagittal planes. As a result, they must rely more heavily on their upper extremities to compensate for this lack of muscular support. This reliance on the upper extremities necessitates the use of more supportive assistive devices such as Lofstrand crutches or walkers. Walking remains a physically demanding activity, and thus may be less functional than wheelchair propulsion for long distances. People with lower lesions have more intact motor function around their hips, allowing them to walk with less (or no) reliance on their upper extremities. As a result, walking may be performed using less supportive assistive devices such as standard canes, or even without any assistive devices. Walking is also less physically demanding for people with lower lesions, making community ambulation more feasible.

Therapeutic Strategies

Gait training with standard AFOs should emphasize the development of as normal a gait pattern as possible. A more normal gait pattern is likely to be more energy-efficient than an abnormal pattern, and may place less stress on the patient's joints.

Gait training with standard AFOs should develop the capacity for controlled knee flexion during early stance, knee stability during stance, and toe clearance during swing. Additional areas on which to focus include minimization of weight-bearing through the upper extremities, development of pelvic stability in the frontal plane, development of symmetrical weight-shifts and even cadence, prevention of a strong knee extensor thrust during stance, and swing limb advancement without circumduction or scissoring.

In addition to focusing on normalizing the gait pattern, gait training should address purely functional aspects of the patient's ambulatory ability. These functional aspects include the patient's ability to walk safely and independently for long distances, to walk at speeds that are normal or near normal, and to ambulate over various terrains and obstacles.

A variety of strategies can be employed to develop a more normal gait pattern and to enhance a patient's capacity for functional ambulation. The strategies presented in the discussion of incomplete injuries ("Ambulation and Therapeutic Strategies Following Incomplete Spinal Cord Injury") can be used with people with complete injuries who are learning to walk with standard AFOs.

Floor-Reaction AFOs

Floor-reaction AFOs are occasionally recommended for individuals who have functioning hip flexors but lack the quadriceps strength needed to stabilize their knees during stance. This group includes people with complete L2 and L3 paraplegia. Ambulation is more frequently achieved using KAFOs when neurologic level of injury is this high.

Floor-reaction AFOs provide knee stability during stance by holding the ankles in a slightly plantar flexed position. This ankle position causes the floor reaction force vector to pass anterior to the knee during stance, creating an extension moment that stabilizes the knee in extension.[s]

The knee stability provided by a floor-reaction AFO occurs only while the floor reaction force vector remains anterior to the knee.[63] Thus to ensure knee stability, the person's center of gravity must remain relatively anterior. If the center of gravity is positioned posteriorly (as would occur if the person leaned back on crutches positioned behind her feet), or if the knee is positioned anteriorly (as could occur if the person did not fully extend her knee prior to stepping onto that leg), the ground reaction force is located posterior to the knee. A flexion moment at the knee results. Since the individual's quadriceps are not strong

---

[s] An explanation of floor reaction forces (also called ground reaction forces) and their significance during walking is beyond the scope of this text. The reader is referred to the following sources: 68, 73, 74.

enough to stabilize the knee against this flexion moment, the knee will flex. During gait training with floor-reaction AFOs, the patient must learn to walk in such a way that the floor reaction force remains anterior to the knee whenever the knee is supporting weight.

AMBULATION AND THERAPEUTIC STRATEGIES FOLLOWING INCOMPLETE SPINAL CORD INJURY

The ambulatory capacity of an individual with an incomplete lesion depends largely on the voluntary motor function present below her neurologic level of injury. People who retain *or regain* only sensory function below their lesions (ASIA B) have ambulatory abilities similar to those with complete (ASIA A) injuries. Those who retain motor function below their lesions at the time of injury, and those who experience motor return after their injuries, have a better prognosis for achieving functional ambulation.

When attempting to predict an individual's potential for ambulation, it is important to consider the likelihood that she will experience motor return. In general, people with incomplete injuries, even ASIA B, are more likely to experience functionally useful motor return than are those with complete (ASIA A) injuries.[2, 26, 33, 94, 98] Table 13–16 presents research results that may be useful in predicting ambulatory outcome following spinal cord injury. Clinicians should keep in mind, however, that it is not possible to predict with certainty the level of functional independence that a given individual will achieve.

As is true with complete injuries, voluntary motor function is not the sole determinant of functional outcomes after incomplete spinal cord injuries. Muscle tone is a particularly important consideration when predicting functional potential. Incomplete lesions tend to result in more spasticity than do complete lesions,[48, 78] and severe spasticity can greatly affect walking performance.[45] Sensory sparing and return can also impact on function. Because somatosensory feedback is required for normal motor control, sensory impairments can prevent optimal utilization of musculature that remains or returns after a spinal cord injury. Finally, age can impact on ambulatory outcomes. Among patients with ASIA C tetraplegia, individuals who are over 50 years of age are less likely than their younger counterparts to regain functional ambulation.[13, 33]

Therapeutic Strategies

Ambulation requires the capacity to support the body's weight on a stable lower extremity during stance, advance the limb during swing, and progress the body's center of gravity in the direction of ambulation. Functional ambulation is more feasible for individuals who can perform these tasks safely with minimal or no bracing and with minimal or no weight-bearing through their upper extremities. This capacity requires adequate strength and motor control in the lower extremities, trunk, and (if assistive devices are used) upper extremities.

People with incomplete spinal cord injuries frequently experience neurological return for a year or more after they are injured. With this return comes the potential for greater levels of independence in ambulation. Individuals who experience return can benefit from therapeutic programs to take full advantage of their new motor and sensory capacities as they emerge. It is not practical, however, to continue rehabilitation uninterrupted throughout the time period during which neurological return may occur. A more efficient approach involves rehabilitation in stages. With this approach, patients undergo a series of inpatient, outpatient, or home health therapeutic programs. These programs are interspersed with periods of independent work at home. During the structured therapeutic intervention programs, patients work with therapists to maximize their level of independence within the constraints of their current impairments. They also develop functional skill techniques and home programs aimed at enabling them to continue to improve their motor abilities.[10]

The therapeutic program at each stage in the rehabilitation process should be based on a careful examination and evaluation of the individual's impairments and ambulatory abilities. The therapist should identify the factors that are contributing to the patient's inability or impaired ability to walk and perform related activities such as sit-to-stand. If the individual is unable to walk, the therapist should identify the factors causing this inability. If the patient is able to walk, the therapist should identify gait deviations, functional limitations, and factors causing these problems. There are multiple possible causes for any problem. For example, excessive knee flexion during stance could be caused by weakness in the quadriceps or plantar flexors, limited knee extension range of motion, elevated muscle tone in the hamstrings, impaired proprioception in the knee, or use of ineffective motor strategies. The therapist should examine the

TABLE 13-16.   FACTORS ASSOCIATED WITH FUTURE AMBULATORY POTENTIAL

Factor	Subjects	Outcomes
Complete versus incomplete, and paraplegia versus tetraplegia	246 patients with complete paraplegia, and incomplete paraplegia and tetraplegia[93]	Complete paraplegia: 5% community ambulators at 1 year Incomplete paraplegia: 76% community ambulators at 1 year Incomplete tetraplegia: 46% community ambulators at 1 year
Initial ASIA classification	118 patients with tetraplegia[33]	Tetraplegia, ASIA A: 0% ambulatory at 1 year Tetraplegia, ASIA B: 47% ambulatory at 1 year Tetraplegia, motor incomplete (ASIA C & D): 87% ambulatory at 1 year
Initial ASIA classification	41 patients with tetraplegia, all 50 years of age or older[2]	Tetraplegia, ASIA A: 0% ambulatory at follow-up Tetraplegia, ASIA B: 20% ambulatory at follow-up Tetraplegia, ASIA C: 85% ambulatory at follow-up Tetraplegia, ASIA D: 90% ambulatory at follow-up *Mean time of follow-up: 5.5 years after injury.*
Initial ASIA classification and age	105 patients with incomplete tetraplegia, ASIA C and D[13]	Tetraplegia, ASIA C, <50 years old: 91% ambulatory by discharge from inpatient rehabilitation Tetraplegia, ASIA C, ≥50 years old: 42% ambulatory by discharge from inpatient rehabilitation Tetraplegia, ASIA D: 100% ambulatory by discharge from inpatient rehabilitation, regardless of age
Lower Extremity Motor Score (LEMS)[a] at one month to 60 days post injury	54 patients with incomplete paraplegia due to trauma[94]	LEMS 0: 33% community ambulators at 1 year LEMS 1–9: 70% community ambulators at 1 year LEMS ≥10: 100% community ambulators at 1 year
LEMS measured 0.5 to 0.7 years after injury	36 patients with complete and incomplete paraplegia and incomplete tetraplegia, *all with sufficient preserved lower extremity motor function to ambulate and adequate trunk extension strength to allow independent sitting without the use of the arms for support*[95]	Ambulatory performance at time of study (0.5 to 0.7 years after injury) LEMS ≤20: 100% household ambulators; most relied on 2 KAFOs and 2 crutches LEMS ≥30: 100% community ambulators
Preservation of hip flexor or quadriceps function at 30 to 60 days post injury	54 patients with incomplete paraplegia due to trauma[94]	All with ≥2/5 initial hip flexor *or* knee extensor strength were community ambulators at 1 year
Quadriceps strength at 2 months postinjury	17 patients with ASIA C injuries, C4-T10[19]	≥3/5 in strongest quadriceps: 100% household or community ambulators at 1 year post injury <3/5 in strongest quadriceps: 25% household or community ambulators at 1 year post injury

TABLE 13–16. *(Continued)*

Factor	Subjects	Outcomes
Sparing of pin sensation below neurological level of injury, tested within 72 hours of injury	27 patients with ASIA B paraplegia and tetraplegia resulting from trauma[20]	Pin sensation spared: 88% recovered ability to walk independently ≥200 feet by discharge from rehabilitation
		Light touch spared but pin sensation absent: 11% recovered ability to walk independently ≥200 feet by discharge from rehabilitation
Pattern of injury	38 patients with cervical Brown-Séquard and Brown-Séquard-plus syndromes resulting from trauma[81]	"Pure" Brown-Sequard: 20% independent ambulators at time of discharge from rehabilitation
		Brown-Sequard-plus: 85% independent ambulators at time of discharge from rehabilitation
		Upper limb weaker than lower limb: more likely to walk at discharge

KAFOs, knee-ankle-foot orthoses.

[a] LEMS is explained in Chapter 8.

patient and analyze the findings to determine which of the possible factors are contributing to the patient's gait problems. The therapeutic program should then be based on this analysis.

The therapeutic approaches used to restore ambulation following incomplete spinal cord injury are not unique to this population. Therapists can often employ strategies that they use with people who have similar impairments and functional limitations resulting from other pathologies. For example, a patient who has asymmetrical paralysis resulting from Brown-Séquard syndrome may have a clinical picture that resembles hemiplegia due to a stroke or head injury. Many therapeutic activities aimed at developing improved locomotor capability after a stroke or head injury could be employed with this individual.[t]

Gait training. Gait training following incomplete spinal cord injury should work toward the development of as normal a gait pattern as possible, within the limits of the individual's impairments. Weight-bearing on the upper extremities should be minimized to the extent possible without compromising safety. This normalization of

gait pattern and minimization of upper extremity weight-bearing will lead to a more energy-efficient gait.

Gait training should be directed at developing the capacity to walk independently, safely, and over functional distances. The patient should practice walking forward, backward, and to the side, because daily activities include walking in each of these directions. Walking practice can take place on even surfaces at first, with progression to ambulation over uneven surfaces and obstacles as the individual's skills develop.

In many instances, patients benefit from therapeutic activities that develop component skills used in ambulation. Examples of such activities include practice of the following skills: shifting weight while maintaining knee stability, maintaining knee stability in stance without hyperextending the knee, progressing the body's weight forward to step past the stance foot, and stepping forward with proper placement of the foot.[11, 84]

Some patients may benefit from therapeutic activities that develop more basic skills. Examples of such therapeutic activities include dynamic balance while standing with the feet in different positions or on various surfaces; practice stabilizing and moving in different postures such as standing, modified plantigrade, kneeling, quadruped, bridging and hooklying; and practice balancing and moving while supported on a therapeutic ball.[11, 70, 82] Each of these activities is intended to develop a

---

[t] A comprehensive description of strategies for developing ambulation skills of people with neurological disabilities is beyond the scope of this book. The reader is encouraged to find additional information in the following references: 11, 15, 21, 27, 70, 82, 84.

foundation of balance and coordinated motor control to undergird the individual's capacity to walk.

Aquatic therapy. Aquatic therapy can be a useful adjunct to "land therapy" in developing ambulation skills. The buoyant force that water exerts on people as they stand partially immersed in water supports a portion of their weight. The percentage of their weight supported depends in part on the depth of water in which they stand; standing in deeper water increases the buoyant force, effectively reducing the weight borne through the lower extremities. Patients who have limited voluntary motor function in their trunk and lower extremities may be able to practice standing and walking in shoulder-high water. The support provided by the water at this depth makes walking possible for some people who are nonambulatory on land.[9] As their strength and walking ability improve, they can practice walking in progressively more shallow water, accepting more of their weight on their lower extremities.

Orthotic considerations. Orthotic prescription should be based on a careful analysis of the patient's biomechanical needs. Orthoses are frequently designed to compensate for functional deficits such as the inability to support the body's weight during stance or the inability to clear the foot during swing. Alternatively or in addition, orthoses may be designed to provide joint protection. For example, people who habitually thrust their knees into extension with excessive force during stance (knee extension thrust) may damage their knees over time, leading to pain and diminished function. When a knee extension thrust persists despite therapeutic attempts to eliminate this gait deviation, orthotic stabilization may be indicated to protect the knee.

Because neurological return is likely to occur during the first year or more after an incomplete injury, an individual's needs for orthotic stabilization are likely to change with time. This change in biomechanical needs may be accommodated with orthotic changes such as conversion of a KAFO to an AFO, or alteration of the control provided at the ankle joint.[u]

Muscle strength, range of motion, and muscle tone. In addition to gait training, the thera-

peutic program should address muscle strength, range of motion, and muscle tone.

Muscle strength. The strengthening program should address innervated muscles involved in walking. The therapist should analyze the patient's strength deficits in relation to her ambulatory ability and gait pattern, and develop a strengthening program accordingly. Although lower extremity musculature is an obvious focus for strengthening to enhance ambulatory ability, trunk musculature is also important. Adequate strength is required in the trunk to stabilize the upper body on the pelvis during gait. Patients who utilize assistive devices also require strength in their upper extremities, particularly in their triceps and shoulder girdle depressors.

Strength can be developed through progressive resistive exercises, proprioceptive neuromuscular facilitation techniques, isometric exercises, isokinetic exercise, and electrical stimulation.[22, 50, 55, 76, 87, 88] The strengthening program will better prepare the patient for the demands of walking if it includes open- and closed-chain activities, as well as exercises involving both concentric and eccentric contractions.

Range of motion. As is true for all other functional skills, range of motion is critical for ambulation. The therapeutic program should restore or maintain normal joint range and muscle flexibility to enhance ambulation.

Muscle tone. Elevated muscle tone is common among people with incomplete spinal cord injuries. When severe, it can interfere with ambulation in a variety of ways. Elevated tone in the hip extensors, hip adductors, quadriceps, or plantar flexors can impede swing limb advancement by preventing the normal sequence of motions that make it possible to clear the floor and progress the leg forward. During stance, hyperactivity in the quadriceps or plantar flexors can interfere with the knee and ankle motions that allow for a smooth transfer of weight onto the lower extremity, and can cause a knee extension thrust or genu recurvatum later in stance. Elevated muscle tone in the trunk or upper extremities can also interfere with ambulation. Involuntary spasms in the trunk musculature can interfere with balance, and elevated tone in the upper extremities can interfere with balance and utilization of assistive devices. Although elevated muscle tone often interferes with ambulation, at times it can help. For example, involuntary muscle contractions may aug-

---

[u] Additional principles of orthotic prescription are presented earlier in this chapter.

ment the ability to stabilize the knees in standing when voluntary contractions do not provide adequate force.

Strategies for treating elevated muscle tone are presented in Chapter 3. When planning therapies to reduce muscle tone, the rehabilitation team should take into consideration its influence on function: will the individual be more or less functional if spasticity is reduced? This question is not always possible to answer without actually reducing the patient's muscle tone and noting the effect that this change has on her ability to walk and perform other activities. Finding the optimal level of spasticity reduction may take a period during which various medications and dosages are tried and evaluated.

Body-weight support treadmill training. In recent years, an alternative method of locomotor training has emerged. Using this approach, patients with spinal cord injuries walk on treadmills while their body weight is partially supported by harnesses. During early training, therapists can assist with foot placement to ensure that patients utilize a proper gait pattern.[6, 7, 23–25, 30, 103] This approach has been shown to improve the ambulatory capabilities of people with long-standing incomplete[v] cervical or thoracic injuries, as well as those with relatively recent injuries. A follow-up study done 6 months to 6.5 years after training revealed that the functional improvements (in non-treadmill walking) were maintained over time in most cases.[102] Although treadmill training with body weight support remains experimental, it shows promise of being an effective means of restoring walking ability to people with incomplete spinal cord lesions.

FUNCTIONAL ELECTRICAL STIMULATION

No chapter on ambulation after spinal cord injury would be complete without a mention of functional electrical stimulation (FES).[w] Since the mid-seventies, research has been done on eliciting contractions in paralyzed musculature for ambulation. Using FES and assistive devices, people with complete spinal cord lesions have been able to walk over even surfaces, over mild inclines,

and to ascend and descend stairs.[40, 44, 51, 71, 90] FES has also been used to augment ambulation with mechanical orthoses.[36, 54, 86, 101]

To date, the use of FES for functional ambulation following spinal cord injury remains limited. A variety of problems remain to be solved, including the development of fatigue in electrically stimulated muscles, the relative complexity of FES systems, and the continued need for assistive devices and mechanical orthoses. [31, 38, 41, 44, 52, 85, 92] Moreover, like ambulation with mechanical orthoses, ambulation using FES has high energy requirements, making it a physically demanding activity. For these reasons, FES is not a viable alternative to wheelchairs for functional mobility for people with complete lesions.[17, 29, 31, 32, 40, 44, 63, 85] This is also true of hybrid systems that combine FES with RGOs.[36, 89]

FES has also been utilized to enhance ambulatory ability in people who have incomplete spinal cord injuries.[4, 5, 46, 104] Although the energy demands of FES-assisted walking for this population have yet to be determined, this intervention shows promise.

SUMMARY

- Walking is a skill that is of high priority to many patients because of its psychological and social significance. The high energy costs of ambulation with orthoses and assistive devices, however, make ambulation following spinal cord injury prohibitively difficult for many people.

- A person with a complete spinal cord injury who wishes to walk functionally must utilize assistive devices, lower extremity orthoses, and compensatory strategies for this activity. This chapter presents descriptions of lower extremity orthoses commonly used for people with spinal cord injuries, principles of orthotic prescription, and compensatory techniques that can be used for ambulation.

- The orthotic requirements and methods of ambulation possible for a person with an incomplete spinal cord injury will depend largely on the extent of motor sparing or return below her lesion. If she has little or no voluntary motor function below her lesion, she is likely to walk using orthoses and gait patterns similar to those used by people with complete injuries. If she has more significant motor function in her trunk and lower extremities, she

---

[v] The patients in this study all had some voluntary motor function in their lower extremities, including quadriceps function.
[w] FES is also called FNS, or functional neuromuscular stimulation.

may be able to walk with less orthotic support and with a more normal gait pattern.

- During rehabilitation, the therapist and patient work together to discover the movement strategies that will enable the patient to walk and perform other ambulation-related skills such as donning and doffing the orthoses and coming to stand. The therapeutic program then consists of activities directed at developing the strength, range of motion, and skill needed to perform these functional tasks. This chapter presents a variety of strategies for developing the skills involved.

- The therapist and patient should take appropriate precautions during gait training to prevent motion of unstable vertebrae, skin abrasions and pressure ulcers, and injury from falls.

References

Chapter 1

1. Atrice, M., Gonter, M., Griffin, D., Morrison, S., & McDowell, S. (1995). Traumatic spinal cord injury. In: D. Umphred (Ed.), *Neurological Rehabilitation*, 3rd ed. (pp. 484–532). St. Louis: Mosby.
2. Donovan, W.; Carter, R.; Bedbrook, G.; Young, J.; & Griffiths, E. (1984). Incidence of medical complications in spinal cord injury: patients in specialised, compared with non-specialised centres. *Paraplegia*, 22(5), 282–290.
3. Duncan, P. (1994). Stroke disability. *Physical Therapy*, 74(5), 300–407.
4. Guccione, A. (1991). Physical therapy diagnosis and the relationship between impairments and function. *Physical Therapy*, 71(7), 499–503.
5. Jette, A. (1994). Physical disablement concepts for physical therapy research and practice. *Physical Therapy*, 74(5), 380–386.
6. Marino, R. & Stineman, M. (1996). Functional assessment in spinal cord injury. *Topics in Spinal Cord Injury Rehabilitation*, 1(4), 32–45.
7. Nagi, S. (1991). Disability concepts revisited: implications for prevention. In: A. Pope & A. Tarlov (Eds.), *Disability in America: Toward a National Agenda for Prevention* (pp. 309–327). Washington, DC: National Academy Press.
8. Nagi, S. (1969). *Disability and Rehabilitation: Legal, Clinical, and Self-Concepts and Measurement*. Columbus, OH: Ohio State University Press.
9. Nagi, S. (1965). Some conceptual issues in disability and rehabilitation. In: M. Sussman (Ed.), *Sociology and Rehabilitation*. Washington, DC: American Sociological Association (pp. 100–113).
10. National Institutes of Health. (1993). *Research Plan for the National Center of Medical Rehabilitation Research*. (NIH Publication No. 93-3509). Washington, DC: U.S. Department of Health and Human Services.
11. Oakes, D.; Wilmot, C.; Hall, K.; & Sherck, J. (1990). Benefits of early admission to a comprehensive trauma center for patients with spinal cord injury. *Archives of Physical Medicine and Rehabilitation*, 71(9), 637–643.
12. Pope, A. & Tarlov, A. (Eds.). (1991). *Disability in America: Toward a National Agenda for Prevention*. Washington, DC: National Academy Press.
13. Rothstein, J. (Ed.). (1997). Guide to physical therapy practice. *Physical Therapy*, 77(11), 1163–1650.
14. Tator, C.; Duncan, E.; Edmonds, V.; Lapczak, L.; & Andrews, D. (1995). Neurological recovery, mortality and length of stay after acute spinal cord injury associated with changes in management. *Paraplegia*, 33, 254–262.

Chapter 2

1. Achong, M. (1986). Urinary tract infections in the patient with a neurogenic bladder. In: R. Bloch & M. Basbaum (Eds.), *Management of Spinal Cord Injuries* (pp. 164–179). Baltimore: Williams & Wilkins.
2. Allen, B. (1989). Recognition of injuries to the lower cervical spine. In: H. Sherk, E. Dunn, & F. Eismont (Eds.), *The Cervical Spine* (pp. 286–298). Philadelphia: J.B. Lippincott.
3. American Spinal Injury Association. (1989). *Standards for Neurological Classification of Spinal Injury Patients*. Chicago: American Spinal Injury Association.
4. American Spinal Injury Association. (2000). *International Standards for Neurological Classification of Spinal Cord Injury*. Chicago: American Spinal Injury Association. (Available from the American Spinal Injury Association, 2020 Peachtree Road NW, Atlanta, GA 30309 USA.)
5. Anderson, P. (1998). Spinal cord injury and lower cervical spine injuries. In: H. An (Ed.), *Principles and Techniques of Spine Surgery* (pp. 295–330). Baltimore: Williams & Wilkins.
6. Anson, C. & Shepherd, C. (1996). Incidence of secondary complications in spinal cord injury. *Inter-*

national Journal of Rehabilitation Research, 19(1), 55–66.

7. Anthes, D.; Theriault, E.; & Tator, C. (1996). Ultrastructural evidence for arteriolar vasospasm after spinal cord trauma. *Neurosurgery*, 39(4), 804–814.

8. Atkinson, P. & Atkinson, J. (1996). Spinal shock. *Mayo Clinic Proceedings*, 71(4), 384–389.

9. Balentine, J. (1988). Spinal cord trauma: In search of the meaning of granular axoplasm and vesicular myelin. *Journal of Neuropathology and Experimental Neurology*, 47(2), 77–92.

10. Banik, N.; Matzelle, D.; Gantt-Wilford, G.; Osborne, A.; & Hogan, E. (1997). Increased calpain content and progressive degradation of neurofilament protein in spinal cord injury. *Brain Research*, 752(1–2), 301–306.

11. Banik, N.; Shields, D.; Ray, S.; Davis, B.; Matzelle, D.; Wilford, G.; & Hogan, E. (1998). Role of calpain in spinal cord injury: effects of calpain and free radical inhibitors. *Annals of New York Academy of Sciences*, 844, 131–137.

12. Bauman, W.; Adkins, R.; Spungen, A.; Kemp, B.; & Waters, R. (1998). The effect of residual neurological deficit on serum lipoproteins in individuals with chronic spinal cord injury. *Spinal Cord*, 36(1), 13–17.

13. Bauman, W.; Garland, D.; & Schwartz, E. (1997). Calcium metabolism and osteoporosis in individuals with spinal cord injury. *Topics in Spinal Cord Injury Rehabilitation*, 2(4), 84–95.

14. Bauman, W.; Raza, M.; Spungen, A.; & Machac, J. (1994). Cardiac stress testing with thallium-201 imaging reveals silent ischemia in individuals with paraplegia. *Archives of Physical Medicine and Rehabilitation*, 75(9), 446–450.

15. Bauman, W.; Spungen, A.; Raza, M.; Rothstein, J. et al. (1992). Coronary artery disease: metabolic risk factors and latent disease in individuals with paraplegia. *Mount Sinai Journal of Medicine*, 59(2), 163–168.

16. Bedbrook, G. (1981). *The Care and Management of Spinal Cord Injuries*. New York: Springer-Verlag.

17. Berczeller, P., & Bezkor, M. (1986). *Medical Complications of Quadriplegia*. Chicago: Year Book Medical Publishers.

18. Beric, A., Dimitrijevic, M., & Light, J. (1987). A clinical syndrome of rostral and caudal spinal injury: neurological, neurophysiological and urodynamic evidence for occult sacral lesion. *Journal of Neurology, Neurosurgery, and Psychiatry*, 50, 600–606.

19. Berman, S.; Young, R.; Sarkarati, M.; & Shefner, J. (1996). Injury zone denervation in traumatic quadriplegia in humans. *Muscle and Nerve*, 19(6), 701–706.

20. Bethea, J.; Castro, M.; Keane, R.; Lee, T.; Dietrich, W.; & Yezierski, R. (1998). Traumatic spinal cord injury induces nuclear factor-kB activation. *Journal of Neuroscience*, 18(9), 3251–3260.

21. Bloch, R. (1986). Autonomic dysfunction. In: R. Bloch & M. Basbaum (Eds.), *Management of Spinal Cord Injuries* (pp. 149–163). Baltimore: Williams & Wilkins.

22. Bohlman, H., & Boada, E. (1989). Fractures and dislocations of the lower cervical spine. In: Sherk, H., Dunn, F., & Eismont, J. (Eds.), *The Cervical Spine* (2nd ed.). Philadelphia: J.B. Lippincott.

23. Braddom, R. & Rocco, J. (1991). Autonomic dysreflexia: a survey of current treatment. *American Journal of Physical Medicine and Rehabilitation*, 70(5), 234–241.

24. Buchanan, L. (1987). Emergency care. In: L. Buchanan & D. Nawoczenski (Eds.), *Spinal Cord Injury: Concepts and Management Approaches* (pp. 21–34). Baltimore: Williams & Wilkins.

25. Buchanan, L., & Ditunno, J. (1987). Acute care: medical/surgical management. In: L. Buchanan & D. Nawoczenski (Eds.), *Spinal Cord Injury: Concepts and Management Approaches* (pp. 35–60). Baltimore: Williams & Wilkins.

26. Bullock, B., & Rosendahl, P. (1988). *Pathophysiology: Adaptations and Alterations in Function* (2nd ed.). Boston: Scott, Foresman & Company.

27. Burt, A. (1993). *Textbook of Neuroanatomy*. Philadelphia: W. B. Saunders.

28. Cardenas, D.; Farrell-Roberts, L.; Sipski, M.; & Rubner, D. (1995). Management of gastrointestinal, genitourinary, and sexual function. In: S. Stover, J. De Lisa, & G. Whiteneck (Eds.), *Spinal Cord Injury: Clinical Outcomes from the Model Systems* (pp. 120–144). Gaithersburg, MD: Aspen.

29. Cardus, D.; Ribas-Cardus, F.; & McTaggart, W. (1992). Coronary risk in spinal cord injury: assessment following a multivariate approach. *Archives of Physical Medicine and Rehabilitation*, 73(10), 930–933.

30. Carlson, S.; Parrish, M.; Springer, J.; Doty, K.; & Dossett, L. (1998). Acute inflammatory response in spinal cord following impact injury. *Experimental Neurology*, 151(1), 77–88.

31. Choi, D., & Rothman, S. (1990). The role of glutamate neurotoxicity in hypoxic-ischemic neuronal death. *Annual Review of Neurosciences*, 13, 171–182.

32. Cohen, M.; Sheehan, T.; & Herbison, G. (1996). Content validity and reliability of the International Standards for Neurological Classification of Spinal Cord Injury. *Topics in Spinal Cord Injury Rehabilitation*, 1(4), 15–31.

33. Colachis, S. (1997). Autonomic hyperreflexia with spinal cord injury. *Topics in Spinal Cord Injury Rehabilitation*, 3(1), 71–81.

34. Cole, J. (1988). The pathophysiology of the autonomic nervous system in spinal cord injury. In: L. Illis (Ed.), *Spinal Cord Dysfunction: Assessment* (pp. 201–235). New York: Oxford University Press.

35. Consortium for Spinal Cord Medicine. (1997). *Spinal Cord Medicine Clinical Practice Guidelines: Prevention of Thromboembolism in Spinal Cord Injury*. Washington, DC: Paralyzed Veterans of America.

36. Consortium for Spinal Cord Medicine. (1998). *Spinal Cord Medicine Clinical Practice Guidelines: Neurogenic Bowel Management in Adults with Spinal Cord Injury*. Washington, DC: Paralyzed Veterans of America.

37. Consortium for Spinal Cord Medicine. (1998). *Spinal Cord Medicine Clinical Practice Guidelines: Acute Management of Autonomic Dysreflexia*. Washington, DC: Paralyzed Veterans of America.

38. Coogler, C. (1985). Clinical decision making among neurologic patients: spinal cord injury. In: S. Wolf (Ed.), *Clinical Decision Making in Physical Therapy* (pp. 149–170). Philadelphia: F.A. Davis.

39. Cook, P. (1988). Radiology of the spine and spinal cord injury. In: L. Illis (Ed.), *Spinal Cord Dysfunction: Assessment* (pp. 41–103). New York: Oxford University Press.

40. Cotman, C., & Nieto-Sampedro, M. (1985). Progress in facilitating the recovery of function after central nervous system trauma. *Annals of the New York Academy of Sciences*, 457, 83–104.

41. Crawford, P., & Shepherd, D. (1989). Hyperextension injuries to the cervical cord in the elderly. *British Medical Journal*, 299(6700), 669–670.

42. Crowell, R., Edwards, T., & White, A. (1989). Mechanisms of injury in the cervical spine: experimental evidence and biomechanical modeling. In: Sherk, H., Dunn, E., Eismont, F. (Eds.), *The Cervical Spine* (pp. 70–90). Philadelphia: J.B. Lippincott.

43. Curt, A.; Nitsche, B.; Rodic, B.; Schurch, B.; & Dietz, V. (1997). Assessment of autonomic dysreflexia in patients with spinal cord injury. *Journal of Neurology, Neurosurgery and Psychiatry*, 62(5), 473–477.

44. Dalyan, M.; Sherman, A.; & Cardenas, D. (1998). Factors associated with contractures in acute spinal cord injury. *Spinal Cord*, 36(6), 405–408.

45. da Paz, A.; Beraldo, P.; Almeida, M.; Neves, E.; Alves, C.; & Khan, P. (1992). Traumatic injury to the spinal cord: prevalence in Brazilian hospitals. *Paraplegia*, 30(9), 636–640.

46. Davis, G. (1993). Exercise capacity of individuals with paraplegia. *Medical Science in Sports and Exercise*, 25(4), 423–432.

47. Dearwater, S.; Laporte, R.; Robertson, R.; Brenes, G.; Adams, L.; & Becker, D. (1986). Activity in the spinal cord-injured patient: an epidemiologic analysis of metabolic parameters. *Medicine and Science in Sports and Exercise*, 18(5), 541–544.

48. deGroot, J., & Chusid, J. (1988). *Correlative Neuroanatomy* (20th ed.). East Norwalk, CT: Appleton & Lange.

49. De Looze, D.; Van Laere, M.; De Muynck, M.; Beke, R.; & Elewaut, A. (1998). Constipation and other chronic gastrointestinal problems in spinal cord injury patients. *Spinal Cord*, 36(1), 63–66.

50. Demediuk, P., Daly, M., & Faden, A. (1989). Effect of impact trauma on neurotransmitter and non-neurotransmitter amino acids in rat spinal cord. *Journal of Neurochemistry*, 52(5), 1529–1536.

51. Demirel, G.; Yilmaz, H.; Paker, N.; & Onel, S. (1998). Osteoporosis after spinal cord injury. *Spinal Cord*, 36(12), 822–825.

52. Denis, F. (1983). The three column spine and its significance in the classification of acute thoracolumbar spinal injuries. *Spine*, 8(8), 817–831.

53. Derenne, J.; Macklem P.; & Roussos, C. (1978). The respiratory muscles: mechanics, control, and pathophysiology, part III. *American Review of Respiratory Disease*, 118, 581–601.

54. DeVivo, M.; Black, K.; & Stover, S. (1993). Causes of death during the first 12 years after spinal cord injury. *Archives of Physical Medicine and Rehabilitation*, 74(3), 248–254.

55. DeVivo, M., Kartus, P., Stover, S., Rutt, R., & Fine, P. (1989). Cause of death for patients with spinal cord injuries. *Archives of Internal Medicine*, 149(8), 1761–1766.

56. DeVivo, M. & Stover, S. (1995). Long-term survival and causes of death. In: S. Stover, J. DeLisa, & G. Whiteneck (Eds.), *Spinal Cord Injury: Clinical Outcomes from the Model Systems* (pp. 289–316). Gaithersburg, MD: Aspen.

57. Dijkers, M. (1999). Spinal cord injury caused by interpersonal violence: epidemiologic data from the National Spinal Cord Injury Database. *Topics in Spinal Cord Injury Rehabilitation*, 4(3), 1–22.

58. Ditunno, J.; Cohen, M.; Formal, C.; & Whiteneck, G. (1995). Functional outcomes. In: S. Stover, J. DeLisa, & G. Whiteneck (Eds.), *Spinal Cord Injury: Clinical Outcomes from the Model Systems* (pp. 170–184). Gaithersburg, MD: Aspen.

59. Ditunno, J. & Formal, C. (1994). Chronic spinal cord injury. *New England Journal of Medicine*, 330(8), 550–556.

60. Ditunno, J.; Sipski, M.; Posuniak, E.; Chen, Y.; Staas, W.; & Herbison, G. (1987). Wrist extensor recovery in traumatic quadriplegia. *Archives of Physical Medicine and Rehabilitation*, 68(5), 287–290.

61. Ditunno, J.; Stover, S.; Freed, M.; & Ahn, J. (1992). Motor recovery of the upper extremities in traumatic quadriplegia: a multicenter study. *Archives of Physical Medicine and Rehabilitation*, 73(5), 431–436.

62. Eide, P. (1998). Pathophysiological mechanisms of central neuropathic pain after spinal cord injury. *Spinal Cord*, 36(9), 601–612.

63. Emery, E.; Aldana, P.; Bunge, M.; Puckett, W.; Srinivasan, A.; Keane, R.; Bethea, J.; & Levi, A. (1998). Apoptosis after traumatic human spinal cord injury. *Journal of Neurosurgery*, 89(6), 911–920.

64. Faden, A., & Simon, R. (1987). A potential role for excitotoxins in the pathophysiology of spinal cord injury. *Annals of Neurology*, 23(6), 623–626.

65. Farmer, J.; Vaccaro, A.; Albert, T.; Malone, S.; Balderston, R.; & Cotler, J. (1998). Neurologic deterioration after cervical spinal cord injury. *Journal of Spinal Disorders*, 11(3), 192–196.

66. Figoni, S. (1993). Exercise responses and quadriplegia. *Medicine and Science in Sports and Exercise* 25(4), 433–441.

67. Fine, P.; Kuhlemeier, K.; DeVivo, M.; & Stover, S. (1979). Spinal cord injury: an epidemiological perspective. *Paraplegia*, 17, 237–250.

68. Fredericks, C. (1996). Clinical presentations in disorders of motor function. In: C. Fredericks & L. Saladin (Eds.), *Pathophysiology of the Motor Systems: Principles and Clinical Presentations* (pp. 257–288). Philadelphia: F. A. Davis.

69. Fredericks, C. (1996). Disorders of the spinal cord. In: C. Fredericks & L. Saladin (Eds.), *Pathophysiology of the Motor Systems: Principles and Clinical Presentations* (pp. 394–423). Philadelphia: F. A. Davis.

70. Freebourn, T.; Barber, D.; & Able, A. (1999). The treatment of immature heterotopic ossification in spinal cord injury with combination surgery, radi-

ation therapy, and NSAID. *Spinal Cord*, 37(1), 50–53.

71. Frost, F. (1993). Role of rehabilitation after spinal cord injury. *Urologic Clinics of North America*, 20(3), 549–559.

72. Frost, F. (1998). Spinal cord injury: gastrointestinal implications and management. *Topics in Spinal Cord Injury Rehabilitation*, 4(2), 56–80.

73. Galli, R., Spaite, D., & Simon, R. (1989). *Emergency Orthopedics: The Spine*. Norwalk, CT: Appleton & Lange.

74. Gellman, H.; Sie, I.; & Waters, R. (1988). Late complications of the weight-bearing upper extremity in the paraplegic patient. *Clinical Orthopaedics and Related Research*, 233, 132–135.

75. Glenn, M. & Bergman, S. (1997). Cardiovascular changes following spinal cord injury. *Topics in Spinal Cord Injury Rehabilitation*, 2(4), 47–53.

76. Go, B.; DeVivo, M.; & Richards, J. (1995). The epidemiology of spinal cord injury. In: S. Stover, J. DeLisa, & G. Whiteneck (Eds.), *Spinal Cord Injury: Clinical Outcomes from the Model Systems* (pp. 21–55). Gaithersburg, MD: Aspen.

77. Graziani, V.; Crozier, K.; & Selby-Silverstein, L. (1996). Lower extremity function following spinal cord injury. *Topics in Spinal Cord Injury Rehabilitation*, 1(4), 46–55.

78. Grimm, D.; de Meersman, R.; Almenoff, P.; Spungen, A.; & Bauman, W. (1997). Sympathovagal balance of the heart in subjects with spinal cord injury. *American Journal of Physiology*, 272(2 Pt. 2), H835–H842.

79. Hall, M.; Hackler, R.; Zampieri, T.; & Zampieri, J. (1989). Renal calculi in spinal cord-injured patient: association with reflux, bladder stones, and Foley catheter drainage. *Urology*, 34(4), 126–128.

80. Harris, J.; Edeiken-Monroe, B.; Kopaniky, D. (1986). A practical classification of acute cervical spine injuries. *Orthopedic Clinics of North America*, 17(1), 15–30.

81. Hooker, S. & Wells, C. (1989). Effect of low- and moderate- intensity training in spinal cord-injured persons. *Medicine and Science in Sports and Exercise*, 21(1), 18–22.

82. Hopman, M.; Oeseburg, B.; & Binkhorst, R. (1992). Cardiovascular responses in paraplegic subjects during arm exercise. *European Journal of Applied Physiology*, 65(1), 73–78.

83. Hughes, J. (1988). Pathological changes after spinal cord injury. In: L. Illis (Ed.), *Spinal Cord Dysfunction: Assessment* (pp. 34–40). New York: Oxford University Press.

84. Iizuka, H.; Yamamoto, H.; Iwasaki, Y.; Yamamoto, T.; & Konno, H. (1987). Evolution of tissue damage in compressive spinal cord injury in rats. *Journal of Neurosurgery*, 66(4), 595–603.

85. Illis, L. (1988). Clinical evaluation and pathophysiology of the spinal cord in the chronic stage. In: L. Illis (Ed.), *Spinal Cord Dysfunction: Assessment* (pp. 107–128). New York: Oxford University Press.

86. Imai, K.; Kadowaki, T.; Aizawa, Y.; & Fukutomi, K. (1994). Morbidity rates of complications in persons with spinal cord injury according to the site of injury and with special reference to hypertension. *Paraplegia*, 32(4), 246–252.

87. Isaac, L. & Pejic, L. (1995). Secondary mechanisms of spinal cord injury. *Surgical Neurology*, 43(5), 484–485.

88. Jacobs, S.; Yeaney, N.; Herbison, G.; & Ditunno, J. (1995). Future ambulation prognosis as predicted by somatosensory evoked potentials in motor complete and incomplete quadriplegia. *Archives of Physical Medicine and Rehabilitation*, 76, 635–641.

89. Johnson, R.; Gerhart, A.; McCray, J.; Menconi, J.; & Whiteneck, G. (1998). Secondary conditions following spinal cord injury in a population-based sample. *Spinal Cord*, 36 (1), 45–50.

90. Kannisto, M.; Alaranta, H.; Merikanto, J.; Kroger, H.; & Karkkainen, J. (1998). Bone mineral status after pediatric spinal cord injury. *Spinal Cord*, 36, 641–646.

91. Kennedy, E., Stover, S., & Fine, P. (Eds). (1986). *Spinal Cord Injury: The Facts and Figures*. Birmingham, AL: The University of Alabama Spinal Cord Injury Statistical Center.

92. Kessler, K.; Pina, I.; Green, B.; Burnett, B.; Laighold, M.; Bilsker, M.; Palomo, A.; & Myerburg, R. (1986). Cardiovascular findings in quadriplegic and paraplegic patients and in normal subjects. *American Journal of Cardiology*, 58(6), 525–530.

93. Kim, N.; Lee, H.; & Chun, I. (1999). Neurologic injury and recovery in patients with burst fracture of the thoracolumbar spine. *Spine*, 24(3), 290–293.

94. King, M.; Lichtman, S.; Pellicone, J.; Close, R.; & Lisanti, P. (1994). Exertional hypotension in spinal cord injury. *Chest*, 106(4), 1166–1171.

95. Kiwerski, J. (1993). Factors contributing to the increased threat to life following spinal cord injury. *Paraplegia*, 31(12), 793–799.

96. Knutsdottir, S. (1993). Spinal cord injuries in Iceland 1973–1989. A follow up study. *Paraplegia*, 31(1), 68–72.

97. Kocina, P. (1997). Body composition of spinal cord injured adults. *Sports Medicine*, 23(1), 48–60.

98. Lal, S.; Hamilton, B.; Heinemann, A.; & Betts, H. (1989). Risk factors for heterotopic ossification in spinal cord injury. *Archives of Physical Medicine and Rehabilitation*, 70(5), 387–390.

99. Leybaert, L. & de Hemptinne, A. (1996). Changes in intracellular free calcium following mechanical injury in a spinal cord slice preparation. *Experimental Brain Research*, 112(3), 392–402.

100. Lehmann, K.; Lane, J.; Piepmeier, J.; & Batsford, W. (1987). Cardiovascular abnormalities accompanying acute spinal cord injury in humans: incidence, time course and severity. *Journal of the American College of Cardiology*, 10(1), 46–52.

101. Levi, R.; Hultling, C.; & Seiger, A. (1995). The Stockholm spinal cord injury study: 2. Associations between clinical patient characteristics and post-acute medical problems. *Paraplegia*, 33(10), 585–594.

102. Little, J.; Ditunno, J.; Stiens, S.; & Harris, R. (1999). Incomplete spinal cord injury: neuronal mechanisms of motor recovery and hyperreflexia. *Archives of Physical Medicine and Rehabilitation*, 80(5), 587–599.

103. Little, J.; Micklesen, P.; Umlauf, R.; & Britell, C. (1989). Lower extremity manifestations of spastic-

ity in chronic spinal cord injury. *American Journal of Physical Medicine and Rehabilitation*, 68(1), 32–36.

104. Lou, J.; Lenke, L.; Ludwig, F.; & O'Brien, M. (1998). Apoptosis as a mechanism of neuronal cell death following acute experimental spinal cord injury. *Spinal Cord*, 36(10), 683–690.

105. Lu, W.; Rhoney, D.; Boling, W.; Johnson, J.; & Smith, T. (1997). A review of stress ulcer prophylaxis in the neurosurgical intensive care unit. *Neurosurgery*, 41(2), 416–426.

106. Mackenzie, C. & Ducker, T. (1986). Cervical spinal cord injury. In: J. Matjasko & J. Katz (Eds.), *Clinical Controversies in Neuroanesthesia and Neurosurgery* (pp. 77–134). New York: Grune & Stratton.

107. Mange, K.; Ditunno, J.; Herbison, G.; & Jaweed, M. (1990). Recovery of strength at the zone of injury in motor complete and motor incomplete cervical spinal cord injured patients. *Archives of Physical Medicine and Rehabilitation*, 71(8), 562–565.

108. Marieb, E. (1995). *Human Anatomy and Physiology* (3rd ed.). Redwood City, CA: Benjamin/Cummings.

109. Martini, F. (1998). *Fundamentals of Anatomy and Physiology* (4th ed.). Upper Saddle River, NJ: Prentice Hall.

110. Mayer, N. (1997). Clinicophysiologic concepts of spasticity and motor dysfunction in adults with an upper motoneuron lesion. *Muscle and Nerve*, 20(Suppl. 6), S1–S13.

111. Maynard, F.; Karunas, R.; Adkins, R.; Richards, J.; & Waring, W. (1995). Management of the neuromusculoskeletal systems. In: S. Stover, J. DeLisa, & G. Whiteneck (Eds.), *Spinal Cord Injury: Clinical Outcomes from the Model Systems* (pp. 145–169). Gaithersburg, MD: Aspen.

112. Maynard, F.; Karunas, R.; & Waring, W. (1990). Epidemiology of spasticity following traumatic spinal cord injury. *Archives of Physical Medicine and Rehabilitation*, 71(8), 566–569.

113. McCagg, C. (1986). Postoperative management and acute rehabilitation of patients with spinal cord injuries. *Orthopedic Clinics of North America*, 17(1), 171–182.

114. McCullen, G.; Yuan, H.; & Fredrickson, B. (1998). Thoracolumbar spine injuries. In: H. An (Ed.), *Principles and Techniques of Spine Surgery* (pp. 359–384). Baltimore: Williams & Wilkins.

115. McGuire, T. & Kumar, N. (1986). Autonomic dysreflexia in the spinal cord-injured: what the physician should know about this medical emergency. *Postgraduate Medicine*, 80(2), 81–89.

116. McLeod, J., & Lance, J. (1989). *Introductory Neurology* (3rd ed.). Boston: Blackwell Scientific Publications.

117. McQueen, J. & Khan, M. (1989). Evaluation of patients with cervical spine lesions. In: Sherk, H., Dunn, E., & Eismont, F. (Eds.), *The Cervical Spine* (pp. 199–211). Philadelphia: J.B. Lippincott.

118. Meyer, P. (Ed.). (1989). *Surgery of Spine Trauma*. New York: Churchill Livingstone.

119. Meyer, P. & Heim, S. (1989). Surgical stabilization of the cervical spine. In: P. Meyer (Ed.), *Surgery of Spine Trauma* (pp. 397–523). New York: Churchill Livingstone.

120. Moore, D. (1998). Helping your patients with spasticity reach maximal function. *Postgraduate Medicine*, 104(2), 123–135.

121. Morgan, M.; Silver, J.; & Williams, S. (1986). The respiratory system of the spinal cord patient. In: R. Bloch & M. Basbaum (Eds.), *Management of Spinal Cord Injuries* (pp. 78–116). Baltimore: Williams & Wilkins.

122. Nakajima, A.; Honda, S.; Yoshimura, S.; Ono, Y.; Kawamura, J.; & Moriai, N. (1989). The disease pattern and causes of death of spinal cord injured patients in Japan. *Paraplegia*, 27(3), 163–171.

123. Nash, M. (1998). Exercise reconditioning of the heart and peripheral circulation after spinal cord injury. *Topics in Spinal Cord Injury Rehabilitation*, 3(3), 1–15.

124. Naso, F. (1992). Cardiovascular problems in patients with spinal cord injury. *Physical Medicine and Rehabilitation Clinics in North America*, 3(4), 741–749.

125. National Spinal Cord Injury Statistical Center. (1999). Spinal Cord Injury: Facts and Figures at a Glance. Available from: www.spinalcord.uab.edu/docs/factsfig.htm.

126. Nitsche, B.; Perschak, H.; Curt, A.; & Dietz, V. (1996). Loss of circadian blood pressure variability in complete tetraplegia. *Journal of Human Hypertension*, 10(5), 311–317.

127. Nobunaga, A. (1998). Orthostatic hypotension in spinal cord injury. *Topics in Spinal Cord Injury Rehabilitation*, 4(1), 73–80.

128. Northrup, B. & Alderman, J. (1989). Nonsurgical treatment. In: Sherk, H., Dunn, E., & Eismont, F. (Eds.), *The Cervical Spine* (2nd ed.). Philadelphia: J.B. Lippincott.

129. O'Brien, M.; Lenke, L.; Lou, J.; Bridwell, K.; & Joyce, M. (1994). Astrocyte response and transforming growth factor-beta localization in acute spinal cord injury. *Spine*, 19(20), 2321–2329.

130. Pang, D. & Pollack, I. (1989). Spinal cord injury without radiologic abnormality in children—the SCIWORA syndrome. *Journal of Trauma*, 29(5), 654–664.

131. Paynton, A.; O' Farrell, D.; Shannon, F.; Murray, P.; McManus, F.; & Walsh, M. (1997). Sparing of sensation of pin prick predicts recovery of motor segment after injury to the spinal cord. *Journal of Bone and Joint Surgery* (British), 79(6), 952–954.

132. Pentland, W. & Twomey, L. (1994). Upper limb function in persons with long term paraplegia and implications for independence: Part I. *Paraplegia*, 32(4), 211–218.

133. Peterson, D., & Altman, K. (1989). Central cervical spinal cord syndrome due to minor hyperextension injury. *Western Journal of Medicine*, 150(6), 691–694.

134. Phillips, W.; Kiralti, B.; Sarkarati, M.; Weraarchakul, G.; Meyers, J.; Franklin, B.; Parkash, I.; & Froelicher, V. (1998). Effect of spinal cord injury on the heart and cardiovascular fitness. *Current Problems in Cardiology*, 23(11), 649–716.

135. Piepmeier, J. & Jenkins, R. (1988). Late neurological changes following traumatic spinal cord injury. *Journal of Neurosurgery*, 69, 399–402.

136. Ragnarsson, K; Hall, K.; Wilmot, C.; & Carter, E. (1995). Management of pulmonary, cardiovascular, and metabolic conditions after spinal cord injury. In: S. Stover, J. De Lisa, & G. Whiteneck (Eds.), *Spinal Cord Injury: Clinical Outcomes from the Model Systems* (pp. 79–99). Gaithersburg, MD: Aspen.

137. Rasmussen, P.; Rabin, M.; Mann, D.; Perl, J.; Lorenz, J.; & Vrbos, L. (1994). Reduced transverse spinal area secondary to burst fractures: is there a relationship to neurologic injury? *Journal of Neurotrauma*, 11(6), 711–720.

138. Rieser, T., Mudiyam, R., & Waters, R. (1985). Orthopedic evaluation of spinal cord injury and management of vertebral fractures. In: H. Adkins (Ed.), *Spinal Cord Injury* (pp. 1–35). New York: Churchill Livingstone.

139. Roberts, D.; Lee, W.; Cuneo, R.; Wittmann, J.; Ward, G.; Flatman, R.; McWhinney, B.; & Hickman, P. (1998). Longitudinal study of bone turnover after acute spinal cord injury. *Journal of Clinical Endocrinology and Metabolism*, 83(2), 415–422.

140. Robinson, C.; Kett, N.; & Bolam, J. (1988). Spasticity in spinal cord injured patients: 2. Initial measures and long-term effects of surface electrical stimulation. *Archives of Physical Medicine and Rehabilitation*, 69(10), 862–868.

141. Rodriguez, G.; Claus-Walker, J.; Kent, M.;, & Garza, H. (1989). Collagen metabolite excretion as a predictor of bone- and skin-related complications in spinal cord injury. *Archives of Physical Medicine and Rehabilitation*, 70(6), 442–444.

142. Rogers, L. (1989). Radiologic assessment of acute neurologic and vertebral injuries. In: P. Meyer (Ed.), *Surgery of Spine Trauma* (pp. 185–263). New York: Churchill Livingstone.

143. Rosse, C. & Gaddum-Rosse, P. (1997). *Hollinshead's Textbook of Anatomy* (5th ed.). Philadelphia: Lippincott/Raven.

144. Roth, E.; Lawler, M.; & Yarkony, G. (1990). Traumatic central cord syndrome: clinical features and functional outcomes. *Archives of Physical Medicine and Rehabilitation*, 71(1), 18–23.

145. Roth, E.; Park, T.; Pang, T.; Yarkony, G.; & Lee, M. (1991). Traumatic cervical Brown-Séquard and Brown-Séquard-plus syndromes: the spectrum of presentations and outcomes. *Paraplegia*, 29, 582–589.

146. Seaton, T. & Hollingworth, R. (1986). Gastrointestinal complications in spinal cord injuries. In: R. Bloch & M. Basbaum (Eds.), *Management of Spinal Cord Injuries* (pp. 134–148). Baltimore: Williams & Wilkins.

147. Shackelford, M; Farley, T.; & Vines, C. (1998). A comparison of women and men with spinal cord injury. *Spinal Cord*, 36(5), 337–339.

148. Shuman, S.; Bresnahan, J.; & Beattie, M. (1997). Apoptosis of microglia and oligodendrocytes after spinal cord contusion in rats. *Journal of Neuroscience Research*, 50(5), 798–808.

149. Sie, I.; Waters, R.; Adkins, R.; & Gellman, H. (1992). Upper extremity pain in the postrehabilitation spinal cord injured patient. *Archives of Physical Medicine and Rehabilitation*, 73(1), 44–48.

150. Silfverskiold, J. & Waters, R. (1991). Shoulder pain and functional disability in spinal cord injury patients. *Clinical Orthopaedics and Related Research*, 272, 141–145.

151. Soderstrom, G. & Ducker, T. (1985). Increased susceptibility of patients with cervical cord lesions to peptic gastrointestinal complications. *Journal of Trauma*, 25(11), 1030–1038.

152. Springer, J.; Azbill, R.; Mark, R.; Begley, J.; Waeg, G.; & Mattson, M. (1997). 4-Hydroxynonenal, a lipid peroxidation product, rapidly accumulates following traumatic spinal cord injury and inhibits glutamate uptake. *Journal of Neurochemistry*, 68(6), 2469–2476.

153. Stein, A.; Pomerantz, F.; & Schechtman, J. (1997). Evaluation and management of spasticity in spinal cord injury. *Topics in Spinal Cord Injury Rehabilitation*, 2(4), 70–83.

154. Stjernberg, L., Blumberg, H., & Wallin, G. (1986). Sympathetic activity in man after spinal cord injury. *Brain*, 109, 695–715.

155. Stys, P. (1998). Anoxic and ischemic injury of myelinated axons in CNS white matter: from mechanistic concepts to therapeutics. *Journal of Cerebral Blood Flow and Metabolism*, 18(1), 2–25.

156. Szollar, S.; Martin, E.; Sartoris, D.; Parthemore, J.; & Deftos, L. (1998). Bone mineral density and indexes of bone metabolism in spinal cord injury. *American Journal of Physical Medicine and Rehabilitation*, 77(1), 28–35.

157. Tator, C. (1998). Biology of neurological recovery and functional restoration after spinal cord injury. *Neurosurgery*, 42(4), 696–707.

158. Tator, C. & Fehlings, M. (1991). Review of the secondary injury theory of acute spinal cord trauma with emphasis on vascular mechanisms. *Journal of Neurosurgery*, 75, 15–26.

159. Tator, C. & Koyangi, I. (1997). Vascular mechanisms in the pathophysiology of human spinal cord injury. *Journal of Neurosurgery*, 86(3), 483–492.

160. Thelan, L.; Davie, J.; & Urden, L. (1990). *Textbook of Critical Care Nursing: Diagnosis and Management*. Baltimore: C.V. Mosby.

161. Turpie, A. (1986). Thrombosis prevention and treatment in spinal cord injured patients. In: R. Bloch & M. Basbaum (Eds.), *Management of Spinal Cord Injuries* (pp. 212–240). Baltimore: Williams & Wilkins.

162. Vapnek, J. (1997). Autonomic dysreflexia. *Topics in Spinal Cord Injury Rehabilitation*, 2(4), 54–69.

163. Wang, A.; Jaeger, R.; Yarkony, G.; & Turba, R. (1997). Cough in spinal cord injured patients: the relationship between motor level and peak expiratory flow. *Spinal Cord*, 35(5), 299–302.

164. Waring, W. & Karunas, R. (1991). Acute spinal cord injuries and the incidence of clinically occurring thromboembolic disease. *Paraplegia*, 29(1), 8–16.

165. Washburn, R. & Figoni, S. (1998). Physical activity and chronic cardiovascular disease prevention in spinal cord injury: a comprehensive literature review. *Topics in Spinal Cord Injury Rehabilitation*, 3(3), 16–32.

166. Waters, R.; Adkins, R.; Yakura, J.; & Sie, I. (1994). Motor and sensory recovery following incomplete

paraplegia. *Archives of Physical Medicine and Rehabilitation*, 75, 67–72.

167. Waters, R.; Adkins, R.; Yakura, J.; & Sie, I. (1994). Motor and sensory recovery following incomplete tetraplegia. *Archives of Physical Medicine and Rehabilitation*, 75, 306–311.

168. Waters, R.; Sie, I.; Adkins, R.; & Yakura, J. (1999). The neuropathology of violence-induced spinal cord injury. *Topics in Spinal Cord Injury Rehabilitation*, 4(5), 23–28.

169. Waters, R.; Sie, I.; Adkins, R.; & Yakura, J. (1995). Injury pattern effect on motor recovery after traumatic spinal cord injury. *Archives of Physical Medicine and Rehabilitation*, 76(5), 440–443.

170. Waxman, S. (1989). Demyelination in spinal cord injury. *Journal of Neurological Sciences*, 91(1–2), 1–14.

171. Weaver, L.; Cassam, A.; Krassioukov, A.; & Llewellyn-Smith, I. (1997). Changes in immunoreactivity for growth associated protein-43 suggest reorganization of synapses on spinal sympathetic neurons after cord transection. *Neuroscience*, 81(2), 535–551.

172. Widerstrom-Noga, E.; Felipe-Cuervo, E.; Broton, J.; Duncan, R.; & Yezierski, R. (1999). Perceived difficulty in dealing with consequences of spinal cord injury. *Archives of Physical Medicine and Rehabilitation*, 80(5), 580–586.

173. Wu, L.; Marino, R.; Herbison, G.; & Ditunno, J. (1992). Recovery of zero-grade muscles in the zone of partial preservation in motor complete quadriplegia. *Archives of Physical Medicine and Rehabilitation*, 73, 40–43.

174. Wynsberghe, D.; Noback, C.; & Carola, R. (1995). *Human Anatomy and Physiology* (3rd ed.). New York: McGraw-Hill.

175. Yanase, M.; Sakou, T.; & Fukuda, T. (1995). Role of N-methyl-D-aspartate receptor in acute spinal cord injury. *Journal of Neurosurgery*, 83(5), 884–888.

176. Yarkony, G. & Heinemann, A. (1995). Pressure ulcers. In: S. Stover, J. De Lisa & G. Whiteneck (Eds.), *Spinal Cord Injury: Clinical Outcomes from the Model Systems* (pp. 100–119). Gaithersburg, MD: Aspen.

177. Yashon, D. (1986). *Spinal Injury* (2nd ed.). Norwalk, CT: Appleton Century Crofts.

178. Yekutiel, M.; Brooks, M.; Ohry, A.; Yarom, J.; & Carel, R. (1989). The prevalence of hypertension, ischemic heart disease and diabetes in traumatic spinal cord injured patients and amputees. *Paraplegia*, 27(1), 58–62.

179. Young, J., Burns, P., Bowen, A., & McCutchen, R. (1982). *Spinal Cord Injury Statistics: Experience of the Regional Spinal Cord Injury Systems*. Phoenix, AZ: Good Samaritan Medical Center.

180. Young, R. & Shahani, B. (1986). Spasticity in spinal cord injured patients. In: R. Bloch & M. Basbaum (Eds.), *Management of Spinal Cord Injuries* (pp. 241–283). Baltimore: Williams & Wilkins.

181. Young, W. (1993). Secondary injury mechanisms in acute spinal cord injury. *Journal of Emergency Medicine*, 11 (Suppl. 1), 13–22.

182. Young, W. & Ransohoff, J. (1989). Acute spinal cord injuries: experimental therapy, pathophysiological mechanisms, and recovery of function. In: Sherk, H., Dunn, E., & Eismont, F. (Eds.), *The Cervical Spine* (2nd ed., pp. 464–495). Philadelphia: J.B. Lippincott.

183. Zhang, Z.; Krebs, C.; & Guth, L. (1997). Experimental analysis of progressive necrosis after spinal cord trauma in the rat: etiological role of the inflammatory response. *Experimental Neurology*, 143(1), 141–152.

184. Zhang, Z. & Guth, L. (1997). Experimental spinal cord injury: Wallerian degeneration in the dorsal column is followed by revascularization, glial proliferation, and nerve regeneration. *Experimental Neurology*, 147(1), 159–171.

185. Zhang, Z.; Guth, L.; & Steward, O. (1998). Mechanisms of motor recovery after subtotal spinal cord injury: insights from the study of mice carrying a mutation (Wld^s) that delays cellular responses to injury. *Experimental Neurology*, 149(1), 221–229.

186. Zhou, G.; Yu, J.; Tang, H.; & Shi, J. (1997). The determination of vasoactive substances during autonomic dysreflexia. *Spinal Cord*, 35(6), 390–393.

Chapter 3

1. American Spinal Injury Association. (2000). *International Standards for Neurological Classification of Spinal Cord Injury*. Chicago, IL: American Spinal Injury Association.

2. Askins, V. & Eismont, J. (1997). Efficacy of five cervical orthoses in restricting cervical motion: A comparison study. *Spine*, 22(11), 1193–1198.

3. Aung, T. & El Masry, W. (1997). Audit of a British centre for spinal injury. *Spinal Cord*, 35(3), 147–150.

4. Axelsson, P.; Johnsson, R.; & Stromqvist, B. (1993). Lumbar orthosis with unilateral hip immobilization. Effect on intervertebral mobility determined by roentgen stereophotogrammetric analysis. *Spine*, 18(7), 876–879.

5. Azouvi, P.; Mane, M.; Thiebaut, J.; Denys, P; Remy-Neris, O.; & Bussel, B. (1996). Intrathecal baclofen administration for control of severe spinal spasticity: functional improvement and long-term follow-up. *Archives of Physical Medicine and Rehabilitation*, 77(1), 35–39.

6. Banovac, K. & Gonzalez, F. (1997). Evaluation and management of heterotopic ossification in patients with spinal cord injury. *Spinal Cord*, 35(3), 158–162.

7. Barker, E. & Higgins, R. (1989). Managing a suspected spinal cord injury. *Nursing*, 19(4), 52–59.

8. Barker, E. & Higgins, R. (1989). Rescuing an SCI victim from a pool. *Nursing*, 19(5), 58–64.

9. Barstow, T.; Scremin, E.; Mutton, D.; Kunkel, C.; Cagle, T.; & Whipp, B. (1996). Changes in gas exchange kinetics with training in patients with spinal cord injury. *Medicine and Science in Sports and Exercise*, 28(10), 1221–1228.

10. Bauman, W.; Garland, D.; & Schwartz, E. (1997). Calcium metabolism and osteoporosis in individuals with spinal cord injury. *Topics in Spinal Cord Injury Rehabilitation*, 2(4), 84–95.

11. Bauman, W.; Spungen, A.; Raza, M.; Rothstein, J.; Zhang, R.; Zhong, Y. et al. (1992). Coronary artery disease: metabolic risk factors and latent disease in individuals with paraplegia. *Mount Sinai Medical Journal*, 59(2), 163–168.

12. BeDell, K.; Scremin, E.; Perell, K.; & Kunkel, C. (1996). Effects of functional electrical stimulation-induced lower extremity cycling on bone density of spinal cord-injured patients. *American Journal of Physical Medicine and Rehabilitation*, 29–34.

13. Benzel, E. & Doezema, D. (1996). Prehospital management of the spinally injured patient. In: R. Narayan, J. Wilberger, & J. Povlishock (Eds.), *Neurotrauma* (pp. 1113–1120). New York: McGraw-Hill.

14. Benzel, E.; Hadden, T.; & Saulsbery, C. (1989). A comparison of the Minerva and halo jackets for stabilization of the cervical spine. *Journal of Neurosurgery*, 70, 411–414.

15. Bloch, R. (1986). Autonomic dysfunction. In: R. Bloch & M. Basbaum (Eds.), *Management of Spinal Cord Injuries* (pp. 149–163). Baltimore: Williams & Wilkins.

16. Bloomfield, S.; Mysiw, W.; & Jackson, R. (1996). Bone mass and endocrine adaptations to training in spinal cord injured individuals. *Bone*, 19(1), 61–68.

17. Botel, U.; Glaser, E.; & Niedeggen, A. (1997). The surgical treatment of acute spinal paralysed patients. *Spinal Cord*, 35(7), 420–428.

18. Botte, M.; Byrne, T.; Abrams, R.; & Garfin, S. (1995). The halo skeletal fixator: current concepts of application and maintenance. *Orthopedics*, 18(5), 463–471.

19. Botte, M.; Garfin, S.; Byrne, T.; Woo, S.; & Nickel, V. (1989). The halo skeletal fixator: principles of application and maintenance. *Clinical Orthopedics and Related Research*, 239, 12–18.

20. Bracken, M. (1992). Pharmacological treatment of acute spinal cord injury: current status and future prospects. *Paraplegia*, 30(2), 102–107.

21. Bracken, M. & Holford, T. (1993). Effects of timing of methylprednisolone or naloxone administration on recovery of segmental and long-tract neurological function in NASCIS 2. *Journal of Neurosurgery*, 79(4), 500–507.

22. Bracken, M.; Shepard, M.; Collins, W.; Holford, T.; Young, W.; Baskin, D. et al. (1990). A randomized, controlled trial of methylprednisolone or naloxone in the treatment of acute spinal-cord injury. *New England Journal of Medicine*, 322(20), 1405–1411.

23. Bracken, M.; Shepherd, M.; Holford, T.; Leo-Summers, L.; Aldrich, E.; Fazi, M. et al. (1997). Administration of methylprednisolone for 24 hours or 48 hours or tirilazad mesylate for 48 hours in the treatment of acute spinal cord injury. *Journal of the American Medical Association*, 277(20), 1597–1604.

24. Braddom, R. & Rocco, J. (1991). Autonomic dysreflexia: a survey of current treatment. *American Journal of Physical Medicine and Rehabilitation*, 70(5), 234–241.

25. Bradford, D. & McBride, G. (1987). Surgical management of thoracolumbar spine fractures with incomplete neurologic deficits. *Clinical Orthopaedics and Related Research*, 218, 201–216.

26. Bregman, B.; Kunkel-Bagden, E.; Schnell, L.; Dal, H.; Gao, D.; & Schwab, M. (1995). Recovery from spinal cord injury mediated by antibodies to neurite growth inhibitors. *Nature*, 378(6556), 498–501.

27. Brown, C. & Chow, G. (1997). Orthoses for spinal trauma and postoperative care. In: B. Goldberg & J. Hsu (Eds.), *Atlas of Assistive Devices* (3rd ed., pp. 251–258). St. Louis: Mosby.

28. Brunette, D. & Rockswold, G. (1987). Neurologic recovery following rapid spinal realignment for complete cervical spinal cord injury. *Journal of Trauma*, 27(4), 445–447.

29. Bucci, M.; Dauser, R.; Maynard, F.; & Hoff, J. (1988). Management of post-traumatic cervical spine instability: operative fusion versus halo vest immobilization: an analysis of 49 cases. *Journal of Trauma*, 28(7), 1001–1006.

30. Buchanan, L., & Ditunno, J. (1987). Acute care: medical/surgical management. In: L. Buchanan & D. Nawoczenski (Eds.), *Spinal Cord Injury: Concepts and Management Approaches* (pp. 35–60). Baltimore: Williams & Wilkins.

31. Capen, D. (1998). Emergency management of spine trauma. In: D. Capen & W. Haye (Eds.), *Comprehensive Management of Spine Trauma* (pp. 33–38). Saint Louis: Mosby.

32. Carvell, J. & Grundy, D. (1994). Complications of spinal surgery in acute spinal cord injury. *Paraplegia*, 32(6), 389–395.

33. Castillo, R. & Bell, J. (1988). Cervical spine injury: stabilization and management. *Postgraduate Medicine*, 83(7), 131–138.

34. Chase, T. (1996). Physical fitness strategies. In: I. Lanig, T. Chase, L. Butt, K. Hulse, & K. Johnson (Eds.), *A Practical Guide to Health Promotion After Spinal Cord Injury* (pp. 243–291). Gaithersburg, MD: Aspen.

35. Chen, T.; Lee, S.; Lui, T.; Wong, C.; Yeh, Y.; Tzaan, W.; & Hung, S. (1997). Efficacy of surgical treatment in traumatic central cord syndrome. *Surgical Neurology*, 48(5), 435–441.

36. Cheng, H.; Cao, Y.; & Olson, L. (1996). Spinal cord repair in adult paraplegic rats: partial restoration of hind limb function. *Science*, 273(5274), 510–513.

37. Chesnut, R. (1996). Emergency management of spinal cord injury. In: R. Narayan, J. Wilberger & J. Povlishock (Eds.), *Neurotrauma* (pp. 1121–1138). New York: McGraw-Hill.

38. Consortium for Spinal Cord Medicine. (1997). *Clinical Practice Guidelines: Acute Management of Autonomic Dysreflexia: Adults with Spinal Cord Injury Presenting to Health-Care Facilities*. Washington, DC: Paralyzed Veterans of America.

39. Consortium for Spinal Cord Medicine. (1997). *Clinical Practice Guidelines: Prevention of Thromboembolism in Spinal Cord Injury*. Washington, DC: Paralyzed Veterans of America.

40. Cook, P. (1988). Radiology of spine and spinal cord injury. In: L. Illis (Ed.), *Spinal Cord Dysfunction: Assessment* (pp. 41–103). New York: Oxford University Press.

41. Cooper, P. (1996). Use of lateral mass plates for stabilization of the lower cervical spine. In: R. Fessler & R. Haid (Eds.), *Current Techniques in Spinal Stabilization* (pp. 129–138). New York: McGraw-Hill.

42. Cowell, L.; Squires, W.; & Raven, P. (1986). Benefits of aerobic exercise for the paraplegic: a brief review. *Medicine and Science in Sports and Exercise*, 18(5), 501–508.

43. Crum, N. (1990). Signs of temporomandibular joint dysfunction in spinal cord injured patients wearing halo braces: a clinical report. *Physical Therapy*, 70(2), 132–137.

44. Curry, K. & Casady, L. (1992). The relationship between extended periods of immobility and decubitus ulcer formation in the acutely spinal cord-injured individual. *Journal of Neuroscience Nursing*, 24(4), 185–189.

45. Dalyan, M.; Sherman, A.; & Cardenas, D. (1998). Factors associated with contractures in acute spinal cord injury. *Spinal Cord*, 36(6), 405–408.

46. de Bruin, E.; Frey-Rindova, F.; Herzog, R.; Dietz, V.; Dambacher, M.; & Stussi, E. (1999). Changes of tibia bone properties after spinal cord injury: effects of early intervention. *Archives of Physical Medicine and Rehabilitation*, 80(2), 214–220.

47. Denis, F. (1983). The three column spine and its significance in the classification of acute thoracolumbar spinal injuries. *Spine*, 8(8), 817–831.

48. De Vivo, M.; Black, K.; & Stover, S. (1993). Causes of death during the first twelve years after spinal cord injury. *Archives of Physical Medicine and Rehabilitation*, 74(3), 248–254.

49. De Vivo, M. & Stover, S. (1995). Long-term survival and causes of death. In: S. Stover, J. De Lisa & G. Whiteneck (Eds.), *Spinal Cord Injury: Clinical Outcomes from the Model Systems* (pp. 289–316). Gaithersburg, MD: Aspen.

50. DeVivo, M.; Kartus, P.; Stover, S.; & Fine, P. (1990). Benefits of early admission to an organized spinal cord injury care system. *Paraplegia*, 28(9), 545–555.

51. DiCarlo, S. (1988). Effect of arm ergometry training on wheelchair propulsion endurance of individuals with quadriplegia. *Physical Therapy*, 68(1), 40–44.

52. Dickman, C. & Zerick, W. (1996). Cervical, thoracic, and lumbar orthoses. In: R. Narayan, J. Wilberger & J. Povlishock (Eds.), *Neurotrauma* (pp. 1139–1147). New York: McGraw-Hill.

53. Ditunno, J. & Formal, C. (1994). Chronic spinal cord injury. *New England Journal of Medicine*, 330(8), 550–556.

54. Donovon, W.; Kopaniky, D.; Stolzmann, E.; & Carter, R. (1987). The neurological and skeletal outcome in patients with closed cervical spinal cord injury. *Journal of Neurosurgery*, 66(5), 690–694.

55. Edie, P. (1998). Pathophysiological mechanisms of central neuropathic pain after spinal cord injury. *Spinal Cord*, 36(9), 601–612.

56. Faden, A. (1996). Pharmacological treatment of central nervous system trauma. *Pharmacology and Toxicology*, 78(1), 12–17.

57. Farmer, J.; Vaccaro, A.; Albert, T.; Malone, S.; Balderston, R.; & Cotler, J. (1998). Neurologic deterioration after cervical spinal cord injury. *Journal of Spinal Disorders*, 11(3), 192–196.

58. Fehlings, M. & Louw, D. (1996). Initial stabilization and medical management of acute spinal cord injury. *American Family Physician*, 54(1), 155–162.

59. Fehlings, M.; Rao, S.; Tator, C.; Skaf, G.; Arnold, P.; & Benzel, E. (1999). The optimal radiologic method for assessing spinal canal compromise and cord compression in patients with cervical spinal cord injury. Part II: results of a multicenter study. *Spine*, 24(6), 605–613.

60. Finkelstein, J. & Anderson, P. (1998). Surgical management of cervical instability. In: D. Capen & W. Haye (Eds.), *Comprehensive Management of Spine Trauma* (pp. 144–184). Saint Louis: Mosby.

61. Fishman, S.; Berger, N.; Edelstein, J.; & Springer, W. (1985). Spinal orthoses. In W. Bunch, R. Keagy, A. Kritter, L. Kruger, M. Letts, J. Lonstein, et al. (Eds.), *Atlas of Orthotics: Biomechanical Principles and Application* (2nd ed., pp. 238–256). Princeton: C. V. Mosby.

62. Fredericks, C. (1996). Clinical presentations in disorders of motor function. In: C. Fredericks & L. Saladin (Eds.), *Pathophysiology of the Motor Systems: Principles and Clinical Presentations* (pp. 257–288). Philadelphia: F. A. Davis.

63. Freebourn, T.; Barber, D.; & Able, A. (1999). The treatment of immature heterotopic ossification in spinal cord injury with combination surgery, radiation therapy, and NSAID. *Spinal Cord*, 37(1), 50–53.

64. Frost, F. (1993). Role of rehabilitation after spinal cord injury. *Urologic Clinics of North America*, 20(3), 549–558.

65. Garfin, S.; Botte, M.; Triggs, K.; & Nickel, V. (1988). Subdural abscess associated with halo-pin traction. *Journal of Bone and Joint Surgery*, 70-A(9), 1338–1340.

66. Garfin, S.; Botte, M.; Waters, R.; & Nickel, V. (1986). Complications in the use of the halo fixation device. *Journal of Bone and Joint Surgery*, 68-A(3), 320–325.

67. Geisler, F. (1998). Clinical trials of pharmacotherapy for spinal cord injury. *Annals of the New York Academy of Science*, 845, 374–381.

68. Geisler, F. (1993). GM-1 Ganglioside and motor recovery following human spinal cord injury. *The Journal of Emergency Medicine*, 11(Suppl 1), 49–55.

69. Gellman, H.; Sie, I.; & Waters, R. (1988). Late complications of the weight-bearing upper extremity in the paraplegic patient. *Clinical Orthopaedics and Related Research*, 233, 132–135.

70. Gianino, J. (1993). Intrathecal baclofen for spinal spasticity: implications for nursing practice. *Journal of Neuroscience Nursing*, 25(4), 254–264.

71. Gimenez, Y.; Ribotta, M.; & Privat, A. (1998). Biological interventions for spinal cord injury. *Current Opinion in Neurology*, 11(6), 647–654.

72. Glaser, R. (1994). Functional neuromuscular stimulation: exercise conditioning of spinal cord injured patients. *International Journal of Sports Medicine*, 15(3), 142–148.

73. Glaser, J.; Jaworski, B.; Cuddy, B.; Albert, T.; Hollowell, J.; McLain, R.; & Bozzette, S. (1998). Varia-

tion in surgical opinion regarding management of selected cervical spine injuries. *Spine*, 23(9), 975–983.

74. Glaser, J.; Whitehill, R.; Stamp, W.; & Jane, J. (1986). Complications associated with the halo-vest: a review of 245 cases. *Journal of Neurosurgery*, 65(6), 762–769.

75. Graber, M. & Kathol, M. (1999). Cervical spine radiographs in the trauma patient. *American Family Physician*, 59(2), 331–342.

76. Gracies, J.; Elovic, E.; McGuire, J.; & Simpson, D. (1997a). Traditional pharmacological treatments for spasticity. Part I: local treatments. *Muscle and Nerve*, (Suppl 6), S61–S91.

77. Gracies, J.; Elovic, E.; McGuire, J.; & Simpson, D. (1997b). Traditional pharmacological treatments for spasticity. Part II: General and regional treatments. *Muscle and Nerve*, (Suppl 6), S92–S120.

78. Graziano, G. & Charles, L. (1998). Spinal orthoses. In: H. An (Ed.), *Principles and Techniques of Spine Surgery* (pp. 641–652). Baltimore: Williams & Wilkins.

79. Graziano, A.; Scheidel, E.; Cline, J.; & Baer, L. (1987). A radiographic comparison of prehospital cervical immobilization methods. *Annals of Emergency Medicine*, 16(10), 1127–1131.

80. Grundy, D.; Swain, A.; & Russell, J. (1986). ABC of spinal cord injury: early management and complications I. *British Medical Journal*, 292(6512), 44–47.

81. Guth, L.; Zhang, Z.; & Roberts, E. (1994). Key role for pregnenolone in combination therapy that promotes recovery after spinal cord injury. *Proceedings of the National Academy of Science, U S A*, 91(25), 12308–12312.

82. Hansebout, R. (1986). The neurosurgical management of cord injuries. In: R. Bloch & M. Basbaum (Eds.), *Management of Spinal Cord Injuries* (pp. 1–27). Baltimore: Williams & Wilkins.

83. Hardcastle, P.; Bedbrook G.; & Curtis K. (1987). Long-term results of conservative and operative management in complete paraplegics with spinal cord injuries between T10 and L2 with respect to function. *Clinical Orthopedics and Related Research*, 224, 88–96.

84. Harms, J. & Tabasso, G. (1999). *Instrumented Spinal Surgery: Principles and Technique*. New York: Thieme.

85. Hart, A.; Malone, T.; & English, T. (1998). Shoulder function and rehabilitation implications for the wheelchair racing athlete. *Topics in Spinal Cord Injury Rehabilitation*, 3(3), 50–65.

86. Heary, R.; Vaccaro, A.; Mesa, J.; Northrup, B.; Albert, T.; Balderston, R.; & Cotler, J. (1997). Steroids and gunshot wounds to the spine. *Neurosurgery*, 41(3), 576–583.

87. Hoffman, M. (1986). Cardiorespiratory fitness and training in quadriplegics and paraplegics. *Sports Medicine*, 3(5), 312–330.

88. Hooker, S.; Scremin, E.; Mutton, D.; Kunkel, C.; & Cagle, G. (1995). Peak and submaximal physiologic responses following electrical stimulation leg cycle ergometer training. *Journal of Rehabilitation Research and Development*, 32(4), 361–366.

89. Hooker, S. & Wells, C. (1989). Effects of low- and moderate-intensity training in spinal cord-injured persons. *Medicine and Science in Sports and Exercise*, 21(1), 18–22.

90. Hughes, S. (1998). How effective is the Newport/Aspen collar? A prospective radiographic evaluation in healthy adult volunteers. *Journal of Trauma*, 45(2), 374–378.

91. Janssen, T.; Glaser, R.; & Shuster, D. (1998). Clinical efficacy of electrical stimulation exercise training: effects on health, fitness, and function. *Topics in Spinal Cord Injury Rehabilitation*, 3(3), 33–49.

92. Johnson, R.; Hart, D.; Simmons, E.; Ramsby, G.; & Southwick, W. (1977). Cervical orthoses. A study comparing their effectiveness in restricting cervical motion in normal subjects. *Journal of Bone and Joint Surgery*, 59-A(3), 332–339.

93. Kalfas, I. (1996). Cervical spine stabilization: surgical techniques. In: R. Narayan, J. Wilberger & J. Povlishock (Eds.), *Neurotrauma* (pp. 1179–1192). New York: McGraw-Hill.

94. Karbi, O.; Caspari, D.; & Tator, C. (1988). Extrication, immobilization, and radiologic investigation of patients with cervical spine injuries. *Canadian Medical Association Journal*, 139(7), 617–621.

95. Kirshblum, S.; Druin, E.; & Planten, K. (1997). Musculoskeletal conditions in chronic spinal cord injury. *Topics in Spinal Cord Injury Rehabilitation*, 2(4), 23–35.

96. Kiwerski, J. (1993). Neurological outcome from conservative or surgical treatment of cervical spinal cord injured patients. *Paraplegia*, 31(3), 192–196.

97. Kulkarni, M.; McArdle, C.; Kopanicky, D.; Miner, M.; Cotler, H.; Lee, K.; & Harris, J. (1987). Acute spinal cord injury: MR imaging at 1.5 T. *Radiology*, 164(3), 837–843.

98. Kunkel, C.; Scremin, A.; Eisenberg, B.; Garcia, J.; Roberts, S.; & Martinez, S. (1993). Effect of "standing" on spasticity, contracture, and osteoporosis in paralyzed males. *Archives of Physical Medicine and Rehabilitation*, 74(1), 73–78.

99. Laskin, J.; James, S.; & Cantwell, B. (1997). A fitness and wellness program for people with spinal cord injury. *Topics in Spinal Cord Injury Rehabilitation*, 3(1), 16–33.

100. Lee, T.; Green, B.; & Petrin, D. (1998). Treatment of stable burst fractures of the atlas (Jefferson Fracture) with rigid cervical collar. *Spine*, 23(18), 1963–1967.

101. Leeds, E.; Klose, J.; Ganz, W.; Serafini, A.; & Green, B. (1990). Bone mineral density after bicycle ergometry training. *Archives of Physical Medicine and Rehabilitation*, 71(3), 207–209.

102. Lehman, L. (1987). Injury of the cervical spine: some fundamentals of management. *Postgraduate Medicine*, 82(2), 193–200.

103. Linares, H.; Mawson, A.; Suarez, E.; & Biundo, J. (1987). Association between pressure sores and immobilization in the immediate post-injury period. *Orthopedics*, 10(7), 571–573.

104. Loubser, P. & Donovan, W. (1996). Chronic pain associated with spinal cord injury. In R. Narayan, J. Wilberger & J. Povlishock (Eds.), *Neurotrauma* (pp. 1311–1322). New York: McGraw-Hill.

105. Lu, W.; Rhoney, D.; Boling, W.; Johnson, J.; & Smith, T. (1997). A review of stress ulcer prophylaxis in the neurosurgical intensive care unit. *Neurosurgery*, 41(2), 416–425.

106. Lu, J. & Waite, P. (1999). Advances in spinal cord regeneration. *Spine*, 24(9), 926–930.

107. Maddox, S. (1987). *Spinal Network*. Boulder, CO: Spinal Network.

108. Maher, A. (1985). Dealing with head and neck injuries. *RN*, 48(3), 43–46.

109. Marion, D. (1998). Head and spinal cord injury. *Neurologic Clinics of North America*, 16(2), 485–502.

110. Marshall, S.; Marshall, L.; Vos, H.; & Chesnut, R. (1990). *Neuroscience Critical Care: Pathophysiology and Patient Management*. Philadelphia: W.B. Saunders Company.

111. Matthews, P. & Carlson, C. (1987). *Spinal Cord Injury: A Guide to Rehabilitation Nursing*. Rockville, MD: Aspen Publishers.

112. Mayer, N. (1997). Clinicophysiologic concepts of spasticity and motor dysfunction in adults with an upper motor neuron lesion. *Muscle and Nerve*, 20(Suppl. 6), S1–S13.

113. Maynard, F.; Karunas, R.; Adkins, R.; Richards, J.; & Waring, W. (1995). Management of the neuromusculoskeletal systems. In: S. Stover, J. DeLisa, & G. Whiteneck (Eds.), *Spinal Cord Injury: Clinical Outcomes from the Model Systems* (pp. 145–169). Gaithersburg, MD: Aspen.

114. McBride, D. & Rodts, G. (1994). Intensive care of patients with spinal trauma. *Neurosurgery Clinics of North America*, 5(4), 755–766.

115. McCagg, C. (1986). Postoperative management and acute rehabilitation of patients with spinal cord injuries. *Orthopedic Clinics of North America*, 17(1), 171–182.

116. McGuire, R.; Green, B.; Eismont, F.; & Watts, C. (1988). Comparison of stability provided to the unstable spine by the kinetic therapy table and Stryker frame. *Neurosurgery*, 22(5), 842–845.

117. McGuire, R.; Neville, S.; Green, B.; & Watts, C. (1987). Spinal instability and the log-rolling maneuver. *Journal of Trauma*, 27(5), 525–531.

118. McLain, R. & Benson, D. (1998). Missed cervical dissociation—recognizing and avoiding potential disaster. *The Journal of Emergency Medicine*, 16(2), 179–183.

119. Meiners, T.; Abel, R.; Bohm, V.; & Gerner, H. (1997). Resection of heterotopic ossification of the hip in spinal cord injured patients. *Spinal Cord*, 35(7), 443–445.

120. Meyer, P. (1989). *Surgery of Spine Trauma*. New York: Churchill Livingstone.

121. Meyer, P., & Heim, S. (1989). Surgical stabilization of the cervical spine. In: P. Meyer (Ed.), *Surgery of Spine Trauma* (pp. 397–523). New York: Churchill Livingstone.

122. Millington, P.; Ellingsen, J.; Hauswirth, B.; & Fabian, P. (1987). Thermoplastic minerva body jacket—a practical alternative to current methods of cervical spine stabilization. *Physical Therapy*, 67(2), 223–225.

123. Mirza, S.; Krengel, W.; Chapman, J.; Anderson, P.; Bailey, J.; Grady, M.; & Yuan, H. (1999). Early versus delayed surgery for acute cervical spinal cord injury. *Clinical Orthopaedics and Related Research*, 359, 104–114.

124. Mirvis, S.; Geisler, F.; Jelinek, J.; Joslyn, J.; & Gellad, F. (1988). Acute cervical spine trauma: evaluation with 1.5-T imaging. *Radiology*, 166(3), 807–816.

125. Moore, D. (1998). Helping your patients with spasticity reach maximal function. *Postgraduate Medicine*, 104(2), 123–135.

126. Muhr, M.; Seabrook, D.; & Wittwer, L. (1999). Paramedic use of a spinal injury clearance algorithm reduces spinal immobilization in the out-of-hospital setting. *Prehospital Emergency Care*, 3(1), 1–6.

127. Nash, M. (1998). Exercise reconditioning of the heart and peripheral circulation after spinal cord injury. *Topics in Spinal Cord Injury Rehabilitation*, 3(3), 1–15.

128. Naso, F. (1992). Cardiovascular problems in patients with spinal cord injury. *Physical Medicine and Rehabilitation Clinics of North America*, 3(4), 741–749.

129. Nawoczenski, D.; Rinehart, M.; Duncanson, P.; & Brown, B. (1987). Physical management. In: L. Buchanan & D. Nawoczenski (Eds.), *Spinal Cord Injury: Concepts and Management Approaches* (pp. 123–184). Baltimore: Williams & Wilkins.

130. Needham-Shropshire, B.; Broton, J.; Klose, K.; Lebwohl, N.; Guest, R.; & Jacobs, P. (1997). Evaluation of a training program for persons with SCI paraplegia using the Parastep 1 ambulation system: part 3. Lack of effect on bone mineral density. *Archives of Physical Medicine and Rehabilitation*, 78(8), 799–803.

131. Nelson, R. (1998). Nonsurgical management of cervical spine instability. In: D. Capen & W. Haye (Eds.), *Comprehensive Management of Spine Trauma* (pp. 134–143). Saint Louis: Mosby.

132. Nesathurai, S. (1998). Steroids and spinal cord injury: revisiting the NASCIS 2 and NASCIS 3 trails. *The Journal of Trauma: Injury, Infection and Critical Care*, 45(6), 1088–1093.

133. New York University. (1983). *Spinal Orthotics*. New York: New York University Post-Graduate Medical School.

134. Nikas, D. (1986). Resuscitation of patients with central nervous system trauma. *Nursing Clinics of North America*, 21(4), 693–704.

135. Parry, H.; Delargy, M.; & Burt, A. (1988). Early mobilization of patients with cervical cord injury using the halo device. *Paraplegia*, 26(4), 226–232.

136. Pentland, W. & Twomey, L. (1994). Upper limb function in persons with long term paraplegia and implications for independence: part I. *Paraplegia*, 32(4), 211–218.

137. Phillips, W.; Kiralti, B.; Sarkarati, M.; Weraarchakul, G.; Meyers, J.; Franklin, B.; Parkash, I.; & Froelicher, V. (1998). Effect of spinal cord injury on the heart and cardiovascular fitness. *Current Problems in Cardiology*, 23(11), 649–716.

138. Pitts, L.; Ross, A.; Chase, G.; & Faden, A. (1995). Treatment with thyrotropin-releasing hormone (TRH) in patients with traumatic spinal cord injuries. *Journal of Neurotrauma*, 12(3), 235–243.

139. Prendergast, M.; Saxe, J.; Ledgerwood, A.; Lucas, C.; & Lucas, W. (1994). Massive steroids do not reduce the zone of injury after penetrating spinal cord injury. *The Journal of Trauma*, 37(4), 576–579.

140. Priebe, M.; Sherwood, A.; Thornby, J.; Kharas, N.; & Markowski, J. (1996). Clinical assessment of spasticity in spinal cord injury: a multidimensional problem. *Archives of Physical Medicine and Rehabilitation*, 77(7), 713–716.

141. Prod'hom, G.; Leuenberger, P.; Koerfer, J.; Blum, A.; Chiolero, R.; Schaller, M.; Perret, C.; Spinnler, O.; Blondel, J.; Siegrist, H. et al. (1994). Nosocomial pneumonia in mechanically ventilated patients receiving antacid, ranitidine, or sucralfate as prophylaxis for stress ulcer. A randomized controlled trail. *Annals of Internal Medicine*, 120(8), 653–662.

142. Przybylski, G. & Marion, D. (1996). Injury to the vertebrae and spinal cord. In: D. Feliciano, E. Moore, & K. Mattox (Eds.), *Trauma* (3rd ed., pp. 307–327). Stamford, CT: Appleton & Lange.

143. Quencer, R.; Nunez, D.; & Green, B. (1997). Controversies in imaging acute cervical spine trauma. *American Journal of Neuroradiology*, 18(10), 1866–1868.

144. Ragnarsson, K.; Stein, A. & Kirshblum, S. (1998). Rehabilitation and comprehensive care of the person with spinal cord injury. In: D. Capen & W. Haye (Eds.), *Comprehensive Management of Spine Trauma* (pp. 365–413). Saint Louis: Mosby.

145. Rodts, G. & Haid, R. (1996). Intensive care management of spinal cord injury. In: R. Narayan, J. Wilberger & J. Povlishock (Eds.), *Neurotrauma* (pp. 1201–1212). New York: McGraw-Hill.

146. Romeo, J. (1988). The critical minutes after spinal cord injury. *RN*, 51(4), 61–67.

147. Roth, E. (1994). Pain in spinal cord injury. In: G. Yarkony (Ed.), *Spinal Cord Injury: Medical Management and Rehabilitation* (pp. 141–158). Gaithersburg, MD: Aspen.

148. Sandler, A.; Dvorak, J.; Humke, T.; Grob, D.; & Daniels, W. (1996). The effectiveness of various cervical orthoses. An in vivo comparison of the mechanical stability provided by several widely used models. *Spine*, 21(14), 1624–1629.

149. Shaffrey, C.; Shaffrey, M.; Whitehill, R.; & Nockels, R. (1997). Surgical treatment of thoracolumbar fractures. *Neurosurgery Clinics of North America*, 8(4), 519–540.

150. Shen, W. & Shen, Y. (1999). Nonsurgical treatment of three-column thoracolumbar junction burst fractures without neurological deficit. *Spine*, 24(4), 412–415.

151. Sie, I.; Waters, R.; Adkins, R.; & Gellman, H. (1992). Upper extremity pain in the postrehabilitation spinal cord injured patient. *Archives of Physical Medicine and Rehabilitation*, 73(1), 44–48.

152. Silfverskiold, J. & Waters, R. (1991). Shoulder pain and functional disability in spinal cord injury patients. *Clinical Orthopedics and Related Research*, 272, 141–145.

153. Simpson, R., Venger, B., & Narayan, R. (1989). Treatment of acute penetrating injuries of the spine: a retrospective analysis. *Journal of Trauma*, 29(1), 42–46.

154. Slabaugh, P. & Nickel, V. (1978). Complications with use of the Stryker frame. *Journal of Bone and Joint Surgery*, 60-A(8), 1111–1112.

155. Soderstrom, C. & Brumback, R. (1986). Early care of the patient with cervical spine injury. *Orthopedic Clinics of North America*, 17(1), 3–13.

156. Stein, A.; Pomerantz, F.; & Schnechtman, J. (1997). Evaluation and management of spasticity in spinal cord injury. *Topics in Spinal Cord Injury Rehabilitation*, 2(4), 70–83.

157. Stiens, S.; Johnson, M.; & Lyman, P. (1995). Cardiac rehabilitation in patients with spinal cord injuries. *Physical Medicine and Rehabilitation Clinics in North America*, 6(2), 263–296.

158. Swain, A.; Grundy, D.; & Russell, J. (1985a). ABC of spinal cord injury: at the accident. *British Medical Journal*, 291(6508), 1558–1560.

159. Swain, A.; Grundy, D.; & Russell, J. (1985b). ABC of spinal cord injury: evacuation and initial management at the hospital. *British Medical Journal*, 291(6509), 1623–1625.

160. Tator, C. (1998). Biology of neurological recovery and functional restoration after spinal cord injury. *Neurosurgery*, 42(4), 696–708.

161. Tator, C. & Fehlings, M. (1991). Review of the secondary injury theory of acute spinal cord trauma with emphasis on vascular mechanisms. *Journal of Neurosurgery*, 75(1), 15–26.

162. Tator, C.; Fehlings, M.; Thorpe, K.; & Taylor, W. (1999). Current use and timing of spinal surgery for management of acute spinal cord injury in North America: results of a retrospective multicenter study. *Journal of Neurosurgery*, 91(Suppl1), 12–18.

163. Thelan, L.; Davie, J.; & Urden, L. (1990). *Textbook of Critical Care Nursing: Diagnosis and Management*. Baltimore: C.V. Mosby.

164. Tryba, M. (1987). Risk of acute stress bleeding and nosocomial pneumonia in ventilated intensive care unit patients: sucralfate versus antacids. *American Journal of Medicine*, 83(3B), 117–124.

165. Tryba, M. & Cook, D. (1997). Current guidelines on stress ulcer prophylaxis. *Drugs*, 54(4), 581–596.

166. Turpie, A. (1986). Thrombosis prevention and treatment in spinal cord injured patients. In: R. Bloch & M. Basbaum (Eds.), *Management of Spinal Cord Injuries* (pp. 212–240). Baltimore: Williams & Wilkins.

167. Vaccaro, A.; Lavernia, C.; Botte, M.; Bergmann, K.; & Garfin, S. (1998a). Spinal orthoses in the management of spine trauma. In: A. Levine, F. Eismont, S. Garfin, & J. Zigler (Eds.), *Spine Trauma* (pp. 171–194). Philadelphia: W. B. Saunders.

168. Vaccaro, A.; Silveri, C.; & Balderston, R. (1998b). Nonsurgical and surgical management of fractures at the thoracolumbar junction. In: D. Capen & W. Haye (Eds.), *Comprehensive Management of Spine Trauma* (pp. 199–213). Saint Louis: Mosby.

169. Vale, F.; Burns, J.; Jackson, A.; & Hadley, M. (1997). Combined medical and surgical treatment after acute spinal cord injury: results of a prospective pilot study to assess the merits of aggressive medical resuscitation and blood pressure management. *Journal of Neurosurgery*, 87(2), 239–246.

170. Vapnek, J. (1997). Autonomic dysreflexia. *Topics in Spinal Cord Injury Rehabilitation*, 2(4), 54–69.

171. Wang, G.; Moskal, J.; Albert, T.; Pritts, C.; Schuch, C.; & Stamp, W. (1988). The effect of halo-vest length on stability of the cervical spine. *Journal of Bone and Joint Surgery*, 70-A(3), 357–360.

172. Wang, J. & Delamarter, R. (1998). Lumbar fractures of the spine. In: D. Capen & W. Haye (Eds.), *Comprehensive Management of Spine Trauma* (pp. 214–234). Saint Louis: Mosby.

173. Washburn, R. & Figoni, S. (1998). Physical activity and chronic cardiovascular disease prevention in spinal cord injury: a comprehensive literature review. *Topics in Spinal Cord Injury Rehabilitation*, 3(3), 16–32.

174. Waters, R.; Apple, D.; Meyer, P.; Cotler, J.; & Adkins, R. (1995). Emergency and acute management of spine trauma. In S. Stover, J. DeLisa, & G. Whiteneck (Eds.), *Spinal Cord Injury: Clinical Outcomes from the Model Systems* (pp. 56–78). Gaithersburg, MD: Aspen.

175. Wells, J. & Nicosia, S. (1993). The effects of multidisciplinary team care for acute spinal cord injury patients. *Journal of the American Paraplegia Society*, 16(1), 23–29.

176. Whitehill, R.; Richman, J.; & Glaser, J. (1986). Failure of immobilization of the cervical spine by the halo vest. A report of five cases. *Journal of Bone and Joint Surgery*, 68-A(3), 326–332.

177. Wilberger, J. (1998). Athletic spinal cord and spine injuries. *Clinics in Sports Medicine*, 17(1), 111–120.

178. Wolf, A. & Wilberger, J. (1996). Timing of surgical intervention after spinal cord injury. In: R. Narayan, J. Wilberger & J. Povlishock (Eds.), *Neurotrauma* (pp. 1193–1199). New York: McGraw-Hill.

179. Yakura, J.; Waters, R.; & Adkins, R. (1990). Changes in ambulation parameters in spinal cord injury individuals following rehabilitation. *Paraplegia*, 28(6), 364–370.

180. Yarkony, G. (1994). Medical and physical complications in spinal cord injury. In: G. Yarkony (Ed.), *Spinal Cord Injury: Medical Management and Rehabilitation* (pp. 17–25). Gaithersburg, MD: Aspen.

181. Yu, D. (1998). A crash course in spinal cord injury. *Postgraduate Medicine*, 104(2), 109–120.

182. Zompa, E.; Cain, L.; Everhart, A.; Moyer, M.; & Hulsebosch, C. (1997). Transplant therapy: recovery of function after spinal cord injury. *Journal of Neurotrauma*, 14(8), 479–506.

Chapter 4

1. Auvenshine, C. & Noffsinger, A. (1984). *Counseling: An Introduction For the Health and Human Services*. Baltimore: University Park Press.

2. Bach, J. & Tilton, M. (1994). Life satisfaction and well-being measures in ventilator assisted individuals with traumatic tetraplegia. *Archives of Physical Medicine and Rehabilitation*, 75(6), 626–632.

3. Bracken, M.; Shepard, M.; & Webb, S. (1981). Psychological response to acute spinal cord injury: an epidemiological study. *Paraplegia*, 19, 271–283.

4. Brockopp, D.; Hayko, D.; Davenport, W.; & Winscott, S. (1989). Personal control and the needs for hope and information among adults diagnosed with cancer. *Cancer Nursing*, 12(2), 112–116.

5. Brown, M.; Gordon, W.; & Ragnarsson, K. (1987). Unhandicapping the disabled: what is possible? *Archives of Physical Medicine and Rehabilitation*, 68, 206–209.

6. Brown, R. & Hughson, E. (1987). *Behavioral and Social Rehabilitation and Training*. New York: Wiley.

7. Carlson, C. (1979). Conceptual style and life satisfaction following spinal cord injury. *Archives of Physical Medicine and Rehabilitation*, 60, 346–352.

8. Chesler, M. & Chesney, B. (1988). Self-help groups: empowerment attitudes and behaviors of disabled or chronically ill persons. In: H. Yuker (Ed.), *Attitudes toward Persons with Disabilities* (pp. 230–245). New York: Springer Publishing.

9. Cobb, S. (1976). Social support as a moderator of life stress. *Psychosomatic Medicine*, 38(5), 300–313.

10. Cogswell, B. (1977). Self-socialization: readjustment of paraplegics in the community. In: R. Marinelli & A. Dell Orto (Eds.), *The Psychological and Social Impact of Physical Disability* (pp. 151–159). New York: Springer Publishing.

11. Consortium for Spinal Cord Medicine. (1998). *Depression Following Spinal Cord Injury: A Clinical Practice Guideline for Primary Care Physicians*. Washington, DC: Paralyzed Veterans of America.

12. Corbet, B. (1987). Options revisited. In: S. Maddox (Ed.), *Spinal Network* (pp. 12–19). Boulder, CO: Spinal Network.

13. Corbet, B. (1980). *Options: Spinal Cord Injury and the Future*. Denver, CO: A. B. Hirschfeld Press.

14. Craig, A.; Hancock, K.; Chang, E.; & Dickson, H. (1998). Immunizing against depression and anxiety after spinal cord injury. *Archives of Physical Medicine and Rehabilitation*, 79(4), 375–377.

15. Craig, A.; Hancock, K.; & Dickson, H. (1999). Improving the long-term adjustment of spinal cord injured persons. *Spinal Cord*, 37(5), 345–350.

16. Craig, A.; Hancock, K.; Dickson, H.; & Chang, E. (1997). Long-term psychological outcomes in spinal cord injured persons: results of a controlled trial using cognitive behavior therapy. *Archives of Physical Medicine and Rehabilitation*, 78(1), 33–38.

17. Crewe, N. (1996). Gains and losses due to spinal cord injury: views across 20 years. *Topics in Spinal Cord Injury Rehabilitation*, 2(2), 46–57.

18. Crossman, M. (1996). Sensory deprivation in spinal cord injury—an essay. *Spinal Cord*, 34(10), 573–577.

19. Cushman, L. & Hassett, J. (1992). Spinal cord injury: 10 and 15 years after. *Paraplegia*, 30(10), 690–696.

20. Daverat, P.; Petit, H.; Kemoun, G.; Dartigues, J.; & Barat, M. (1995). The long term outcome in 149 patients with spinal cord injury. *Paraplegia*, 33(11), 665–668.

21. Decker, N. (1984). Brief psychotherapy of chronic illness. In: D. Krueger (Ed.), *Emotional Rehabilita-

tion of *Physical Trauma and Disability* (pp. 195–218). New York: SP Medical & Scientific Books.

22. DeJong, G. (1979). Independent living: from social movement to analytic paradigm. *Archives of Physical Medicine and Rehabilitation*, 60, 435–446.

23. DeJong, G.; Branch, L.; & Corcoran, P. (1984). Independent living outcomes in spinal cord injury: multivariate analyses. *Archives of Physical Medicine and Rehabilitation*, 65, 66–73.

24. DeSantis, N. & Becker, B. (1999). Building a durable relationship: avoiding catastrophe between the therapeutic team and the patient with a new spinal cord injury. *Topics in Spinal Cord Injury Rehabilitation*, 4(3), 29–35.

25. DeVivo, M. & Fine, P. (1982). Employment status of spinal cord injured patients 3 years after injury. *Archives of Physical Medicine and Rehabilitation*, 63, 200–203.

26. Dijkers, M. (1999). Correlates of life satisfaction among persons with spinal cord injury. *Archives of Physical Medicine and Rehabilitation*, 80(8), 867–876.

27. Dijkers, M. (1998). Community integration: conceptual issues and measurement approaches in rehabilitation research. *Topics in Spinal Cord Injury Rehabilitation*, 4(1), 1–15.

28. Dijkers, M. (1997). Quality of life after spinal cord injury: a meta analysis of the effects of disablement components. *Spinal Cord*, 35(12), 829–840.

29. Dijkers, M.; Abela, M.; Gans, B.; & Gordon, W. (1995). The aftermath of spinal cord injury. In: S. Stover, J. DeLisa, & G. Whiteneck (Eds.), *Spinal Cord Injury: Clinical Outcomes from the Model Systems* (pp. 185–212). Gaithersburg, MD: Aspen.

30. Ducharme, S. & Ducharme, J. (1984). Psychological adjustment to spinal cord injury. In: D. Krueger (Ed.), *Emotional Rehabilitation of Physical Trauma and Disability* (pp. 149–156). New York: SP Medical & Scientific Books.

31. El Ghatit, A. & Hanson, R. (1979). Educational and training levels and employment of the spinal cord injured patient. *Archives of Physical Medicine and Rehabilitation*, 60, 405–406.

32. Elliott, T. & Frank, R. (1996). Depression following spinal cord injury. *Archives of Physical Medicine and Rehabilitation*, 77(8), 816–823.

33. Elliott, T. & Jackson, W. (1996). Psychologic assessment in spinal cord injury rehabilitation: benefiting patient, treatment team, and health care delivery system. *Topics in Spinal Cord Injury Rehabilitation*, 2(2), 34–45.

34. English, R. (1977). Combating stigma toward physically disabled persons. In: R. Marinelli & A. Dell Orto (Eds.), *The Psychological and Social Impact of Physical Disability* (pp. 183–193). New York: Springer Publishing.

35. Fichten, C. (1988). Students with physical disabilities in higher education: attitudes and beliefs that affect integration. In: H. Yuker (Ed.), *Attitudes toward Persons with Disabilities* (pp. 171–186). New York: Springer Publishing.

36. Flynn, R. (1981). Normalization, social integration, and sex behavior: a service approach and evaluation method for improving rehabilitation programs. In: A. Sha'ked (Ed.), *Human Sexuality and Rehabilitation Medicine: Sexual Functioning Following Spinal Cord Injury* (pp. 37–66). Baltimore: Williams & Wilkins.

37. Frank, R.; Elliott, T.; Buckelew, S.; & Haut, A. (1988). Age as a factor in response to spinal cord injury. *American Journal of Physical Medicine and Rehabilitation*, 67(3), 128–131.

38. French, D.; McDowell, R.; & Keith, R. (1977). Participant observation as a patient in a rehabilitation hospital. In: R. Marinelli & A. Dell Orto (Eds.), *The Psychological and Social Impact of Physical Disability* (pp. 289–296). New York: Springer Publishing.

39. Fuhrer, M.; Rintala, D.; Hart, K.; Clearman, R.; & Young, M. (1992). Relationship of life satisfaction to impairment, disability, and handicap among persons with spinal cord injury living in the community. *Archives of Physical Medicine and Rehabilitation*, 73(6), 552–557.

40. Fuhrer, M.; Rossi, D.; Gerken, L.; Nosek, M.; & Richards, L. (1990). Relationships between independent living centers and medical rehabilitation programs. *Archives of Physical Medicine and Rehabilitation*, 71(7), 519–522.

41. Gellman, W. (1977). Projections in the field of physical disability. In: R. Marinelli & A. Dell Orto (Eds.), *The Psychological and Social Impact of Physical Disability* (pp. 34–48). New York: Springer Publishing.

42. Gerhart, K. (1997). Quality of life: the danger of differing perceptions. *Topics in Spinal Cord Injury Rehabilitation*, 2(3), 78–84.

43. Gerhart, K.; Johnson, R.; & Whiteneck, G. (1992). Health and psychosocial issues of individuals with incomplete and resolving spinal cord injuries. *Paraplegia*, 30(4), 282–287.

44. Gerhart, K.; Weitzenkamp, D.; Kennedy, P.; Glass, C.; & Charlifue, S. (1999). Correlates of stress in long–term spinal cord injury. *Spinal Cord*, 37(3), 183–190.

45. Geskie, M. & Salasek, J. (1988). Attitudes of health care personnel toward persons with disabilities. In: H. Yuker (Ed.), *Attitudes toward Persons with Disabilities* (pp. 187–200). New York: Springer Publishing.

46. Gilliland, B. & James, R. (1988). *Crisis Intervention Strategies*. Pacific Grove, CA: Brooks/Cole Publishing.

47. Glass, C.; Jackson, H.; Dutton, J.; Charlifue, S.; & Orritt, C. (1997). Estimating social adjustment following spinal trauma—II: population trends and effects of compensation on adjustment. *Spinal Cord*, 35(6), 349–357.

48. Goldberg, R. & Freed, M. (1982). Vocational development of spinal cord injury patients: an 8-year follow-up. *Archives of Physical Medicine and Rehabilitation*, 63, 207–210.

49. Gorman, C.; Kennedy, P.; & Hamilton, L. (1998). Alterations in self-perceptions following childhood onset of spinal cord injury. *Spinal Cord*, 36(3), 181–185.

50. Green, B.; Pratt, C.; & Grigsby, T. (1984). Self-concept among persons with long-term spinal cord

injury. *Archives of Physical Medicine and Rehabilitation*, 65(12), 751–754.

51. Hall, K.; Harper, B.; & Whiteneck, G. (1997). Follow-up study of individuals with high tetraplegia (C1 - C4) 10 to 21 years postinjury. *Topics in Spinal Cord Injury Rehabilitation*, 2(3), 107–117.

52. Halstead, L.; Rintala, D.; Kanellos, M.; Griffin, B.; Higgins, L.; Rheinecker, S.; Whiteside, W.; & Healy, J. (1986). The innovative rehabilitation team: an experiment in team building. *Archives of Physical Medicine and Rehabilitation*, 67, 357–361.

53. Hammell, K. (1994). Psychosocial outcome following spinal cord injury. *Paraplegia*, 32(11), 771–779.

54. Haney, M. & Rabin, B. (1984). Modifying attitudes toward disabled persons while resocializing spinal cord injured patients. *Archives of Physical Medicine and Rehabilitation*, 65, 431–436.

55. Hansen, N.; Forchheimer, M.; Tate, D.; & Luera, G. (1998). Relationships among community reintegration, coping strategies, and life satisfaction in a sample of persons with spinal cord injury. *Topics in Spinal Cord Injury Rehabilitation*, 4(1), 56–72.

56. Hartkopp, A.; Bronnum-Hansen, H.; Seidenschnur, A.; & Biering-Sorensen, F. (1998). Suicide in a spinal cord injured population: its relation to functional status. *Archives of Physical Medicine and Rehabilitation*, 79(11), 1356–1361.

57. Heinemann, A.; Donohue, R.; & Schnoll, S. (1988). Alcohol use by persons with recent spinal cord injury. *Archives of Physical Medicine and Rehabilitation*, 69, 619–624.

58. Hoff, L. (1989). *People in Crisis: Understanding and Helping*. Redwood City, CA: Addison-Wesley Publishing.

59. Holicky, R. (1997). What consumers tell us. *Topics in Spinal Cord Injury Rehabilitation*, 2(3), 118–123.

60. Hooper, E. (1989). If the cure came tomorrow, would I want it? *Spinal Network*, Spring 1989, 50–52.

61. Horne, M. (1988). Modifying peer attitudes toward the handicapped: procedures and research issues. In: H. Yuker (Ed.), *Attitudes toward Persons with Disabilities* (pp. 203–222). New York: Springer Publishing.

62. Howell, T.; Fullerton, D.; Harvey, R.; & Klein, M. (1981). Depression in spinal cord injured patients. *Paraplegia*, 19, 284–288.

63. Jaques, M., & Patterson, K. (1977). The self-help group model: a review. In: R. Marinelli & A. Dell Orto (Eds.), *The Psychological and Social Impact of Physical Disability* (pp. 270–281). New York: Springer Publishing.

64. Johnson, R.; Gerhart, K.; McCray, J.; Menconi, J.; & Whiteneck, G. (1998). Secondary conditions following spinal cord injury in a population-based sample. *Spinal Cord*, 36(1), 45–50.

65. Judd, F. & Brown, D. (1988). The psychosocial approach to rehabilitation of the spinal cord injured patient. *Paraplegia*, 26, 419–424.

66. Judd, F. & Brown, D. (1987). Psychiatry in the spinal injuries unit. *Paraplegia*, 25, 254–257.

67. Kemp, B. & Krause, J. (1999). Depression and life satisfaction among people aging with post-polio and spinal cord injury. *Disability and Rehabilitation*, 21(5–6), 241–249.

68. Kerr, N. (1977). Staff expectations for disabled persons: helpful or harmful. In: R. Marinelli & A. Dell Orto (Eds.). *The Psychological and Social impact of Physical Disability* (pp. 342–350). New York: Springer Publishing.

69. Kishi, Y.; Robinson, R.; & Forrester, A. (1995). Comparison between acute and delayed onset major depression after spinal cord injury. *Journal of Nervous and Mental Disease*, 183(5), 286–292.

70. Krause, J. (1998). Aging and life adjustment after spinal cord injury. *Spinal Cord,* 36(5), 320–328.

71. Krause, J. (1992). Employment after spinal cord injury. *Archives of Physical Medicine and Rehabilitation*, 73(2), 163–169.

72. Krause, J. (1992). Longitudinal changes in adjustment after spinal cord injury: A 15-year study. *Archives of Physical Medicine and Rehabilitation*, 73(6), 564–568.

73. Krause, J. & Anson, C. (1996). Employment after spinal cord injury: relation to selected participant characteristics. *Archives of Physical Medicine and Rehabilitation*, 77(8), 737–743.

74. Kreuter, M.; Sullivan, M.; Dahllof, A.; & Siosteen, A. (1998). Partner relationships, functioning, mood and global quality of life in persons with spinal cord injury and traumatic brain injury. *Spinal Cord*, 36(4), 252–261.

75. Krueger, D. (1984). Emotional rehabilitation: an overview. In: D. Krueger (Ed.), *Emotional Rehabilitation of Physical Trauma and Disability* (pp. 3–12). New York: SP Medical & Scientific Books.

76. Krueger, D. (1984). Psychological rehabilitation of physical trauma and disability. In: D. Krueger (Ed.), *Rehabilitation Psychology: A Comprehensive Textbook* (pp. 3–13). Rockville, MD: Aspen Publishers.

77. Lasky, R.; Dell Orto, A.; & Marinelli, R. (1977). Structured experimental therapy: a group approach to rehabilitation. In: R. Marinelli & A. Dell Orto (Eds.), *The Psychological and Social Impact of Physical Disability* (pp. 319–333). New York: Springer Publishing.

78. Lawson, N. (1978). Significant events in the rehabilitation process: the spinal cord patient's point of view. *Archives of Physical Medicine and Rehabilitation*, 59, 573–579.

79. Lindemann, J. (1981). *Psychological and Behavioral Aspects of Physical Disability: A Manual for Health Practitioners*. New York: Plenum Press.

80. Lys, K. & Pernice, R. (1995). Perceptions of positive attitudes toward people with spinal cord injury. *International Journal of Rehabilitation Research*, 18(1), 35–43.

81. MacDonald, M.; Nielson, W.; & Cameron, M. (1987). Depression and activity patterns of spinal cord injured persons living in the community. *Archives of Physical Medicine and Rehabilitation*, 68, 339–342.

82. Macleod, A. (1988). Self-neglect of spinal injured patients. *Paraplegia*, 26, 340–349.

83. Macleod, L. & Macleod, G. (1998). Control cognitions and psychological disturbance in people with contrasting physically disabling conditions. *Disability and Rehabilitation*, 20(12), 448–456.

84. Mader, J. (1988). The importance of hope. *RN*, 51(12), 17–18.

85. Maddox, S. (1987). *Spinal Network*. Boulder, CO: Spinal Network.

86. Malec, J. & Neimeyer, R. (1983). Psychological prediction of duration of inpatient spinal cord injury rehabilitation and performance of self-care. *Archives of Physical Medicine and Rehabilitation*, 64, 359–363.

87. McCarthy, H. (1988). Attitudes that affect employment opportunities for persons with disabilities. In: H. Yuker (Ed.), *Attitudes toward Persons with Disabilities* (pp. 246–261). New York: Springer Publishing.

88. McColl, M. & Skinner, H. (1995). Assessing inter- and intrapersonal resources: social support and coping among adults with a disability. *Disability and Rehabilitation*, 17(1), 24–34.

89. McGowan, M. & Roth, S. (1987). Family functioning and functional independence in spinal cord injury adjustment. *Paraplegia*, 25, 357–365.

90. Moeller, T. & Hartman, D. (1984). The group psychotherapy process in rehabilitation settings. In: D. Krueger (Ed.), *Emotional Rehabilitation of Physical Trauma and Disability* (pp. 219–233). New York: SP Medical & Scientific Books.

91. Morgan, D. (1980). Not all sadness can be treated with antidepressants. *West Virginia Medical Journal*, 76(6), 136–137.

92. Moses, K. (Speaker). (1989). Shattered dreams and growth: a workshop on helping and being helped (Cassette Recording). Evanston, IL: Resource Networks, Inc.

93. Nichols, S. & Brasile, F. (1998). The role of recreational therapy in physical medicine. *Topics in Spinal Cord Injury Rehabilitation*, 3(3), 89–98.

94. Northouse, P. & Northouse, L. (1985). *Health Communication: A Handbook for Health Professionals*. Englewood Cliffs, NJ: Prentice-Hall.

95. Nosek, M.; Parker, R.; & Larsen, S. (1987). Psychosocial independence and functional abilities: their relationship in adults with severe musculoskeletal impairments. *Archives of Physical Medicine and Rehabilitation*, 68(12), 840–845.

96. Noyes, R. (1984). The existential crisis of serious illness. In: D. Krueger (Ed.), *Emotional Rehabilitation of Physical Trauma and Disability* (pp. 51–61). New York: SP Medical & Scientific Books.

97. Osterweis, M.; Solomon, F.; & Green, M. (1984). *Bereavement: Reactions, Consequences, and Care*. Washington, DC: National Academy Press.

98. Park, L. (1977). Barriers to normality for the handicapped adult in the United States. In: R. Marinelli & A. Dell Orto (Eds.), *The Psychological and Social Impact of Physical Disability* (pp. 25–33). New York: Springer Publishing.

99. Pinkerton, A. & Griffin, M. (1983). Rehabilitation outcomes in females with spinal cord injury: a follow-up study. *Paraplegia*, 21, 166–175.

100. Post, M.; de Witte, L.; van Asbeck, F.; van Dijk, A.; & Shrijvers, J. (1998). Predictors of health status and life satisfaction in spinal cord injury. *Archives of Physical Medicine and Rehabilitation*, 79(4), 395–401.

101. Quigley, M. (1995). Impact of spinal cord injury on the life roles of women. *American Journal of Occupational Therapy*, 49(8), 780–786.

102. Richards, J. (1986). Psychologic adjustment to spinal cord injury during first postdischarge year. *Archives of Physical Medicine and Rehabilitation*, 67, 362–365.

103. Richards, J.; Seitz, M.; & Eisele, W. (1986). Auditory processing in spinal cord injury: a preliminary investigation from a sensory deprivation perspective. *Archives of Physical Medicine and Rehabilitation*, 67, 115–117.

104. Rogers, M. (1986). *Living with Paraplegia*. Boston: Faber & Faber.

105. Rohrer, K.; Adelman, B.; Puckett, J.; Toomey, B.; Talbert, D.; & Johnson, E. (1980). Rehabilitation in spinal cord injury: use of a patient–family group. *Archives of Physical Medicine and Rehabilitation*, 61, 225–229.

106. Roush, S. (1986). Health professionals as contributors to attitudes toward persons with disabilities. A special communication. *Physical Therapy*, 66(10), 1551–1554.

107. Russell, M. (1994). Malcolm teaches us, too. In: B. Shaw (Ed.), *The Ragged Edge: The Disability Experience from the Pages of the First Fifteen Years of* The Disability Rag (pp. 11–14). Louisville, KY: The Avocado Press.

108. Sammallahti, P.; Kannisto, M.; & Aalberg, V. (1996). Psychological defenses and psychiatric symptoms in adults with pediatric spinal cord injuries. *Spinal Cord*, 34(11), 669–672.

109. Schneider, J. (1984). *Stress, Loss, and Grief: Understanding Their Origins and Growth Potential*. Baltimore: University Park Press.

110. Scivoletto, G; Petrelli, A.; Di Lucente, L.; & Castellano, V. (1997). Psychological investigation of spinal cord injury patients. *Spinal Cord*, 35(8), 516–520.

111. Servoss, A. & Krueger, D. (1984). Normal vs. pathological grief and mourning: some precursors. In: D. Krueger (Ed.), *Emotional Rehabilitation of Physical Trauma and Disability* (pp. 45–49). New York: SP Medical & Scientific Books.

112. Stewart, R. & Bhagwanjee, A. (1999). Promoting group empowerment and self-reliance through participatory research: a case study of people with physical disability. *Disability and Rehabilitation*, 21(7), 338–345.

113. Stubbins, J. (1988). The politics of disability. In: H. Yuker (Ed.), *Attitudes toward Persons with Disabilities* (pp. 22–32). New York: Springer Publishing.

114. Tate, D. & Forchheimer, M. (1998). Enhancing community reintegration after inpatient rehabilitation for persons with spinal cord injury. *Topics in Spinal Cord Injury Rehabilitation*, 4(1), 42–55.

115. Trieschmann, R. (1988). *Spinal Cord Injuries: Psychological, Social, and Vocational Rehabilitation*. New York: Demos.

116. Trieschmann, R. (1986). The psychosocial adjustment to spinal cord injury. In: R. Bloch & M. Basbaum (Eds.), *Management of Spinal Cord Injuries* (pp. 302–319). Baltimore: Williams & Wilkins.

117. Tunks, E.; Bahry, N.; & Basbaum, M. (1986). The resocialization process after spinal cord injury. In:

R. Bloch & M. Basbaum (Eds.), *Management of Spinal Cord Injuries* (pp. 387–409). Baltimore: Williams & Wilkins.

118. Urey, J. & Henggeler, S. (1987). Marital adjustment following spinal cord injury. *Archives of Physical Medicine and Rehabilitation*, 68, 69–74.

119. Ville, I. & Ravaud, J. (1996). Work, non-work and consequent satisfaction after spinal cord injury. *International Journal of Rehabilitation Research*, 19(3), 241–252.

120. Weinberg, N. (1988). Another perspective: attitudes of persons with disabilities. In: H. Yuker (Ed.), *Attitudes toward Persons with Disabilities* (pp. 141–153). New York: Springer Publishing.

121. Weitzenkamp, D.; Gerhart, K.; Charlifue, S.; Whiteneck, G.; & Savic, G. (1997). Spouses of spinal cord injury survivors: the added impact of caregiving. *Archives of Physical Medicine and Rehabilitation*, 78(8), 822–827.

122. Westgren, N. & Levi, R. (1998). Quality of life and traumatic spinal cord injury. *Archives of Physical Medicine and Rehabilitation*, 79(11), 1433–1439.

123. Wolfensberger, W. & Glenn, L. (1978). *PASS (Program Analysis of Service Systems: A Method for the Quantitative Evaluation of Human Services— Field Manual)* (3rd ed.). Toronto: National Institute on Mental Retardation.

124. Wolfensberger, W. & Thomas, S. (1983). *PASSING (Program Analysis of Service Systems' Implementation of Normalization Goals)* (2nd ed.). Toronto: National Institute on Mental Retardation.

125. Wolfensberger, W. & Tullman, S. (1982). A brief outline of the principle of normalization. *Rehabilitation Psychology*, 27(3), 131–145.

126. Worden, J. (1982). *Grief Counseling and Grief Therapy: A Handbook for the Mental Health Practitioner*. New York: Springer Publishing.

127. Wright, B. (1988). Attitudes and the fundamental negative bias: conditions and corrections. In: H. Yuker (Ed.), *Attitudes toward Persons with Disabilities* (pp. 3–21). New York: Springer Publishing.

128. Young, M.; Rintala, D.; Rossi, D.; Hart, K.; & Fuhrer, M. (1995). Alcohol and marijuana use in a community-based sample of persons with spinal cord injury. *Archives of Physical Medicine and Rehabilitation*, 76(6), 525–532.

129. Yuker, H. (1988). The effects of contact on attitudes toward disabled persons: some empirical generalizations. In: H. Yuker (Ed.), *Attitudes toward Persons with Disabilities* (pp. 262–274). New York: Springer Publishing.

130. Zola, I. (1982). Social and cultural disincentives to independent living. *Archives of Physical Medicine and Rehabilitation*, 63, 394–397.

Chapter 5

1. Althof, S. & Levine, S. (1993). Clinical approach to the sexuality of patients with spinal cord injury. *Urologic Clinics of North America*, 20(3), 527–534.

2. Anderson, C. (1997). Psychosocial and sexuality issues in pediatric spinal cord injury. *Topics in Spinal Cord Injury Rehabilitation*, 3(2), 70–78.

3. Atterbury, J. & Groome, L. (1998). Pregnancy in women with spinal cord injuries. *Nursing Clinics of North America*, 33(4), 603–613.

4. Baker, E. & Cardenas, D. (1996). Pregnancy in spinal cord injured women. *Archives of Physical Medicine and Rehabilitation*, 77(5), 501–507.

5. Berard, E. (1989). The sexuality of spinal cord injured women: physiology and pathophysiology. A review. *Paraplegia*, 27(2), 99–112.

6. Boller, F. & Frank, E. (1982). *Sexual Dysfunction in Neurological Disorders: Diagnosis, Management, and Rehabilitation*. New York: Raven Press.

7. Bonwich, E. (1985). Sex role attitudes and role reorganization in spinal cord injured women. In: Deegan M. J., Brooks N. A. (Eds.), *Women and Disability: The Double Handicap* (pp. 56–67). New Brunswick, NJ: Transaction Books.

8. Brackett, N.; Nash, M.; & Lynne, C. (1996). Male fertility following spinal cord injury: facts and fiction. *Physical Therapy*, 76(11), 1221–1231.

9. Brashear, D. (1978). Integrating human sexuality into rehabilitation practice. *Sexuality and Disability*, 1(3), 190–199.

10. Bregman, S. & Hadley, R. G. (1976). Sexual adjustment and feminine attractiveness among spinal cord injured women. *Archives of Physical Medicine and Rehabilitation*, 57, 448–450.

11. Brindley, G. (1980). Electroejaculation and the fertility of paraplegic men. *Sexuality and Disability*, 3(3), 223–229.

12. Cardenas, D.; Farrell-Roberts, L.; Sipski, M.; & Rubner, D. (1995). Management of gastrointestinal, genitourinary, and sexual function. In: S. Stover, J. DeLisa, & G. Whiteneck (Eds.), *Spinal Cord Injury: Clinical Outcomes from the Model Systems* (pp. 120–144). Gaithersburg, MD: Aspen.

13. Charlifue, S.; Gerhart, K.; Menter, R.; Whiteneck, G.; & Manley, M. (1992). Sexual issues of women with spinal cord injuries. *Paraplegia*, 30(3), 192–199.

14. Chen, D.; Hartwig, D.; & Roth, E. (1999). Comparison of sperm quantity and quality in antegrade V retrograde ejaculates obtained by vibratory penile stimulation in males with spinal cord injury. *American Journal of Physical Medicine and Rehabilitation*, 78(1), 46–51.

15. Chen, S.; Shieh, J.; Wang, Y.; Chang, H.; Ho, H.; & Yang, Y. (1998). Pregnancy achieved by intracytoplasmic sperm injection using cryopreserved vasal-epididymal sperm from a man with spinal cord injury. *Archives of Physical Medicine and Rehabilitation*, 79(2), 218–221.

16. Chung, P.; Verkauf, B.; Eichberg, R.; Casady, L.; Sanford, E.; & Maroulis, G. (1996). Electroejaculation and assisted reproductive techniques for anejaculatory infertility. *Obstetrics and Gynecology*, 87(1), 22–26.

17. Chung, P.; Verkauf, B.; Mola, R.; Skinner, L.; Eichberg, R.; & Maroulis, G. (1997). Correlation between semen parameters of electroejaculates and achieving pregnancy by intrauterine insemination. *Fertility and Sterility*, 67(1), 129–132.

18. Cole, T. (1979). Sexuality and the spinal cord injured. In: Green R. (Ed.), *Human Sexuality: A Health Practitioner's Text* (pp. 243–263). Baltimore: Williams & Wilkins.

19. Cole, T. (1975). Sexuality and physical disabilities. *Archives of Sexual Behavior, 4*(4), 389–403.

20. Cole, T. & Cole, S. (1981). Sexual attitude reassessment programs for spinal cord injured adults, their partners and health care professionals. In: Sha'ked A. (Ed.), *Human Sexuality and Rehabilitation Medicine* (pp. 80–90). Baltimore: Williams & Wilkins.

21. Cole, T. & Cole, S. (1978). The handicapped and sexual health. In: Comfort A. (Ed.), *Sexual Consequences of Disability* (pp. 37–43). Philadelphia: George F. Stickley Company.

22. Cole, T. & Stevens, M. (1975). Rehabilitation professionals and sexual counseling for spinal cord injured adults. *Archives of Sexual Behavior, 4*(6) 631–638.

23. Collins, K. & Hackler, R. (1988). Complications of penile prostheses in the spinal cord injury population. *The Journal of Urology,* 140, 984–985.

24. Conine, T. (1984). Sexual rehabilitation: Roles of allied health professional. In: Krueger D. (Ed.), *Rehabilitation Psychology: A Comprehensive Textbook* (pp. 81–87). Rockville, MD: Aspen Publishers.

25. Corbet, B. (1980). *Options: Spinal Cord Injury and the Future.* Denver, CO: A. B. Hirschfeld Press.

26. Corbet, B.; Dobbs, J.; & Bonin, B., Eds. (1998). *Spinal Network: The Total Wheelchair Resource Book* (3rd ed.).Malibu, CA: Miramar Communications.

27. Courtois, F.; Charvier, K.; Leriche, A.; & Raymond, D. (1993a). Sexual function in spinal cord injury men. I. Assessing sexual capability. *Paraplegia,* 31(12), 771–784.

28. Courtois, F.; Charvier, K.; Leriche, A.; Raymond, D.; & Eyssette, M. (1995). Clinical approach to erectile dysfunction in spinal cord injured men. A review of clinical and experimental data. *Paraplegia,* 33(11), 628–635.

29. Courtois, F.; Gonnaud, P.; Charvier, K.; Leriche, A.; & Raymond, D. (1998). Sympathetic skin responses and psychogenic erections in spinal cord injured men. *Spinal Cord,* 36(2), 125–131.

30. Courtois, F.; MacDougall, J.; & Sachs, B. (1993b). Erectile mechanism in paraplegia. *Physiology and Behavior,* 53(4), 721–726.

31. Craig, D. (1990). The adaptation to pregnancy of spinal cord injured women. *Rehabilitation Nursing,* 15(1), 6–9.

32. Crenshaw, R.; Martin, D.; Warner, H.; & Crenshaw, T. (1978). Organic impotence. In: Comfort A. (Ed.), *Sexual Consequences of Disability* (pp. 25–35). Philadelphia: George F. Stickley Company.

33. Denil, J.; Kuczyk, A.; Schultheiss, D.; Jibril, S.; Kupker, W.; Fischer, R.; Jonas, U.; Schlosser, H.; & Diedrich, K. (1996a). Use of assisted reproductive techniques for treatment of ejaculatory disorders. *Andrologia,* 28(Suppl. 1), 43–51.

34. Denil, J.; Ohl, D.; & Smythe, C. (1996b). Vacuum erection device in spinal cord injured men: patient and partner satisfaction. *Archives of Physical Medicine and Rehabilitation,* 77(8), 750–753.

35. Denys, P.; Mane, M.; Azouvi, P.; Chartier-Kastler, E.; Thiebaut, J.; & Bussel, B. (1998). Side effects of chronic intrathecal baclofen on erection and ejaculation in patients with spinal cord lesions. *Archives of Physical Medicine and Rehabilitation,* 79(5), 494–496.

36. Derry, F.; Dinsmore, W.; Fraser, M.; Gardner, B.; Glass, C.; Maytom, M.; & Smith, M.(1998). Efficacy and safety of oral sildenafil (Viagra) in men with erectile dysfunction caused by spinal cord injury. *Neurology,* 51(6), 1629–1633.

37. Donovon, W. (1985). Sexuality and sexual function. In: Bedbrook G. M. (Ed.), *Lifetime Care of the Paraplegic Patient* (pp. 149–161). New York: Churchill Livingstone.

38. Dunn, M.; Lloyd, E. E.; & Phelps, G. H. (1979). Sexual assertiveness in spinal cord injury. *Sexuality & Disability,* 2(4), 293–300.

39. Eiesland, N. (1995). Potent creativity. *Topics in Spinal Cord Injury Rehabilitation,* 1(2), 65–67.

40. Eisenberg, M. & Rustad, L. (1976). Sex education and counseling program on a spinal cord injury service. *Archives of Physical Medicine and Rehabilitation,* 57, 135–140.

41. Fitzpatrick, W. (1974). Sexual function in the paraplegic patient. *Archives of Physical Medicine and Rehabilitation,* 55, 221–227.

42. Gatens, C. (1984). Sexuality and disability. In: Woods N. F. (Ed.), *Human Sexuality in Health and Illness* (3rd ed., pp. 370–398). St. Louis: C. V. Mosby.

43. Geiger, R. (1979). Neurophysiology of sexual response in spinal cord injury. *Sexuality & Disability,* 2(4), 257–266.

44. Giuliano, F.; Rampin, O.; Benoit, G.; & Jardin, A. (1995). Neural control of penile erection. *Urologic Clinics of North America,* 22(4), 747–766.

45. Go, B.; DeVivo, M.; & Richards, J. (1995). The epidemiology of spinal cord injury. In: S. Stover, J. DeLisa, & G. Whiteneck (Eds.), *Spinal Cord Injury: Clinical Outcomes from the Model Systems* (pp. 21–55). Gaithersburg, MD: Aspen.

46. Gott, L. (1981). Anatomy and physiology of male sexual response and fertility as related to spinal cord injury. In: Sha'ked A. (Ed.), *Human Sexuality and Rehabilitation Medicine* (pp. 67–73). Baltimore: Williams & Wilkins.

47. Green, B.; Killorin, W.; Foote, J.; Bennett, J.; & Sloan, S. (1995). Complications of penile implants in spinal cord injured patients. *Topics in Spinal Cord Injury Rehabilitation,* 1(2), 44–52.

48. Griffith, E.; Tomko, M.; and Timms, R. (1973). Sexual function is spinal cord-injured patients: a review. *Archives of Physical Medicine and Rehabilitation,* 54, 539–543.

49. Griffith, E. & Trieschmann, R. (1975). Sexual functioning in women with spinal cord injury. *Archives of Physical Medicine and Rehabilitation,* 56, 18–21.

50. Griffith, E.; Trieschmann, R.; Hohmann, G.; Cole, T.; Tobis, J.; & Cummings, V. (1975). Sexual dysfunctions associated with physical disabilities. *Archives of Physical Medicine and Rehabilitation,* 56, 8–13.

51. Guyton, A. (1987). *Human Physiology and Mechanisms of Disease* (4th ed.). Philadelphia: W. B. Saunders Company.

52. Hale, G. (Ed.). (1979). *The Source Book for the Disabled: An Illustrated Guide to Easier More Independent Living for Physically Disabled People, Their Families and Friends.* New York: Paddington Press.

53. Halstead, L. (1984). Sexuality and disability. In: Krueger D. W. (Ed.), *Emotional Rehabilitation of Physical Trauma and Disability* (pp. 235–252). New York: Spectrum Publications.

54. Halstead, L.; VerVoort, S.; & Seager, S. (1987). Rectal probe electrostimulation in the treatment of anejaculatory spinal cord injured men. *Paraplegia*, 25, 120–129.

55. Harrison, J.; Glass, C.; Owens, R.; & Soni, B. (1995). Factors associated with sexual functioning in women following spinal cord injury. *Paraplegia*, 33(12), 687–692.

56. Higgins, G. (1984). Sexuality and the spinal cord injured: treatment approaches. In: Krueger D. W. (Ed.), *Emotional Rehabilitation of Physical Trauma and Disability* (pp. 253–265). New York: Spectrum Publications.

57. Hirsch, I. (1995). Spermatogenesis following spinal cord injury. *Topics in Spinal Cord Injury Rehabilitation*, 1(2), 27–43.

58. Iwatsubo, E.; Tanaka, M.; Takahashi, K.; & Akatsu, T. (1986). Non-inflatable penile prosthesis for the management of urinary incontinence and sexual disability of patients with spinal cord injury. *Paraplegia*, 24, 307–310.

59. Kenney, L. (1987). Meet Ellen Stohl. *Playboy*, 34(7), 68–75.

60. Killien, M. (1984). Sexuality and contraception. In: Woods N. F. (Ed.), *Human Sexuality in Health and Illness* (3rd ed., pp. 204–221). St. Louis: C. V. Mosby Company.

61. Kirk, S. (1977). Society and sexual deviance. In: Gochros H. L., & Gochros J. S. (Eds.), *The Sexually Oppressed* (pp. 28–37). New York: Association Press.

62. Kobayashi, A.; Mizobe, T.; Tojo, H.; & Hashimoto, S. (1995). Autonomic hyperreflexia during labour. *Canadian Journal of Anaesthesia*, 42(12), 1134–1136.

63. Komisaruk, B.; Gerdes, C.; & Whipple, B. (1997). 'Complete' spinal cord injury does not block perceptual responses to genital self-stimulation in women. *Archives of Neurology*, 54(12), 1513–1520.

64. Kreuter, M.; Sullivan, M.; Dahllöf, A.; & Siösteen, A. (1998). Partner relationships, functioning, mood and global quality of life in persons with spinal cord injury and traumatic brain injury. *Spinal Cord*, 36(4), 252–261.

65. Kreuter, M.; Sullivan, M.; & Siösteen, A. (1996). Sexual adjustment and quality of relationships in spinal paraplegia: a controlled study. *Archives of Physical Medicine and Rehabilitation*, 77(6), 541–548.

66. Kreuter, M.; Sullivan, M.; & Siösteen, A. (1994). Sexual adjustment after spinal cord injury (SCI) focusing on partner experiences. *Paraplegia*, 32(4), 225–235.

67. Kroll, K. & Klein, E. (1992). *Enabling Romance: A Guide to Love, Sex, and Relationships for the Disabled (And the People Who Care About Them).* Bethesda, MD: Woodbine House.

68. Kuhr, C.; Heiman, J.; Cardenas, D.; Bradley, W.; & Berger, R. (1995). Premature emission after spinal cord injury. *Journal of Urology*, 153(2), 429–431.

69. Langtry, H. & Markham, A. (1999). Sildenafil: a review of its use in erectile dysfunction. *Drugs*, 57(6), 967–989.

70. Larsen, E. & Hejgaard, N. (1984). Sexual dysfunction after spinal cord or cauda equina lesions. *Paraplegia*, 22, 66–74.

71. Levi, R.; Hultling, C.; Nash, M.; & Seiger, A. (1995). The Stockholm Spinal Cord Injury Study: 1: medical problems in a regional SCI population. *Paraplegia*, 33(6), 308–315.

72. Lloyd, L. & Brown, J. (1995). Management of erectile dysfunction in spinal cord injury with intracavernous pharmacotherapy. *Topics in Spinal Cord Injury Rehabilitation*, 1(2), 53–61.

73. Löchner-Ernst, D.; Mandalka, B.; Kramer, G.; & Stöhrer, M. (1997). Conservative and surgical semen retrieval in patients with spinal cord injury. *Spinal Cord*, 35(7), 463–468.

74. Matthews, G.; Gardner, T.; & Eid, F. (1996). In vitro fertilization improves pregnancy rates for sperm obtained by rectal probe ejaculation. *Journal of Urology*, 155(6), 1934–1937.

75. McAlonan, S. (1996). Improving sexual rehabilitation services: the patient's perspective. *American Journal of Occupational Therapy*, 50(10), 826–834.

76. Miller, S.; Szasz, G.; & Anderson, L. (1981). Sexual health care clinician in an acute spinal cord injury unit. *Archives of Physical Medicine and Rehabilitation*, 62, 315–320.

77. Monga, M.; Bernie, J.; & Rajasekaran, M. (1999). Male infertility and erectile dysfunction in spinal cord injury: a review. *Archives of Physical Medicine and Rehabilitation*, 80(10), 1331–1339.

78. National Spinal Cord Injury Statistical Center. (1999). *Spinal Cord Injury: Facts and Figures at a Glance.* Available from: www.spinalcord.uab.edu/docs/factsfig/htm.

79. Nehra, A.; Werner, M.; Bastuba, M.; Title, C.; & Oates, R. (1996). Vibratory stimulation and rectal probe electroejaculation as therapy for patients with spinal cord injury: semen parameters and pregnancy rates. *Journal of Urology*, 155(2), 554–559.

80. Ohl, D.; McCabe, M.; Sonksen, J.; Randolph, J.; & Menge, A. (1996a). Management of infertility in spinal cord injury. *Topics in Spinal Cord Injury Rehabilitation*, 1(3), 65–75.

81. Ohl, D.; Menge, A.; & Sonksen, J. (1996b). Penile vibratory stimulation in spinal cord injured men: optimized vibration parameters and prognostic factors. *Archives of Physical Medicine and Rehabilitation*, 77(9), 903–905.

82. Ohl, D.; Sonksen, J.; Menge, A.; McCabe, M.; & Keller, L. (1997). Electroejaculation versus vibratory stimulation in spinal cord injured men: sperm quality and patient preference. *Journal of Urology*, 157(6), 2147–2149.

83. Pryor, J.; LeRoy, S.; Nagel, T.; & Hensleigh, H. (1995). Vibratory stimulation for treatment of ane-

jaculation in quadriplegic men. *Archives of Physical Medicine and Rehabilitation*, 76(1), 59–64.

84. Rampin, O.; Bernabe, J.; & Giuliano, F. (1997). Spinal control of penile erection. *World Journal of Urology*, 15(1), 2–13.

85. Ray, C. & West, J. (1984). Social, sexual, and personal implications of paraplegia. *Paraplegia*, 22, 75–86.

86. Rivas, D.; King, S.; & Chancellor, M. (1996). Male and female sexual dysfunction. *Topics in Spinal Cord Injury Rehabilitation*, 1(3), 55–64.

87. Romano, M. (1977). The physically handicapped. In: Gochros H. L., & Gochros J. S. (Eds.), *The Sexually Oppressed* (pp. 257–267). New York: Association Press.

88. Romano, M. & Lassiter, R. (1972). Sexual counseling with the spinal-cord injured. *Archives of Physical Medicine and Rehabilitation*, 53, 568–572.

89. Rutkowski, S.; Geraghty, T.; Hagen, D.; Bowers, D.; Craven, M.; & Middleton, J. (1999). A comprehensive approach to the management of male infertility following spinal cord injury. *Spinal Cord*, 37(7), 508–514.

90. Rutkowski, S.; Middleton, J.; Truman, G.; Hagen, D.; & Ryan, J. (1995). The influence of bladder management on fertility in spinal cord injured males. *Paraplegia*, 33(5), 263–266.

91. Saeger, S. & Halstead, L. (1993). Fertility options and success after spinal cord injury. *Urologic Clinics of North America*, 20(3), 543–548.

92. Sedor, J. & Hirsch, I. (1995). Evaluation of sperm morphology of electroejaculates of spinal cord-injured men by strict criteria. *Fertility and Sterility*, 63(5), 1125–1127.

93. Siösteen, A.; Forssman, L.; Steen, Y.; Sullivan, L.; & Wickström, I. (1990a). Quality of semen after repeated ejaculation treatment in spinal cord injury men. *Paraplegia*, 28, 96–104.

94. Siösteen, A.; Lundqvist, C.; Blomstrand, C.; Sullivan, L.; & Sullivan, M. (1990b). Sexual ability, activity, attitudes and satisfaction as part of adjustment in spinal cord-injured subjects. *Paraplegia*, 28(5), 285–295.

95. Sipski, M. & Alexander, C. (1995). Female sexuality after spinal cord injury: Current knowledge and future directions. *Topics in Spinal Cord Injury Rehabilitation*, 1(2), 1–10.

96. Sipski, M.; Alexander, C.; & Rosen, R. (1997). Physiologic parameters associated with sexual arousal in women with incomplete spinal cord injuries. *Archives of Physical Medicine and Rehabilitation*, 78(3), 305–313.

97. Sipski, M.; Alexander, C.; & Rosen, R. (1995a). Orgasm in women with spinal cord injuries: a laboratory-based assessment. *Archives of Physical Medicine and Rehabilitation*, 76(12), 1097–1102.

98. Sipski, M.; Alexander, C.; & Rosen, R. (1995b). Physiological parameters associated with psychogenic sexual arousal in women with complete spinal cord injuries. *Archives of Physical Medicine and Rehabilitation*, 76(9), 811–818.

99. Sipski, M.; Rosen, R.; & Alexander, C. (1996). Physiological parameters associated with the performance of a distracting task and genital self-stimulation in women with complete spinal cord

injuries. *Archives of Physical Medicine and Rehabilitation*, 77(5), 419–424.

100. Smith, E. & Bodner, D. (1993). Sexual dysfunction after spinal cord injury. *Urologic Clinics of North America*, 20(3), 535–542.

101. Sonksen, J.; Sommer, P.; Biering-Sorensen, F.; Ziebe, S.; Lindhard, A.; Loft, A.; Andersen, A.; & Kristensen, J. (1997). Pregnancy after assisted ejaculation procedures in men with spinal cord injury. *Archives of Physical Medicine and Rehabilitation*, 78(10), 1059–1061.

102. Steger, J. & Brockway, J. (1980). Sexual enhancement in spinal cord injured patients: behavioral group treatment. *Sexuality and Disability*, 3(2), 84–96.

103. Stein, R. (1992). Sexual dysfunctions in the spinal cord injured. *Paraplegia*, 30(1), 54–57.

104. Szasz, G. (1987). Sexual management. In: Ford J. & Duckworth B. (Eds.), *Physical Management for the Quadriplegic Patient* (2nd ed., pp. 377–396). Philadelphia: F. A. Davis Company.

105. Tay, H.; Juma, S.; & Joseph, A. (1996). Psychogenic impotence in spinal cord injury patients. *Archives of Physical Medicine and Rehabilitation*, 77(4), 391–393.

106. Taylor, Z.; Molloy, D.; Hill, V.; & Harrison, K. (1999). Contribution of the assisted reproductive technologies to fertility in males suffering spinal cord injury. *Australian and New Zealand Journal of Gynaecology*, 39(1), 84–87.

107. Teal, J. & Athelstan, G. T. (1975). Sexuality and spinal cord injury: some psychosocial considerations. *Archives of Physical Medicine & Rehabilitation*, 56, 264–268.

108. Thews, G. & Vaupel, P. (1985). *Autonomic Functions in Human Physiology*. New York: Springer-Verlag.

109. Thornton, C. (1979). Sexuality counseling of women with spinal cord injuries. *Sexuality & Disability*, 2(4), 267–277.

110. Verduyn, W. (1986). Spinal cord injured women, pregnancy and delivery. *Paraplegia*, 24, 231–220.

111. Vick, R. (1984). *Contemporary Medical Physiology*. Reading, MA: Addison-Wesley Publishing.

112. Wanner, M.; Rageth, C.; & Zach, G. (1987). Pregnancy and autonomic hyperreflexia in patients with spinal cord lesions. *Paraplegia*, 25, 482–490.

113. Watkins, W.; Lim, T.; Bourne, H.; Baker, H.; & Wutthiphan, B. (1996). Testicular aspiration of sperm for intracytoplasmic sperm injection: an alternative treatment to electro-emission: case report. *Spinal Cord*, 34(11), 696–698.

114. Weiss, H. (1978). The physiology of human penile erection. In: Comfort A. (Ed.), *Sexual Consequences of Disability* (pp. 11–24). Philadelphia: George F. Stickley.

115. Westgren, N.; Hultling, C.; Levi, R.; Seiger, A.; & Westgren, M. (1997). Sexuality in women with traumatic spinal cord injury. *Acta Obstetrica et Gynecologica Scandinavia*, 76(10), 977–983.

116. White, M.; Rintala, D.; Hart, K.; Young, M.; & Fuhrer, M. (1992). Sexual activities, concerns and interests of men with spinal cord injury. *American Journal of Physical Medicine and Rehabilitation*, 71(4), 225–231.

117. White, M.; Rintala, D.; Hart, K.; & Fuhrer, M. (1993). Sexual activities, concerns and interests of women with spinal cord injury living in the community. *American Journal of Physical Medicine and Rehabilitation*, 72(6), 372–378.

118. Widerstrom-Noga, E.; Felipe-Cuervo, E.; Broton, J.; Duncan, R.; & Yezierski, R. (1999). Perceived difficulty in dealing with consequences of spinal cord injury. *Archives of Physical Medicine and Rehabilitation*, 80(5), 580–586.

119. Yamamoto, M.; Momose, H.; & Yamada, K. (1997). Fathering of a child with the assistance of electroejaculation in conjunction with intracytoplasmic sperm injection: case report. *Spinal Cord*, 35(3), 179–180.

120. Yarkony, G. & Gittler, M. (1996). Vibratory ejaculation for spinal-cord-injured men. *Topics in Spinal Cord Injury Rehabilitation*, 1(3), 82–87.

121. Zasler, N. & Katz, G. (1989). Synergist erection system in the management of impotence secondary to spinal cord injury. *Archives of Physical Medicine and Rehabilitation*, 70, 712–716.

Chapter 6

1. Abramowicz, M. (Ed.). (1990). Treatment of pressure ulcers. *Medical Letter on Drugs and Therapeutics*, 32, 17–18.

2. Akers, T. & Gabrielson, A. (1984). The effect of high voltage galvanic stimulation on the rate of healing of decubitus ulcers. *Biomedical Science Instrumentation*, 20, 99–100.

3. Anson, C. & Shepherd, C. (1996). Incidence of secondary complications in spinal cord injury. *International Journal of Rehabilitation Research*, 19(1), 55–66.

4. Aung, T. & El Masry, W. (1997) Audit of a British Centre for spinal injury. *Spinal Cord*, 35(3), 147–150.

5. Basta, S. (1991). Pressure sore prevention education with the spinal cord injured. *Rehabilitation Nursing*, 16(1), 6–8.

6. Bates-Jensen, B. (1998). Management of exudate and infection. In: Sussman, C. & Bates-Jensen, B. (Eds.), *Wound Care: A Collaborative Practice Manual for Physical Therapists and Nurses* (pp. 159–177). Gaithersburg, MD: Aspen Publishers.

7. Bates-Jensen, B. (1998). Pressure ulcers: pathophysiology and prevention. In: Sussman, C. & Bates-Jensen, B. (Eds.), *Wound Care: A Collaborative Practice Manual for Physical Therapists and Nurses* (pp. 235–270). Gaithersburg, MD: Aspen Publishers.

8. Bates-Jensen, B. (1997). The pressure sore status tool a few thousand assessments later. *Advances in Wound Care*, 10(5), 65–73.

9. Baynham, S.; Kohlman, P.; & Katner, H. (1999). Treating stage IV pressure ulcers with negative pressure therapy: a case report. *Ostomy Wound Management*, 45(4), 28–32, 34–35.

10. Bergstrom, N.; Allman, R.; Alvarez, O. et al. (1995). Pressure ulcer treatment: quick reference guide for clinicians. *Advances in Wound Care*, 8(2), 22–44.

11. Bergstrom, N.; Allman, R.; Carlson, C.; et al. (1992). *Pressure Ulcers in Adults: Prediction and Prevention. Clinical Practice Guideline, Number 3*. Rockville, MD: U.S. Department of Health and Human Services. Public Health Service, Agency for Health Care Policy and Research. AHCPR Publication No. 92-0047.

12. Bergstrom, N.; Bennett, M.; Carlson, C.; et al. (1994). *Treatment of Pressure Ulcers. Clinical Practice Guideline, Number 15*. Rockville, MD: U.S. Department of Health and Human Services. Public Health Service, Agency for Health Care Policy and Research. AHCPR Publication No. 95-0652.

13. Black, J. & Black, S. (1987). Surgical management of pressure ulcers. *Nursing Clinics of North America*, 22(2), 429–438.

14. Bobel, L. (1987). Nutritional implications in the patient with pressure sores. *Nursing Clinics of North America*, 22(2), 379–390.

15. Brienza, D. & Karg, P. (1998). Seat cushion optimization: a comparison of interface pressure and tissue stiffness characteristics for spinal cord injured and elderly patients. *Archives of Physical Medicine and Rehabilitation*, 79(4), 388–394.

16. Bristow, J.; Goldfarb, E.; & Green, M. (1987). Clinitron therapy: Is it effective? *Geriatric Nursing*, 8(3), 120–124.

17. Brylinsky, C. (1995). Nutrition and wound healing: An overview. *Ostomy/Wound Management*, 41(10), 14–24.

18. Brubaker, C. (1990). Ergonomic considerations. *Journal of Rehabilitation Research and Development*, Clinical Supplement #2, 37048.

19. Buchanan, L. & Ditunno, J. (1987). Acute care: Medical/surgical management. In: Buchanan, L. & Nawoczenski, D. (Eds.), *Spinal Cord Injury: Concepts and Management Approaches* (pp. 35–60). Baltimore: Williams & Wilkins.

20. Burns, S. & Betz, K. (1999). Seating pressures with conventional and dynamic wheelchair cushions in tetraplegia. *Archives of Physical Medicine and Rehabilitation*, 80(5), 566–571.

21. Burr, R.; Chem, C.; Clift-Peace, L.; & Nuseibeh, I. (1993). Haemoglobin and albumin as predictors of length of stay of spinal injured patients in a rehabilitation centre. *Paraplegia*, 31(7), 473–478.

22. Byrne, D. & Salzberg, C. (1996). Major risk factors for pressure ulcers in the spinal cord disabled: A literature review. *Spinal Cord*, 34(5), 255–263.

23. Carley, P. & Wainapel, S. (1985). Electrotherapy for acceleration of wound healing: Low intensity direct current. *Archives of Physical Medicine and Rehabilitation*, 66(7), 443–446.

24. Carvell, J. & Grundy, D. (1994). Complications of spinal surgery in acute spinal cord injury. *Paraplegia*, 32(6), 389–395.

25. Cassell, B. (1986). Treating pressure sores by stage. *RN*, 49, 36–40.

26. Cochran, G. & Palmieri, V. (1980). Development of test methods for evaluation of wheelchair cushions. *Bulletin of Prosthetics Research*, 17(1), 9–30.

27. Cooper, P.; Gray, D.; & Mollison, J. (1998). A randomised controlled trial of two pressure-reducing surfaces. *Journal of Wound Care*, 7(8), 374–376.

28. Cooper, R. (1998). *Wheelchair Selection and Configuration*. New York: Demos Medical Publishing.

29. Cuddigan, J. & Frantz, R. (1998). Pressure ulcer research: pressure ulcer treatment. A monograph from the National Pressure Ulcer Advisory Panel. *Advances in Wound Care*, 11(6), 294–300.

30. Curry, K. & Casady, L. (1992). The relationship between extended periods of immobility and decubitus ulcer formation in the acutely spinal cord-injured individual. *Journal of Neuroscience Nursing*, 24(4), 185–189.

31. Dabnichki, P. & Taktak, D. (1998). Pressure variation under the ischial tuberosity during a push cycle. *Medical Engineering and Physics*, 20(4), 242–256.

32. da Paz, A.; Beraldo, P., Almeida, M.; Neves, E.; Alves, C.; & Khan, P. (1992). Traumatic injury to the spinal cord. Prevalence in Brazilian hospitals. *Paraplegia*, 30(9), 636–640.

33. Dealey, C. (1994). *The Care of Wounds: A Guide for Nurses*. Cambridge, MA: Blackwell Science.

34. DeVivo, M.; Kartus, P.; Stover, S.; & Fine, P. (1990). Benefits of early admission to an organized spinal cord injury care system. *Paraplegia*, 28(9), 545–555.

35. DeVivo, M.; Kartus, P.; Stover, S.; Rutt, R.; & Fine, P. (1989). Cause of death for patients with spinal cord injuries. *Archives of Internal Medicine*, 149(8), 1761–1766.

36. Disa, J.; Carlton, J.; & Goldberg, N. (1992). Efficacy of operative cure in pressure sore patients. *Plastic and Reconstructive Surgery*, 89(2), 272–278.

37. Ditunno, J. & Formal, C. (1994). Chronic spinal cord injury. *New England Journal of Medicine*, 330(8), 550–556.

38. Dover, H.; Pickard, W.; Swain, I.; & Grundy, D. (1992). The effectiveness of a pressure clinic in preventing pressure sores. *Paraplegia*, 30(4), 267–272.

39. Dumurgier, C.; Pujol, G.; Chevalley, J.; Bassoulet, H.; Ucla, E.; & Stchepinsky, P. (1991). Pressure sore carcinoma: A late but fulminant complication of pressure sores in spinal cord injury patients: Case reports. *Paraplegia*, 29(6), 390–395.

40. Economides, N.; Skoutakis, V.; Carter, C.; & Smith, V. (1995). Evaluation of the effectiveness of two support surfaces following myocutaneous flap surgery. *Advances in Wound Care*, 8(1), 49–53.

41. Feedar, J. (1995). Clinical management of chronic wounds. In McCulloch, J., Kloth, L., & Feedar, J. (Eds.), *Wound Healing: Alternatives in Management* (2nd ed; pp. 137–176). Philadelphia: F. A. Davis Co.

42. Ferguson-Pell, M. (1990). Seat cushion selection. *Journal of Rehabilitation Research and Development*, Clinical Supplement #2, 47–73.

43. Ferrell, B. (1997). The Sessing Scale for measurement of pressure ulcer healing. *Advances in Wound Care*, 19(5), 78–80.

44. Fine, C. (1996). Utilizing a day hospital program as part of a pressure ulcer management program continuum. *Topics in Spinal Cord Injury Rehabilitation*, 2(1), 42–50.

45. Fletcher, J. (1996). Types of pressure-relieving equipment available: 1. *British Journal of Nursing*, 5(11), 694,696, 700–701.

46. Fowler, E. (1987). Equipment and products used in management and treatment of pressure ulcers. *Nursing Clinics of North America*, 22(2), 449–460.

47. Frost, F. (1993). Role of rehabilitation after spinal cord injury. *Urologic Clinics of North America*, 20(3), 549–559.

48. Fuhrer, M.; Garber, S.; Rintala, D.; Clearman, R.; & Hart, K. (1993). Pressure ulcers in community-resident persons with spinal cord injury: prevalence and risk factors. *Archives of Physical Medicine and Rehabilitation*, 74(11), 1172–1177.

49. Garber, S. (1985). Wheelchair cushions: A historical review. *American Journal of Occupational Therapy*, 39(7), 453–459.

50. Garg, M.; Rubayi, S.; & Montgomerie, J. (1992). Postoperative wound infections following myocutaneous flap surgery in spinal injury patients. *Paraplegia*, 30, 734–739.

51. Gault, W. & Gatens, P. (1976). Use of low intensity direct current in management of ischemic skin ulcers. *Physical Therapy*, 56(3), 265–269.

52. Gilsdorf, P.; Patterson, R.; & Fisher, S. (1991). Thirty-minute continuous sitting force measurements with different support surfaces in the spinal cord injured and able-bodied. *Journal of Rehabilitation Research and Development*, 28(4), 33–38.

53. Gogia, P. (1995). Low-energy laser in wound management. In: Gogia, P. (Ed.), *Clinical Wound Management* (pp. 165–172). Thorofare, NJ: SLACK Incorporated.

54. Goldstein, B.; Sanders, J.; & Benson, E. (1996). Pressure ulcers in SCI: Does tension stimulate wound healing? *American Journal of Physical Medicine and Rehabilitation*, 75(2), 130–133.

55. Goode, P. & Allman, R. (1989). The prevention and management of pressure ulcers. *Medical Clinics of North America*, 73(6), 1511–1524.

56. Gosnell, D. (1987). Assessment and evaluation of pressure sores. *Nursing Clinics of North America*, 22(2), 399–416.

57. Griffin, J.; Tooms, R.; Mendius, R.; Clifft, J.; Vander Zwaag, R; & El-Zeky, F. (1991). Efficacy of high voltage pulsed current for healing of pressure ulcers in patients with spinal cord injury. *Physical Therapy*, 71(6), 433–442, (discussion) 442–444.

58. Grundy, D.; Swain, A.; & Russell, J. (1986). ABC of spinal cord injury: Early management and complications I. *British Medical Journal*, 292(6512), 44–47.

59. Grundy, D.; Swain, A.; & Russell, J. (1986). ABC of spinal cord injury: Early management and complications II. *British Medical Journal*, 292(6513), 123–125.

60. Gunnewicht, B. (1996). Management of pressure sores in a spinal injuries unit. *Journal of Wound Care*, 5(1), 36–39.

61. Gunnewicht, B. (1995). Pressure sores in patients with acute spinal cord injury. *Journal of Wound Care*, 4(10), 452–454.

62. Hammond, M.; Bozzacco, V.; Stiens, S.; Buhrer, R.; & Lyman, P. (1994). Pressure ulcer incidence on a spinal cord injury unit. *Advances in Wound Care*, 7(6), 57–60.

63. Henderson, C.; Ayello, E.; Sussman, C.; et al. (1997). Draft definition of stage I pressure ulcers:

Inclusion of persons with darkly pigmented skin. *Advances in Wound Care*, 10(5), 16–19.

64. Henderson, J.; Price, S.; Brandstater, M.; & Mandac, B. (1994). Efficacy of three measures to relieve pressure in seated persons with spinal cord injury. *Archives of Physical Medicine and Rehabilitation*, 75(5), 535–539.

65. Hess, C. (1995). *Wound Care: Nurse's Clinical Guide*. Springhouse, PA: Springhouse Corporation.

66. Hobson, D. (1992). Comparative effects of posture on pressure and shear at the body-seat interface. *Journal of Rehabilitation Research and Development*, 29(4), 21–31.

67. Johnson, R.; Gerhart, K.; McCray, J.; Menconi, J.; & Whiteneck, G. (1998). Secondary conditions following spinal cord injury in a population-based sample. *Spinal Cord*, 36(1), 45–50.

68. Karp, G. (1998). *Choosing a Wheelchair: A Guide for Optimal Independence*. Sebastopol, CA: O'Reilly & Associates.

69. Kennedy, E.; Stover, S.; & Fine, P. (Eds.). (1986). *Spinal Cord Injury: The Facts and Figures*. Birmingham, AL: The University of Alabama Spinal Cord Injury Statistical Center.

70. Kernozek, T. & Lewin, J. (1998). Seat interface pressures of individuals with paraplegia: influence of dynamic wheelchair locomotion compared with static seated measurements. *Archives of Physical Medicine and Rehabilitation*, 79(3), 313–316.

71. Kierney, P.; Cardenas, D.; Engrav, L.; Grant, J.; & Rand, R. (1998). Limb-salvage in reconstruction of recalcitrant pressure sores using the inferiorly based rectus abdominis myocutaneous flap. *Plastic and Reconstructive Surgery*, 102(1), 111–116.

72. King, T.; Temkin, A.; & Vesmarovich, S. (1996). Taking charge: A proactive nursing approach to skin management. *Topics in Spinal Cord Injury Rehabilitation*, 2(1), 21–25.

73. Kirk, P. (1996). Pressure ulcer management following spinal cord injury. *Topics in Spinal Cord Injury Rehabilitation*, 2(1), 9–20.

74. Kloth, L. & Feedar, J. (1988). Acceleration of wound healing with high voltage, monophasic, pulsed current. *Physical Therapy*, 68(4), 503–508. (Erratum: *Physical Therapy*, 69(8), 702.)

75. Knight, A. (1988). Medical management of pressure sores. *Journal of Family Practice*, 27(1), 95–100.

76. Knutsdottir, S. (1993). Spinal cord injuries in Iceland 1973–1989. A follow up study. *Paraplegia*, 31(1), 68–72.

77. Koo, T.; Mak, A.; & Lee, Y. (1996). Posture effect on seating interface biomechanics: Comparison between two seating cushions. *Archives of Physical Medicine and Rehabilitation*, 77(1), 40–47.

78. Krasner, D. (1997). Wound Healing Scale, Version 1.0: A proposal. *Advances in Wound Care*, 10(5), 82–85.

79. Krause, J. (1998). Skin sores after spinal cord injury: Relationship to life adjustment. *Spinal Cord*, 36(1), 51–56.

80. Krouskop, T.; Williams, R.; Noble, P.; & Brown, J. (1986). Inflation pressure effect on performance of air-filled wheelchair cushions. *Archives of Physical Medicine and Rehabilitation*, 67, 126–128.

81. Lehman, C. (1995). Risk factors for pressure ulcers in the spinal cord injured in the community. *SCI Nursing*, 12(4), 110–114.

82. Levine, S.; Kett, R.; Cederna, P.; & Brooks, S. (1990). Electric muscle stimulation for pressure sore prevention: Tissue shape variation. *Archives of Physical Medicine and Rehabilitation*, 71(3), 210–215.

83. Levine, S.; Kett, R.; Gross, M.; Wilson, B.; Cederna, P.; & Juni, J. (1990). Blood flow in the gluteus maximus of seated individuals during electrical muscle stimulation. *Archives of Physical Medicine and Rehabilitation*, 71(9), 682–686.

84. Linares, H.; Mawson, A.; Suarez, E.; & Biundo, J. (1987). Association between pressure sores and immobilization in the immediate post-injury period. *Orthopedics*, 10(4), 571–573.

85. Ljungberg, S. (1998). Comparison of dextranomer paste and saline dressings for management of decubital ulcers. *Clinical Therapeutics*, 20(4), 737–743.

86. Loehne, H. (1998). Pulsatile lavage with concurrent suction. In Sussman, C. & Bates-Jensen, B. (Eds.), *Wound Care: A Collaborative Practice Manual for Physical Therapists and Nurses* (pp. 389–403). Gaithersburg, MD: Aspen Publishers.

87. Macklebust, J. (1987). Pressure ulcers: Etiology and prevention. *Nursing Clinics of North America*, 22(2), 359–377.

88. Matthews, P. & Carlson, C. (1987). *Spinal Cord Injury: A Guide to Rehabilitation Nursing*. Rockville, MD: Aspen Publishers.

89. Mawson, A.; Siddiqui, F.; & Biundo, J. (1993). Enhancing host resistance to pressure ulcers: A new approach to prevention. *Preventive Medicine*, 22(3), 433–450.

90. Mayall, J. & Desharnais, G. (1995). *Positioning in a Wheelchair: A Guide for Professional Caregivers of the Disabled Adult* (2nd ed.). Thorofare, NJ: Slack.

91. McBride, D. & Rodts, G. (1994). Intensive care of patients with spinal trauma. *Neurosurgical Intensive Care*, 5(4), 755–766.

92. McCagg, C. (1986). Postoperative management and acute rehabilitation of patients with spinal cord injuries. *Orthopedic Clinics of North America*, 17(1), 171–182.

93. McGlinchey-Berroth, R.; Morrow, L.; Ahlquist, M.; Sarkarati, M.; & Minaker, K. (1995). Late-life spinal cord injury and aging with a long term injury: Characteristics of two emerging populations. *Journal of Spinal Cord Medicine*, 18(3), 183–193.

94. McGuire, R.; Green, B.; Eismont, F. & Watts, C. (1988). Comparison of stability provided to the unstable spine by the kinetic therapy table and Stryker frame. *Neurosurgery*, 22(5), 842–845.

95. McLeod, A. (1997). Principles of alternating pressure surfaces. *Advances in Wound Care*, 10(7), 30–36.

96. Menter, R. & Hudson, L. (1995). Effects of age at injury and the aging process. In: Stover, S., De Lisa, J., & Whiteneck, J. (Eds.), *Spinal Cord Injury:*

Clinical Outcomes from the Model Systems (pp. 272–288). Gaithersburg, MD: Aspen.

97. Montgomerie, J. (1997). Infections in patients with spinal cord injuries. *Clinical Infectious Diseases*, 25(6), 1285–1290.

98. Montgomerie, J.; Chan, E.; Gilmore, D.; Canawati, H.; & Sapico, F. (1991). Low mortality among patients with spinal cord injury and bacteremia. *Reviews of Infectious Diseases*, 13(5), 867–871.

99. Morykwas, M.; Argenta, L.; Shelton-Brown, E.; & McGuirt, W. (1997). Vacuum-assisted closure: A new method for wound control and treatment: Animal studies and basic foundation. *Annals of Plastic Surgery*, 38(6), 553–562.

100. Nakajima, A.; Honda, S.; Yoshimura, S.; Ono, Y.; Kawamura, J.; & Moriai, N. (1989). The disease pattern and causes of death of spinal cord injured patients in Japan. *Paraplegia*, 27(3), 163–171.

101. National Pressure Ulcer Advisory Panel. (1989). Pressure ulcers prevalence, cost and risk assessment: Consensus development conference statement. *Decubitus*, 2(2), 24–28.

102. Nawoczenski, D. (1987). Pressure sores: Prevention and management. In: Buchanan, L. & Nawoczenski, D. (Eds.), *Spinal Cord Injury: Concepts and Management Approaches* (pp. 99–121). Baltimore: Williams & Wilkins.

103. Nelson, A.; Malassigne, P.; Cors, M.; Amerson, T; Bonifay, R.; & Schnurr, E. (1996). Patient evaluation of prone carts used in spinal cord injury. *SCI Nursing*, 13(2), 39–44.

104. Niazi, Z.; Salzberg, A.; Byrne, D.; & Viehbeck, M. (1997). Recurrence of initial pressure ulcer in persons with spinal cord injuries. *Advances in Wound Care*, 10(3), 38–42.

105. Nikas, D. (1986). Resuscitation of patients with central nervous system trauma. *Nursing Clinics of North America*, 21(4), 693–704.

106. Nixon, V. (1985). *Spinal Cord Injury: A Guide to Functional Outcomes in Physical Therapy Management*. Rockville, MD: Aspen Publishers.

107. Nussbaum, E.; Biemann, I.; & Mustard, B. (1994). Comparison of ultrasound/ultraviolet-C and laser for treatment of pressure ulcers in patients with spinal cord injury. *Physical Therapy*, 74(9), 812–823.

108. Palmieri, V.; Haelen, G.; & Cochran, G. (1980). A comparison of sitting pressures on wheelchair cushions as measured by air cell transducers and miniature electronic transducers. *Bulletin of Prosthetics Research*, 17(1), 5–8.

109. Patterson, R. & Fisher, S. (1986). Sitting pressure-time patterns in patients with quadriplegia. *Archives of Physical Medicine and Rehabilitation*, 67(11), 812–814.

110. Pena, M.; Drew, G.; & Smith, S. (1992). The inferiorly based rectus abdominis myocutaneous flap for reconstruction of recurrent pressure sores. *Plastic Reconstructive Surgery*, 89(1), 90–95.

111. Peters, J. & Johnson, G. (1990). Proximal femurectomy for decubitus ulceration in the spinal cord injury patient. *Paraplegia*, 28(1), 55–61.

112. Peterson, M. & Adkins, H. (1982). Measurement and redistribution of excessive pressures during wheelchair sitting. *Physical Therapy*, 62(7), 990–994.

113. Petrie, L. & Hummel, R. (1990). A study of interface pressure for pressure reduction and relief mattresses. *Journal of Enterostomal Therapy*, 17(5), 212–216.

114. Pires, M. & Adkins, R. (1996). Pressure ulcers and spinal cord injury: Scope of the problem. *Topics in Spinal Cord Injury Rehabilitation*, 2(1), 1–8.

115. Ragnarsson, K. (1990). Prescription considerations and a comparison of conventional and lightweight wheelchairs. *Journal of Rehabilitation Research and Development*, Clinical Supplement #2, 8–16.

116. Rao, D.; Sane, P.; & Georgiev, E. (1975). Collagenase in the treatment of dermal and decubitus ulcers. *Journal of the American Geriatric Society*, 23(1), 22–30.

117. Rischbieth, H.; Jelbart, M.; & Marshall, R. (1998). Neuromuscular electrical stimulation keeps a tetraplegic subject in his chair: A case study. *Spinal Cord*, 36, 443–445.

118. Rochon, P.; Beaudet, M.; McGlinchey-Berroth, R.; Morrow, L.; Ahlquist, M.; Young, R.; & Minaker, K. (1993). Risk assessment for pressure ulcers: an adaptation of the National Pressure Ulcer Advisory Panel risk factors to spinal cord injured patients. *Journal of the American Paraplegia Society*, 16(3), 169–177.

119. Rodeheaver, G.; Baharestani, M.; Brabec, M.; Byrd, H.; Salzberg, C.; Scherer, P.; & Vogelpohl, T. (1994). Wound healing and wound management: focus on debridement. An interdisciplinary round table, September 18, 1992, Jackson Hole, WY. *Advances in Wound Care*, 7(1), 22–24, 26–29, 32–36.

120. Rodriguez, G.; Claus-Walker, J.; Kent, M.; & Garza, H. (1989). Collagen metabolite excretion as a predictor of bone- and skin-related complications in spinal cord injury. *Archives of Physical Medicine and Rehabilitation*, 70(6), 442–444.

121. Rodriguez, G. & Garber, S. (1994). Prospective study of pressure ulcer risk in spinal cord injury patients. *Paraplegia*, 32(3), 150–158.

122. Salcido, R. (Ed.). (1999). Defining products by generic categories. *Advances in Wound Care*, 12(4), 164–174.

123. Salzberg, C.; Byrne, D.; Cayten, G.; Kabir, R. et al. (1998). Predicting and preventing pressure ulcers in adults with paralysis. *Advances in Wound Care*, 11(5), 237–246.

124. Salzberg, C.; Byrne, D.; Cayten, C.; van Nieuwerburgh, P.; Murphy, J.; & Viehbeck, M. (1996). A new pressure ulcer risk assessment scale for individuals with spinal cord injury. *American Journal of Physical Medicine and Rehabilitation*, 75(2), 96–104.

125. Salzberg, C.; Cooper-Vastola, S.; Perez, F.; Viehbeck, M.; & Byrne, D. (1995). The effects of non-thermal pulsed electromagnetic energy on wound healing of pressure ulcers in spinal cord-injured patients: A randomized, double-blind study. *Ostomy Wound Management*, 41(3), 42–4, 46, 48.

126. Salzberg, C.; Gray, B.; Petro, J.; & Salisbury, R. (1990). The perioperative antimicrobial management of pressure ulcers. *Decubitus*, 3(2), 24–26.

127. Sapountzi-Krepia, D.; Soumilas, A.; Papadakis, G.; Nomicos, J.; Theodossopoulou, E.; & Dimitriadou, A. (1998). Post traumatic paraplegics living in Athens: The impact of pressure sores and UTIs on everyday life activities. *Spinal Cord*, 36(6), 432–437.

128. Seiler, W.; Allen, S.; & Stahelin, H. (1986). Influence of the 30 laterally inclined position and the "super soft" 3-piece mattress on skin oxygen tension on areas of maximum pressure—implications for pressure sore prevention. *Gerontology*, 32, 158–166.

129. Seymour, R. & Lacefield, W. (1985). Wheelchair cushion effect on pressure and skin temperature. *Archives of Physical Medicine and Rehabilitation*, 66(2), 103–108.

130. Shenaq, S. & Dinh, T. (1990). Decubitus ulcers: How to prevent them—and intervene should prevention fail. *Postgraduate Medicine*, 87(4), 91–95.

131. Sprigle, S.; Chung, K.; & Brubaker, C. (1990). Reduction of sitting pressure with custom contoured cushions. *Journal of Rehabilitation Research and Development*, 27(2), 135–140.

132. Stewart, P. & Wharton, G. (1976). Bridging: An effective and practical method of preventive skin care for the immobilized person. *Southern Medical Journal*, 69(11), 1469–1473.

133. Sumiya, T.; Kawamura, K.; Tokuhiro, A.; Takechi, H.; & Ogata, H. (1997). A survey of wheelchair use by paraplegic individuals in Japan. Part 2: Prevalence of pressure sores. *Spinal Cord*, 35(9), 595–598.

134. Sussman, C. (1998). Whirlpool. In: Sussman, C. & Bates-Jensen, B. (Eds.), *Wound Care: A Collaborative Practice Manual for Physical Therapists and Nurses* (pp.447–460). Gaithersburg, MD: Aspen Publishers.

135. Sussman, C. & Swanson, G. (1997). Utility of the Sussman Wound Healing Tool in predicting wound healing outcomes in physical therapy. *Advances in Wound Care*, 10(5), 74–77.

136. Sussman, G. (1998). Management of the wound environment. In: Sussman, C. & Bates-Jensen, B. (Eds.), *Wound Care: A Collaborative Practice Manual for Physical Therapists and Nurses* (pp. 201–213). Gaithersburg, MD: Aspen Publishers.

137. Takechi, H. & Tokuhiro, A. (1998). Evaluation of wheelchair cushions by means of pressure distribution mapping. *Acta Medica Okayama*, 52(5), 245–254.

138. Thomas, D. (1997). Existing tools: Are they meeting the challenges of pressure ulcer healing? *Advances in Wound Care*, 10(5), 86–90.

139. Thomas, D.; Rodeheaver, G.; Bartolucci, A.; Franz, R.; Sussman, C.; Ferrell, B.; Cuddigan, J.; Stotts, N.; & Maklebust, J. (1997). Pressure ulcer scale for healing: Derivation and validation of the PUSH tool. *Advances in Wound Care*, 10(5), 96–101.

140. Uveges, J. (1996). Psychosocial correlates of pressure ulcers. *Topics in Spinal Cord Injury Rehabilitation*, 2(1), 51–56.

141. Vidal, J. & Sarrias, M. (1991). An analysis of the diverse factors concerned with the development of pressure sores in spinal cord injured patients. *Paraplegia*, 29(4), 261–267.

142. Vohra, R. & McCollum, C. (1994). Pressure sores. *British Medical Journal*, 309(6958), 853–857.

143. Wagner, D.; Fox, M.; & Ellis, E. (1994). Developing a successful interdisciplinary seating program. *Ostomy/Wound Management*, 40(1), 32–41.

144. Whittle, H.; Fletcher, C.; Hoskin, A.; & Campbell, K. (1996). Nursing management of pressure ulcers using a hydrogel dressing protocol: Four case studies. *Rehabilitation Nursing*, 21(5), 239–242.

145. Willey, T. (1989). High-tech beds and mattress overlays: A decision guide. *American Journal of Nursing*, 89(9), 1142–1145.

146. Williams, C. (1998). RoHo dry flotation system: An alternative means of pressure relief. *British Journal of Nursing*, 7(22), 1400, 1402–1404.

147. Wilson, A. (1992). *How to Select and Use Manual Wheelchairs*. Topping, VA: Rehabilitation Press.

148. Xakellis, G. & Chrischilles, E. (1992). Hydrocolloid versus saline-gauze dressings in treating pressure ulcers: A cost-effective analysis. *Archives of Physical Medicine and Rehabilitation*, 73(5), 463–469.

149. Xakellis, G. & Frantz, R. (1997). Pressure ulcer healing: what is it? What influences it? How is it measured? *Advances in Wound Care*, 10(5), 20–26.

150. Yarkony, G. (1994). Pressure ulcers: A review. *Archives of Physical Medicine and Rehabilitation*, 75(8), 908–917.

151. Yarkony, G. & Heinemann, A. (1995). Pressure ulcers. In: Stover, S., De Lisa, J., & Whiteneck, G. (Eds.), *Spinal Cord Injury: Clinical Outcomes from the Model Systems* (pp. 100–119). Gaithersburg, MD: Aspen Publishers.

152. Yob, S.; Wagner, D.; Casson, H.; & Leclerc, J. (1990). Skin management of the SCI patient. In: *Dawn of a New Decade: Spinal Cord Injury in the 1990's*. Symposium sponsored by National Rehabilitation Hospital, Washington, DC.

153. Young, J.; Burns, P.; Bowen, A.; & McCutchen, R. (1982). *Spinal Cord Injury Statistics: Experience of the Regional Spinal Cord Injury Systems*. Phoenix, AZ: Good Samaritan Medical Center.

Chapter 7

1. Alvarez, S.; Peterson, M.; & Lunsford, B. (1981). Respiratory treatment of the adult patient with spinal cord injury. *Physical Therapy*, 61(12), 1737–1745.

2. Bach, J. (1991). New approaches in the rehabilitation of the traumatic high level quadriplegic. *American Journal of Physical Medicine and Rehabilitation*, 70(1), 13–19.

3. Bach, J. (1993). A comparison of long-term ventilatory support alternatives from the perspective of the patient and care giver. *Chest*, 104, 1702–1706.

4. Bach, J. (1993). Inappropriate weaning and late onset ventilatory failure of individuals with traumatic spinal cord injury. *Paraplegia*, 31(7), 430–438.

5. Bach, J. (1993). Mechanical insufflation-exsufflation: Comparison of peak expiratory flows with manually assisted and unassisted coughing techniques. *Chest*, 104, 1553–1562.

6. Bach, J. (1994). Update and perspectives on non-invasive respiratory muscle aids, part 1: The inspiratory aids. *Chest*, 105, 1230–1240.

7. Bach, J. (1994). Update and perspectives on non-invasive respiratory muscle aids, part 2: The expiratory aids. *Chest*, 105, 1538–1544.

8. Bach, J. (1995). Respiratory muscle aids for the prevention of pulmonary morbidity and mortality. *Seminars in Neurology*, 15(1), 72–81.

9. Bach, J. (1997). Noninvasive alternatives for tracheostomy for managing respiratory muscle dysfunction in spinal cord injury. *Topics in Spinal Cord Injury Rehabilitation*, 2(3), 49–58.

10. Bach, J. & Alba, A. (1990). Noninvasive options for ventilatory support of the traumatic high level quadriplegic patient. *Chest*, 98(3), 613–619.

11. Bach, J. & Alba, A. (1991). Intermittent abdominal pressure ventilator in a regimen of noninvasive ventilatory support. *Chest*, 99(3), 630–636.

12. Bach, J.; Alba, A.; & Saporito, L. (1993). Intermittent positive pressure ventilation via the mouth as an alternative to tracheostomy for 257 ventilator users. *Chest*, 103, 174–182.

13. Bach, J.; Smith, W.; Michaels, J.; Saporito, L.; Alba, A.; Dayal, R.; & Pan, J. (1993). Airway secretion clearance by mechanical exsufflation for post-poliomyelitis ventilator-assisted individuals. *Archives of Physical Medicine and Rehabilitation*, 74, 170–177.

14. Bach, J. & Wang, T. (1994). Pulmonary function and sleep disordered breathing in patients with traumatic tetraplegia: A longitudinal study. *Archives of Physical Medicine and Rehabilitation*, 75, 279–284.

15. Bluechardt, M.; Wiens, M.; Thomas, S.; & Plyley, M. (1992). Repeated measurements of pulmonary function following spinal cord injury. *Paraplegia*, 30(11), 768–774.

16. Brannon, F.; Foley, M.; Starr, J.; & Saul, L. (1998). *Cardiopulmonary Rehabilitation: Basic Theory and Application* (3rd ed). Philadelphia: F. A. Davis.

17. Brownlee, S. & Williams, S. (1987). Physiotherapy in the respiratory care of patients with high spinal injury. *Physiotherapy*, 73(3), 148–152.

18. Buchanan, L. & Ditunno, J. (1987). Acute care: Medical/surgical management. In: Buchanan, L. & Nawoczenski, D. (Eds.), *Spinal Cord Injury: Concepts and Management Approaches* (pp. 35–60). Baltimore: Williams & Wilkins.

19. Burkett, L.; Chisum, J.; Stone, W.; & Fernhall, B. (1990). Exercise capacity of untrained spinal cord injured individuals and the relationship of peak oxygen uptake to level of injury. *Paraplegia*, 28, 512–521.

20. Butler, S. (1996). Clinical assessment of the cardiopulmonary system. In: Frownfelter, D. & Dean, E. (Eds.), *Principles and Practice of Cardiopulmonary Physical Therapy* (3rd ed.; pp. 209–228). St. Louis: Mosby.

21. Chen, C.; Lien, I.; & Wu, M. (1990). Respiratory function in patients with spinal cord injuries: effects of posture. *Paraplegia*, 28(2), 81–86.

22. Clough, P.; Lindenauer, D.; Hayes, M.; & Zekany, B. (1986). Guidelines for routine respiratory care of patients with spinal cord injury. *Physical Therapy*, 66(9), 1395–1402.

23. Dean, E. & Hobson, L. (1996). Cardiopulmonary anatomy. In Frownfelter, D. & Dean, E. (Eds.), *Principles and Practice of Cardiopulmonary Physical Therapy* (3rd ed.; pp. 23–51). St. Louis: Mosby.

24. Derenne, J.; Macklem P.; & Roussos, C. (1978). The respiratory muscles: Mechanics, control, and pathophysiology, part I. *American Review of Respiratory Disease*, 118, 119–133.

25. Derenne, J.; Macklem P.; & Roussos, C. (1978). The respiratory muscles: Mechanics, control, and pathophysiology, part II. *American Review of Respiratory Disease*, 118, 373–390.

26. Derenne, J.; Macklem P.; & Roussos, C. (1978). The respiratory muscles: Mechanics, control, and pathophysiology, part III. *American Review of Respiratory Disease*, 118, 581–601.

27. Derrickson, J.; Ciesla, N.; Simpson, N.; & Imle, P. (1992). A comparison of two breathing exercise programs for patients with quadriplegia. *Physical Therapy*, 72(11), 763–769.

28. De Vivo, M.; Black, K.; & Stover, S. (1993). Causes of death during the first 12 years after spinal cord injury. *Archives of Physical Medicine and Rehabilitation*, 74, 248–254.

29. DeVivo, M. & Ivie, C. (1995). Life expectancy of ventilator-dependent persons with spinal cord injuries. *Chest*, 108(1), 226–232.

30. De Vivo, M.; Kartus, P.; Stover, S.; Rutt, R.; & Fine, P. (1989). Cause of death for patients with spinal cord injuries. *Archives of Internal Medicine*, 149(8), 1761–1766.

31. De Vivo, M. & Stover, S. (1995). Long-term survival and causes of death. In: Stover, S., De Lisa, J., & Whiteneck, G. (Eds.), *Spinal Cord Injury: Clinical Outcomes from the Model Systems* (pp. 298–316). Gaithersburg, MD: Aspen Publishers.

32. De Vivo, M.; Stover, S.; & Black, K. (1992). Prognostic factors for 12-year survival after spinal cord injury. *Archives of Physical Medicine and Rehabilitation*, 73, 156–162.

33. Douglas, W.; Rehder, K.; Beynen, F.; Sessler, A.; & Marsh, M. (1977). Improved oxygenation in patients with acute respiratory failure: The prone position. *American Review of Respiratory Disease*, 115, 559–566.

34. Esclarin, A.; Bravo, P.; Arroyo, O.; Mazaira, J.; Garrido, H.; & Alcaraz, M. (1994). Tracheostomy ventilation versus diaphragmatic pacemaker ventilation in high spinal cord injury. *Paraplegia*, 32(10), 687–693.

35. Esteban, A. et al. (1995). A comparison of four methods of weaning patients from mechanical ventilation. *New England Journal of Medicine*, 332(6), 345–350.

36. Estenne, M. & De Troyer, A. (1987). Mechanism of the postural dependence of vital capacity in tetraplegic subjects. *American Review of Respiratory Disease*, 135(2), 367–371.

37. Estenne, M.; Knoop, C.; Vanvaerenbergh, J.; Heilporn, A.; & Troyer, A. (1989). The effect of pectoralis muscle training in tetraplegic subjects. *American Review of Respiratory Disease*, 139, 1218–1222.

38. Figoni, S. (1993). Exercise responses and quadriplegia. *Medicine and Science in Sports and Exercise, 25*(4), 433–441.

39. Frownfelter, D. (1996). Pulmonary function tests. In: Frownfelter, D. & Dean, E. (Eds.), *Principles and Practice of Cardiopulmonary Physical Therapy* (3rd ed.; pp. 145–152). St. Louis: Mosby.

40. Frownfelter, D. (1996). Arterial blood gasses. In: Frownfelter, D. & Dean, E. (Eds.), *Principles and Practice of Cardiopulmonary Physical Therapy* (3rd ed.; pp. 153–158). St. Louis: Mosby.

41. Gerold, K. & Nussbaum, E. (1994). Understanding mechanical ventilation. *Physical Therapy Practice, 3*(2), 81–91.

42. Gilgoff, I.; Barras, D.; Jones, M.; & Adkins, H. (1988). Neck breathing: A form of voluntary respiration for the spine injured ventilator-dependent quadriplegic child. *Pediatrics, 82*(5), 741–745.

43. Glenn, M. & Bergman, S. (1997). Cardiovascular changes following spinal cord injury. *Topics in Spinal Cord Injury Rehabilitation, 2*(4), 47–53.

44. Gross, D.; Ladd, H.; Riley, E.; Macklem, P.; & Grassino, A. (1980). The effect of training on strength and endurance of the diaphragm in quadriplegia. *The American Journal of Medicine, 68*, 27–35.

45. Grundy, D.; Swain, A.; & Russell, J. (1986). ABC of spinal cord injury: Early management and complications I. *British Medical Journal, 292*(6512), 44–47.

46. Haas, F.; Axen, K.; Pineda, H.; Gandino, D.; & Haas, A. (1985). Temporal pulmonary function changes in cervical cord injury. *Archives of Physical Medicine and Rehabilitation, 66*, 139–144.

47. Hall, K.; Harper, B.; & Whiteneck, G. (1997). Follow-up study of individuals with high tetraplegia (C1-C4) 10 to 21 years postinjury. *Topics in Spinal Cord Injury Rehabilitation, 2*(3), 107–116.

48. Hislop, H. & Montgomery, J. (1995). *Daniels and Worthingham's Muscle Testing: Techniques of Manual Examination* (6th ed). Philadelphia: W. B. Saunders Company.

49. Hopman, M.; Nommensen, E.; van Asten, W.; Oeseburg, B.; & Binkhorst, R. (1994). Properties of the venous vascular system in the lower extremities of individuals with paraplegia. *Paraplegia, 32*, 810–816.

50. Jackson, A. & Groomes, T. (1994). Incidence of respiratory complications following spinal cord injury. *Archives of Physical Medicine and Rehabilitation, 75*, 270–275.

51. Jaeger, R.; Turba, R.; Yarkony, G. & Roth, E. (1993). Cough in spinal cord injured patients: Comparison of three methods to produce cough. *Archives of Physical Medicine and Rehabilitation, 74*, 1358–1361.

52. Johnson, K.; Grant, T.; & Peterson, P. (1997). Ventilator weaning for the patient with high-level tetraplegia. *Topics in Spinal Cord Injury Rehabilitation, 2*(3), 11–20.

53. Keen, M. (1994.) Management of the ventilator-dependent patient with quadriplegia. In: Yarkony, G. (Ed.), *Spinal Cord Injury: Medical Management and Rehabilitation* (pp. 129–135). Gaithersburg, MD: Aspen Publishers.

54. Kendall, F.; McCreary, E.; & Provance, P. (1993). *Muscles: Testing and Function* (4th ed). Baltimore: Williams & Wilkins.

55. Kennedy, E.; Stover, S.; & Fine, P. (Eds.). (1986). *Spinal Cord Injury: The Facts and Figures.* Birmingham, AL: The University of Alabama Spinal Cord Injury Statistical Center.

56. Kiwerski, J. (1993). Factors contributing to the increased threat to life following spinal cord injury. *Paraplegia, 31*(12), 793–799.

57. Langer, M.; Mascheroni, D.; Marcolin, R.; & Gattinoni, L. (1988). The prone position in ARDS patients: A clinical study. *Chest, 94*, 103–107.

58. Lanig, I. & Lammertse, D. (1992). The respiratory system in spinal cord injury. *Physical Medicine and Rehabilitation Clinics of North America, 3*(4), 725–740.

59. Ledsome, J. & Sharp, J. (1981). Pulmonary function in acute spinal cord injury. *American Review of Respiratory Disease, 124*(1), 41–44.

60. Lehman, K.; Lane, J.; Piepmeier, J. & Batsford, W. (1987). Cardiovascular abnormalities accompanying acute spinal cord injury in humans: Incidence, time course and severity. *Journal of the American College of Cardiology, 10*(1), 46–52.

61. Lemons, V. & Wagner, F. (1994). Respiratory complications after spinal cord injury. *Spine, 19*(20), 2315–2320.

62. Lin, V.; Singh, H.; Chitkara, R.; & Perkash, I. (1998). Functional magnetic stimulation for restoring cough in patients with tetraplegia. *Archives of Physical Medicine and Rehabilitation, 79*, 517–522.

63. Linder, S. (1993). Functional electrical stimulation to enhance cough in quadriplegia. *Chest, 103*(1), 166–169.

64a. Loveridge, B.; Badour, M.; & Dubo, H. (1989). Ventilatory muscle endurance training in quadriplegia: effects on breathing pattern. *Paraplegia, 27*, 329–339.

64b. Madama, V. (1993). *Pulmonary Function Testing and Cardiopulmonary Stress Testing.* Albany, NY: Delmar Publishers.

65. Mansel, J. & Norman, J. (1990). Respiratory complications and management of spinal cord injuries. *Chest, 97*, 1446–1452.

66. Marshall, S.; Marshall, L.; Vos, H.; & Chesnut, R. (1990). *Neuroscience Critical Care: Pathophysiology and Patient Management.* Philadelphia: W.B. Saunders Company.

67. Martini, F. (1998). *Fundamentals of Anatomy and Physiology* (4th ed). Upper Saddle River, NJ: Prentice Hall.

68. Massery, M. (1994). What's positioning got to do with it? *Neurology Report, 18*(3), 11–14.

69. Massery, M. (1996). Manual breathing and coughing aids. *Physical Medicine and Rehabilitation Clinics of North America, 7*(2), 407–422.

70. Massery, M. (1996). The patient with neuromuscular or musculoskeletal dysfunction. In: Frownfelter, D. & Dean, E. (Eds.), *Principles and Practice of Cardiopulmonary Physical Therapy* (3rd ed.; pp. 679–702). St. Louis: Mosby.

71. Massery, M. & Frownfelter, D. (1996). Body mechanics—the art of positioning and moving

patients. In: Frownfelter, D. & Dean, E. (Eds.), *Principles and Practice of Cardiopulmonary Physical Therapy* (3rd ed.; pp. 737–748). St. Louis: Mosby.

72. Massery, M. & Frownfelter, D. (1996). Facilitating airway clearance with coughing techniques. In: Frownfelter, D. & Dean, E. (Eds.), *Principles and Practice of Cardiopulmonary Physical Therapy* (3rd ed.; pp. 367–382). St. Louis: Mosby.

73a. Massery, M. & Frownfelter, D. (1996c). Facilitating ventilation patterns and breathing strategies. In: Frownfelter, D. & Dean, E. (Eds.), *Principles and Practice of Cardiopulmonary Physical Therapy* (3rd ed.;, pp. 383–416). St. Louis: Mosby.

73b. McArdle, W.; Katch, F.; & Katch, V. (2000). *Essentials in Exercise Physiology* (2nd ed.). Philadelphia: Lippincott Williams & Wilkins.

74. McBride, D. & Rodts, G. (1994). Intensive care of patients with spinal trauma. *Neurosurgery Clinics of North America*, 5(4), 755–766.

75. McCagg, C. (1986). Postoperative management and acute rehabilitation of patients with spinal cord injuries. *Orthopedic Clinics of North America*, 17(1), 171–182.

76. McCool, F.; Pichurko, B.; Slutsky, A.; Sarkarati, M.; Rossier, A.; & Brown, R. (1986). Changes in lung volume and rib cage configuration with abdominal binding in quadriplegia. *Journal of Applied Physiology*, 60(4), 1198–1202.

77. McMinn, R. (1994). *Last's Anatomy: Regional and Applied* (9th ed.). New York: Churchill Livingstone.

78. Mengelkoch, L.; Martin, D.; & Lawler, J. (1994). A review of the principles of pulse oximetry and accuracy of pulse oximeter estimates during exercise. *Physical Therapy*, 74(1), 40–49.

79. Meyer, P. (1989). Surgical stabilization of the cervical spine. In: Meyer, P. (Ed.), *Surgery of Spine Trauma* (pp. 397–523). New York: Churchill Livingstone.

80. Miller, H.; Thomas, E.; & Wilmot, C. (1988). Pneumobelt use among high quadriplegic population. *Archives of Physical Medicine and Rehabilitation*, 69, 369–372.

81. Moore, K. (1992). *Clinically Oriented Anatomy*. Baltimore: Williams & Wilkins.

82. Morgan, M.; Silver, J.; & Williams, S. (1986). The respiratory system of the spinal cord patient. In: Bloch, R. & Basbaum, M. (Eds.), *Management of Spinal Cord Injuries* (pp. 78–116). Baltimore: Williams & Wilkins.

83. Naso, F. (1992). Cardiovascular problems in patients with spinal cord injury. *Physical Medicine and Rehabilitation Clinics of North America*, 3(4), 741–749.

84. Nikas, D. (1986). Resuscitation of patients with central nervous system trauma. *Nursing Clinics of North America*, 21(4), 693–704.

85. Pappert, D.; Rossaint, R.; Slama, K.; Gruning, T.; & Falke, K. (1994). Influence of positioning on ventilation-perfusion relationships in adult respiratory distress syndrome. *Chest*, 106, 1511–1516.

86. Peterson, P.; Brooks, C.; Mellick, D. & Whiteneck, G. (1997). Protocol for ventilator management in high tetraplegia. *Topics in Spinal Cord Injury Rehabilitation*, 2(3), 101–106.

87. Peterson, W.; Charlifue, W.; Gerhart, A.; & Whiteneck, G. (1994). Two methods of weaning persons with quadriplegia from mechanical ventilators. *Paraplegia*, 32(2), 98–103.

88. Ragnarsson, K.; Hall, K.; Wilmot, C.; & Carter, E. (1995). Management of pulmonary, cardiovascular, and metabolic conditions after spinal cord injury. In: Stover, S., De Lisa, J., & Whiteneck, G. (Eds.), *Spinal Cord Injury: Clinical Outcomes from the Model* Systems (pp. 79–90). Gaithersburg, MD: Aspen Publishers.

89. Rinehart, M. & Nawoczenski, D. (1987). Respiratory care. In: Buchanan, L. & Nawoczenski, D. (Eds.), *Spinal Cord Injury: Concepts and Management Approaches* (pp. 61–79). Baltimore: Williams & Wilkins.

90. Rosse, C. & Gaddum-Rosse, P. (1997). *Hollinshead's Textbook of Anatomy* (5th ed.). Philadelphia: Lippincott-Raven.

91. Roth, E.; Lu, A.; Primack, S.; Oken, J.; Nussbaum, S.; Berkowitz, M.; & Powley, S. (1997). Ventilatory function in cervical and high thoracic spinal cord injury: Relationship to level of injury and tone. *American Journal of Physical Medicine and Rehabilitation*, 76(4), 262–267.

92. Roth, E.; Nussbaum, S.; Berkowitz, M.; Primack, S.; Oken, J.; Powley, S.; & Lu, A. (1995). Pulmonary function testing in spinal cord injury: Correlation with vital capacity. *Paraplegia*, 33(8), 454–457.

93. Rutchik, A.; Weissman, A.; Almenoff, P.; Spungen, A.; Bauman, W.; & Grimm, D. (1998). Resistive inspiratory muscle training in subjects with chronic cervical spinal cord injury. *Archives of Physical Medicine and Rehabilitation*, 79, 293–297.

94. Scanlon, P.; Loring, S.; Pichurko, B.; McCool, F.; Slutsky, A.; Sarkarati, M. & Brown, R. (1989). Respiratory mechanics in acute quadriplegia: Lung and chest wall compliance and dimensional changes during respiratory maneuvers. *American Review of Respiratory Disease*, 139(3), 615–620.

95. Silva, A.; Neder, J.; Chiurciu, M.; Pasqualin, D.; da Silva, R.; Fernandez, A.; Lauro, F.; de Mello, M.; & Tufik, S. (1998). Effect of aerobic training on ventilatory muscle endurance of spinal cord injured men. *Spinal Cord*, 36(4), 240–245.

96. Snell, R. (1995). *Clinical Anatomy for Medical Students* (5th ed). Boston: Little, Brown and Company.

97. Vander, A.; Sherman, J.; & Luciano, D. (1998). *Human Physiology: The Mechanisms of Body Function* (7th ed). Boston, MA: McGraw-Hill.

98. Vincken, W. & Corne, L. (1987). Improved arterial oxygenation by diaphragmatic pacing in quadriplegia. *Critical Care Medicine*, 15(9), 872–873.

99. Voss, D.; Ionta, M.; & Myers, B. (1985). *Proprioceptive Neuromuscular Facilitation* (3rd ed.). Philadelphia: Harper & Row.

100. Wang, A.; Jaeger, R.; Yarkony, G.; & Turba, R. (1997). Cough in spinal cord injured patients: The relationship between motor level and peak expiratory flow. *Spinal Cord*, 35(5), 299–302.

101. Wetzel, J. (1985). Respiratory evaluation and treatment. In: Adkins, H. (Ed.), *Spinal Cord Injury* (pp. 75–98). New York: Churchill Livingstone.

102. Wetzel, J.; Lunsford, B.; Peterson, M.; & Alvarez, S. (1995). Respiratory rehabilitation of the patient with a spinal cord injury. In: Irwin, S. & Tecklin, J. (Eds.), *Cardiopulmonary Physical Therapy* (3rd ed.; pp. 579–603). St. Louis: Mosby.

103. Wicks, A. & Menter, R. (1986). Long-term outlook in quadriplegic patients with initial ventilator dependency. *Chest*, 90, 406–410.

104. Yarkony, G. & Jaeger, R. (1995). Phrenic nerve pacemakers for tetraplegia. *Topics in Spinal Cord Injury Rehabilitation*, 1(1), 77–82.

105. Yarkony, G.; Jaeger, R.; & Gittler, M. (1997). Cough in tetraplegia. *Topics in Spinal Cord Injury Rehabilitation*, 3(1), 67–70.

106. Yashon, D. (1986). *Spinal Injury* (2nd ed.). Norwalk, CT: Appleton, Century, Crofts.

107. Zupan, A.; Savrin, R.; Erjavec, T.; Kralj, A.; Karcnik, T.; Skorjanc, T.; Benko, H.; & Obreza, P. (1997). Effects of respiratory muscle training and electrical stimulation of abdominal muscles on respiratory capabilities in tetraplegic patients. *Spinal Cord*, 35(8), 540–545.

Chapter 8

1. American Spinal Injury Association. (2000). *International Standards for Neurological Classification of Spinal Cord Injury*. Chicago: American Spinal Injury Association.

2. Atrice, M.; Gonter, M.; Griffin, D.; Morrison, S.; & McDowell, S. (1995). Traumatic spinal cord injury. In: Umphred, D. (Ed.), *Neurological Rehabilitation* (3rd ed.; pp. 484–534.). St. Louis: Mosby.

3. Basmajian, J., Ed. (1994). *Physical Rehabilitation Outcome Measures*. Toronto, Ontario: Canadian Physiotherapy Association.

4. Bohannon, R. & Smith, M. (1987). Interrator reliability of a modified Ashworth scale of muscle spasticity. *Physical Therapy*, 67(2), 206–207.

5. Boss, B.; Pecanty, L.; McFarland, S.; & Sasser, L. (1995). Self-care competence among persons with spinal cord injury. *Spinal Cord Injury Nursing*, 12(2), 48–53.

6. Burgess, C. (1998). Managed care and its effects on how we deliver services. *Topics in Spinal Cord Injury Rehabilitation*, 3(4), 17–27.

7. Catz, A.; Itzkovich, M.; Agranov, E.; Ring, H.; & Tamir, A. (1997). SCIM—Spinal Cord Independence Measure: A new disability scale for patients with spinal cord lesions. *Spinal Cord*, 35(12), 850–856.

8. Consortium for Spinal Cord Medicine. (1999). *Outcomes Following Traumatic Spinal Cord Injury: Clinical Practice Guidelines for Health-Care Professionals*. Washington, DC: Paralyzed Veterans of America.

9. Corbet, B. (1980). *Options: Spinal Cord Injury and the Future*. Denver, CO: A.B. Hirschfeld Press.

10. Daverat, P.; Petit, H.; Kemoun, G.; Dartigues, J.; & Barat, M. (1995). The long term outcome in 149 patients with spinal cord injury. *Paraplegia*, 33, 665–668.

11. DeJong, G. & Sutton, J. (1998). Managed care and catastrophic injury: The case of spinal cord injury. *Topics in Spinal Cord Injury Rehabilitation*, 3(4), 1–16.

12. Deutsch, A.; Braun, S.; & Granger, C. (1997). The Functional Independence Measure (FIM Instrument). *Journal of Rehabilitation Outcomes Measures*, 1(2), 67–71.

13. Dittmar, S. (1997). Overview: A functional approach to measurement of rehabilitation outcomes. In: Dittmar, S. & Gresham, G. (Ed.), *Functional Assessment and Outcome Measures for the Rehabilitation Health Professional* (pp. 1–15). Gaithersburg, MD: Aspen Publishers.

14. Dittmar, S. & Gresham, G. (Eds.) (1997). *Functional Assessment and Outcome Measures for the Rehabilitation Health Professional*. Gaithersburg, MD: Aspen Publishers.

15. Ditunno, J.; Cohen, M.; Formal, C.; & Whiteneck, G. (1995). Functional outcomes. In: Stover, S., DeLisa, J., & Whiteneck, G. (Eds.), *Spinal Cord Injury: Clinical Outcomes from the Model Systems* (pp. 170–184). Gaithersburg, MD: Aspen Publishers.

16. Ditunno, J.; Graziani, V.; & Tessler, A. (1997). Neurological assessment in spinal cord injury. *Advances in Neurology*, 72: 325–333.

17. Ditunno, J.; Sipski, M.; Posuniak, E.; Chen, Y.; Staas, W.; & Herbison, G. (1987). Wrist extensor recovery in traumatic quadriplegia. *Archives of Physical Medicine and Rehabilitation*, 68(5), 287–290.

18. Finkbeiner, K. & Russo, S. (1990). *Physical Therapy Management of Spinal Cord Injury: Accent on Independence*. Fishersville, VA: Woodrow Wilson Rehabilitation Center.

19. Fredericks, C. & Saladin, L. (1996). Clinical presentations in disorders of motor function. In: Fredericks, C. & Saladin, L. (Eds.), *Pathophysiology of the Motor Systems: Principles and Clinical Presentations* (pp. 257–288). Philadelphia: F.A. Davis.

20. Ford, J. & Duckworth, B. (1987). *Physical Management for the Quadriplegic Patient* (2nd ed.). Philadelphia: F. A. Davis.

21. Graziani, V.; Crozier, K.; & Selby-Silverstein, L. (1996). Lower extremity function following spinal cord injury. *Topics in Spinal Cord Injury Rehabilitation*, 1(4), 46–55.

22. Grover, J.; Gellman, H.; & Waters, R. (1996). The effect of a flexion contracture of the elbow on the ability to transfer in patients who have quadriplegia at the sixth cervical level. *Journal of Bone and Joint Surgery* (American), 78(9), 1397–1400.

23. Lazar, R.; Yarkony, G.; Ortolano, D.; Heinemann, A.; Perlow, E.; Lovell, L.; & Meyer, P. (1989). Prediction of functional outcome by motor capability after spinal cord injury. *Archives of Physical Medicine and Rehabilitation*, 70(11), 819–822.

24. Little, J.; Micklessen, P.; Umlauf, R.; & Britell, C. (1989). Lower extremity manifestations of spasticity in chronic spinal cord injury. *American Journal of Physical Medicine and Rehabilitation*, 68(1), 32–36.

25. Mange, K.; Ditunno, J.; Herbison, G.; & Jaweed, M. (1990). Recovery of strength at the zone of injury in motor complete and motor incomplete cervical spinal cord injured patients. *Archives of Physical Medicine and Rehabilitation*, 71(8), 562–565.

26. Marino, R. & Stineman, M. (1996). Functional assessment in spinal cord injury. *Topics in Spinal Cord Injury Rehabilitation*, 1(4):32–45.

27. Maynard, F.; Karunas, R.; Adkins, R.; Richards, J.; & Waring, W. (1995). Management of the neuromusculoskeletal systems. In: Stover, S., DeLisa, J., & Whiteneck, G. (Eds.), *Spinal Cord Injury: Clinical Outcomes from the Model Systems* (pp. 145–169). Gaithersburg, MD: Aspen Publishers.

28. McClay, I. (1983). Electric wheelchair propulsion using a hand control in C4 quadriplegia. *Physical Therapy*, 63(2), 221–223.

29. Nixon, V. (1985). *Spinal Cord Injury: A Guide to Functional Outcomes in Physical Therapy Management*. Rockville, MD: Aspen Publishers.

30. Ota, T.; Akaboshi, K.; Nagata, M.; Sonoda, S.; Domen, K.; Seki, M.; & Chino, N. (1996). Functional assessment of patients with spinal cord injury: Measured by the Motor Score and the Functional Independence Measure. *Spinal Cord*, 34(9), 531–535.

31. Parke, B.; Penn, R.; Savoy, S.; & Corcos, D. (1989). Functional outcome after delivery of intrathecal baclofen. *Archives of Physical Medicine and Rehabilitation*, 70(1), 30–32.

32. Parsons, K. (1998). Impact of managed care on spinal cord injury physicians and their patients. *Topics in Spinal Cord Injury Rehabilitation*, 3(4), 28–35.

33. Penrod, L.; Hegde, S.; & Ditunno, J. (1990). Age effect on prognosis for functional recovery in acute, traumatic central cord syndrome. *Archives of Physical Medicine and Rehabilitation*, 71(11), 963–968.

34. Peterson, M. (1985). Ambulation and orthotic management. In: Adkins, H. (Ed.), *Spinal Cord Injury* (pp. 199–217). New York: Churchill Livingstone.

35. Priebe, M.; Sherwood, A.; Thornby, J.; Kharas, N.; & Markowski, J. (1996). Clinical assessment of spasticity in spinal cord injury: A multidimensional problem. *Archives of Physical Medicine & Rehabilitation*, 77(7), 713–716.

36. Robinson, C.; Kett, N.; & Bolam, J. (1988). Spasticity in spinal cord injured patients: 2. Initial measures and long-term effects of surface electrical stimulation. *Archives of Physical Medicine and Rehabilitation*, 69(10), 862–868.

37. Roth, E.; Lawler, M.; & Yarkony, G. (1990). Traumatic central cord syndrome: Clinical features and functional outcomes. *Archives of Physical Medicine and Rehabilitation*, 71(1), 18–23.

38. Rothstein, J. (Ed.). (1997). Guide to physical therapist practice. *Physical Therapy*, 77 (11), 1163–1650.

39. Rymer, Z. (1997). Spasticity: Pathophysiology and implications for measurement. *Neurology Report*, 21(3), 73–75.

40. Saboe, L.; Darrah, J.; Pain, K.; & Guthrie, J. (1997). Early predictors of functional independence 2 years after spinal cord injury. *Archives of Physical Medicine and Rehabilitation*, 78(6), 644–650.

41. Stevenson, V.; Playford, E.; Langdon, D.; & Thompson, A. (1996). Rehabilitation of incomplete spinal cord pathology: Factors affecting prognosis and outcome. *Journal of Neurology*, 243, 644–647.

42. Waters, R. (1996). Functional prognosis of spinal cord injuries. *Journal of Spinal Cord Medicine*, 19(2), 89–92.

43. Waters, R.; Adkins, R.; Yakura, J.; & Sie, I. (1993). Motor and sensory recovery following complete tetraplegia. *Archives of Physical Medicine and Rehabilitation*, 74(3), 242–247.

44. Waters, R.; Adkins, R.; Yakura, J.; & Sie, I. (1994). Motor and sensory recovery following incomplete paraplegia. *Archives of Physical Medicine and Rehabilitation*, 75(1), 67–72.

45. Waters, R.; Adkins, R.; Yakura, J.; & Sie, I. (1994). Motor and sensory recovery following incomplete tetraplegia. *Archives of Physical Medicine and Rehabilitation*, 75(3), 306–311.

46. Waters, R. & Miller, L. (1987). A physiologic rationale for orthotic prescription in paraplegia. *Clinical Prosthetics and Orthotics*, 11(2), 66–73.

47. Waters, R.; Yakura, J.; Adkins, R.; & Barnes, G. (1989). Determinants of gait performance following spinal cord injury. *Archives of Physical Medicine and Rehabilitation*, 70(11), 811–818.

48. Welch, R.; Lobley, S.; O'Sullivan, S.; & Freed, M. (1986). Functional independence in quadriplegia: critical levels. *Archives of Physical Medicine and Rehabilitation*, 67(4), 235–240.

49. Yarkony, G. & Heinemann, A. (1995). Pressure ulcers. In: Stover, S., DeLisa, J., & Whiteneck, G. (Eds.) *Spinal Cord Injury: Clinical Outcomes from the Model Systems* (pp. 100–119). Gaithersburg, MD: Aspen Publishers.

50. Yarkony, G.; Roth, E.; Heinemann, A.; Lovell, L.; & Wu, Y. (1988). Functional skills after spinal cord injury rehabilitation: Three-year longitudinal follow-up. *Archives of Physical Medicine and Rehabilitation*, 69(2), 111–114.

51. Yavuz, N.; Tezyurek, M. & Akyuz, M. (1998). A comparison of two functional tests in quadriplegia: The Quadriplegia Index of Function and the Functional Independence Measure. *Spinal Cord*, 36, 832–837.

52. Young, W. & Ransohoff, J. (1989). Acute spinal cord injuries: Experimental therapy, pathophysiological mechanisms, and recovery of function. In: Sherk H., Dunn, F., Eismont, F. (eds.), *The Cervical Spine* (2nd ed.; pp. 464–495).Philadelphia: J. B. Lippincott.

Chapter 9

1. Allison, L. (1995). Balance disorders. In: Umphred, D. (Ed.), *Neurological Rehabilitation* (2nd ed.; pp. 802–837). St. Louis: Mosby.

2. Bohannon, R. (1994). Orthopaedic problems in the neurologic patient. In: Donatelli, R. & Wooden, M. (Eds.), *Orthopaedic Physical Therapy* (2nd ed.; pp. 675–695). New York: Churchill Livingstone.

3. Crutchfield, C.; Shumway-Cook, A.; & Horak, F. (1989). Balance and coordination training. In: Scully, R. & Barnes, M. (Eds.), *Physical Therapy* (pp. 825–843). Philadelphia: J.B. Lippincott.

4. Delitto, A.; Snyder-Mackler, L; & Robinson, A. (1995). Electrical stimulation of muscle: Techniques and applications. In: Robinson, J. & Snyder-Mackler, L. (Eds.), *Clinical Electrophysiology: Electrotherapy and Electrophysiologic Testing* (2nd ed.; pp. 121–153). Baltimore: Williams & Wilkins.

5. Ditunno, J., Cohen, M., Formal, C., & Whiteneck, G. (1995). Functional outcomes. In: Stover, S., DeLisa, J., & Whiteneck, G. (Eds.), *Spinal Cord Injury: Clinical Outcomes from the Model Systems* (pp. 170–184). Gaithersburg, MD: Aspen.

6. Ditunno, J.; Sipski, M.; Posuniak, E.; Chen, Y.; Staas, W.; & Herbison, G. (1987). Wrist extensor recovery in traumatic quadriplegia. *Archives of Physical Medicine and Rehabilitation*, 68(5), 287–290.

7. Ditunno, J.; Stover, S.; Freed, M. & Ahn, J. (1992). Motor recovery of the upper extremities in traumatic quadriplegia: A multicenter study. *Archives of Physical Medicine and Rehabilitation*, 73(5), 431–436.

8. Fredericks, C. (1996). Skeletal muscle: The somatic effector. In: Fredericks, C. & Saladin, L. (Eds.), *Pathophysiology of the Motor Systems: Principles and Clinical Presentations* (pp. 30–61). Philadelphia: F.A. Davis.

9. Hislop, H. & Montgomery, J. (1995). *Daniels and Worthingham's Muscle Testing: Techniques of Manual Examination*. Philadelphia: W. B. Saunders Company.

10. Kahn, J. (1989). Physical agents: Electrical, sonic, and radiant modalities. In: Scully, R. & Barnes, M. (Eds.), *Physical Therapy* (pp. 876–900). Philadelphia: J.B. Lippincott.

11. Kendall, F.; McCreary, E.; & Provance, P. (1993). *Muscles: Testing and Function* (4th ed.). Baltimore: Williams & Wilkins.

12. Mange, K.; Ditunno, J.; Herbison, G. & Jaweed, M. (1990). Recovery of strength at the zone of injury in motor complete and motor incomplete cervical spinal cord injured patients. *Archives of Physical Medicine and Rehabilitation*, 71(8), 562–565.

13. Mange, K.; Marino, R.; Gregory, P.; Herbison, G.; & Ditunno, J. (1992). Course of motor recovery in the zone of partial preservation in spinal cord injury. *Archives of Physical Medicine and Rehabilitation*, 73(5), 437–441.

14. Mangine, R.; Heckman, T.; & Eldridge, V. (1989). Improving strength, endurance, and power. In: Scully, R. & Barnes, M. (Eds.), *Physical Therapy* (pp. 739–762). Philadelphia: J.B.Lippincott.

15. Marciello, M.; Herbison, G.; Cohen, M.; & Schmidt, R. (1995). Elbow extension using anterior deltoids and upper pectorals in spinal cord-injured subjects. *Archives of Physical Medicine and Rehabilitation*, 76(5), 426–432.

16. Maynard, F.; Karunas, R.; Adkins, R.; Richards, J.; & Waring, W. (1995). Management of the neuromusculoskeletal system. In: Stover, S., DeLisa, J., & Whiteneck, G. (Eds.), *Spinal Cord Injury: Clinical Outcomes from the Model Systems* (pp. 145–169). Gaithersburg, MD: Aspen.

17. McCulloch, K. & Nelson, C. (1995). Electrical stimulation and electromyographic biofeedback: Applications for neurologic dysfunction. In: Umphred, D. (Ed.), *Neurological Rehabilitation* (3rd ed.;pp. 852–871). St. Louis: Mosby.

18. Nawoczenski, D.; Rinehart, M.; Duncanson, P.; & Brown, B. (1987). Physical management. In: Buchanan, L. & Nawoczenski, D. (Eds.), *Spinal Cord Injury: Concepts and Management Approaches* (pp. 123–184). Baltimore: Williams & Wilkins.

19. Nicholson, D. (1996). Motor learning. In: Fredericks, C. & Saladin, L. (Eds.), *Pathophysiology of the Motor Systems: Principles and Clinical Presentations* (pp. 238–254). Philadelphia: F.A. Davis.

20. O'Sullivan, S. (1994). Strategies to improve motor control and motor learning. In: O'Sullivan, S. & Schmitz, T. (Eds.), *Physical Rehabilitation: Assessment and Treatment* (pp. 225–249). Philadelphia: F.A. Davis.

21. Redford, J. (1980). Principles of orthotic devices. In: Redford, J. (Ed.), *Orthotics Etcetera* (2nd ed.; pp. 1–21). Baltimore: Williams & Wilkins.

22. Schmidt, R. (1991). Motor learning principles for physical therapy. In: Lister, M. (Ed.). *Contemporary Management of Motor Control Problems: Proceedings of the II STEP Conference* (pp. 49–63). Fredericksburg, VA: Foundation for Physical Therapy.

23. Schmidt, R. & Lee, T. (1999). *Motor Control and Learning: A Behavioral Emphasis* (2nd ed.). Champaign, IL: Human Kinetics.

24. Shumway-Cook, A. & Woollacott, M. (1995). *Motor Control: Theory and Application*. Baltimore: Williams & Wilkins.

25. Sullivan, P. & Minor, M. (1987). *Clinical Procedures in Therapeutic Exercise*. Norwalk, CT: Appleton & Lange.

26. Sullivan, P.; Markos, P.; & Minor, M. (1982). *An Integrated Approach to Therapeutic Exercises: Theory and Clinical Application*. Reston, VA: Reston.

27. Winstein, C. (1991). Designing practice for motor learning: clinical implications. In: Lister, M. (Ed.). *Contemporary Management of Motor Control Problems: Proceedings of the II STEP Conference* (pp. 65–76). Fredericksburg, VA: Foundation for Physical Therapy.

28. Young, W. & Ransohoff, J. (1989). Acute spinal cord injuries: Experimental therapy, pathophysiological mechanisms, and recovery of function. In Sherk, H., Dunn, E., & Eismont, F. (Eds.), *The Cervical Spine* (2nd ed., pp. 464–495). Philadelphia: J.B. Lippincott.

29. Zachazewski, J. (1989). Improving flexibility. In: Scully, R. & Barnes, M. (Eds.), *Physical Therapy* (pp. 698–738). Philadelphia: J.B. Lippincott.

Chapter 10

1. Kendall, F.; McCreary, E.; & Provance, P. (1993). *Muscles: Testing and Function* (4th ed.). Baltimore: Williams & Wilkins.

2. Little, J.; Micklessen, P.; Umlauf, R.; & Britell, C. (1989). Lower extremity manifestations of spasticity in chronic spinal cord injury. *American Jour-

nal of Physical Medicine and Rehabilitation, 68(1), 32–36.

3. Martini, F. (1998). *Fundamentals of Anatomy and Physiology* (4th ed.). Upper Saddle River, NJ: Prentice Hall.

4. Maynard, F.; Karunas, R.; Adkins, R.; Richards, J.; & Waring, W. (1995). Management of the neuromusculoskeletal systems. In: Stover, S, DeLisa, J & Whiteneck, G. (Eds.), *Spinal Cord Injury: Clinical Outcomes from the Model Systems* (pp. 145–169). Gaithersburg, MD: Aspen Publishers.

5. McCoy, J. & Van Sant, A. (1993.) Movement patterns of adolescents rising from a bed. *Physical Therapy*, 73(3), 182–193.

6. McMinn, R. (1994). *Last's Anatomy* (9th ed.). New York: Churchill Livingstone.

7. Moore, K. (1992). *Clinically Oriented Anatomy*. Baltimore: Williams & Wilkins.

8. O'Sullivan, S. & Schmitz, T. (1998.) *Physical Laboratory Manual: Focus on Functional Training*. Philadelphia: F. A. Davis.

9. Richter, R.; Van Sant, A.; & Newton, R. (1989.) Description of adult rolling movements and hypothesis of developmental sequences. *Physical Therapy*, 69(1), 63–71.

10. Robinson, C.; Kett, N.; & Bolam, J. (1988). Spasticity in spinal cord injured patients: 2. Initial measures and long–term effects of surface electrical stimulation. *Archives of Physical Medicine and Rehabilitation*, 69(10), 862–868.

11. Rosse, C. & Gaddum-Rosse, P. (1997). *Hollinshead's Textbook of Anatomy* (5th ed.). Philadelphia: Lippincott-Raven.

12. Shumway–Cook, A. & Woollacott, M. (1995.) *Motor Control: Theory and Practical Applications*. Baltimore: Williams & Wilkins.

Chapter 11

1. Behrman, A.; Sawyer, K.; & Tomlinson, S. (1993). "I want to walk": An approach to physical therapy management of the individual with an incomplete spinal cord injury. *Neurology Report* 17(2), 7–12.

2. Burgess, C. (1998). Managed care and its effects on how we deliver services. *Topics in Spinal Cord Injury Rehabilitation*, 3(4), 17–27.

3. Ditunno, J.; Cohen, M.; Formal, C.; & Whiteneck, G. (1995). Functional outcomes. In: Stover, S., DeLisa, J. & Whiteneck, G. (Eds.), *Spinal Cord Injury: Clinical Outcomes from the Model Systems* (pp. 170–184). Gaithersburg, MD: Aspen Publishers.

4. Gefen, J.; Gelmann, A.; Herbison, G.; Cohen, M.; & Schmidt, R. (1997). Use of shoulder flexors to achieve isometric elbow extension in C6 tetraplegic patients during weight shift. *Spinal Cord*, 35, 308–313.

5. Graziani, V.; Crozier, K.; & Selby-Silverstein, L. (1996). Lower extremity function following spinal cord injury. *Topics in Spinal Cord Injury Rehabilitation*, 1(4), 46–55.

6. Kendall, F.; McCreary, E.; & Provance, P. (1993). *Muscles: Testing and Function* (4th ed.). Baltimore: Williams & Wilkins.

7. Little, J.; Micklessen, P.; Umlauf, R.; & Britell, C. (1989). Lower extremity manifestations of spasticity in chronic spinal cord injury. *American Journal of Physical Medicine and Rehabilitation*, 68(1), 32–36.

8. Marciello, M; Herbison, G.; Cohen, M.; & Schmidt, R. (1995). Elbow extension using anterior deltoids and upper pectorals in spinal cord-injured subjects. *Archives of Physical Medicine and Rehabilitation*, 76, 426–432.

9. Martini, F. (1998). *Fundamentals of Anatomy and Physiology* (4th ed.). Upper Saddle River, NJ: Prentice Hall.

10. Maynard, F.; Karunas, R.; Adkins, R.; Richards, J.; & Waring, W. (1995). Management of the neuromusculoskeletal systems. In: Stover, S, DeLisa, J. & Whiteneck, G. (Eds.), *Spinal Cord Injury: Clinical Outcomes from the Model Systems* (pp. 145–169). Gaithersburg, MD: Aspen Publishers.

11. McMinn, R. (1994). *Last's Anatomy* (9th ed.). New York: Churchill Livingstone.

12. Moore, K. (1992). *Clinically Oriented Anatomy*. Baltimore: Williams & Wilkins.

13. O'Sullivan, S. & Schmitz, T. (1999). *Physical Rehabilitation Laboratory Manual: Focus on Functional Training*. Philadelphia: F. A. Davis.

14. Perry, J.; Gronley, J.; Newsam, C.; Reyes, M.; & Mulroy, S. (1996). Electromyographic analysis of the shoulder muscles during depression transfers in subjects with low-level paraplegia. *Archives of Physical Medicine and Rehabilitation*, 77, 350–355.

15. Robinson, C.; Kett, N.; & Bolam, J. (1988). Spasticity in spinal cord injured patients: 2. Initial measures and long-term effects of surface electrical stimulation. *Archives of Physical Medicine and Rehabilitation*, 69(10), 862–868.

16. Rosse, C. & Gaddum-Rosse, P. (1997). *Hollinshead's Textbook of Anatomy* (5th ed.). Philadelphia: Lippincott-Raven.

17. Schmitz, T. (1994). Preambulation and gait training. In: O'Sullivan, S. & Schmitz, T. (Eds.), *Physical Rehabilitation: Assessment and Treatment* (3rd ed; pp. 251–276). Philadelphia: F. A. Davis.

18. Shumway-Cook, A. & Woollacott, M. (1995). *Motor Control: Theory and Practical Applications*. Baltimore: Williams & Wilkins.

Chapter 12

1. Axelson, P.; Minkel, J.; & Chesney, D. (1994). *A Guide to Wheelchair Selection: How to Use the ANSI/RESNA Wheelchair Standards to Buy a Wheelchair*. Washington, DC: Paralyzed Veterans of America.

2. Boninger, M.; Cooper, R.; Robertson, R.; & Shimada, S. (1997). Three-dimensional pushrim forces during two speeds of wheelchair propulsion. *American Journal of Physical Medicine and Rehabilitation*, 76(5), 420–426.

3. Brubaker, C. (1990). Ergonomic considerations. *Journal of Rehabilitation Research and Development*, Clinical Supplement #2, 37–48.

4. Buchanan, L. & Ditunno, J. (1987). Acute care: Medical/surgical management. In: Buchanan, L. &

Nawoczenski, D. (Eds), *Spinal Cord Injury: Concepts and Management Approaches* (pp. 35–60). Baltimore: Williams & Wilkins.

5. Cappozzo, A.; Felici, F.; Figura, F.; Marchetti, M.; & Ricci, B. (1991). Prediction of ramp traversability for wheelchair dependent individuals. *Paraplegia*, 29(7), 470–478.

6. Chase, T. (1996). Physical fitness strategies. In: Lanig, I., Chase, T., Butt, L., Hulse, K., & Johnson, K. (Eds), *A Practical Guide to Health Promotion after Spinal Cord Injury* (pp. 243–291). Gaithersburg, MD: Aspen Publishers.

7. Cole, J. (1988). The pathophysiology of the autonomic nervous system in spinal cord injury. In: Illis, L. (Ed.), *Spinal Cord Dysfunction: Assessment* (pp. 201–235). New York: Oxford University Press.

8. Cooper, R. (1998). *Wheelchair Selection and Configuration*. New York: Demos Medical Publishing.

9. Curtis, K.; Roach, K.; Applegate, E.; Amar, T.; Benbow, C.; Genecco, T.; & Gualano, J. (1995). Development of the Wheelchair User's Shoulder Pain Index (WUSPI). *Paraplegia*, 33(5), 290–293.

10. Dallmeijer, A.; Kappe, Y.; Veeger, D.; Janssen, T.; & van der Woude, L. (1994). Anaerobic power output and propulsion technique in spinal cord injured subjects during wheelchair ergometry. *Journal of Rehabilitation Research and Development*, 31(2), 120–128.

11. Dallmeijer, A.; van der Woude, L.; Veeger, D.; & Hollander, A. (1998). Effectiveness of force application in manual wheelchair propulsion in persons with spinal cord injuries. *American Journal of Physical Medicine and Rehabilitation*, 77(3), 213–221.

12. DiCarlo, S. (1988). Effect of arm cycle ergometry training on wheelchair propulsion endurance of individuals with quadriplegia. *Physical Therapy*, 68(1), 40–44.

13. Gaal, R.; Rebholtz, N.; Hotchkiss, R.; & Pfaelzer, P. (1997). Wheelchair rider injuries: Causes and consequences for wheelchair design and selection. *Journal of Rehabilitation Research and Development*, 34(1), 58–71.

14. Gellman, H.; Sie, I.; & Waters, R. (1988). Late complications of the weight bearing extremity in the paraplegic patient. *Clinical Orthopaedics and Related Research*, 233, 132–135.

15. Gerhart, K.; Bergstrom, E.; Charlifue, S.; Menter, R.; & Whiteneck, G. (1993). Long-term spinal cord injury: Functional changes over time. *Archives of Physical Medicine and Rehabilitation*, 74, 1030–1034.

16. Gilsdorf, P.; Patterson, R.; & Fisher, S. (1991). Thirty-minute sitting force measurements with different support surfaces in the spinal cord injured and able-bodied. *Journal of Rehabilitation Research and Development*, 28(4), 33–38.

17. Graziani, V.; Crozier, K.; & Selby-Silverstein, L. (1996). Lower extremity function following spinal cord injury. *Topics in Spinal Cord Injury Rehabilitation*, 1(4), 46–55.

18. Heinneman, A.; Magiera-Planey, R. Schiro-Geist, C. & Gimines, G. (1987). Mobility for persons with spinal cord injury: An evaluation of two systems.

Archives of Physical Medicine and Rehabilitation, 68, 90–93.

19. Henderson, J.; Price, S.; Brandstater, M.; & Mandac, B. (1994). Efficacy of three measures to relieve pressure in seated persons with spinal cord injury. *Archives of Physical Medicine and Rehabilitation*, 75(5), 535–539.

20. Hilbers, P. & White, T. (1987). Effects of wheelchair design on metabolic and heart rate responses during propulsion by persons with paraplegia. *Physical Therapy*, 67(9), 1355–1358.

21. Hughes, C.; Weimar, W.; Sheth, P.; & Brubaker, C. (1992). Biomechanics of wheelchair propulsion as a function of seat position and user-to-chair interface. *Archives of Physical Medicine and Rehabilitation*, 73(3), 263–269.

22. Karp, G. (1998). *Choosing a Wheelchair: A Guide of Optimal Independence*. Sebastopol, CA: O'Reilly & Associates.

23. Kendall, F.; McCreary, E.; & Provance, P. (1993). *Muscles: Testing and Function* (4th ed.). Baltimore: Williams & Wilkins.

24. Kirby, R.; Ackroyd-Stolarz, S.; Brown, M.; Kirkland, S.; & MacLeod, D. (1994). Wheelchair-related accidents caused by tips and falls among noninstitutionalized users of manually propelled wheelchairs in Nova Scotia. *American Journal of Physical Medicine and Rehabilitation*, 73(5), 319–330.

25. Kirby, R.; McLean, A.; & Eastwood, B. (1992). Influence of caster diameter on the static and dynamic forward stability of occupied wheelchairs. *Archives of Physical Medicine and Rehabilitation*, 73, 73–77.

26. Kirby, R.; Sampson, M.; Thoren, F.; & MacLeod, D. (1995). Wheelchair stability: Effect of body position. *Journal of Rehabilitation Research and Development*, 32(4), 367–372.

27. Kirshblum, S.; Druin, E.; & Planten, K. (1997). Musculoskeletal conditions in chronic spinal cord injury. *Topics in Spinal Cord Injury Rehabilitation*, 2(4), 23–35.

28. Koo, T.; Mak, A.; & Lee, Y. (1996). Posture effect on seating interface biomechanics: Comparison between two seating cushions. *Archives of Physical Medicine and Rehabilitation*, 77(1), 40–47.

29. Krause, J. (1995). Changes in wheelchair technology: a consumer commentary. *Topics in Spinal Cord Injury Rehabilitation*, 1(1), 66–70.

30. Kreutz, D. (1995). Manual wheelchairs: Prescribing for function. *Topics in Spinal Cord Injury Rehabilitation*, 1(1), 1–16.

31. Kulig, K.; Rao, S.; Mulroy, S.; Newsam, C.; Gronley, J.; Bontrager, E.; & Perry, J. (1998). Shoulder joint kinetics during the push phase of wheelchair propulsion. *Clinical Orthopedics*, 354, 132–143.

32. Lehman, K.; Lane, J.; Piepmeier, J.; & Batsford, W. (1987). Cardiovascular abnormalities accompanying acute spinal cord injury in humans: Incidence, time course and severity. *Journal of the American College of Cardiology*, 10(1), 46–52.

33. Leonard, R. (1995). To tilt or recline? *Topics in Spinal Cord Injury Rehabilitation*, 1(1), 17–22.

34. McClay, I. (1983). Electric wheelchair propulsion using a hand control in C4 quadriplegia. *Physical Therapy*, 63(2), 221–223.

35. Little, J.; Micklessen, P.; Umlauf, R.; & Britell, C. (1989). Lower extremity manifestations of spasticity in chronic spinal cord injury. *American Journal of Physical Medicine and Rehabilitation*, 68(1), 32–36.

36. Martini, F. (1998). *Fundamentals of Anatomy and Physiology* (4th ed.). Upper Saddle River, NJ: Prentice Hall.

37. Mayall, J. & Desharnais, G. (1995). *Positioning in a Wheelchair: A Guide for Professional Caregivers of the Disabled Adult* (2nd ed). Thorofare, NJ: Slack.

38. Maynard, F.; Karunas, R.; Adkins, R.; Richards, J.; & Waring, W. (1995). Management of the neuromusculoskeletal systems. In: Stover, S., DeLisa, J., & Whiteneck, G. (Eds.), *Spinal Cord Injury: Clinical Outcomes from the Model Systems* (pp. 145–169). Gaithersburg, MD: Aspen Publishers.

39. McMinn, R. (1994). *Last's Anatomy* (9th ed.). New York: Churchill Livingstone.

40. Moore, K. (1992). *Clinically Oriented Anatomy.* Baltimore: Williams & Wilkins.

41. Newsam, C.; Mulroy, S.; Gronley, J.; Bontrager, E.; & Perry, J. (1996). Temporal-spatial characteristics of wheelchair propulsion: Effects of level of spinal cord injury, terrain, and propulsion rate. *American Journal of Physical Medicine and Rehabilitation*, 75(4), 292–299.

42. O'Neil, L. & Seelye, R. (1990) Power wheelchair training for patients with marginal upper extremity function. *Neurology Report*, 14(3), 19–20.

43. Parziale, J. (1991). Standard v lightweight wheelchair propulsion in spinal cord injured patients. *American Journal of Physical Medicine and Rehabilitation*, 70(2), 76–80.

44. Pentland, W. & Twomey, L. (1994). Upper limb function in persons with long term paraplegia and implications for independence: Part I. *Paraplegia* 32(4), 211–218.

45. Peterson, M. & Adkins, H. (1982). Measurement and redistribution of excessive pressures during wheelchair sitting: A clinical report. *Physical Therapy* 62(7), 990–994.

46. Ragone, D. (1987). Is it worth it? A personal perspective. In: Buchanan, L. & Nawoczenski, D. (Eds.), *Spinal Cord Injury: Concepts and Management Approaches* (pp. 249–265). Baltimore: Williams & Wilkins.

47. Robertson, R.; Boninger, M.; Cooper, R.; & Shimada, S. (1996). Pushrim forces and joint kinetics during wheelchair propulsion. *Archives of Physical Medicine and Rehabilitation* 77(9), 856–864.

48. Robinson, C.; Kett, N.; & Bolam, J. (1988). Spasticity in spinal cord injured patients: 2. Initial measures and long-term effects of surface electrical stimulation. *Archives of Physical Medicine and Rehabilitation*, 69(10), 862–868.

49. Rodgers, M.; Gayle, G.; Figoni, S.; Kobayashi, M.; Lieh, J.; & Glaser, R. (1994). Biomechanics of wheelchair propulsion during fatigue. *Archives of Physical Medicine and Rehabilitation*, 75(1), 85–93.

50. Rosse, C. & Gaddum-Rosse, P. (1997). *Hollinshead's Textbook of Anatomy* (5th ed.). Philadelphia: Lippincott-Raven.

51. Scherer, M. (1996). Outcomes of assistive technology use on quality of life. *Disability and Rehabilitation*, 18(9), 439–448.

52. Sie, I.; Waters, R.; Adkins, R.; & Gellman, H. (1992). Upper extremity pain in the postrehabilitation spinal cord injured patient. *Archives of Physical Medicine and Rehabilitation*, 73(1), 44–48.

53. Swarts, A.; Krouskop, T.; & Smith, D. (1988). Tissue pressure management in the vocational setting. *Archives of Physical Medicine and Rehabilitation*, 69, 97–99.

54. Tahamont, M.; Knowlton, R.; Sawka, M. & Miles, D. (1986). Metabolic responses of women to exercise attributable to long term use of a manual wheelchair. *Paraplegia*, 24, 311–317.

55. Taylor, S. (1987). Evaluating the client with physical disabilities for wheelchair seating. *American Journal of Occupational Therapy*, 41(11), 711–716.

56. Taylor, S. (1995). Powered mobility evaluation and technology. *Topics in Spinal Cord Injury Rehabilitation*, 1(1), 23–36.

57. Tomlinson, J. (1990). Maximizing manual wheelchair propulsion for the marginal user. *Neurology Report*, 14(3), 14–18.

58. Veeger, D.; van der Woude, L.; & Rozendal, R. (1989). The effect of rear wheel camber in manual wheelchair propulsion. *Journal of Rehabilitation Research and Development*, 26(2), 37–46.

59. Waters, R. & Lunsford, B. (1985). Energy costs of paraplegic locomotion. *Journal of Joint and Bone Surgery*, 67-A(8), 1245–1250.

60. Waters, R. & Miller, L. (1987). A physiologic rationale for orthotic prescription in paraplegia. *Clinical Prosthetics and Orthotics*, 11(2), 66–73.

61. Wilson, A. (1986). *Wheelchairs: A Prescription Guide.* Charlottesville, VA: Rehabilitation Press.

62. Wilson, A. (1992). *How to Select and Use Manual Wheelchairs.* Topping, VA: Rehabilitation Press.

63. Wolfe, G.; Waters, R.; & Hislop, H. (1977). Influence of floor surface on the energy cost of wheelchair propulsion. *Physical Therapy* 57(9), 1022–1027.

64. Yashon, D. (1986). *Spinal Injury* (2nd ed.), Norwalk, CT: Appleton, Century, Crofts.

Chapter 13

1. Adams, J. & Perry, J. (1994). Gait analysis: clinical application. In: Rose, J. & Gamble, J. (Eds.), *Human Walking* (2nd ed., pp. 139–164). Baltimore: Williams & Wilkins.

2. Alander, D.; Parker, J.; & Stauffer, E. (1997). Intermediate-term outcome of cervical spinal cord-injured patients older than 50 years of age. *Spine*, 22 (11), 1189–1192.

3. Baardman, G.; Ijzerman, M.; Hermens, H.; Veltink, P.; Boom, H.; & Zilvold, G. (1997). The influence of the reciprocal hip joint link in the advanced reciprocating gait orthosis on standing performance in paraplegia. *Prosthetics and Orthotics International*, 21(3), 201–221.

4. Bajd, T.; Andrews, B.; Kralj, A.; & Katakis, J. (1985). Restoration of walking in patients with

incomplete spinal cord injuries by use of surface electrical stimulation—preliminary results. *Prosthetics and Orthotics International*, 9(2), 109–111.

5. Bajd, T.; Stefancic, M; Matjacic, Z.; Kralj, A.; Savrin, R.; Benko, H.; Karcnik, T.; & Obreza, P. (1997). Improvement in step clearance via calf muscle stimulation. *Medical and Biological Engineering and Computing*, 35(2), 113–116.

6. Barbeau, H.; Ladouceur, M.; Norman, K.; Pepin, A.; & Leroux, A. (1999). Walking after spinal cord injury: evaluation, treatment, and functional recovery. *Archives of Physical Medicine and Rehabilitation*, 80(2), 225–235.

7. Barbeau, H. & Rossignol, S. (1994). Enhancement of locomotor recovery following spinal cord injury. *Current Opinion in Neurology*, 7, 517–524.

8. Barnett, S.; Bagley, A.; & Skinner, H. (1993). Ankle weight effect on gait: orthotic implications. *Orthopedics*, 16(10), 1127–1131.

9. Bates, A. & Hanson, N. (1996). *Aquatic Exercise Therapy.* Philadelphia: W. B. Saunders Company.

10. Behrman, A.; Sawyer, K.; & Tomlinson, S. (1993). "I want to walk": An approach to physical therapy management of the individual with an incomplete spinal cord injury. *Neurology Report*, 17(2), 7–12.

11. Bennett, S. & Karnes, J. (1998). *Neurological Disabilities: Assessment and Treatment.* Philadelphia: Lippincott.

12. Bernardi, M.; Canale, I.; Castellano, V.; Di Filippo, L.; Felici, F.; & Marchetti, M. (1995). The efficiency of walking of paraplegic patients using a reciprocating gait orthosis. *Paraplegia*, 33(7), 409–415.

13. Burns, S.; Golding, D.; Rolle, W.; Graziani, V.; & Ditunno, J. (1997). Recovery of ambulation in motor-incomplete tetraplegia. *Archives of Physical Medicine and Rehabilitation*, 78(11), 1169–1172.

14. Campbell, J. & Moore, T. (1997). Lower extremity orthoses for spinal cord injury. In: B. Goldberg, B. & Hsu, J. (Eds.), *Atlas of Orthoses and Assistive Devices* (3rd ed.; pp. 391–400). St. Louis: Mosby.

15. Carr, J. & Shepherd, R. (1998). *Neurological Rehabilitation: Optimizing Motor Performance.* London: Butterworth-Heinemann Medical.

16. Cerny, K.; Waters, R.; Hislop, H.; & Perry, J. (1980). Walking and wheelchair energetics in persons with paraplegia. *Physical Therapy*, 60(9), 1133–1139.

17. Chaplin, E. (1996). Functional neuromuscular stimulation for mobility in people with spinal cord injuries—the Parastep system. *The Journal of Spinal Cord Medicine*, 19(2), 99–105.

18. Consortium for Spinal Cord Medicine. (1999). *Outcomes Following Traumatic Spinal Cord Injury.* Washington, DC: Paralyzed Veterans of America.

19. Crozier, K.; Cheng, L.; Graziani, V.; Zorn, G.; Herbison, G.; & Ditunno, J. (1992) Spinal cord injury: prognosis for ambulation based on quadriceps recovery. *Paraplegia*, 30(11), 762–767.

20. Crozier, K.; Graziani, V.; Ditunno, J.; & Herbison, G. (1991). Spinal cord injury: prognosis for ambulation based on sensory examination in patients who are initially motor complete. *Archives of Physical Medicine and Rehabilitation*, 72(2), 119–121.

21. Davies, P. (1991). *Steps to Follow: A Guide to the Treatment of Adult Hemiplegia* (2nd ed.). New York: Springer-Verlag.

22. Delitto, A., Snyder-Mackler, L, & Robinson, A. (1995). Electrical stimulation of muscle: Techniques and applications. In: Robinson, J. & Snyder-Mackler, L. (Eds.), *Clinical Electrophysiology: Electrotherapy and Electrophysiologic Testing* (2nd ed.; pp. 121–153). Baltimore: Williams & Wilkins.

23. Dietz, V.; Colombo, G.; & Jensen, L. (1994). Locomotor activity in spinal man. *Lancet,* 344(8932), 1260–1263.

24. Dietz, V.; Colombo, G.; Jensen, L.; & Baumgartner, L. (1995). Locomotor capacity of spinal cord in paraplegic patients. *Annals of Neurology*, 37(5), 574–582.

25. Dietz, V.; Wirz, M.; & Jensen, L. (1997). Locomotion in patients with spinal cord injuries. *Physical Therapy*, 77(5), 508–516.

26. Ditunno, J.; Cohen, M.; Formal, C.; & Whiteneck, G. (1995). Functional Outcomes. In: Stover, S., DeLisa, J., & Whiteneck, G. (Eds.). *Spinal Cord Injury: Clinical Outcomes from the Model Systems* (pp. 170–184). Gaithersburg, MD: Aspen Publishers.

27. Fisher, B. & Woll, S. (1995). Considerations in the Restoration of Motor Control. In: Montgomery, J. (Ed.), *Physical Therapy for Traumatic Brain Injury* (pp. 55–78). New York: Churchill Livingstone.

28. Franceschini, M.; Baratta, S.; Zampolini, M.; Loria, D.; & Lotta, S. (1997). Reciprocating gait orthoses: A multicenter study of their use by spinal cord injured patients. *Archives of Physical Medicine and Rehabilitation*, 78(6), 582–586.

29. Gallien, P.; Brissot, R.; Eyssette, M.; Tell, L.; Barat, M.; Wiart, L.; & Petit, H. (1995). Restoration of gait by functional electrical stimulation for spinal cord injured patients. *Paraplegia*, 33(11), 660–664.

30. Gardner, M.; Holden, M.; Leikauskas, J.; & Richard, R. (1998). Partial body weight support with treadmill locomotion to improve gait after incomplete spinal cord injury: a single-subject experimental design. *Physical Therapy*, 78(4) 361–374.

31. Graupe, D. & Kohn, K. (1997). Transcutaneous functional neuromuscular stimulation of certain traumatic complete thoracic paraplegics for independent short-distance ambulation. *Neurological Research*, 19(3), 323–333.

32. Graupe, D. & Kohn, K. (1998). Functional neuromuscular stimulator for short-distance ambulation by certain thoracic-level spinal-cord-injured paraplegics. *Surgical Neurology*, 50(3), 202–207.

33. Graziani, V.; Crozier, K.; & Selby-Silverstein, L. (1996). Lower extremity function following spinal cord injury. *Topics in Spinal Cord Injury Rehabilitation*, 1(4), 46–55.

34. Hawran, S. & Biering-Sorensen, F. (1996). The use of long leg calipers for paraplegic patients: a follow-up study of patients discharged 1973–1982. *Spinal Cord*, 34(11), 666–668.

35. Heinneman, A.; Magiera-Planey, R.; Schiro-Geist, C.; & Gimines, G. (1987). Mobility for persons with

spinal cord injury: An evaluation of two systems. *Archives of Physical Medicine and Rehabilitation*, 68, 90–93.

36. Hirokawa, S.; Solomonow, M.; Baratta, R.; & D'Ambrosia, R. (1996). Energy expenditure and fatiguability in paraplegic ambulation using reciprocating gait orthosis and electric stimulation. *Disability and Rehabilitation*, 18(3), 115–122.

37. Jacobs, S.; Yeaney, N.; Herbison, G.; & Ditunno, J. (1995). Future ambulation prognosis as predicted by somatosensory evoked potentials in motor complete and incomplete quadriplegia. *Archives of Physical Medicine and Rehabilitation*, 76, 635–641.

38. Jaeger, R. (1996). Principles underlying functional electrical stimulation techniques. *The Journal of Spinal Cord Medicine*, 19(2), 93–96.

39. Kendall, F.; McCreary, E.; & Provance, P. (1993). *Muscles: Testing and Function* (4th ed.). Baltimore: Williams & Wilkins.

40. Kobetic, R.; Marsolias, E.; Samame, P.; & Borges, G. (1994). The next step: Artificial walking. In: Rose, J. & Gamble, J. (Eds.), *Human Walking* (2nd ed.; pp. 225–252.) Baltimore: Lippincott Williams & Wilkins.

41. Kobetic, R.; Triolo, R.; & Marsolias, B. (1997). Muscle selection and walking performance of multichannel FES systems for ambulation in paraplegia. *IEEE Transactions on Rehabilitation Engineering*, 5(1), 23–29.

42. Kohlmeyer, K. & Yarkony, G. (1994). Functional Outcome after Spinal Cord Injury Rehabilitation. In: Yarkony, G. (Ed.), *Spinal Cord Injury: Medical Management and Rehabilitation* (pp. 9–14). Rockville, MD: Aspen Publishers.

43. Kralj, A.; Bajd, T.; & Turk, R. (1988). Enhancement of gait restoration in spinal injured patients by functional electrical stimulation. *Clinical Orthopaedics and Related Research*, 233, 34–43.

44. Kralj, A. & Jaeger, R. (1994). Functional electrical stimulation for spinal cord injury. In: Yarkony, G. (Ed.)., *Spinal Cord Injury: Medical Management and Rehabilitation* (pp. 175–182). Rockville, MD: Aspen Publishers.

45. Krawetz, P. & Nance, P. (1996). Gait analysis of spinal cord injured subjects: Effects of injury level and spasticity. *Archives of Physical Medicine and Rehabilitation*, 77(7), 635–638.

46. Ladouceur, M.; Pepin, A.; Norman, K.; & Barbeau, H. (1997). Recovery of walking after spinal cord injury. *Advances in Neurology*, 72, 249–255.

47. Lehmann, J. (1986). Lower limb orthotics. In: Redford, J. (Ed.), *Orthotics Etcetera* (3rd ed.; pp. 278–351). Baltimore: Williams & Wilkins.

48. Little, J.; Micklessen, P.; Umlauf, R.; & Britell, C. (1989). Lower extremity manifestations of spasticity in chronic spinal cord injury. *American Journal of Physical Medicine and Rehabilitation*, 68(1), 32–36.

49. Lunsford, T. & Wallace, J. (1997). The orthotic prescription. In: Goldberg, B. & Hsu, J. (Eds.), *Atlas of Orthoses and Assistive Devices* (3rd ed.; pp. 3–14). St. Louis, Mosby.

50. Mangine, R., Heckman, T., & Eldridge, V. (1989). Improving strength, endurance, and power. In:

Scully, R. & Barnes, M. (Eds.), *Physical Therapy* (pp. 739–762). Philadelphia: J.B. Lippincott.

51. Marsolias, E., & Kobetic, R. (1987). Functional electrical stimulation for walking with paraplegia. *The Journal of Bone and Joint Surgery*, 69-A(5), 728–733.

52. Marsolias, E., & Kobetic, R. (1988). Development of a practical electrical stimulation system for restoring gait in the paralyzed patient. *Clinical Orthopaedics and Related Research*, 233, 64–74.

53. Martini, F. (1998). *Fundamentals of Anatomy and Physiology* (4th ed.). Upper Saddle River, NJ: Prentice Hall.

54. McClelland, M.; Andrews, B.; Patrick, J.; Freeman, P.; & El Masri, W. (1987). Augmentation of the Owestry ParaWalker orthosis by means of surface electrical stimulation: Gait analysis of three patients. *Paraplegia*, 25, 32–38.

55. McCulloch, K. & Nelson, C. (1995). Electrical stimulation and electromyographic biofeedback: applications for neurologic dysfunction. In: Umphred, D. (Ed.), *Neurological Rehabilitation* (3rd ed.; pp. 852–871). St. Louis: Mosby.

56. McMinn, R. (1994). *Last's Anatomy* (9th ed.). New York: Churchill Livingstone.

57. Merkel, K.; Miller, N.; & Merritt, J. (1985). Energy expenditure in patients with low-, mid-, or high-thoracic paraplegia using Scott-Craig knee-ankle-foot orthoses. *Mayo Clinic Proc*, 60(3), 165–168.

58. Michael, J. (1997). Lower limb orthoses. In: Goldberg, B. & Hsu, J. (Eds.), *Atlas of Orthoses and Assistive Devices* (3rd ed.; pp 209–224). St. Louis: Mosby.

59. Miller, P. (1997). Orthoses for the pelvic and hip region. In: Nawoczenski, D. & Epler, M. (Eds.), *Orthotics in Functional Rehabilitation of the Lower Limb* (pp. 15–29). Philadelphia: W.B. Saunders.

60. Moore, K. (1992). *Clinically Oriented Anatomy*. Baltimore: Williams & Wilkins.

61. Nawoczenski, D. (1997). Introduction to orthotics: Rationale for treatment. In Nawoczenski, D. & Epler, M. (Eds.), *Orthotics in Functional Rehabilitation of the Lower Limb* (pp. 1–13). Philadelphia: W.B. Saunders.

62. Nawoczenski, D.; Rinehart, M.; Duncanson, P.; & Brown, B. (1987). Physical management. In Buchanan, L. &. Nawoczenski, D. (Eds.), *Spinal Cord Injury: Concepts and Management Approaches* (pp. 123–184). Baltimore: Williams & Wilkins.

63. Nene, A.; Hermens, H.; & Zilvold, G. (1996). Paraplegic locomotion: A review. *Spinal Cord*, 34(9), 507–524.

64. New York University. (1986). *Lower Limb Orthotics*. New York: New York University Post-Graduate Medical School.

65. Nixon, V. (1985). *Spinal Cord Injury: A Guide to Functional Outcomes in Physical Therapy Management*. Rockville, MD: Aspen Publishers.

66. Noreau, L.; Richards, C.; Comeau, F.; & Tardif, D. (1995). Biomechanical analysis of swing-through gait in paraplegic and non-disabled individuals. *Journal of Biomechanics*, 28(6), 689–700.

67. Noreau, L. & Shephard, R. (1995). Spinal cord injury, exercise and quality of life. *Sports Medicine*, 20(4), 226–250.

68. Norkin, C. & Levangie, P. (1992). *Joint Structure and Function: A Comprehensive Analysis* (2nd ed.). Philadelphia: F. A. Davis.

69. O'Daniel, B. & Krapfl, B. (1989). Spinal cord injury. In Payton, O. (Ed.), *Manual of Physical Therapy* (pp. 69–172). New York: Churchill Livingstone.

70. O'Sullivan, S. & Schmitz, T. (1999). *Physical Rehabilitation Laboratory Manual: Focus on Functional Training.* Philadelphia: F. A. Davis.

71. Peckham, P. (1987). Functional electrical stimulation: Current status and future prospects of applications to the neuromuscular system in spinal cord injury. *Paraplegia*, 25, 279–288.

72. Penrod, L.; Hegde, S.; & Ditunno, J. (1990). Age effect on prognosis for functional recovery in acute, traumatic central cord syndrome. *Archives of Physical Medicine and Rehabilitation*, 71, 963–968.

73. Perry, J. (1992). *Gait Analysis: Normal and Pathological Function.* Thorofare, NJ: Slack.

74. Perry, J. (1997). Normal and pathological gait. In: Goldberg, B. & Hsu, J. (Eds.), *Atlas of Orthoses and Assistive Devices* (3rd ed.; pp. 67–91). St. Louis: Mosby.

75. Peterson, M. (1985). Ambulation and orthotic management. In: Adkins, H. (Ed.), *Spinal Cord Injury* (pp. 199–217). New York: Churchill Livingstone.

76. Prentice, W. (1998). Proprioceptive neuromuscular facilitation techniques. In: Prentice, W. (Ed.), *Therapeutic Modalities for Allied Health Professionals.* New York: McGraw-Hill.

77. Rancho Los Amigos Medical Center. (1996). *Observational Gait Analysis.* Downey, CA: Rancho Los Amigos Medical Center.

78. Robinson, C.; Kett, N.; & Bolam, J. (1988). Spasticity in spinal cord injured patients: 2. Initial measures and long-term effects of surface electrical stimulation. *Archives of Physical Medicine and Rehabilitation*, 69, 862–868.

79. Rosse, C. & Gaddum-Rosse, P. (1997). *Hollinshead's Textbook of Anatomy* (5th ed.). Philadelphia: Lippincott-Raven.

80. Roth, E.; Lawler, M.; & Yarkony, G. (1990). Traumatic central cord syndrome: clinical features and functional outcomes. *Archives of Physical Medicine and Rehabilitation*, 71, 18–23.

81. Roth, E.; Park, T.; Pang, T.; Yarkony, G.; & Lee, M. (1991). Traumatic cervical Brown-Sequard and Brown-Sequard-plus syndromes: the spectrum of presentations and outcomes. *Paraplegia*, 29, 582–589.

82. Schmitz, T. (1994). Preambulation and gait training. In: O'Sullivan, S. & Schmitz, T. (Eds.), *Physical Rehabilitation: Assessment and Treatment* (3rd ed.; pp. 251–276). Philadelphia: F. A. Davis.

83. Seleski, S. (1996). Orthotic prescription principles. *The Journal of Spinal Cord Medicine*, 19(2), 97–98.

84. Shumway-Cook, A. & Woollacott, M. (1995). *Motor Control: Theory and Practical Applications.* Baltimore: Williams & Wilkins.

85. Smith, B. (1997). Functional electrical stimulation. *Topics in Spinal Cord Injury Rehabilitation*, 3(2), 56–69.

86. Stallard, J. & Major, R. (1995). The influence of orthosis stiffness on paraplegic ambulation and its implications for functional electrical stimulation (FES) walking systems. *Prosthetics and Orthotics International*, 19(2), 108–114.

87. Sullivan, P., & Markos, P. (1987). *Clinical Procedures in Therapeutic Exercise.* Norwalk, CT: Appleton & Lange.

88. Sullivan, P.; Markos, P.; & Minor, M. (1982). *An Integrated Approach to Therapeutic Exercise: Theory and Clinical Application.* Reston, VA: Reston Publishing Company.

89. Sykes, L.; Ross, E.; Powell, E.; & Edwards, J. (1996). Objective measurement of use of the reciprocating gait orthosis (RGO) and the electrically augmented RGO in patients with spinal cord lesions. *Prosthetics and Orthotics International*, 20(3), 182–190.

90. Thoma, H.; Frey, M.; Holle, J.; Kern, H.; Mayr, W.; Schwanda, G.; & Stohr, H. (1987). State of the art of implanted multichannel devices to mobilize paraplegics. *International Journal of Rehabilitation Research*, 10(4) (Suppl. 5), 86–90.

91. Vogel, L. & Lubicky, J. (1995). Ambulation in children and adolescents with spinal cord injuries. *Journal of Pediatric Orthopaedics*, 15, 510–516.

92. Vogel, L. & Lubicky, J. (1997). Pediatric spinal cord injury issues: ambulation. *Topics in Spinal Cord Injury Rehabilitation*, 3(2), 37–47.

93. Waters, R. (1996). Functional prognosis of spinal cord injuries. *The Journal of Spinal Cord Medicine*, 19(2), 89–92.

94. Waters, R.; Adkins, R.; Yakura, J.; & Sie, I. (1994). Motor and sensory recovery following incomplete paraplegia. *Archives of Physical Medicine and Rehabilitation*, 75, 67–72.

95. Waters, R.; Adkins, R.; Yakura, J.; & Vigil, D. (1994). Prediction of ambulatory performance based on motor scores derived from standards of the American Spinal Injury Association. *Archives of Physical Medicine and Rehabilitation*, 75, 756–760.

96. Waters, R., & Lunsford, B. (1985). Energy costs of paraplegic locomotion. *Journal of Joint and Bone Surgery*, 67-A(8), 1245–1250.

97. Waters, R. & Miller, L. (1987). A physiologic rationale for orthotic prescription in paraplegia. *Clinical Prosthetics and Orthotics*, 11(2), 66–73.

98. Waters, R.; Sie, I.; & Adkins, R. (1995). Rehabilitation of the patient with a spinal cord injury. *Orthopedic Clinics of North America*, 26(1), 117–122.

99. Waters, R.; Yakura, J.; & Adkins, R. (1993). Gait performance after spinal cord injury. *Clinical Orthopaedics and Related Research*, 288, 87–96.

100. Waters, R.; Yakura, J.; Adkins, R.; & Barnes, G. (1989). Determinants of gait performance following spinal cord injury. *Archives of Physical Medicine and Rehabilitation*, 70, 811–818.

101. Watkins, E.; Edwards, D.; & Patrick, J. (1987). ParaWalker paraplegic walking. *Physiotherapy*, 73(2), 99–100.

102. Wernig, A.; Nanassy, A.; & Muller, S. (1998). Maintenance of locomotor abilities following Laufband (treadmill) therapy in para- and tetraplegic persons: Follow-up studies. *Spinal Cord*, 36(11), 744–749.

103. Wickelgren, I. (1998). Teaching the spinal cord to walk. *Science,* 279, 319–321.

104. Wieler, M.; Stein, R.; Ladouceur, M.; Whittaker, M.; Smith, A.; Naaman, S.; Barbeau, H.; Bugaresti, J.; & Aimone, E. (1999). Multicenter evaluation of electrical stimulation systems for walking. *Archives of Physical Medicine and Rehabilitation,* 80(5), 495–500.

105. Winchester, P.; Carollo, J.; Parekh, R.; Lutz, L.; & Aston, W. (1993). A comparison of paraplegic gait performance using two types of reciprocating gait orthoses. *Prosthetics and Orthotics International,* 17(2), 101–106.

106. Yakura, J.; Waters, R.; & Adkins, R. (1990). Changes in ambulation parameters in spinal cord injury individuals following rehabilitation. *Paraplegia,* 28(6), 364–370.

107. Yang, L.; Condie, D.; Granat, M.; Paul, J.; & Rowley, D. (1996). Effects of joint motion constraints on the gait of normal subjects and their implications on the further development of hybrid FES orthosis for paraplegic persons. *Journal of Biomechanics,* 29(2), 217–226.

108. Yarkony, G.; Roth, E.; Heinemann, A.; Lovell, L.; & Wu, Y. (1988). Functional skills after spinal cord injury rehabilitation: three-year longitudinal follow-up. *Archives of Physical Medicine and Rehabilitation,* 69, 111–114.

109. Zablotny, C. (1997). Use of orthoses for the adult with neurological involvement. In: Nawoczenski, D. & Epler, M. (Eds.), *Orthotics in Functional Rehabilitation of the Lower Limb* (pp. 205–243). Philadelphia: W.B. Saunders.

Index

Flexion injuries (*cont.*)
  lumbar, 18
  thoracic, 16, 17
Flexion with distraction injuries, lumbar, 18, 19
Flexion with rotation injuries
  cervical, 13
  lumbar, 18
  thoracic, 17
Floor-reaction AFOs, 354, 400–401
Floor transfers, 246–250, 267–268. *See also* Uneven
      transfers
  back approach, 249–250, 252
  front approach, 248–249, 250
  side approach, 247–248, 249
Follow-up, postdischarge, 54, 69, 159
Footrests, wheelchair, adjustments, 283
Four-point gait, 364–365, 367
Fracture management, 40–46, 47
  emergency, 38–40
  nonsurgical, 40–41
  orthotic, 46, 47
  surgical, 41–42
Fractures
  burst, 13, 17, 19
  clay-shoveler, 12
  flexion teardrop, 12
  relationship to osteoporosis, 34
  wedge, 12, 15, 16, 18
Frankel grading scale, 28
Functional electrical stimulation (FES), 405
Functional evaluation, 150–154, 155
Functional independence measure (FIM), 151, 152,
      154, 155
Functional limitations
  defined, 1
  in NAGI Model, 1–2
Functional potentials, 156–159
  ambulation, 358, 359–362, 400, 401, 402–403
  mat skills, 186
  transfers, 231–232
  wheelchair skills, 287–289
Functional rehabilitation, 164–182
  equipment selection, 179–181
  movement strategies, 164–168
  physical prerequisites, 168, 170–171
  precautions, 175–179. *See also* Precautions
  strategies for functional training, 68, 171–175
Functional skills, 3–4
Functional training, 171–179

G

Gait patterns
  drag-to, 368–370
  four-point, 364–365, 367
  swing-through, 365–366, 368
  swing-to, 366–368, 369
Gait training, 387–403. *See also* Ambulation; Ambula-
      tion over even surfaces; Ambulation over
      obstacles
  following incomplete injury, 403

  with ankle-foot orthoses, 400–401
  with knee-ankle-foot orthoses, 387–393
Gastrointestinal care, 46–47
Gastrointestinal complications, 35
Genital function
  following injury, 32, 76
    females, 80–82
    males, 76–80
  neurological control
    females, 74–76
    males, 73–74, 75
Glossopharyngeal breathing, 137
Goal setting, 2–3, 144, 159–162
Gray matter, 8–9
Grieving, 58, 59
Gross mobility in sitting, 200–201, 204
  with incomplete injury, 226
  physical prerequisites, 204
  skill descriptions, 200–201, 226
  skill prerequisites, 204
  therapeutic strategies, 201–202, 205
    control pelvis using head-hips relationship, 260
    in long-sitting
      lift or unweight buttocks and move laterally,
          262–263
      lift or unweight buttocks by leaning forward on
          extended arms, 259–260, 261–262
      move buttocks forward and back, 221
      prop forward on extended arms, 259
    tolerate upright sitting position, 318
Growth
  during psychosocial adjustment, 60, 69
  rehabilitative strategies for, 61
Guarding, during gait training, 389–390
Gunshot wounds, 20

H

Halo orthosis, 43–44
Handrims, 278, 292. *See also* Propulsion of manual
      wheelchair with pegged handrims; Propulsion
      of manual wheelchair with standard handrims
Head-hips relationship, 168, 170, 260
Health care environment, 5–6, 64–65
Health maintenance, 4. *See also* Complications, Educa-
      tion
Health professionals
  constructive practices, 63–66
  destructive practices, 61–63
  influence of, 2, 70
  negative attitudes, 57, 58, 62
Heterotopic ossification, 31, 34, 51–52
HGO (Hip Guidance Orthoses), 357
High-lesion skills: positioning in wheelchair and
      power wheelchair propulsion
  physical prerequisites, 291
  skill descriptions
    driving power wheelchair, 292–293
    positioning in wheelchair, 290
    pressure reliefs, 290
  skill prerequisites, 291